THE WOMEN'S GUIDE TO HOMEOPATHY

Dr Andrew Lockie was born in Glasgow. He graduated in medicine from Aberdeen University, then studied at the Royal London Homeopathic Hospital. He is a member of the Royal College of Practitioners. Dr Lockie is a homeopathic consultant to the *Journal of Alternative & Complementary Medicine* and has written numerous articles for both the medical and lay press. He has been the guest doctor on *The Peter Murray Show* on LBC, and has made other radio and TV appearances. He is also the author of the bestselling *The Family Guide to Homeopathy*. Dr Lockie is married to an acupuncturist. They have four children and live in Surrey.

Dr Nicola Geddes studied medicine at Edinburgh University and then undertook postgraduate training in nutrition and homeopathy. She worked with Dr Lockie in Guildford, at the Tunbridge Wells Homeopathic Hospital and at the Bramblefield Complementary Centre at Kemsley, Sittingbourne. She has now returned to Edinburgh, where she runs her own homeopathic practice.

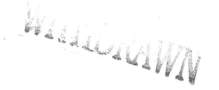

THE WOMEN'S GUIDE TO HOMEOPATHY

The Natural Way to a Healthier Life for Women

Dr Andrew Lockie and
Dr Nicola Geddes

HAMISH HAMILTON · LONDON

*To M, who planted the seed that is growing into a forest
(AL)*

To my parents and the forester (NG)

HAMISH HAMILTON LTD

Published by the Penguin Group
Penguin Books Ltd, 27 Wrights Lane, London W8 5TZ, England
Penguin Books USA Inc., 375 Hudson Street, New York, New York 10014, USA
Penguin Books Australia Ltd, Ringwood, Victoria, Australia
Penguin Books Canada Ltd, 10 Alcorn Avenue, Toronto, Ontario, Canada M4V 3B2
Penguin Books (NZ) Ltd, 182–190 Wairau Road, Auckland 10, New Zealand

Penguin Books Ltd, Registered Offices: Harmondsworth, Middlesex, England

First published in hardback by Hamish Hamilton Ltd 1992
First published in paperback by Hamish Hamilton Ltd 1993
10 9 8 7 6 5 4 3 2 1

Filmset in Linotron Palatino
Printed in Great Britain by Butler and Tanner Ltd, Frome and London

A CIP catalogue record for this book is available from the British Library
ISBN 0-241-13344-0

Contents

Acknowledgements

THE authors would like to thank Alleysa Wint for permission to reprint, with captions, her notes on childbirth; Foresight, and in particular Mrs Belinda Barnes, for help with the pre-conceptual section; Michael Thomson for his considerable help with MacRepertory which saved hours of frustration; Kate Theobald for her advice with the introduction; Margaret Royle for information on the Alexander Technique; Barbara Lockie for her invaluable research; Sandra Dawn for beauty material; Lesley Holloway for putting thoughts on to a word processor; Chris, Marjorie, Clare and Jackie for keeping the practice going; GMB for information on tenosynovitis; Pam Dix for her understanding and her attention to detail.

Dr Lockie should also like to thank David, Kirsty, Alastair and Sandy for their help, encouragement and patience; Keith Taylor, for his advice on some structural problems; and Dr Nuria Booth, Dr Michael Callender, Dr David Curtin, Mr Christopher Sutton and Dr Jane Winfield for their helpful comments and suggestions.

Also, many thanks to those who helped with those parts of *The Family Guide to Homeopathy* which have been incorporated into this book.

Introduction

THANK you for acquiring this book. The authors feel that as the twenty-first century draws near, medicine exhibits a male-dominated, aggressive approach to therapeutics. Women, on the whole, favour a more gentle, holistic approach to health, which homeopathy epitomizes. We offer this book to support you in this aim by providing a safe, clinical framework within which you can operate.

Women as healers

Women have always played a pivotal role in health, both within the family and in society in general. (By healing, we mean anything which helps to make the person whole or well, whether it be homeopathy, spiritual healing, dietary change, use of herbs or acupuncture, drugs or surgery.) The fortunes of women in the healing arts, like the fortunes of women in society in general, have fluctuated throughout history. According to *Encyclopaedia Britannica*, medicine was a female vocation in pre-scientific ages and cultures. It was part of the domestic craft passed from mother to daughter. Healing the sick and wounded accords well with the creation of new life.

During the Middle Ages, women's healing gifts were regarded with suspicion and mistrust by men. Women who treated the sick and used herbs were denounced as witches, tortured, and put to death. With the advent of the Industrial Revolution and the opening up of society in the nineteenth century, things began to change. Women began to assert themselves in medicine, mainly as midwives and nurses, and finally as doctors. They were considerably put down at first, because men believed that they would be unreliable, due to their menstrual cycle, pregnancies and child-rearing. Since the 1900s, due to the publication of self-help literature, women have been in a better position to exert their healing force.

This innate, intuitive aspect of the feminine attitude to healing is in marked contrast to the masculine, aggressive attitude of 'Burn the tumour' and 'Cut out the disease'. A useful analogy is with politics – you can negotiate and use diplomacy, tact, understanding and persuasion to end a crisis, or you can declare war. War often has an unfortunate habit of creating new problems.

In medicine, life is the final arbiter. It is better to have surgery, or to be on a drug for the rest of your life, than to die without it. Even the greatest scientist in the world cannot yet create a human life. Whilst we have labelled orthodox medicine as masculine, and more gentle medicine as feminine, we would like to point out that each sex may, and indeed should, exhibit qualities of its opposite. In general, however, women tend towards using gentler, less aggressive methods of treatment for themselves and their families. It is these women that the authors wish to support.

The ages of woman

In adolescence there are, fortunately, rarely major health problems. It is, however, an extremely turbulent time as young women work out their new-found sexuality and place in the world. The inevitable challenges that go hand in hand with these changes are difficult to manage. With the help, we hope, of various sections in this book – blushing, shyness and acne, for example – these challenges can be successfully met. It keeps things in perspective if you bear in mind that most people are not as self-confident and assured as they appear to be.

As women reach their 20s and 30s, there is the trauma of the workplace and establishing a career, proving to yourself that you can succeed. Do try and make sure of your motivation – are you working for yourself, or are you trying to prove yourself to someone else? Typical medical conditions that may be encountered at this stage include pre-menstrual syndrome, period problems, thrush, cystitis and chronic fatigue syndrome.

If you are thinking of starting a family please read the section on pre-conceptual care. Having a baby will bring great changes and adjustments, especially if you have been single-mindedly pursuing a career. Pregnancy is as dramatic in its effects as puberty. Many women find pregnancy and childbirth deeply satisfying and feel happily in tune with their changing body. However, if you are concerned or unhappy with any aspect of your pregnancy, read the chapters on fertility and pregnancy, and childbirth and postnatal problems.

Having children is a whole new experience. One of the most difficult aspects – having recovered sufficiently from sleepless nights to be able to think – is the apparent loss of the ability to concentrate. Mostly, however, it is not a total loss of concentration; it is more that a different set of concentration skills are required. When you were just working, you could concentrate on one thing at a time in great depth. As a mother and house-wife, perhaps still pursuing your career, you have to keep tabs on a lot of different things at once, without necessarily thinking too deeply about any one of them. We hope that reading the sections on fatigue, stress, and infants will be helpful.

If you have chosen to stay at home while your children are small there may be a dilemma about returning to work, whether it be full- or part-time. Whilst there are more opportunities for women to return to the workplace and compete with men on more or less equal terms, there are still the children to look after and the household to run, either with or without a partner willing to participate. Much of the stress for a working mother comes from having to think of too many things at once, something many men still do not always appreciate. Whilst ultimately resolution of this conflict requires further change in attitude and in work practice, homeopathic treatment – especially constitutional – can help women to fulfil their potential. Bear in mind that the real source of stress lies behind the thinking about rather than the doing of the multiplicity of tasks that you face.

In the menopause, and beyond, metabolism slows down, there is a tendency to put on weight, the skin begins to lose its elasticity and wrinkles appear. Remember that the part of you that you call 'me' never changes; it is still at peace, deep inside. It is difficult to keep external changes, which may alter how you think of yourself, in perspective. Being more conscientious about diet and exercise is important, in order to keep in shape. If you are at peace within yourself, that quality will shine through, and help you to grow old with dignity. We hope that the sections on the menopause and beauty care will be helpful.

Women and homeopathy

Whilst this book is loosely based on Ruddock's *Lady's Manual of Homoeopathic treatment*, an early twentieth-century guide to the use of homeopathy by women, we have tried to make it completely relevant to the needs of women at the close of the twentieth and beginning of the twenty-first centuries. The information and advice contained within *The Women's Guide to Homeopathy* ranges from ancient knowledge, through advances made in the last 150 years, up to state of the art technology. It is now recognized by most health care professionals that no one medical system has

all the answers for all the ills that afflict women. The main problem is to know which is the most appropriate treatment for any particular woman. Obviously, the less life-threatening and more chronic the condition, the more sense it makes to use homeopathy and other non-toxic and immune-system-boosting therapies first, and only to progress to potentially harmful methods if these fail or the situation becomes more critical. In the case of acute, serious illness we still have to rely heavily on proven orthodox methods, at least until we have had more experience of using alternative or complementary therapies in these situations.

This is the spirit in which this book has been written. It is offered to assist you in helping yourself in minor accidents and ailments and to tell you when to stop. It is also to support you when facing more serious situations. It tells you who to call and how quickly to act, and also what you can do whilst waiting for assistance.

Do bear in mind that prevention of health problems should always be your priority, and you will find an extensive section on this in *The Family Guide to Homeopathy*.

The heart of the book you will find in PART 2, 'Ailments and Conditions'. Here we have tried to consider in as much detail as we can those major health and life problems that will arise at some time in any woman's life. In addition we have included a chapter, 'Special problems in infants', since for those women who have children, the first year in their lives is crucial.

PART 3 lists in alphabetical order other con-ditions which you may have to contend with. Some are associated with problems outlined in PART 2.

Please read the opening chapters carefully, especially PART 1, and the opening remarks to PART 2, before attempting to use the book; so that you are familiar with the philosophy of homeopathy, and with the way the book is constructed. Please pay particular attention to the meaning of the symbols used for determining how to get assistance. Please note that throughout this book, when you are referred to a 'homeopath' this means a medically qualified homeopathic physician. If a medically qualified homeopathic physician is not available in your area and you wish to consult a registered non-medically qualified homeopath, the authors advise that you do this under the continuing observation of your own GP. (See 'Finding a homeopathic practitioner', p. 21).

We hope that when you have done all this and used the remedies for yourself, you will agree with us that homeopathy goes a long way to-wards meeting Lord Colwyn's criteria for an ideal medical system. These are that it should be effective, have minimal or no risk for the patient, strengthen the constitution (increase well being and the ability to live life to the full) and not just palliate, not be expensive, be accessible and understood by all members of the public and be linked to the general ecological good.

Finally, please remember that no book can be a substitute for a good and caring physician and so, if you are in doubt, CALL YOUR DOCTOR!

Introduction for health care practitioners

Anyone who has read *The Family Guide to Homeopathy* will recognize elements of it in this new book. We make no apologies for this, as much of this material remains entirely valid. The core of this book, however, PART 2, 'Ailments and Conditions', is based on entirely new research. For this reason we have not considered First Aid or the role of prevention in any depth here – see *The Family Guide to Homeopathy* for sections on these subjects. Women suffering from each condition were identified using the age–sex register in our own practice. Their details were analysed using the MacRepertory computer programme. The symptoms listed under each remedy represent the actual symptoms presented by patients, with a few 'typical' textbook additions. The remedies in the sections on specific ailments are a result of our original research.

As with *The Family Guide to Homeopathy*, we have included comprehensive repertories, or Remedy Finders, to help women choose the best remedy for the totality of the case. These have also been derived from the MacRepertory.

We hope that by giving strict rules and duration guides we will succeed in encouraging women to ask for help when their condition is not suitable for self care. This is always a difficult balance to achieve and we would, again, welcome any comments you may have on whether this has been achieved. We also hope we can be forgiven for using the American spelling of Homeopathy, which has been done for the sake of simplicity.

We offer this book to our colleagues in general practice and hospital medicine in the hope that it may inspire them to experiment with this remarkably safe addition to their therapeutic armamentarium. We hope they will be as satisfied with it as we have become over the years. If they wish to take it further, we can assure them of a warm welcome at the courses run in various parts of the country. Simply phone the education secretary at the nearest homeopathic hospital and ask for details of the postgraduate curriculum. For addresses and phone numbers see p. 338.

PART 1
HOMEOPATHY

What is Homeopathy?

HOMEOPATHY is an exceptionally safe form of medicine which treats the whole individual. It is equally concerned with maintaining good health and aiding recovery from ill health, and like all forms of medicine – even those which use powerful drugs and high technology surgery – relies for its effects on the body's own powers of self-regulation and self-healing. Since its development nearly two hundred years ago homeopathy has benefited millions of people, young and old, from all walks of life, in countries all over the world.

The word 'homeopathy' (also spelt 'homoeopathy') comes from two Greek words, *omio* meaning 'same' and *pathos* meaning 'suffering'. A homeopathic remedy is one which produces the same symptoms as those the sick person complains of, and in doing so sharply provokes the body into throwing them off. 'Like may be cured by like', also expressed as *similia similibus curentur*, is the basic principle of homeopathic therapeutics. The opposite therapeutic approach is 'allopathy', which is defined as a system of therapeutics in which diseases are treated by producing a condition incompatible with or antagonistic to the condition to be cured or alleviated.

The idea that remedies and symptoms sharing certain key features might interact in such a way as to banish illness, and the implied corollary that two similar states of discomfort cannot exist in the same body, was not new even two centuries ago. The great achievement of Samuel Hahnemann, the founder of homeopathy, was that he systematically studied, for himself, all the orthodox medical remedies of his day, noted their effects on healthy people, and then used this knowledge to give very specific and safe treatment to sick people. This was revolutionary in an age when medicines were indiscriminately prescribed, often in poisonous quantities.

Homeopathy is a naturopathic form of medicine – it seeks to assist Nature rather than bludgeon her, to assist the body's own healing energies rather than override them. The 'disease' is not only the virus or the bacteria – these are merely the organisms which move in when the body's defences are low. The discovery of legions of microorganisms since Hahnemann's time has done nothing to alter this fundamental truth. The fever, the inflammation, the diarrhoea, the headache – these are not the disease either, but the body's attempt to return to normality. Such ideas may be difficult to adjust to if one has been brought up in the belief that both attack and cure come from the outside, but they are ideas which have been accepted by humanistic physicians since the time of Hippocrates.

Another tenet of naturopathic and therefore of homeopathic philosophy is that every person is different. The same remedy, the same diet, the same general advice does not necessarily help everyone with the same ailment. Indeed there is no such thing as the same ailment; the course of a particular kind of cancer in one person will not be the same as that in another. Accordingly, homeopathy has the most flexible system of remedy prescribing of any system of therapeutics, as this book demonstrates. The most effective remedy is always the one which matches three things: the physical symptoms, the mental and emotional symptoms, and the general sensitivities of the person concerned. It is also taken in the least possible dose for the least possible time.

If homeopathy is, or becomes, your first line of health care you will probably want to consult a professional homeopath from time to time. Indeed his or her skills should complement and guide your own. The purpose of this book is to enable you to decide on a sensible course of action for ailments and diseases already diagnosed. It will also enable you to treat homeopathically the symptoms which do not add up to any particular diagnosis, symptoms which general practitioners see most of and find hardest to treat.

Homeopathy is also a rational system of medicine. If the body's defence systems are handicapped by poor diet, bad habits, destructive emotions, and environmental stresses, it stands to reason that homeopathic remedies, of themselves, will be of limited benefit. If you consult a homeopath, he or she may suggest a change of diet or lifestyle before prescribing any remedy. Homeopathy is not a system for those in search of instant, easy answers, although it can act very swiftly in acute conditions. It requires careful self-monitoring and a willingness to stick to a course of action. The prize is higher vitality and greater resistance to all disease processes.

The beginnings of homeopathy

The 'father' of homeopathy was Samuel Christian Hahnemann, born in Dresden, Germany, in 1755. Despite his humble background – his father worked in a porcelain factory – he acquired a good education, became fluent in eight languages, and studied chemistry and medicine. He then set up in practice as a physician. But the accepted medical customs of his day, which included excessive purging, blood-letting, and cavalier prescribing of drugs which often caused more suffering than they cured, gnawed at his conscience, and after a few years he turned to translating rather than doctoring to earn his living.

It was while he was translating a treatise on herbs by a Dr Cullen of Edinburgh that he came across the tiny seed which was to flower into a whole new system of medicine. Cullen stated that quinine, an astringent substance purified from the bark of the cinchona tree (*Cinchona calisaya*), was a good treatment for malaria because it was an astringent. Why, Hahnemann wondered, should quinine have an effect on malaria when other, more powerful, astringents did not? He decided to investigate. For several days he dosed himself with quinine and noted down his reactions in great detail. It seemed that in a healthy person, himself, quinine produced all the symptoms of malaria – fever, sweating, shivering, weakness. Was this why it also cured malaria?

Fascinated, Hahnemann repeated the quinine tests, which he called 'provings', on his acquaintances, again noting their reactions in meticulous detail. He then went on to test other substances in widespread use, such as arsenic, belladonna, and mercury. There were strict requirements for the people involved in these provings. They had to be healthy in mind and body; they could not take anything which might confuse the results, such as alcohol, tea, coffee, or spicy foods; and they were to avoid 'all disturbing passions'.

Hahnemann found that people's responses varied. Some of his volunteers showed one or two mild symptoms in response to a particular substance, but others experienced vigorous reactions with many and varied symptoms. The symptoms most commonly found for each substance he called 'first line' or 'keynote' symptoms. 'Second line' symptoms were less common, and 'third line' symptoms rare or idiosyncratic. Together these symptoms added up to a 'drug picture' of the substance concerned.

Using the results of his provings, Hahnemann went on to test various substances on sick people.

But before he did so he questioned them thoroughly about their symptoms, general health, way of life, and attitudes, and gave them a physical examination. From each interview and examination he built up what he called a 'symptom picture', then prescribed the substance whose drug picture most closely matched it. The closer the match, the more successful the treatment. What he had suspected from his early experiments with quinine was indeed proving to be the case: a remedy and a disease which produce the same symptoms cancel each other out in some way. The adage *similia similibus curentur*, 'like may be cured by like', was true. In his first essay on the subject, *A New Principle for Ascertaining the Curative Powers of Drugs and Some Examination of the Previous Principles*, published in 1796, he stated: 'One should imitate Nature, which at times heals a chronic illness by another additional one. One should apply in the disease to be healed, particularly if it is chronic, that remedy which is able to simulate another artificially produced disease, as similar as possible, and the former will be healed...' The name he gave to this new principle of healing was 'homeopathy'.

This was not the end of the story, however. To Hahnemann's dismay some of his patients reported that their symptoms actually got worse before they got better. To prevent such 'aggravations', as he called them, Hahnemann started to dilute his remedies. First he made a tincture of the substance concerned, leaving it to stand in a solvent, usually pure alcohol, for one month. He then strained off the liquid, the 'mother tincture'. Then he took one drop of mother tincture and added it to 99 drops of pure alcohol, a dilution factor of 1:100. To mix the one drop with the 99 thoroughly he 'succussed' the mixture by repeatedly banging it on a hard surface for a specific length of time. The dilution process could be repeated again and again, with each successive dilution having one hundredth the strength of the preceding dilution. If the substance was insoluble, it was triturated, or ground up, before being dissolved into solution.

To Hahnemann's surprise, diluted remedies not only forestalled 'aggravations' but seemed to act much faster and more effectively. They were, paradoxically, weaker but more potent. The process of successive dilution and succussion 'potentized' the original substance in a way which is difficult to explain.

Today, in Britain, most homeopathic remedies are available in centesimal potencies, that is successively diluted by a factor of 100. It is also possible to obtain some of them in decimal potencies, successively diluted by a factor of 10, or as mother tinctures. In this book 6c is the potency recommended for most acute or self-limiting ailments, and 30c the potency recommended in chronic conditions or emergencies. 6c means that the remedy has been diluted six times by a factor of 100, and 30c that it has been diluted 30 times by a factor of 100. This means that 30c remedies are many, many times more potent in homeopathic terms, although they contain much less original substance. A small range of remedies can be bought in most ordinary chemists, mail order companies offer a wider range, and homeopathic pharmacies and hospitals the widest range of all (see Useful Addresses, p. 333–8). Many of the commonest remedies are sold as lactose (milk sugar) pilules which have been impregnated with potentized solution; these are taken by dissolving them on the tongue. Others are available as solutions which can be dropped directly on the tongue (the recommended method if you are allergic to lactose) or on to lactose pilules. Some can be obtained in lactose powder form, others as creams or ointments, and a few as injections, although only medically qualified homeopaths are allowed to give such injections. Suggestions for building a home medicine chest appear on p. 24.

However, before we return to Hahnemann's work, it is important to point out that there is no such thing as a 'homeopathic remedy'. This is not a perverse statement. A remedy can be prepared homeopathically, by successive dilution and succussion and in accordance with standards laid down by the Medicines Act, but it will not *act* homeopathically unless its drug picture matches the symptom picture of the person taking it. Herein lies the art of homeopathic prescribing. An over-the-counter product which commends itself to a thoroughly miserable hay fever sufferer because it says 'for hay fever' may indeed work, but only fortuitously. A remedy specially selected to match the sufferer's constitution and personality as well as his or her most distressing hay fever symptoms would be a surer route to eventual cure. A fundamental tenet of homeopathy, and of all the healing arts, is that there is no such thing as a disease purely of the mind or body. Mind and body are one. Influence one and you influence the other. Stress one and you stress the other. The beauty of homeopathy is that its prescribing system, although complex, takes full account of the physical and the mental.

It is not difficult to imagine the scorn which Hahnemann's contemporaries poured upon his claim that weaker remedies produced stronger effects. This ran, and still runs, completely counter to the principles of clinical pharmacology. At dilutions above the eleventh or twelfth centesimal potency, does even one molecule of the original substance remain in solution? Modern physics affords a glimmer of an explanation why the energies of the original substance persist through successive dilutions and succussions, but how did Hahnemann answer his critics two centuries ago? Then, as today, the cures achieved by homeopathy are real. They cannot be dismissed because the mechanism of cure is not fully understood.

Being a chemist, Hahnemann knew that whatever active principles his dilute remedies contained, they could only be present in infinitesimal quantities. And yet the merest trace of them was enough to produce a strong effect. At some level in the body, he reasoned, there must be something which responds to such tiny hints, an extremely subtle something capable of switching the body from sickness to health, and vice versa. He called that something the 'Vital Force'.

It was this force which was responsible for the orderly and therefore healthy running of the body, and for coordinating the body's defences against disease. In fact Hahnemann thought of the Vital Force as a form of electromagnetic energy or vibration. If this coherent energy became jangled and disturbed by stress, poor diet, lack of exercise, inherited constitutional problems, or climatic change, illness would result. The signs and symptoms of the illness were the body's attempts to restore order.

Most of the ailments doctors see are 'acute' – they onset quickly, run a fairly well-defined course, and then clear up of their own accord with or without treatment. Hahnemann's rationale for prescribing homeopathic remedies in such cases was that they hastened recovery. The Vital Force, temporarily depressed, was more than equal to bouncing back. He discovered that in outbreaks of acute infection – measles for example – where the basic symptoms are usually the same for most people, the same remedy could be routinely prescribed for those afflicted; he also prescribed the same remedy as a preventive.

By contrast, 'chronic' or long-standing illnesses represent a series of minor victories and capitulations on the part of the Vital Force. Though relapses may be followed by remissions, the general trend is downwards. In his writing Hahnemann likened this process to a wearying civil war, with both sides alternately losing and winning battles. In such circumstances, the Vital Force stands sorely in need of mercenaries, or rather correctly prescribed homeopathic remedies.

Perhaps a less bellicose analogy is better suited to the spirit of homeopathy today. Let's imagine, instead, that the Vital Force is a trampoline and that the stresses which beset us all from time to time are stones dropped on to it at random from a great height. If the Vital Force is flowing strongly, the trampoline will be taut; any stone falling on to it, even quite a big one, will be flung off. A homeopathic remedy will merely provoke a quicker recoil.

But if the Vital Force is weak and confused, the trampoline will sag; it will not have the recoil energy to fling off the stones, so the stones will settle and make it sag even more. The only way to provoke a recoil sufficient to throw off the stones is to bounce something much heavier on to the trampoline, in the hope that the recoil will be fierce enough to throw off the stones along with the heavy object. This, essentially, is what homeopathic remedies do in cases of chronic illness; they are the stimuli which energize the Vital Force.

Although Hahnemann did not understand the immune system or the intricacies of homeostasis (the body's ever vigilant self-steadying mechanism) as we understand them today, or appreciate that where infection is present so are viruses, bacteria and other microorganisms, his intuition that it is some quality or energy in the individual which makes for health or illness is difficult to quarrel with.

Hahnemann gradually re-established himself as a physician, using his new homeopathic methods. However, it was not long before he realized that certain patients, whom he had treated for acute conditions, were returning to him complaining of new sets of symptoms. These often seemed to declare themselves after stressful events. As the years passed, it became clear to him that such patients were treading a descending spiral of health, despite intervals of feeling reasonably well. Were their episodes of acute illness a manifestation of some deeper malaise? In treating the symptoms of each acute episode, was he not repressing the fundamental, underlying problem or 'miasm'? 'Miasm', meaning 'taint', was the word Hahnemann used to describe these putative, deep-seated tendencies.

Hahnemann recognized various miasms, some of which we now know to be mediated by specific microorganisms which can indeed provoke repeated episodes of deepening illness if treatment is inappropriate or delayed; among them were syphilis, gonorrhea, tuberculosis, and cholera. Another was 'psora', which manifested itself in skin eruptions. Modern public health measures have made such taints less frequent, but the miasm concept continues to be useful and is much discussed among homeopaths. We now know that many bacteria and viruses, including those associated with measles, chickenpox, influenza, and AIDS, seem to create, in predisposed people, a vulnerability to all sorts of seemingly unconnected ailments. Depression and anxiety seem to underlie a host of conditions, from migraine to cancer. Hereditary conditions also have a miasmatic character. The task of the homeopath is to look for and recognize such disease patterns and attempt to treat them. By diligent research, mainly with sick people, Hahnemann developed remedies which seemed to work at the deeper miasmatic level. He also gave strict advice on the sort of diet and lifestyle his patients should follow – no perfumes or scented waters, no tooth powders, no snuff, sparing use of tobacco, no woollen underwear, no excessive bathing, no card playing, only occasional visits to the theatre, only moderate studying, and no madcap riding or cab-driving.

The first edition of *An Organon of Rational Healing*, the best-known and most comprehensive of all Hahnemann's writings on the nature of health, disease, and homeopathic healing, was published in 1810. He revised the book five times before his death in 1843, each time searching for greater understanding of the potency of homeopathic remedies and the nature of the Vital Force. At the time of writing it is still in print.

The spread of homeopathy

During the nineteenth century Hahnemann's ideas spread quickly from Germany across Europe and then to the Americas, and also eastwards to Asia. Today homeopathy is well respected in many countries, notably in Britain, France, Germany, The Netherlands, Greece, India (where it is recognized and supported by the state), Italy, Israel, South Africa and South America, but mistrusted in others.

Homeopathy 'arrived' in Britain in 1832 when a Dr Harvey Quin began to minister to fashionable society from premises at 19 King Street in London's West End. Quin had travelled to Germany to consult Hahnemann on his own account and learned homeopathy from the Leipzig homeopaths. Later Quin became the first President of the British Homeopathic Society, founded in 1844. Thereafter, despite opposition from orthodox physicians, homeopathy steadily grew in popularity. Quin set up the first homeopathic hospital in London in 1850. The first royal patron of homeopathy was Queen Adelaide, consort of William IV, who, from 1835 until her death in 1849, was the patient of Dr Ernst Stapf, one of Samuel Hahnemann's closest colleagues. Three very distinguished homeopathic physicians have served the present Queen in the past, Dr John Weir, Dr Margery Blackie, and Dr Charles Elliott. Currently, Dr Ronald Davey holds this honour.

In the United States the fire of homeopathy was lit by Dr Constantine Hering (b.1800). As well as formulating the Laws of Cure summarized below, he pioneered the use of 'nosodes', remedies made not from plants or minerals but from diseased tissue or from bodily secretions. In 1838 he and his colleagues used a homeopathic preparation of infected sheep's spleen to cure anthrax, at one time an almost certainly fatal disease.

Materia medicas and repertories

Hahnemann originally published the results of his provings in the form of a book called a materia medica. This listed, under each remedy, the symptoms that the remedy produced in healthy people. Later work has increased the number of substances used as remedies to 3,000, although not all of these have been tested with the same thoroughness as Hahnemann's original investigations. The materia medicas of today contain not only details of symptoms from provings, but also the effects of poisons from the science of toxicology and details of symptoms from clinical observations.

Most of the remedies found in materia medicas nowadays were discovered in the last century or in the early part of this century. Many homeopaths agree that there is an urgent need to update the information, in order to find out if the twentieth-century environment has changed people's responses to remedies. Some work has been done – in England, in mainland Europe and in the USA – but there is still much to do.

Materia medicas are used to find out which symptoms a remedy might cause. Homeopaths have also developed remedy finders or repertories. In a repertory, there is a series of headings concerned with parts or systems of the body, such as mental, vertigo, head, eyes, nose and so on down to toes. Under each heading there is a list of symptoms, such as pain, redness or swelling. Alongside each symptom are printed all the remedies known to produce that symptom, together with any factors which may affect it. The symptoms are graded, the most well proven being given in bold type, the second in italic and the third in plain roman. In our repertory, or General Remedy Finder, we have stuck to a single grading system for simplicity.

Homeopathic laws

The 'Laws of Cure' were partly devised by the physician who established homeopathy in America, Dr Constantine Hering. They state that cure takes place from the top of the body downwards, from the inside outwards and from the most important organs to the least important.

Cure takes place in reverse order to the onset of symptoms. Therefore, for example, an ill person will start to feel better emotionally before the physical symptoms disappear and a long-standing complaint will take longer to disappear than a recent one.

Other homeopathic laws state:

1. Small stimuli encourage living systems, medium stimuli impede them and strong stimuli tend to stop or destroy them altogether. (Arndt's law.)
2. The quantity of action necessary to effect a change in nature is the least possible, and the decisive amount is always the minimum – perhaps an infinitesimal amount.
3. Functional symptoms are produced by the Vital Force in exact proportion to the profundity of the disturbance, and functional symptoms come before structural change.

The preventive role of homeopathy

At the deepest level, homeopathy is preventive in intent. Homeopathic remedies do not wade in and 'zap' offending organisms, leaving the immune system less able to cope than before. Quite the opposite. They nudge the immune system – not only the white cell populations of the body but also the mental and emotional states which keep those populations healthy – into greater responsiveness and readiness so that disease is kept away or prevented from recurring. In fact, homeopaths are trained to look for diseases *before* they happen. When a homeopath prescribes constitutionally, he or she is prescribing not only for the present ailment but for tendencies which have not yet manifested themselves as medically recognized ailments.

The foetus in the womb can be treated homeopathically to minimize imbalances inherited from the mother and father. Homeopathic treatment of childhood ailments lessens the risk of the latent weaknesses they cause being activated in later life – infants and children, with their newly minted immune systems, respond excellently to homeopathic treatment. Homeopathic immunization against the graver diseases of childhood is not usually offered unless a child is particularly at risk; most homeopaths prefer to take the route of boosting general resistance to disease, rather than exposing a child unnecessarily to the influence of powerful disease organisms. That said, homeopathic immunization has never damaged anyone, although the properly conducted trials that are needed to show that it is as effective as orthodox immunization have not been done.

In adult women, prompt homeopathic treatment of minor illnesses can often prevent persistent, and sometimes serious, complaints developing in later life. At all points in the cycle of development, birth, growth and maturity, subtle symptoms of constitutional weakness can be picked up by careful homeopathic analysis and treated before they burgeon into chronic and entrenched disease.

Unfortunately, no one has yet invented a way of trying out homeopathic and orthodox remedies on the same person and comparing their effects over a lifetime, but the following hypothetical case history shows how a homeopathic physician might approach a case of late-onset asthma.

At nine months old, the future Mrs X develops eczema; the ointment used to treat it leaves her skin very dry. Apart from dry skin and constipation, she is a generally healthy child. At the age of 14, she has a bad fall from a horse. A year later she develops hay fever, which turns into allergic rhinitis (a runny nose all year round). Skin tests show that she is allergic to house dust, house dust mites, grasses and horses. Desensitizing injections clear up her runny nose but leave her feeling unwell for some time afterwards.

In her early 20s she is underweight and suffers from an almost continuous nasal drip (catarrh dripping down the back of the throat). In her late 20s she marries and has two children, both full-term, healthy babies. Apart from dry skin, constipation, occasional nosebleeds and irregular periods, she feels reasonably well throughout her 30s. In her early 40s, she loses two people very close to her, her mother and eldest son. Shortly afterwards, she develops asthma.

She consults a homeopathic physician for the first time. High potency Natrum mur. is prescribed to help her through the grieving process, and she is advised to cut down on salt and carbohydrates. A month later, the asthma has all but disappeared, but she continues to suffer from dry skin, constipation, and catarrh at the back of the throat; if anything, she reports, her throat feels worse than before; and she also feels chilly and irritable, and has had several boils. Hepar sulph. is prescribed. This clears up the boils and the catarrh, but the runny nose remains. Allium and Arnica clear up the runny nose; Sulphur clears up the dry skin and the constipation. At this juncture the eczema she had as a very young child reappears. Since there is a family history of tuberculosis and allergies, she is given Tuberculinum; this clears up the eczema. She is then advised to follow the *twice-a-week eating rule* (see p. 248). She continues in good health, visiting the homeopath at infrequent intervals, until the age of 75 when she dies of pneumonia.

The homeopathic treatment involves a peeling away of layers of illness, removing symptoms in the reverse order in which they appeared, each time reaching farther back into the chain of cause and effect.

There is little doubt that predispositions to certain groups of ailments run in families. Mrs X's Achilles' heel, so to speak, was her respiratory tract. Had she been treated homeopathically from childhood onwards, this vulnerability might have been dispelled. Even from the age of 45 onwards, homeopathic health care prolonged her life and enhanced her quality of life.

Unlike many other modes of 'health care' which swing into action once health has broken down, homeopathy is based upon helping the organism to resist breakdown.

Constitutional prescribing

Most people, when they are ill, suffer not only from the basic diagnostic symptoms of the disease, but also from other symptoms which are specific to each person. In orthodox medicine, these individual symptoms are mostly unimportant. But in homeopathy, they are vital for giving the correct prescription. This is why different patients may receive different remedies for the same disease.

Many homeopaths who worked on the provings, especially the American James Tyler Kent, noticed that different types of people reacted strongly to certain remedies and proposed that people could be placed in different categories, called 'constitutional types'. Homeopaths talk of, for example, 'phosphoric types' (people who react strongly to phosphorus) or 'arsenicum album types' (those who react strongly to arsenicum album). The belief is that people of one type share similarities in terms of body shape, character and personality, and the sorts of diseases from which they suffer. For instance, Natrum mur. women tend to be pear-shaped, have a dark complexion, be fastidious and rigid in personality, keep themselves to themselves, crave salt and suffer from constipation. Lycopodium types tend to be tall, gangly and of stooped appearance, with an anxious expression, a craving for sweets, and a propensity to produce intestinal gas.

Of course, constitutional types have their limitations. In reality, each person is an individual, and so there are as many constitutional types as there are human beings, and account must be taken of the sum total of the person's inherited predispositions, past illnesses, diet, general reactions to the environment, intellectual and emotional features, and general attitude to life. This is what is meant in this book by 'constitutional treatment'.

Finding a homeopathic practitioner

In the UK today there are three basic kinds of people practising homeopathy. One is the medically qualified homeopath. There are about 600 such in Britain. They have studied at an orthodox medical school and later at one of the homeopathic hospitals (see Useful Addresses, p. 333–8). They have access to conventional methods of diagnosis and treatment as well as homeopathic techniques. The second is a registered homeopath, who will have no orthodox qualifications, and thus lacks the medical experience of the full spectrum of disease. However, the training in homeopathy is comprehensive, and high standards are being set by the Society of Homeopaths (address p. 338), who are endeavouring to standardize qualifications between the different Colleges. The third is the lay practitioner, who mainly uses homeopathy for first aid or amongst friends, but who does not wish to set up as a practitioner.

If you wish to contact a homeopath, ask the advice of a National Health Service general practitioner – usually, your own family doctor. If you have any difficulties, contact the British Homeopathic Association (address p. 338) or the Hahnemann Society.

You may be put in touch with a homeopath who uses less conventional methods. There are many concepts which go under the name of homeopathy today. The practitioner is the best guide to the one which will best suit your needs. If you discover that your homeopath's philosophy and practice do not meet your expectations, you are of course free to find another practitioner.

The homeopathic practitioner must put the care and cure of his or her patients above any particular beliefs about which branch of homeopathy is right. As Hahnemann himself said, it is not so much the theories about the causation and treatment of illness that are important, but the results.

The consultation

At your first consultation with a homeopath, there are a great many questions to answer. He or she will want to know about the symptoms of your illness and what affects them, about your medical history from your mother's pregnancy onwards, your appetite, likes and dislikes, and the regularity of your bodily functions.

Some questions are aimed at deciding which constitutional group you fit into. Your activities, occupational and recreational, are discussed, along with your emotional state.

The homeopath will prescribe a remedy, which she may dispense herself or which you can obtain from a homeopathic pharmacist; she may also give you advice on any changes you should make in your lifestyle and on the sort of diet you should follow. Hahnemann stated that nutrition was one of the principal factors which could modify the body's response to disease. He was very strict about what his patients ate, especially those with chronic illness.

In a second consultation where constitutional treatment is concerned the homeopath must interpret your response to the prescription in detail, and decide how to continue treatment.

Controversy and proof

Homeopathy is a living, evolving form of treatment. Throughout its history there have been controversies and arguments. There was a split in the homeopathic world when Hahnemann introduced his theory of the Vital Force and how it could be influenced by remedies diluted, one to 100, perhaps 30 times (30c) or more. Some homeopaths, such as Kent and now Vithoulkas, supported his theory. Others believed that Hahnemann left science behind at this point. One of these was the British homeopath, Richard Hughes. He produced his own materia medica called *The Cyclopedia* (1884–91), based on laboratory findings and low potencies, without regard for the theory of the Vital Force. Those who followed him tended to see homeopathy in more conventional scientific and medical terms. It was as a result of this split that homeopathy foundered in America some years before the introduction of antibiotics. One living homeopath who champions the middle road, using both approaches with great skill and expertise, is the Argentinian Dr Francisco Eizyaga. (For further details see *The Two Faces of Homoeopathy* by Anthony Campbell (see p. 339).)

Does homeopathy stand up to scrutiny by modern medical and scientific methods? Lack of convincing scientific proof is one of the great stumbling blocks to homeopathy's acceptance by the general medical community. Many reasons are quoted for this failure, such as lack of money, lack of time and lack of interest. (Although it should be said that many homeopaths are not interested in providing proof, because they know from their own experience that it works.)

There are three main areas which must be explored in an effort to overcome this lack of evidence. First, tests called clinical trials must prove that homeopathic remedies, as prescribed, actually benefit patients. Second, there must be proof that the highly diluted remedies have a measurable effect on living organisms, to show that they do contain some of the original substance. Third, the theoretical mechanism behind the potentization effect must be explored.

Clinical trials

In conventional medicine, all new drugs must undergo clinical trials before being licensed for prescription by doctors. There have been few well-run clinical trials in homeopathy. In 1854, there was an outbreak of cholera in London. The mortality rates were compared for homeopathic and orthodox hospitals. The former had a mortality rate of 16.4 per cent, while the rate in the latter was 51.8 per cent. The Board of Health at the time attempted to suppress these damning figures. It was only after the matter was raised in Parliament that the figures were duly recorded.

During World War II there were experiments on the homeopathic treatment of mustard gas burns, for the Ministry of Defence. Controlled trials of mustard gas nosode 30c, and a remedy called Rhus tox. 30c, showed a protective effect when these were given as a preventive measure.

A more recent study was conducted in 1980 by Gibson and colleagues, in Glasgow. It compared homeopathic treatment of rheumatoid arthritis with orthodox treatment by the drug aspirin. The results showed that the improvement rate was higher among the former group. However, a combination of aspirin and homeopathic remedies was even more effective.

Smaller trials have shown that Arnica 30c can significantly control pain and bleeding after dental treatment, and that Borax 30c and Candida nosode 30c are effective treatments for vaginal discharge.

In 1986 there was a double-blind study of the homeopathic treatment for hay fever, by Reilly. This showed significantly reduced symptoms in patients taking prescribed homeopathic remedies, compared with those taking a placebo.

Dr Peter Fisher, in conjunction with St Bartholomew's Hospital, published a trial showing that Rhus tox. was effective in the treatment of fibromyalgia (muscle ache), provided that the remedy was only given when properly indicated. Perhaps the most convincing clinical evidence is now beginning to emerge from the veterinary world. Farmers are reported to be buying homeopathic remedies in large quantities because they are far more cost-effective than antibiotics when treating conditions such as mastitis in cows.

A survey of 107 clinical trials in homeopathy published in the *British Medical Journal* in February 1991 showed that 80 per cent were positive in favour of homeopathy. They concluded that while further research was necessary, there was now enough proof to justify the use of homeopathy in certain conditions.

The effects of high dilutions

What about the evidence that living systems can be influenced by substances in high dilution? It is known that animals can be extraordinarily sensitive. For example, salmon in the ocean can detect the 'scent' of their home water at dilutions of one part in 1,000,000. The human nose is capable of detecting the foul-smelling substance mercaptan at concentrations of only one part in 500,000,000,000 parts of air.

In 1940, Dr W E Boyd conducted an important experiment in Edinburgh. He showed that the chemical mercuric chloride, diluted to 60c, had a measurable effect on the rate at which an enzyme, diastase, affected starch. Similar experiments have been done using animal tissues in the laboratory, including frog's heart and rat's uterus. Yeasts and plants have also been tested. All the results demonstrate that substances 'in potency' (diluted to typical homeopathic concentrations) have effects on living tissues. Many other experiments are recorded, but most have not been repeated and have been criticized for their accuracy. However, recently there has been a world-wide standardization of homeopathy, which it is hoped will give future scientific experiments their due credence. Dr Fisher is currently involved in research into the effects of homeopathic remedies on tissue cultures.

The theories behind potentization

When a substance is diluted one to 100, for 12 times (the 12c potency) or more, then it is likely that in any one sample, nothing of the original substance remains – it is pure solvent. Naturally, it is difficult to give a chemical explanation for how such infinitesimally small doses, or even no doses at all, produce their effect.

One possibility is the 'placebo effect'. It has been shown that up to three-quarters of patients will feel better if given a 'treatment' which is actually only a placebo. It appears that, if they think it will cure them, then this belief is enough, and they do improve. But it seems unlikely that babies or animals would respond to this effect – and respond they do, to homeopathic remedies.

It has also been proposed that minute quantities of a remedy may act as a catalyst, a substance that speeds up the chemical workings of the body and so stimulates its innate healing powers. However, the extreme dilutions seem to preclude this.

It may be that physics, rather than chemistry, holds the answer. Experiments have been conducted using Raman lasers and nuclear magnetic resonators (NMR machines, used in medical scanning) to reveal the electromagnetic or vibratory properties of remedies in high dilutions. Evidence indicates that the structure of the solvent molecules may be electrochemically changed by succussion (the violent mixing used when diluting potencies). The solvent molecules may be imprinted and 'remember' the vibratory properties of the original tincture. When the remedy is given to the patient, this 'memory' is communicated to the living system and stimulates the effect that we see.

A recent experiment to demonstrate potencies was carried out in France by Dr Benveniste and its results were published in the prestigious *Nature* magazine. It provoked a flurry of comment and resulted in the rerun of the experiments under the 'scientific' eyes of a fraud detector, a journalist and a magician. The resulting furore has done little to clarify the issue of potentization and much to discredit the objectivity and reputation of the orthodox scientific community.

Homeopathy and conventional medicine

Homeopathic remedies are not exclusive to homeopathy. For example, cis platina is used in the treatment of many types of cancer, in both homeopathic and conventional medicine. Cis platina, in common with many other drugs used in cancer treatment, is itself a 'carcinogen' (cancer-inducing drug). Similar experiments include quinine, digitalis and emetine. Orthodox medicine also employs dilutions of allergens (the allergy-causing substances) to treat the allergies themselves.

It is important that homeopathic physicians use orthodox methods of diagnosis. This permits understanding of how an illness might progress without treatment, which in turn helps in assessing the response to the remedy. Such diagnosis also helps the practitioner to identify symptoms that are characteristic to the individual, rather than the illness – information which is vital to prescribing the correct remedy. And qualified homeopaths are aware when it is necessary to recommend that a patient sees an orthodox physician. In addition the repertories include many examples of orthodox diagnoses.

Conventional surgery is used in conjunction with homeopathy in certain cases. For example, there may be an injury or physical blockage in an internal organ, or an illness may be draining the body's ability to cure itself. Homeopathic remedies also help in the healing of the wound made by the surgeon's knife. And homeopathy interacts with toxicology, the study of the effects of poisons on the body. Although remedies are so dilute that they are not poisonous, their toxic effects must be understood.

There are many similarities between the concepts of homeopathy and the new, expanding fields of immunology and allergy study. Indeed, the homeopathic approach to preventive medicine is reflected by the immunizations of orthodox medicine.

Homeopathy and non-orthodox medicines

There are many complementary, alternative or other non-orthodox medicines which share concepts with homeopathy. In particular, common to many such therapies is the concept of a natural healing force by which the body cures itself, given the right circumstances. In its use of natural remedies, homeopathy resembles herbal medicine and aromatherapy. In its use of subtle diagnosis it resembles iridology and kirlian photography. In its emphasis on the calmness of the mind it has a close harmony with yoga, meditation and relaxation techniques. Homeopathy can be used together with hypnotherapy and psychotherapy. And if structural problems are interfering with the progression of a cure, most homeopaths will send patients for physiotherapy, osteopathy, chiropractic or massage. (See p. 341 for further reading on these subjects, and p. 336 for useful addresses.)

Homeopathic Remedies

There are now more than 3,000 homeopathic remedies in use throughout the world, most of them derived from plants and minerals, some from animal and human tissues or secretions, a few from the microorganisms which multiply during disease processes, and even a few from modern drugs. You will find all the remedies mentioned in this book, some 250 in all, listed on pp. 297–304, with their full Latin names and common names.

Since many of the commonly used abbreviations of remedy names are neither consistently used nor particularly meaningful to the non-homeopath, remedies in this book are generally referred to by the first part of their Latin name, with a suffix if there is any chance of confusion.

For example *Allium cepa* is simply referred to as Allium, whereas *Allium sativa* is Allium sat. *Mercurius solubilis* is simply Mercurius, but *Mercurius corrosivus* is Mercurius corr. *Nux vomica* is simply Nux, but *Nux moschata* is Nux mosch. If in doubt about which remedy is meant, turn to pp. 297–304. More detailed information on 60 of the remedies can be found in Appendix C, p. 305.

For everyday home use a stock of 3 or 4 dozen remedies would be more than adequate. Suggestions for building a home medicine chest appear opposite. To spread the expense, buy the starter remedies, ointments, and mother tinctures first, and add the other remedies later.

Where can I buy homeopathic remedies?

Some chemists and healthfood shops stock a small range of remedies, usually in pilule form and in the 6c potency. However, in emergencies and in many chronic conditions, 30c remedies should be used. Being many times more diluted, they are many times more potent.

A full range of remedies, in various potencies and also as mother tinctures, can be bought from the specialized pharmacies and manufacturers listed on p. 338. If you consult a homeopath, of course, he or she may dispense remedies direct.

Various other items – unmedicated pilules, phials, storage boxes, droppers, etc. – can be purchased from the Homeopathic Supply Company or Trevor Cox, Homeopathy Ltd (addresses p. 338.)

In what forms are homeopathic remedies available?

Most people buy their remedies in the form of lactose (milk sugar) pilules which have been impregnated with a solution of the named remedy; to take the remedy one simply dissolves one or two pilules on the tongue. For babies and small children, there are also granules, which dissolve more quickly on the tongue and are less easy to spit out!

Remedies are also sold in solution form in small glass phials with screw tops. If you are allergic to lactose, one or two drops can be put directly on the tongue. The dropper should be sterilized between uses.

A few remedies are available as ointments, for topical application only, and some are available as mother tinctures, for mixing with water to make lotions for bathing, gargling, etc. Generally speaking, 10 drops of mother tincture to 0.25 litre (½ pint) of boiled cooled water are sufficient.

Can I get homeopathic remedies on the NHS?

Yes, provided they have been prescribed by a homeopath who is also a GP and working

---

Building a home medicine chest

Starter remedies Aconite, Apis, Arnica, Belladonna, Cantharis, Carbo/veg., Hypericum (30c and 6c potency). Buy the 30c first.
Chamomilla, Euphrasia, Ledum, Rhus tox., Ruta (6c potency only)

Other commonly used remedies Bryonia, Ferrum phos. (30c and 6c potency, but buy the 30c first)
Allium, Alumina, Argentum nit., Arsenicum, Calcarea, Colocynth, Gelsemium, Hamamelis, Hepar sulph., Ignatia, Ipecac., Lachesis, Lycopodium, Magnesia phos., Mercurius, Natrum mur., Nux, Phosphorus, Pulsatilla, Silicea, Sulphur, Urtica (6c potency only)

Less common but useful remedies Glonoinum (30c potency), Anacardium, Antimonium, Antimonium tart., Baryta carb., Calcarea phos., Causticum, Chelidonium, China, Dioscorea, Dulcamara, Graphites, Hyoscyamus, Kali carb., Natrum sulph., Opium, Phosphoric ac., Phytolacca, Sepia, Spongia, Staphisagria, Tarentula, Thuja, Veratrum (6c potency)

Mother tinctures Calendula, Hypericum, Euphrasia (used to make up lotions for bathing, gargling, etc.)
To make up a lotion add 10 drops of mother tincture to 0.25 litre (½ pint) boiled cooled water. If using Euphrasia to bathe eyes, add 1 teaspoon salt to solution.

Ointments Calendula ointment (soothing ointment for sore or inflamed skin)
Hypericum and Calendula ointment (antiseptic ointment for treating grazes and wounds)
Arnica, Calendula and Urtica ointment (general purpose soothing ointment for bruises and inflammation – NOT for use on broken or cut skin)

Bach Rescue Remedy (available as a liquid or ointment), for use in emotional emergencies for effects of anguish, examinations, visits to the dentist, etc. For more information about Bach remedies, read Edward Bach's books (see Bibliography p. 342.)

Tissue Salts come singly or in combinations for specific complaints. For information read Gilbert's book on Biochemic Tissue Salts (see p. 342)

within the National Health Service, or by a homeopath working in an NHS homeopathic hospital (see Useful Addresses, p. 338).

When and how should I take homeopathic remedies?

Remedies are best taken in between meals, at least half an hour after eating, and should be dissolved or dropped on to a clean tongue. They should not be taken when your mouth tastes of toothpaste, tobacco, strongly flavoured sweets, spicy food, etc. In emergencies make sure the mouth is thoroughly rinsed before giving a remedy.

What is the correct dosage?

Frequency and duration of dosage are indicated for all the remedies mentioned in PART 2 and PART 3 of this book.

For both adults and children 'a dose' is 1 pilule or 1 drop, or just enough granules to cover the area of the small finger nail. In chronic conditions 6c is usually the most appropriate potency, but in emergencies or in acute conditions 30c may be more appropriate.

In acute conditions, doses should be taken every ½ or 1 hour to begin with, up to a maximum of 10 doses. But as soon as there is some improvement, the interval between doses should be increased to 8 or 12 hours for 2 or 3 days at most. *There is absolutely no point in continuing to take a remedy once the symptoms have started to disappear.*

In chronic conditions 6c remedies are usually taken 3 times a day for up to 14 days, and 30c remedies every 12 hours for a few days. In chronic conditions the stronger the mental and emotional symptoms the higher the potency, and the stronger the physical symptoms the lower the potency.

Remember, the effectiveness of homeopathic remedies depends on matching the symptom picture to the remedy picture as precisely as you can, and then taking the smallest possible dose for the least possible time. Once the remedy has delivered its message, your Vital Force will do the rest.

Can I give homeopathic remedies to babies or very young children?

Yes, but you may find it easier to give granules rather than pilules because granules dissolve more quickly and are more difficult to spit out. If you do not have granules, you can always crush a pilule between two clean spoons, or dissolve it in a small quantity of warm water.

What should I do if the symptoms get worse?

Aggravation, a temporary worsening of symptoms, is not unusual when taking homeopathic remedies. Aggravation is usually a good sign – it means that a remedy is working. If you have simply taken the wrong remedy, it will have no effect. In acute conditions, discomfort may increase for a few minutes, seldom for longer. In chronic conditions, aggravation may last longer, but very rarely for more than a day or two.

The correct thing to do in such circumstances is to stop taking the remedy and wait until your symptoms improve, as they almost certainly will. If improvement continues, there is no need to take the remedy again. If improvement stops, restart the remedy. Where improvement continues for a while, then stops, leaving you with nagging symptoms, take the remedy in a higher potency; if you are taking 6c, take up to 10 doses of 30c.

If worsening symptoms are accompanied by any of the following – a persistent temperature of 39°C [102°F] or over, spitting blood or passing blood in stools or urine, a rigid and painful abdomen, increasing breathlessness or chest pain, confusion or abnormal drowsiness – dial 999. If you have a diagnosed condition which is potentially serious, contact your GP or homeopathic physician at once.

What should I do if some symptoms improve but others don't?

If you feel better in yourself, gradually cut down the remedy dose – the physical symptoms should improve in time. If you get 'stuck', you may need another remedy, probably one that complements the previous one.

If you experience relief from physical symptoms but find that mental symptoms remain troublesome, it may mean you have suppressed symptoms, although this is quite rare with homeopathy. It is more likely that your underlying condition is changing. To be on the safe side, however, antidote whatever remedy you are taking by drinking two cups of black coffee, or by taking the specific antidote (antidotes are given under each remedy described on pp. 305–32).

What should I do if new symptoms appear?

First, stop the remedy. You may be proving it. The symptoms should quickly disappear. If they do not, you may have the wrong diagnosis or remedy. Recheck, and call your GP or homeopath if unsure.

What should I do if the symptoms get neither better nor worse?

Review your symptoms, being as specific as you can, and consult the General Remedy Finder (pp. 269–96) to see if you can find a more appropriate remedy.

Are there any substances I should avoid when taking homeopathic remedies?

Yes. Coffee, alcohol, tobacco, minty flavourings, highly perfumed cosmetics and toiletries, strongly smelling household cleaners, and some essential oils (see list on p. 195) used in aromatherapy all have the ability to antidote homeopathic remedies, and should be avoided completely in acute ailments. If you have a chronic complaint and your symptoms are steadily improving with homeopathic treatment, you could gradually re-introduce some of them, but if improvement suddenly stops they will probably be the reason why.

How should homeopathic remedies be stored?

In a cool, dry, dark place, well away from things that smell, taking care to keep the tops of phials and containers well screwed on. Stored like this, homeopathic remedies remain potent for up to 100 years. Don't transfer remedies from one container to another. And keep them out of reach of children. They aren't poisonous, however much your child may take, but a small child may experience transient diarrhoea from the lactose sugar – and your whole collection could be wiped out at one go!

Can I take homeopathic remedies as well as orthodox drugs?

Homeopathic remedies will not interfere with any drugs your GP has prescribed for you. However, many orthodox drugs – steroids, major and minor tranquillizers, oral contraceptives, sleeping pills, antihistamines – modify or completely block the effects of homeopathic remedies. If you want to come off orthodox drugs, discuss the matter with your GP first. *Do not on any account stop taking a drug without consulting your GP.* If you have occasion to consult a homeopath, be sure to say what drugs you are taking.

How do I decide which is the right homeopathic remedy?

In emergencies, where swift medical attention is necessary and there is no time to choose between alternative remedies, simply give the homeopathic rescue remedy which appears under the appropriate entry in PART 2: 'Ailments and Conditions', or PART 3: 'A–Z of Other Conditions'. Use the Index to find the relevant entry. If the person is in emotional shock, give 4 drops of the Bach Rescue Remedy (see p. 24) as well.

In acute cases which are not emergencies you should have time to choose an appropriate homeopathic remedy from those listed under the relevant entry in PART 2: 'Ailments and Conditions' and cross-check it by consulting the General Remedy Finder. Choose the remedy which seems to suit the symptoms best. If the remedy does not produce some improvement you may have chosen wrong; it pays to spend 5 minutes getting it right the first time!

In all other cases you should have plenty of time to track down the right remedy. This is what you do.

1 Jot down the most noticeable symptoms – these can be physical (swellings, redness, pain), mental (anxiety, irritability, grief), food-related (a dislike of milk, a craving for fatty foods) or environment-related (sensitivity to noise, symptoms which come on after getting wet) but they must be symptoms which are unusual, out-of-the-ordinary for you or for the person you want to treat.

2 Turn to the Index and see if the physical or mental symptoms have an entry in PART 2: 'Ailments and Conditions'. General symptoms such as HEADACHE and ABDOMINAL PAIN for example appear in PART 3, with suggestions as to their possible causes. If you suspect a particular ailment or disease, refer to the Index and look up the relevant entry in PART 2 or PART 3.

3 Carefully read the PART 2 or PART 3 entry which most closely corresponds to the symptoms you have observed. It may advise you to give first aid, dial 999, or see your GP within 2 hours, 12 hours, 24 hours, 48 hours, or as soon as convenient. If the condition is long-standing and poses no immediate or serious threat to health, it may recommend a number of homeopathic remedies for you to try at home or advise you to consult an experienced homeopath.

4 If home homeopathic treatment seems appropriate, select the remedy which most closely matches the symptoms. But if none of the remedies given seems quite right, or if you consider other symptoms to be equally or even more important than those described, consult the General or Specific Remedy Finders. Full instructions on how to use the General and Specific Remedy Finders appear on p. 27.

5 For further clarification, read the remedies in the 60 Remedy Pictures section (p. 305).

Note: The potencies given are only a guide. If a remedy is well indicated but you don't have the potency recommended, use whatever potency you have, obeying the given time limits or until you can obtain the indicated potency.

How to Use This Book

Remedy Finders

There are two sets of Remedy Finders in this book. Under each of the main complaints in PART 2, 'Ailments and Conditions', there is a Specific Remedy Finder. Here you can find the symptoms which relate directly to that complaint. A General Remedy Finder which covers both the complaints in PART 3, and those in PART 4, may be found as Appendix A. The purpose of these Remedy Finders is to give you more information upon which to choose your remedy, once you are sure of your diagnosis. They can also help you find remedies for symptoms which are at variance with normal appearance and functioning, or which reflect a low level of vitality, but which do not yet add up to any specific ailment or disease.

Symptoms in the General Remedy Finder are grouped under three main headings: Body, Environment and Mind and Emotions. Appropriate remedies are listed alphabetically under each symptom. Please note that a remedy may appear under apparently contradictory headings.

Choosing the right remedy once you are sure of the diagnosis

1 Carefully read through all the remedies listed under your particular ailment. Is there one remedy which covers all the main symptoms you are complaining of? If there is, then you can take it according to the instructions. You can get more information about it from the 60 Remedy Pictures section (Appendix C) if it is included in that. Please note that the remedy you choose will almost certainly contain additional symptoms to yours; this does not matter. You do not have to have all of the listed symptoms in order to choose it; in fact it is a good sign if you do not (see Case 1 below).

2 What do you do if there are 4 or 5 remedies which cover your case and you cannot choose between them? If your complaint is in PART 2, use the Specific Remedy Finder to add symptoms not included in the pictures. You can also check your choice by reading it up in 60 Remedy Pictures (see Case 2 below). If your ailment is not in this section you should use the General Remedy Finder. However, if you do have symptoms of conditions appearing in PART 2, you may also use the Specific Remedy Finder for that section. For instance, your main complaint may be of indigestion, but you might have other symptoms which are aggravated pre-menstrually. In this case you should take the remedies for indigestion, but if you need more symptoms to differentiate between them, then take additional remedies using the symptoms listed in the Specific Remedy Finder for Pre-menstrual Syndrome.

3 If you still have not got enough information from the remedies listed in PART 2, and from the Specific Remedy Finder, then use additional symptoms from the General Remedy Finder (see Case 3 below).

4 If you are still not sure and there is one symptom that is bothering you more than the rest, simply look it up in either the Specific or General Remedy Finder and read up the remedies listed under it in 60 Remedy Pictures (see Case 4 below).

5 If you are still stuck, consult your homeopath.

Finding a remedy for non-specific ailments

The General Remedy Finder can also be used to find remedies for general feelings of unwellness, of being out of kilter and under par, provided you can pinpoint at least six out-of-the-ordinary symptoms, six symptoms which are unusual for you or for the person you are treating. You will probably find that most of them are directly or indirectly related to an external event, either one which has just happened or one which is imminent.

Suppose, for example, one of your close girl-friends loses her mother suddenly from a heart attack. She appears to be coping very well for a few months, then she becomes tired and irritable. When you talk to her about it, she eventually admits to being depressed and angry about her mother's death. You want to help by giving her a remedy. From the General Remedy Finder you look up anger, irritability and depression, and ailments brought on by grief, all of which are found under the MIND and EMOTIONS section. You take the main symptom as ailments brought on by grief and note all the remedies down and underneath put a tick when they appear in the other symptoms in a similar way to the tables for the four cases below.

From the Remedy Finder for fatigue you add the remedies for fatigue after grief (note they are the same as ailments brought on by grief). When you count up the ticks, you find the remedy could be either Aurum or Natrum mur. You need more information, so you ask your friend if she has noticed any other things that are unusual for her. She says she is very hungry and especially wants salty foods like crisps. If you turn to the Remedy Finder for Weight Problems and Eating Disorders and take the remedies for increase in appetite and desire for salty things, it will be obvious your friend needs Natrum mur. As a further check, turn to 60 Remedy Pictures (pp. 305–32) and see what the full picture of the remedy shows. If the cross-check is satisfactory, give her the remedy in the 6c potency 3 times a day for up to 14 days until you detect a general upswing. Dosage should then be discontinued.

If the most important symptom only has 1 or 2 remedies, put the remedies for the second most important, and then the third most important, across the top of the table until you have at least 6 remedies to choose from. If the picture which emerges is inconclusive, consult your homeopath.

Two things must be emphasized here. First, the General Remedy Finder is not an invitation to hypochondria, but an aid to treating imbalances before they lower vitality and resistance to the point where medically recognized ailments set in. Second, homeopathic remedies can and do relieve many vague, unspecific ailments, but their effects can be shortlived unless diet, exercise, and mental and emotional factors can be adjusted in the direction of greater vitality. Symptoms which have been present for a long time, for so long that they have become the norm rather than the exception, suggest a deeply-lying imbalance. In such cases it would be better to seek constitutional treatment from an experienced homeopath than attempt to self-prescribe.

Case 1

'You are struck down by an attack of cystitis. The main features are that you have shooting pains in the bladder on passing water, your bladder burns afterwards, and if you ignore the call you leak urine.'

Turn to the chapters on THRUSH and CYSTITIS. You may need to see your GP or homeopath, but in the meantime, if you read through the remedies you will find that Sepia is the only one which covers these particular symptoms. You can also read it up in 60 Remedy Pictures. You then take it according to the instructions. As we have pointed out, if Sepia also has a number of symptoms of cystitis that you do not have, just ignore them.

Case 2

'You are tired, you have a heavy feeling in your head and when you wake up in the morning you do not feel refreshed. Your periods are getting heavier, and the fatigue is worse during your period. You have also noticed lately that your hair is falling out more than usual and that your hand has begun to tremble slightly. You can get a bit breathless at times. Of course, you have been under a lot of stress over the last 6 months getting everything ready for your daughter's wedding, and you did go a little over the top with all the excitement.'

Turn to the section on FATIGUE. You may need to have some tests done, but in the meantime read all the remedies. You will probably find that none of them completely covers your symptoms. The most likely candidates appear to be: Sulphur, Natrum mur., Nux, Lachesis, Nitric ac. and Carbo veg. These cover all the symptoms except for 'worse during periods', 'fatigue worse after over-excitement' and 'unrefreshing sleep'. Put them in a row as in Chart 1. Now turn to the Specific Remedy Finder for Fatigue. Add these symptoms and it becomes clear that Nitric ac. is the remedy of first choice. You can confirm this by reading it up in 60 Remedy Pictures. Take it according to directions.

	Sulphur	Natrum mur	Nux	Lachesis	Nitric ac	Carbo veg
Worse during periods					I	
Fatigue from overexcitement		I	I	I	I	
Unrefreshing sleep					I	I

Case 3

'It is pre-menstrual time again and you are beginning to get wound up. You are spending longer hours at work, and bite people's heads off! You suffer from giddiness and occasional palpitations, and your breasts are becoming tender. Aside from the usual crampy pains below your stomach, you develop a pain in your left ovary which then spreads to the right ovary as well.'

Write down all the remedies under PRE-MENSTRUAL SYNDROME, as in Chart 2. Add your symptoms using the Specific Remedy Finder. As you can see, the answer is inconclusive: it could

be Sepia, Pulsatilla or Lachesis. However, you still have one trick up your sleeve! Remember that the pain started on the left side and moved to the right? Turn to the section LEFT SIDE/RIGHT SIDE on p. 274 in the General Remedy Finder. Under 'symptoms worse on the left side' you find Sepia and Lachesis. However, Lachesis is the only remedy listed under 'worse on the left, then the right', and is therefore your first choice. You can confirm this by reading it up in 60 Remedy Pictures. Take it according to directions.

	Sepia	Calcarea	Lycopodium	Pulsatilla	Sulphur	Lachesis	Natrum mur	Nux	Phosphorus	Graphites	Kali carb	Silica	Belladonna	Causticum
Workaholic	I	I				I			I					
Irritable	I		I	I			I	I						I
Giddy				I		I								
Abdominal cramps	I			I		I					I		I	I
Ovarian pain				I		I							I	
Tender breasts		I												
Palpitations	I						I							

Case 4

'You are in the menopause and you have one big problem. Certainly your periods have become a

bit heavier, although you are not flooding. You tend to perspire on the face more easily. You

	Sepia	Sulphur	Calcarea	Lycopodium	Lachesis	Pulsatilla	Belladonna	Carbo veg	Graphites	Arsenicum	Mercurius	Phosphorus	Bryonia	Causticum	Natrum mur
Dry vagina	I			I					I	I					I
Facial sweats			I	I		I	I	I			I				
Heavy periods	I	I	I			I			I						

have some dryness of the vagina, but nothing that some KY jelly won't cure. No, the thing that is bothering you is that, although you are perfectly healthy otherwise, and have a really good marriage, you have completely lost your sex drive.'

Write down all the remedies listed under MENOPAUSE, as in Chart 3. Add your symptoms using the Special Remedy Finder. As you can see, it is inconclusive. The right remedy for you could be Sepia, Calcarea, Lycopodium, Belladonna or Graphites. You look them up in 60 Remedy Pictures, but none of the pictures rings a bell. Remember, however, that the only real problem is your lack of libido. Turn to the Specific Remedy Finder and under the symptom 'lack of sex drive', you will find the remedy Conium. It is not one of the remedies in 60 Remedy Pictures. Just go ahead and take it according to the instructions at the beginning of the remedies listed under menopause.

PART 2
AILMENTS AND CONDITIONS

How to use this section

Ailments and conditions are divided into sections. Most ailments not dealt with here may be found in *The Family Guide to Homeopathy*. Cross-references in SMALL CAPITALS should be looked up in the Index.

The most likely causes of an ailment or symptoms are underlined.

If specific remedies but not specific symptoms are given, try the remedies in the order listed: the one given first is most likely to be effective.

In cases of sudden or acute illness, prompt action may be necessary. The symbols used in the text are:

(999) Emergency – call GP, but if not immediately available, dial 999 and ask for ambulance

(2) Consult your doctor if there is no improvement in 2 hours

[12] Consult your doctor if there is no improvement in 12 hours

[24] Consult your doctor if there is no improvement in 24 hours

[48] Consult your doctor if there is no improvement in 48 hours

Introduction

BETWEEN puberty and the menopause, a span of some 35 years, a woman ovulates about 400 times, normally at intervals of 28 days. If an egg is fertilized, pregnancy follows; if not, menstruation occurs as the vascular lining of the womb is shed. This remarkable cycle of fertility is maintained by 3 hormone-producing glands, the hypothalamus, pituitary, and ovaries (see diagram, The Menstrual Cycle). The ovaries produce 2 hormones, oestrogen and progesterone, in response to 2 hormones produced by the pituitary, follicle stimulating hormone (FSH) and luteinizing hormone (LH). Oestrogen levels, responding to FSH levels, rise dramatically in the 12 days leading up to ovulation, and are at their lowest during menstruation. The levels of progesterone secreted in response to LH are highest after ovulation, preparing the lining of the uterus (endometrium) for implantation of the egg. If fertilization of the egg does not occur, progesterone levels fall, and are unable to maintain the lining. Menstrual bleeding begins approximately 2 days after progesterone secretions reach their lowest level. Up to 60 ml (2¼ oz) of blood are then lost over 3 to 7 days.

The uterus or womb is a thick-walled, pear-shaped organ about 7.5 cm (3 in) long, with a narrow neck or cervix at its lower end; the mouth of the cervix juts into the top of the vagina. Opening into the bulbous, upper end of the uterus are 2 tubes about 10 cm (4 in) long, the Fallopian tubes. These are lined with tiny waving hairs which transport eggs from the ovaries to the uterus. It is in one or other Fallopian tube that fertilization usually occurs. There is no direct connection between the ovaries and the Fallopian tubes, however; eggs are simply released into the fluid-filled peritoneal cavity and wafted towards their fringed entrances.

The ovaries themselves are almond-shaped and about 3.5 cm (1½ in) long. At birth they contain many millions of immature eggs and follicles, but as already mentioned only about 400 reach maturity. Although several eggs may begin to mature each month under the influence of FSH, only one matures. Once it has been released from its follicle, the follicle turns into a 'corpus luteum' (literally 'yellow body') and proceeds to secrete large amounts of progesterone.

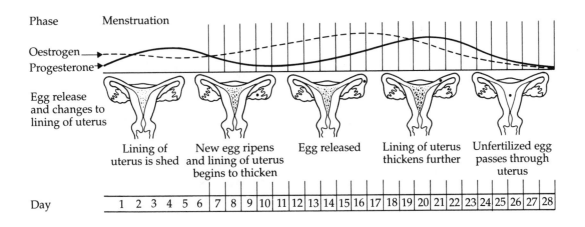

The menstrual cycle

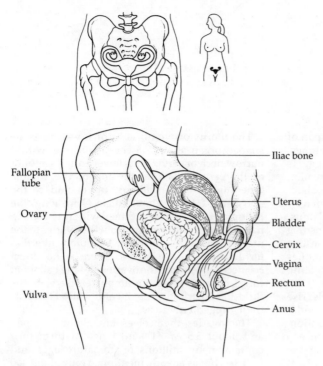

The anatomy of the uterus

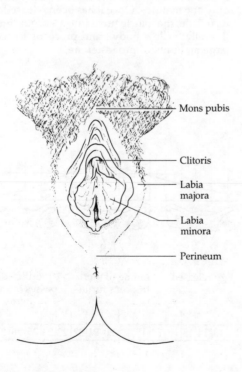

The location of the labia

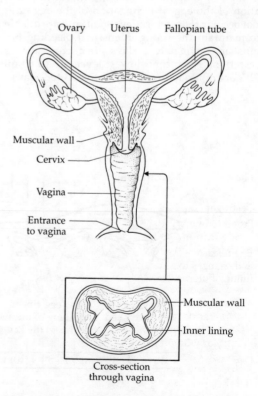

Cross-section
through vagina

The structure of the vagina

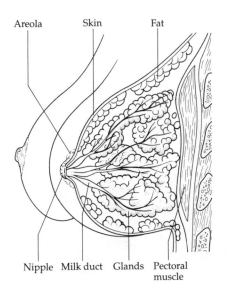

The female breast

The external female genitals, referred to as the vulva, consist of the fleshy inner and outer labia or lips which conceal the entrance to the vagina, and the clitoris, which lies just above the urethral opening where the inner labia meet (see diagram, The Location of the Labia). The clitoris is very sensitive and a focus for many of the sensations which trigger orgasm. The vagina is about 10 cm (4 in) long, expands and lubricates during sexual arousal, and is most sensitive near its entrance (see diagram, The Structure of the Vagina). It is protected from infection by populations of acid-producing bacteria.

Breast development is one of the first signs of puberty. The breasts move with the pectoral muscles underneath and their hang is greatly influenced by posture and the tone of the muscles which brace the shoulders back (see diagram, The Female Breast). Embedded in the fatty tissue of each breast are 15–20 clusters of milk-producing glands whose ducts converge on the nipple. The pigmented area around the nipple, the areola, contains glands which keep the nipple supple.

Weight Problems and Eating Disorders

Obesity

The definition of obesity is an excess of body fat; the definition of overweight is an excess of body weight relative to height. It is important to note that a muscular person may be overweight but have a low fat percentage, so body weight cannot be used alone as an accurate gauge for obesity. Obesity tends to be identified as weight which is greater than 20 per cent over the average desirable weight for women of a given height. Overweight is greater than 10 per cent over the average desirable weight for women of a given height. The body mass index (or BMI) is the most convenient way of expressing body weight, taking into account the individual's height, so BMI equals weight in kilos over height in metres squared. This is expressed as kilos per metre square.

In broad terms there may be considered to be five grades of BMI, although the ranges differ slightly for men and women. Under 19 is underweight, the norm is 19–25, overweight is 25–30, obese is 30–40 and severely obese is 40+.

By these criteria it is estimated that a third of GP patients are overweight, and it is largely agreed that a BMI of over 30 poses a significant health risk. A rough test involves pinching a fold of flesh below the navel and assessing its thickness; if it is an inch or over then you are significantly overweight.

Weight table for women

Which group are you in?
To find out whether you are underweight or normal weight, overweight, or obese, first find your height, then run your finger across to your present weight.

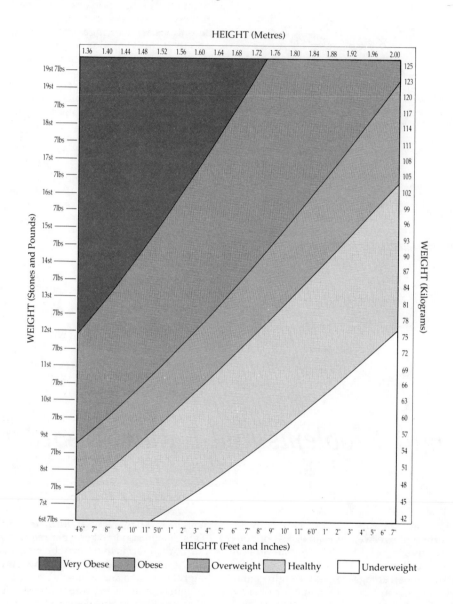

So how many of you are overweight? Obesity is the third most common Western disease after dental caries and coronary artery disease. The Dietary and Nutritional Survey of British adults in 1990 showed a 3-fold increase in clinically obese women since 1984. 50 per cent of British women were dieting, and 50 per cent of these had abandoned the diet before reaching their target weight.

Other findings included the following:

1 Despite the 1983 COMA Report recommending a decrease in fat content in diet from 40 per cent to 35 per cent – or ideally 30 per cent – of total

calories the average was still 40 per cent, with an unacceptably high contribution from saturated, or animal, fat.

2 Consumption of sweets, biscuits, cakes and chocolate, particularly among women, was on the increase.

3 There was also an increasing consumption of alcohol: two-thirds of women drank alcohol every week. This constitutes a consumption of extra 'empty calories' (they have no nutritional value, since they are devoid of micronutrients). At 7 kcals per g the calorific value is relatively high – between fat, which is 9 kcals per g, and protein and carbohydrate, which are 4 kcals per g.

4 There was an increasing number of meals eaten out. This constituted a quarter of women's diet. Foods eaten out tended to be higher in sugar and lower in protein, fibre and vitamins and minerals than the ordinary diet. There was also an increasing consumption of burger, kebab and chip take-aways – foods with a high saturated fat content.

5 Despite a recommended daily intake of fibre of 30–35 g, less than 16 per cent of women were eating as much as 25 g.

6 Average daily exercise was decreasing; 50 per cent of 65-year-olds and older did no activity, 30 per cent of adults did some vigorous activity, but only 6 per cent did enough to have a positive effect on health.

Risks of obesity?

First, mortality. Insurance data from Great Britain and the USA clearly show an increase in mortality related to obesity; for example, a severely obese person has 3 times the risk of dying than a person of average weight. The risk is significantly greater if obesity is associated with smoking. In terms of serious conditions associated with obesity, there is a significantly higher risk of the following:

1 Cardiovascular disease – heart attack, heart failure, high blood pressure and strokes.

2 Diabetes that develops in the older person – recent research shows that the fundamental problem is one of resistance to insulin by the tissues of the body, and the risk is as much as 5 times that for a person of normal weight. There is also new evidence to suggest that infants who are notably underweight at one year have a significantly increased risk of diabetes.

3 Gallstones – fat tissue is a large reservoir of cholesterol, and so obese people have a higher concentration of cholesterol in the bowel with a tendency to precipitation of gallstones.

4 Accidental death from slower movement crossing roads, for example.

5 Complications in pregnancy and reduced fertility.

6 Shortness of breath on exertion, and an increased risk in relation to general anaesthetic for surgery.

7 Osteoarthritis of the weight-bearing joints, especially the back, hips and knees.

8 Malignancy – cancer of the breast, uterus, ovary and cervix – appears to be due to a disturbance of the balance between male and female hormones caused by an enzyme system in fat tissue.

Less serious conditions caused by obesity are mainly associated with low-fibre diets and include piles, varicose veins, diverticulitis and oesophageal reflux.

Fat distribution is relevant, as it has been shown that androids – i.e., apple-shaped people, with a higher waist to hip ratio – have a higher risk of coronary heart disease than gynecoids – i.e., pear shapes.

Possible causes of simple obesity

Obesity occurs when over a period of time net energy intake exceeds net energy output. Thus over-eating and lack of exercise are the most frequent causes. Other underlying causes are relatively rare, e.g., hypothyroidism (see THYROID PROBLEMS). A number of physiological and psychological causes have been put forward for simple obesity; these include the following:

1 *Genetic factors* – Studies of adopted children, for example, show a significant association between the weight status of the child and the biological parents, which cannot be explained on environmental grounds. However, analysis shows that environment plus genetic interaction is more important than true genetic transmission. This implies that a strong family history of obesity is no bar to effective treatment.

2 *Eating habits* – It has been suggested that obese people eat larger and more infrequent meals, and eat more quickly than others. This is a popular misconception.

3 *Reduced metabolic rate* – Do obese people have a reduced metabolic rate? This is clearly not the case since basal metabolic rate is the body's basic 'tick over' speed, and it actually increases with weight.

4 *Inappropriate responses to hunger cues* – Experiments on appetite control show that children possess the ability to adjust their intakes of high and low calorie foods to maintain a relatively constant calorie level, while adults show no such compensatory system. There may be an innate monitoring mechanism present, but this becomes over-ridden to a greater or lesser degree.

5 *Toxin theory* – Another possible cause of

obesity, most often advanced by naturopaths, is delayed transit of faeces and toxins through the bowel. It is not generally appreciated that fat, because it takes a lot of energy to break down, is a convenient dump for all sorts of toxins; more toxins in circulation mean that more fat is laid down to keep them out of circulation. The remedy is a high-fibre diet, and avoidance of as many toxic substances, natural and man-made, as possible.

6 *Psychological factors*

a *Emotional starvation* where food is our sub-conscious compensation.

b *Fear of responsibility* e.g., an adolescent may get fat or thin to avoid being sexually attractive and taking responsibility for relationships.

c *Bereavement* – food may be a form of comfort.

d *Background of over-control* – overeating symbolizes need to break out of dietary strict-ness and overcompensate.

e *'Learned helplessness'* – this engenders a sense of little control over life, including weight e.g., canteen eating gives no choice, and is accepted as such. Food in this way can be used as the substitute answer to a range of emotional problems. This is the basis of compulsive eating suffered by a high proportion of over-weight women, which will be described in more detail later in this chapter.

f *Power of advertising* e.g., sugar and butter are 'good', 'natural' foods. The UK has the highest chocolate consumption in Europe apart from Switzerland, with average intake 17 lb per year. It is notable that in one year the chocolate confectionery industry was observed to spend 20 times the Health Education Authority's expenditure on nutrition messages!

7 *Fatigue* – Lack of sleep leads to impaired ex-cretion of toxins (see 5). Exhausted women may become overweight women as well as the other way round. Increase your sleep!

Psychological factors apart, in basic physio-logical terms there are 4 main factors which contribute to how much fat is stored by the body:

1 The appetite, amount and type of food eaten.
2 The amount of exercise undertaken.
3 The BMR (Basal Metabolic Rate) is the energy expenditure required for activity of the internal organs, and to maintain the body temperature when at rest; it decreases progressively with age. As mentioned earlier, weight gain leads to an increased metabolic rate. However, a reduced calorie diet will result in a lowering of BMR, as the body reacts to what is perceived as starvation conditions. Vigorous and sustained exercise can increase the BMR, not only during the exercise period but for some time after. If, for example, as a

result of vigorous exercise the body temperature is increased by 1 per cent, the BMR can increase by approximately 12 per cent.
4 Thermogenesis can be regarded as the body's ability to metabolize excess calories and produce heat. It may also be increased by exercise and by certain food fuels, which is in addition to the higher BMR induced by exercise and the calories burned off by exercise itself.

Of the above factors the individual has con-siderable control over numbers 1 and 2, and to a lesser extent 3; it is not yet known to what extent 4 may be influenced.

Self-help for number 1 – control of appetite, amount and type of food eaten. In compulsive eaters the signal which triggers eating seems not to be one of physiological hunger, but an emotional one. Eating in response to such emotional cues constitutes a learned behaviour from childhood: food equals comfort, in the sense of being cared for. Although this is a perfectly reasonable reaction for children, for adults the sense of comfort is purely transient, giving way to guilt and self-criticism and repeated attempts between binges to lose, by strict dieting, the gained weight. However, such dieting is doomed to failure in the long term, largely because it is fuelled by an intensely negative self-image. The natural response to severe self-denial in terms of food is to rebel: to binge. In this way, as long as eating remains disassociated with true hunger, a self-perpetuating cycle of dieting and overeating is inevitable. The stricter the self-imposed diet, the greater the kick-back binge is likely to be. It is estimated that over 90 per cent of all successful dieters regain the weight lost plus more. In order to break out of the cycle consider the following:

1 Self-criticism and punitive dieting will not lead to positive permanent changes in eating habits.
2 Diets cannot solve the need to turn to food for reasons other than hunger.
3 Acknowledge the body as it is without nega-tive thoughts, and allow compassion for your need to eat for comfort.
4 Try to face and consider problems and anxieties as they really are, not to 'translate' them into food, which can only provide transitory relief.
5 Get back in touch with physiological hunger instead of eating from emotional cues. More de-tailed advice on how to achieve this can be found in *Overcoming Overeating* by Jane Hirshmann and Carol Munter (see Further Reading, p. 341).

Diets can be useful as a start, but for longer-lasting weight control must be combined with changes in attitudes to foods and eating be-haviour. Weight-loss dietary guidelines are many and varied, but basically fall into two main categories: exclusion and inclusion diets.

Exclusion diets

Particular foods are restricted or excluded, for example chocolate, sugar, potatoes, etc., or more generalized food groups, e.g., low fat or carbohydrate or higher protein and fibre diets.

Low carbohydrate was the basis of many older diets but is now regarded as inappropriate since it inevitably results in increased proportions of energy from protein and fat. Unrefined carbohydrate is the best available source of energy, since it is rich in micronutrients and fibre, and should constitute at least 55 per cent of total calories eaten. It is associated with less fat and sugar and early satiety.

Refined carbohydrate, in contrast, has lost, in the processing, most of its nutrients and fibre. Fibre or Non Starch Polysaccharide (NSP) constitutes a sub-group of carbohydrates; there are 2 types, soluble and insoluble.

1 Insoluble is found in fibre cereals, for example wheatbran and fibrous fruit and vegetables. By absorbing water it contributes to a sense of satiety. It slows down absorption of simple sugars from the gut, thus helping to avert symptoms of HYPOGLYCAEMIA, and decreasing transit times through the bowel; this prevents constipation and diverticulosis, ridding the body of toxins, bile salts, etc.

2 Soluble fibre includes many fruits and vegetables, pulses and oatbran, and can be carried through the bloodstream binding with fat and preventing atherosclerosis.

Other diseases associated with low fibre in the diet include large bowel cancer, coronary artery disease, diabetes, GALLSTONES, PILES and VARICOSE VEINS. The average UK intake of fibre is approximately one eighth that of certain African tribes in which there is virtually no incidence of most of the low-fibre-associated diseases. The latest report from the Committee on Medical Aspects of Food Policy (see Bibliography, p. 341), however, casts doubt on whether this is entirely due to fibre, or whether it may relate more to the levels of starch and animal fats and protein, i.e., a low starch, low fibre, high fat diet; more studies are needed. The average intake of fibre, therefore, should ideally be doubled at least. The fibre content of some foods in g per 100 g of food are as follows:

Bran	44
Wholemeal bread	8.5
White bread	2.7
Rye crispbread	12
Digestive biscuit	6
All Bran	10
Baked beans	8
Dry beans and lentils	up to 25

Low fat diets

Current diets, exclusion and inclusion, will advocate fat reduction. A fat exclusion diet is inappropriate since it will tend also to exclude essential fatty acids which cannot be manufactured by the body. Ideally fat should be reduced to 30 per cent or, even better, 25 per cent of total calories. According to the latest COMA report (see Bibliography, p. 341) percentage of fat should be 33 per cent – too high according to many authorities. It should consist of a poly-unsaturated/mono-unsaturated to saturated fat ratio of $2:1$.

Practical ways of reducing fat include the following:

1 Reduce red meat.
2 Buy leaner meat and trim off the fat; skin poultry.
3 Replace red meat with game meats and fish.
4 Bake or grill or stir fry with a little fat, best done with olive oil which is mono-unsaturated and most stable at high temperatures. A pork chop fried with the fat on contains about 25 g of fat, and grilled with the fat off contains about 8 g.
5 If oil is required use small amounts of sunflower, soya or olive oil.
6 Bake more bean or lentil casseroles with just a little added meat.
7 Reserve roast potatoes for treats, otherwise eat boiled or baked.
8 Cut down on cheese and full cream milk and use substitutes for cream i.e., yoghurt or fromage frais.
9 Beware of fat-dense foods. Typically dietary fat consists of the following:

27 per cent from meat or meat products
25 per cent from butter or margarine
13 per cent from milk
13 per cent from cooking oils and fat
6 per cent from biscuits and cakes, etc.
5 per cent from cheese and cream
11 per cent from other foods

High protein diet

Protein deficiency is virtually unknown in the West. However, a high animal protein diet aimed at weight reduction is inappropriate for the following reasons:

1 It is associated with a high fat content, i.e. there is fat between the muscle fibres of meat, not just around the joint of meat.
2 It contains a relatively high phosphate content, contributing to lost calcium from the bones.

3 It produces a high content of nitrogenous waste, placing extra strain on the kidneys.
4 Unless meat is organically reared, it is likely to contain antibiotic, pesticide and hormone residues.
5 It has a low fibre content.

Although animal protein contains a complete range of amino-acids, it is also possible to achieve the complete range needed by combining 3 or 4 types of vegetable protein, i.e., rice plus tofu plus vegetables, or beans plus rice, or millet and lentils, all with nuts or seeds or products made from them such as nut butters, tahini etc.

N.B. Peanuts are closer to the legume than the nut family and are high in fat.

Typical protein contents include the following:

Chicken 3 oz	28 g
Beef 3 oz	23 g
Fish 3 oz	21 g
Cheddar cheese 3 oz	21 g
Beans with rice 7 oz	17 g
Rice pudding 4 oz	17 g

The average daily requirement for women aged 18–54 is 45–6 g. To sum up, the ideal diet should stick to the following principles: meals high in unrefined foods, foods high in fibre and low in fat, salt and sugar and unnecessary chemicals. For further information, see the *twice-a-week rule* (p. 248).

Inclusion diets

These include *total* energy restriction. This calls for a more 'obsessional' approach since constant calorie counting is required, which can be socially restrictive, boring and time consuming, and not as accurate as it is relied on to be. It is also rather unnatural to try to keep to the same intake day by day, since intake normally varies.

Try to develop a 'calorie' awareness, as this is largely within your own control and not that of a calorie counter. For example fat and sugar are the two most calorie-dense foods. Fibre is an excellent calorie saver as it greatly decreases calorie density, i.e. 2 teaspoons of sugar has the same calorie content as 4 oz peas. Half a pound of chocolates would similarly be equivalent to 5 lb of apples!

Cultivate an eye for calories when eating out, so choose grilled meat or fish, have lots of salad with minimal dressing, largely avoid alcohol and pre-dinner nibbles. Avoid butter on bread and fatty, sugary puddings.

Aim to stick to the low fat and sugar and refined carbohydrate and high fibre principle 90 per cent of the time, allowing for 10 per cent 'treats' without feeling they will rock your dietary foundations.

Rate of weight loss

To achieve significant steady loss most women must decrease their calorie intake to around 1,250 or 1,000 kcals per day, and increase exercise. On undertaking a weight-reducing diet the body cannot be instructed to lose fat alone since energy sources include:

1 Blood glucose.
2 Glycogen stored in muscles and liver.
3 Fat.
4 Protein.

Mobilization of glycogen from the liver at the start of a diet releases water, contributing to a greater weight loss in the first couple of weeks or so. On resumption of normal eating this weight will inevitably be regained. The excess weight in obesity consists of approximately 75 per cent fat and 25 per cent fat-free mass, i.e. other tissue such as muscle which contains protein, glycogen and water. To lose a maximum of fat rather than fat-free mass it is best to eat 1,000 kcals less per day, which will result in a weight loss of 2 lb a week. Remember, however, that as weight is lost the fat-free mass decreases, metabolic rate decreases, and the average daily energy requirement decreases. This means intake must be progressively slightly reduced to maintain steady weight loss, i.e. by around 5 kcals per day for each pound lost.

Very low calorie diets

The very low calorie or 'starvation' diets of around 500 kcals or less – although associated with more impressive initial weight loss – cannot result in a long-term loss for a number of reasons.

1 With a weight loss of greater than 2 lb a week, proportionally more fat-free mass is metabolized. As this results in a decrease in Basal Metabolic Rate, on a return to normal eating it is easier to gain weight than before the diet.
2 Unless specially formulated 'ready-mix' very low calorie diets (VLCDs) are used – i.e. without added micronutrients – very low intake must lead to a deficiency of micronutrients. Depletion of these stores may be associated with triggering of the appetite mechanism, so that HYPOGLYCAEMIA and irresistible bingeing result.
3 Since the 'ready-mix' forms of VLCDs absolve you of responsibility for calorie control of food preparation they lead to no useful change in eating habits.
4 They can possibly lead to unacceptably high losses of fat-free mass, which carries a small risk of sudden death from effects on heart muscle.

VLCDs are only justifiable in the severely obese and those requiring to lose weight urgently, i.e. before surgery. They should not be followed for more than a month without medical supervision, and whilst on the diet any unexpected symptoms should be reported to your GP.

VLCDs are ill-advised if you have gout or porphyria. On stopping such a diet it is essential to adopt healthy eating habits as already described.

Conclusions about diets

Although of some use temporarily, neither exclusion nor inclusion diets are likely to result in permanent weight loss, largely because self-control has been abandoned in favour of dietary rules. Such long-term restriction is more than likely to result in a periodic backlash of unrestrained eating, which then induces guilt and reproach, resulting in starting an even stricter dietary regime. This pattern can be life-long, with cycles of deprivation and indulgence, obsessional weighing and constant mental totalling of each day's food. Re-learning to trust your true hunger results in a restoration of dietary self-control, which in itself is a great sense of relief. There may still be lapses into comfort-type eating. Since strict self-denial leads to backlash binge eating in compensation, craved foods, e.g. chocolate and cakes, are unlikely to remain the most desired foods if eating is actually unrestricted.

New eating habits

These may be aided by the following considerations.

1 Evaluate your reasons for overeating, i.e. boredom, frustration, anger, or habit. Food can potentially be a universal response to all emotions. Try keeping a food diary for a month or so, charting kinds and amounts of food eaten, times of eating, and associated feelings and activity taken. This will give a valuable picture of how much eating is emotional, and how balanced the diet tends to be, and will also supply a useful impression of exercise patterns.
2 Learn to recognize the difference between eating from hunger and from emotional reasons.
3 Try to eat at least 3 meals a day, as skipping meals will simply produce a starvation response from the body so that fat storage increases.
4 Eat without distraction in a relaxing environment.
5 Eat slowly and enjoy all aspects of the food, texture, taste, aroma and colour. Avoid combining eating with reading or watching television.

Anorexia nervosa

This potentially fatal eating disorder was first described in 1874, but is in fact increasingly a disorder of our time, representing perhaps the most dramatic expression of this culture's obsession about regulation of body size. It has shown a marked rise in incidence over the past 20 years or so, and is now said to affect up to 1 : 100 women between 15 and 25, mainly of middle-class background, although it can occur at any age between 12 and 35. Approximately one third of affected women have a history of overweight, and there is a relatively high incidence in diabetics.

Anorexia is characterized by the following features:

1 Self-induced, rigid eating control, and a morbid fear of fatness and associated distorted body image. The sufferer sees herself as much fatter than she really is.
2 An abnormality in reproductive functions generally manifests as amenorrhoea.

Physical effects may include the following:

1 Dry skin and excessive growth of dry, fine, brittle hair over the nape of the neck, cheeks, forearms and thighs called 'lanugo' hair.
2 Cold hands and feet and peripheral oedema.
3 Upset in heart rhythm, and low blood pressure.
4 Constipation.

Other disorders showing some of the same features include: thyrotoxicosis, mal-absorption, and hyperpituitarism, and should be excluded by your doctor.

Possible psychological background

Anorexia nervosa has generally been regarded as a disorder of adolescence, precipitated by a fear of growing up and of sexuality, resulting in an attempt to de-feminize the body. There may also be an association with personality disturbance as a result of a distressed family background. The pre-anorexic personality is generally one of a model of good behaviour, conformity and academic achievement, concealing an underlying sense of self-doubt and ineffectiveness. The onset of the anorexia may well follow exposure to new and vulnerable situations, e.g. starting at a new school, and the need to be liked by being thinner. It may also be linked to a family eating disorder, e.g. anxiety regarding being overweight.

Parental attitudes also appear to be significant, in that parents of anorexics may consciously or unconsciously interfere in their daughter's attempts to establish normal peer relations, perhaps by criticizing her friends, and setting limits in order to keep her close to home. The girl is therefore torn between a fear of separation, and the wish to be accepted by her peers. Changing body shape during puberty adds to a general feeling of lack of control, and controlling her weight becomes the focus for her anxiety. This is further fuelled by cultural messages that only slimness is attractive, and dieting is the solution to the crises of adolescence. There may be a background of rigid order in the home, with each mealtime a potentially serious or tense occasion.

The trigger may be a mainly sociocultural one – there tends to be a high incidence of abnormal attitudes to eating and weight in certain groups, like models and dance students.

Food becomes, in essence, a veritable battle-field, an object of desire yet also of intense anxiety and fear.

Dieting may start relatively inconspicuously, perhaps with dieting during the week and week-ends off, avoiding meals till evening, eating 'slimming' foods, regular fasting etc.

Refusing food and obsessional calorie counting are the mainstay of the anorexic's mode of dietary behaviour. She may even appear to develop an intense interest in food or cooking for others, but refuse to eat herself. There is a perpetual oscillation between shame when 'fattening' foods are eaten, and exhilaration when a new diet is embarked upon. The body thus inevitably becomes an object of intense self-criticism.

A desire not to eat may at times become a total inability to eat, which may be associated with intensive exercise patterns, or interspersed with binges, when anxiety becomes overwhelming. The ultimate goal of 'acceptable' thinness is never resolved, as a result of distorted body image; dieting therefore becomes increasingly rigid, to the extent that severe emaciation may result in a life-threatening condition.

Treatment

This has thankfully moved on from the days of force-feeding and tube-feeding and appetite stimulants, and is now largely a combination of behaviour therapy and, perhaps, also associated family or marital therapy. Hospitalization is a multi-disciplinary approach, generally with one central figure to whom the anorexic can relate well.

Aims

To reach a normal weight range, i.e. equal to a BMI of 19, to re-establish a normal eating pattern, and abolish vomiting, purging and excess exercising.

As a result of her fear of losing control by putting on weight, the anorexia sufferer may well make attempts to sabotage her therapy by being manipulative and untruthful. It is thus essential that at some point she acknowledge that her problem exists, and allow her self-compassion to emerge so that she can accept her feelings. Nutritious food can then cease to be a source of fear and anxiety, and there can be an acceptance of body image.

Self-help organizations outside the NHS include the following: Anorexic-Aid (also for bulimia sufferers), Anorexic Family Aid (also for bulimia sufferers), Samaritans, Relate (see Useful Addresses, p. 333).

Bulimia

This was first described by a psychiatrist, Gerald Russell, in 1979, and may be closely associated with anorexia (40–50 per cent of anorexics may develop bulimia), or it may exist alone. Like anorexia nervosa, its origins appear to be social, cultural and psychological, i.e. as a result of anxieties regarding appearance and sexual attractiveness. Main triggers appear to be anxieties regarding competence to handle responsibility, self-doubt about ability to be liked or loved, and a tendency to want to please others, resulting in lack of identity and purpose.

American studies suggest an association with low levels of beta endorphines – natural body opiates, a raised level of which is known to be associated with jogging or running.

Bulimia is characterized by a morbid fear of fatness, and powerful intractable urges to over-eat. These result in bingeing, with strict dieting between binges, and induced vomiting, purging or use of diuretics to avoid the fattening effects of food. This disorder is estimated to affect 2 per cent of women under 40. A total of 20 per cent under 40, however, are reported to have a less established eating disorder which involves occasional binge eating. Bingeing tends to be precipitated by such triggers as unbearable tension, feelings of inadequacy, or boredom, crises of indecision, and repressed anger. Those suffering from bulimia generally hide the disorder, and will tend to continue until interrupted, or food runs short, or abdominal distension becomes intolerable.

Warning signs of bulimia

These may include the following:

1 Regular avoidance of meals, with the comment 'I'll have something later.'
2 Visits to the bathroom immediately after meals.
3 Inexplicable disappearance of food.
4 Self-criticism of shape.
5 Inexplicably staying up late.

6 Apathy, withdrawal and pessimistic view of life.

Eating and vomiting may become inseparable, so that if vomiting is not possible intense anxiety will result. Bingeing, which generally involves large quantities of refined carbohydrate, produces a transient high, inevitably followed by HYPO-GLYCAEMIA, with possible associated symptoms of sweating, weakness, erratic behaviour or mental confusion. Vomiting provides an enormous sense of relief, as if the body has been rid of its weight of emotional problems, however transiently. It also serves a self-punishment function, a penalty for weak will. Finally, it provides a sense of security, relating to the knowledge that it is possible to overeat without gaining weight. Since a certain proportion of food eaten will be absorbed prior to vomiting or purging, the bulimia sufferer generally does not assume the emaciated appearance of an anorexic.

Physical and emotional side effects

These will depend on the duration of the disorder, the frequency of vomiting or purging, and the quality of nutrition absorbed overall. It will also depend on the body's ability to counteract the resultant chemical imbalance.

Side effects of bingeing

These may include the following:

1 Abdominal distension and pains.
2 Salivary gland swelling.
3 Fatigue, nausea and breathlessness.
4 Dental caries or gum disease from sugary food.

Side effects from vomiting – apart from hypo-glycaemia – will include:

1 Electrolyte imbalance – potassium chlorides and hydrogen ions are lost in vomiting, resulting in the following possible complications:
  a Muscle weakening, with tingling and numbness in fingers and toes.
  b Fatigue.
  c Headaches, confusion and low concentration.
  d Palpitations and low blood pressure.
  e Renal damage.
2 Lack of protein resulting in oedema, i.e., puffy face and ankles.
3 Tooth enamel erosion from vomiting stomach acid.
4 Gastro-intestinal bleeding – vomiting can cause abrasions and tearing of the oesophagus with resultant bleeding and discomfort on swallowing.

Associated problems

These include: depression, a tendency to alcohol addiction or drug dependency, pre-menstrual carbohydrate craving and food allergy. Recently an association between bulimia and POLYCYSTIC OVARIAN SYNDROME has been reported. The emotional aftermath is likely to involve pronounced mood swings, with increasing intolerance, aggression and deceit, resulting in further guilt and self-reproach, and an increasing sense of isolation and despair. In order to break the cycle it is essential for the sufferer to acknowledge that food is serving as a mechanism for coping with stress, and to find alternative ways of dealing with this.

Self-help

The initial avenues of support are similar to those suggested for the anorexic. It may be useful to keep a diary, so that associations between feelings and binges can be acknowledged and accepted with a sense of self-compassion. It is then essential to find a compromise between a strict dieting regime and resultant bingeing. Learning to absorb the occasional slip-up and accept the reasons for it will help.

Psychiatric help as an outpatient is provided, and is likely to consist of psychotherapy and behavioural therapy. The former involves a gradual process of building self-respect, self-confidence and self-discipline, whilst exploring strengths and weaknesses. The latter involves acknowledgement of eating triggers, e.g. loneliness, anger or boredom, and then learning alternative ways of coping with those to regain control of eating. As with anorexia, honesty is a prerequisite for recovery, particularly in view of the fact that bulimics may tend to exaggerate their progress, because of their need to please.

New eating habits

1 Try to leave a little food on the plate.
2 Have plenty of non-fattening snacks in the house.
3 Don't be afraid of an occasional naughty treat.
4 When eating out don't be dictated to by large servings; be aware of your degree of hunger and eat to a comfortable level.

Starting a weight-loss programme

Before starting any programme of weight loss it is sensible to make the following preparations:

1 Keep a food and exercise diary for several weeks, and consider its implications.
2 Look at the range of possible diets to follow, and choose the type which best suits your needs and personality.

3 Select a realistic target weight loss.
4 Consider some support, e.g. a slimming club or regular monitoring by your GP, practice nurse or homeopath.

Best of all, consider those life changes that may need to be made to divest food of its power as your 'comforting enemy', and develop a 'crafty calorie conscious' eye which allows you to trust your own judgement, but also permits you the occasional 'naughty but nice' dietary indiscretion without an associated sense of imminent retribution!

Exercise in weight loss
The additional energy cost of exercise is actually very small compared with energy stores in fat. 1 kg of fat = 9,000 kcals, roughly equivalent to 38 hours of walking. This thought is rather disheartening, but considered over a period of months an effective exercise programme is perfectly possible.

A regular, preferably daily, exercise programme can contribute to maintenance of weight loss by burning off extra calories at the time of exercise and raising the BMR, provided the exercise is sufficiently vigorous and substantial.

Try for 20–30 minutes a day of sustained aerobic exercise, e.g. cycling, swimming, tennis, rebounding at 210 kcals in half an hour, jogging, hill-walking at 300 kcals in half an hour.

Other benefits of exercise are as follows:

1 Raises thermogenesis from food.
2 Lowers appetite for an hour or so after.
3 Produces toning and shaping.
4 Raises muscular strength and stamina.
5 Acts as a natural anti-depressant and anti-stress agent, and promotes sleep.
6 Lowers blood pressure, improves circulation and cardiac capacity, lowers cholesterol, prevents osteoporosis.

N.B. It is important to build up an exercise programme gradually.

Use of drugs in weight loss
Appetite suppressants, e.g. Fenfluranine and Phenteramine are controlled drugs available only on prescription. In the authors' view they are rarely justifiable except to help a severely obese person over an initial weight plateau. They should only be used in the short term, since tolerance develops, and artificial control of hunger is not a long-term answer to an overweight problem.

Research is ongoing into the ideal 'thermogenic' drug, which will ideally raise energy expenditure by approximately 20 per cent, but will not raise intake, also lowering body fat and fat-free mass. Even if such a drug should be produced, the authors' views on the use of drugs in weight loss will remain unchanged.

Homeopathic treatment
Constitutional treatment is recommended.

Specific remedies to be taken in the 30c potency weekly for up to 8 doses.

Please remember to check your choice against the Remedy Pictures (p. 305), where possible.

Calcarea
Eats when worried; panic attacks; depression; dizziness; itchy scalp; craving for sweets; cramping pains; stress incontinence – worse for coughing; thrush; vaginal discharge before periods; swollen breasts before periods; chest pain; stiff neck; clumsiness; eczema.

Generalities: Hot flushes; weakness – worse for not eating regularly; tendency to arthritis.

Lycopodium
Weight goes up when under stress – eats more when anxious; seems to put on weight even when eats only small quantities; weepiness before and after periods; difficulty in concentrating; irritability before periods; dizziness; itchy scalp; hair falling out; painful eyes; craving for sweet things; bloated abdomen before periods; cramping abdominal pains; stress incontinence – worse for coughing; breathlessness; stiff neck; sciatica; swelling of fingers; hot feet.

Generalities: Tendency to arthritis; fatigue worse before period.

Sepia
Weight goes up under stress and during menopause; irritable before periods; difficulty in concentrating; hair falling out; chronic sinusitis; craves sweets; stress incontinence – worse for laughing or coughing; thrush; vaginal discharge before periods; stiff joints; hot sweats.

Generalities: Hot flushes; fatigue – worse before and after periods; tendency to arthritis.

Sulphur
Weight goes up under stress, due to marked increase in appetite; weight gain during the menopause; itchy scalp; hair falling out; chronic sinusitis; craving for sweets, especially before periods; itching in back passage; stiff joints; swollen fingers; hot feet; hot sweats; eczema.

Generalities: Hot flushes; fatigue – worse before periods; tendency to arthritis.

Pulsatilla

Weight goes up due to marked increase in appetite; seems to put on weight even if eats only small quantities – worse during menopause; indecision, weepiness and irritability before periods; dizziness; migraines; craves sweets; bloated abdomen before periods; cramping abdominal pains; stress incontinence – worse for laughing or coughing; thrush; breathlessness; painful chest; swollen fingers; hot feet.

Generalities: Marked fluid retention; hot flushes; fatigue – worse before periods; tendency to arthritis.

Phosphorus

Weight goes up due to marked increase in appetite, by eating even small quantities of food; difficulty in concentrating; panic attacks; weepiness before and after periods; dizziness; fatigue – worse after periods.

Lachesis

Weight gain in menopause; difficulty in concentrating; indecisiveness; depression; hair falling out; sensation of lump in throat; bloated abdomen before periods; breathlessness; stiff neck; painful legs; hot feet; clumsiness.

Generalities: Hot flushes; fatigue – worse before and after periods and if does not eat for a while.

Natrum mur.

Weight gain under stress due to marked increase in appetite; seems to put on weight even if eats only small quantities of food; weepiness and irritability before periods; dizziness; itchy scalp; hair falling out; sore eyes; sensation of lump in throat; stress incontinence – worse for laughing or coughing; thrush.

Generalities: Fatigue and weakness pre-menstrually; tendency to arthritis.

Kali carb.

Weight increase due to stress because eats when anxious; weight seems to increase even if eating only small quantities; panic attacks; hair falling out; migraines; chronic sinusitis; craving for sweets; swollen breasts pre-menstrually; stiff neck.

Generalities: PMS; generally feels worse if she does not eat for a while; tendency to arthritis.

Arsenicum

Eats when worried; depression; panic attacks; craves sweets; thrush; breathlessness; chest pain; stiff joints; swollen fingers; eczema.

Generalities: Marked fluid retention; weakness.

Causticum

Eats when worried; depression; difficulty in concentrating; irritable before periods; migraines; stress incontinence – worse for laughing or coughing; breathlessness; painful chest; stiff neck; stiff joints; hot feet; clumsiness.

Generalities: Hot flushes; tendency to arthritis.

Mercurius

Weight gain from stress; gains weight even though seems to eat only small quantities; panic attacks; painful eyes; craving for sweets; thrush; swollen fingers.

Generalities: Marked fluid retention; fatigue; tendency to arthritis.

Belladonna

Eats when worried; puts on weight even though eating only small quantities; dizziness; cramping pains in abdomen; painful chest; stiff neck; painful legs; clumsiness; hot sweats.

Generalities: Marked fluid retention; weakness pre-menstrually.

Remedy Finder for Weight Problems and Eating Disorders

Goitre (swelling of the thyroid gland in obese patients)
Fucus vesic.

Fat body, thin legs and arms
Ammonium mur.

Obesity in young girls
Antimonium tart.
Badiaga
Calcarea
Capsicum
Ferrum
Kali bichrom.

Overweight during menopause
Graphites

Overweight in old women
Aurum
Kali carb.

Overweight after pregnancies
Kali carb.

Appetite easily satisfied
China
Lycopodium
Platina

Increase in appetite
Abies can.
Ammon. carb.
Argentum
Arsenicum
Calcarea
Calcarea sulph.
Cannabis ind.
China
Cina
Cinnab.
Graphites
Iodum

Lycopodium
Natrum mur.
Nux
Oleander
Petroleum
Phosphorus
Psorinum
Pulsatilla
Sabadilla
Sulphur
Veratrum

Lack of appetite
Arsenicum
Asarum
Calcarea
Chamomilla
Chelidonium
China
Cocculus
Cyclamen
Ferrum
Kali bichrom.
Lycopodium
Natrium mur.
Nux
Phosphorus
Pulsatilla
Rhus tox.
Sepia
Silicea
Sulphur

Lack of appetite despite hunger
Cocculus
Lachesis
Natrum mur.
Nux

Lack of appetite accompanied by thirst
Calcarea
Colchicum
Kali bichrom.
Kali nit.
Phosphorus
Psorinum
Spigelia
Sulphur

Lack of appetite and lack of thirst
Argentum nit.

Ravenous appetite
Ammon. carb.
Argentum
Arsenicum
Arsenicum iod.

Calcarea
Calcarea phos.
Calcarea sulph.
Cannabis ind.
Carbon sulph.
China
Cina
Ferrum
Graphites
Iodum
Lycopodium
Natrum mur.
Nux
Oleander
Petroleum
Phosphorus
Psorinum
Pulsatilla
Sabadilla
Silicea
Sulphur
Veratrum

Eating improves symptoms
Chelidonium
Iodum
Natrum carb.
Phosphorus
Sepia
Spongia

Fasting makes symptoms worse
Calcarea
Crocus
Iodum
Staphisagria

Symptoms worse before eating
Anacardium
Fluoric ac.
Iodum
Laurocerasus
Natrum carb.
Phosphorus

Symptoms worse after eating
Aloe
Arsenicum
Bryonia
Calcarea
Calcarea phos.
Causticum
Colocynth
Conium
Kali bichrom.
Kali carb.

Lachesis
Lycopodium
Natrum mur.
Nux
Phosphorus
Pulsatilla
Rumex
Sepia
Silicea
Sulphur
Zinc

Symptoms improve while eating
Chelidonium
Iodum
Natrum carb.
Phosphorus
Sepia
Spongia

Symptoms get worse while eating
Ammon carb.
Carbo an.
Carbo veg.
Conium
Kali carb.
Nitric ac.
Sulphur

Eating to satiety alleviates symptoms
Arsenicum
Iodum
Medorrhinum
Phosphorus

Eating to satiety makes symptoms worse
Calcarea
Lycopodium
Pulsatilla
Sulphur

Cold drinks alleviate symptoms
Bismuth
Bryonia
Causticum
Phosphorus
Sepia

Cold drinks make symptoms worse
Cantharis
Ferrum
Rhus tox.
Sepia

Warm drinks alleviate symptoms
Arsenicum
Nux
Rhus tox.

Warm drinks make symptoms worse
Rhus tox.

Coffee alleviates symptoms
Chamomilla

Coffee makes symptoms worse
Cantharis
Causticum
Chamomilla
Ignatia
Nux

Tea makes symptoms worse
Selenium
Sepia

Vinegar makes symptoms worse
Antimonium

Aversion to drinks
Belladonna
Cantharis
Ferrum
Hyoscyamus
Nux
Stramonium

Aversion to warm drinks
Phosphorus
Pulsatilla

Aversion to beer
Belladonna
China
Cocculus
Nux

Aversion to coffee
Calcarea
Nux

Aversion to water
Hyoscyamus
Nux
Staphisagria
Stramonium

Aversion to wine
Aconite
Lachesis
Sabadilla

Desire for cold drinks
Aconite
Arsenicum
Bryonia
Chamomilla
China
Cina
Mercurius
Mercurius corr.
Natrum sulph.
Phosphorus
Veratrum

Desire for warm drinks
Bryonia
Lac can.

Desire for alcohol
Arsenicum
Asarum
Capsicum
Crotalus
Hepar sulph.
Lachesis
Nux
Sulphur

Desire for alcohol before periods
Selenium

Desire for beer
Aconite
Nux
Sulphur

Desire for brandy
Lac can.
Lachesis
Lycopodium
Nux
Opium
Ranunculus
Sulphur

Desire for lemonade
Belladonna

Desire for vinegar
Hepar sulph.

Desire for whisky
Lac can.
Sulphur

Thirst makes symptoms worse
Acetic ac.
Aconite
Argentum nit.
Arsenicum
Bryonia
Calcarea
Capsicum

Causticum
Chamomilla
China
Digitalis
Eupatorium
Helleborus
Iodum
Mercurius
Natrum mur.
Opium
Phosphorus
Rhus tox.
Secale
Silicea
Stramonium
Sulphur
Tarentula
Veratrum

Lack of thirst
Antimonium tart.
Apis
China
Colchicum
Gelsemium
Helleborus
Menyanthes
Nux mosch.
Phosphoric ac.
Pulsatilla
Sabadilla

Burning thirst
Acetic ac.
Bryonia
Cannabis ind.
Mercurius
Phosphorus
Tarentula

Thirst for large quantities
Arsenicum
Bryonia
Natrum mur.
Phosphorus
Sulphur
Veratrum

Thirst for large quantities at long intervals
Bryonia

Thirst for small quantities
Arsenicum
Lycopodium

Thirst for small quantities often
Arsenicum

Cold or frozen foods make symptoms worse
Arsenicum
Dulcamara
Lachesis
Lycopodium
Nux
Rhus tox.
Silicea

Raw foods make symptoms worse
Ruta

Starchy foods make symptoms worse
Berberis
Copaiva
Natrum mur.
Natrum sulph.

Fatty foods make symptoms worse, including oily rich foods
Carbo veg.
Cyclamen
Ferrum
Graphites
Pulsatilla
Taraxacum
Tarentula

Flatulent foods like beans and peas make symptoms worse
Bryonia
Lycopodium
Petroleum

Fruit makes symptoms worse
Arsenicum
Bryonia
China
Colocynth
Natrum sulph.
Pulsatilla
Veratrum

Salty foods make symptoms worse
Natrum mur.
Phosphorus

Acidic foods make symptoms worse
Aconite
Antimonium
Carbo veg.

Sweet foods make symptoms worse
Argentum nit.
Ignatia

Bread makes symptoms worse
Bryonia
Pulsatilla

Buckwheat makes symptoms worse
Pulsatilla

Butter makes symptoms worse
Carbo veg.
Pulsatilla

Cabbage makes symptoms worse
Bryonia
Lycopodium
Petroleum

Meat that is going off makes symptoms worse
Arsenicum

Milk makes symptoms worse
Aethusa
Calcarea
Calcarea sulph.
China
Conium
Lac defl.
Magnesia mur.
Natrum carb.
Nitric ac.
Sepia
Staphisagria
Sulphur

Onions make symptoms worse
Lycopodium

Pancakes make symptoms worse
Pulsatilla

Pastry makes symptoms worse
Antimonium
Pulsatilla

Pork makes symptoms worse
Carbo veg.
Cyclamen
Graphites
Pulsatilla
Sepia

Sauerkraut makes symptoms worse
Bryonia
Petroleum

Green vegetables make symptoms worse
Natrum sulph.

Sight of food makes symptoms worse
Colchicum
Sulphur

Smell of food makes symptoms worse
Colchicum

Sensitive to smell of food
Arsenicum
Colchicum
Sepia

Aversion to food despite being hungry
Cocculus
Lachesis
Natrum mur.
Nux

Aversion to warm or hot food
China

Aversion to smell of food
Cocculus
Colchicum
Ipecac.
Sepia

Aversion to sight of food
Arsenicum

Aversion to food until she tastes it then ravenous
Lycopodium

Aversion to food in general
Arnica
Arsenicum
Belladonna
Bryonia
China
Cocculus
Colchicum
Ferrum
Ipecac.
Lilium
Natrum mur.
Nux
Pulsatilla
Sepia

Aversion to fats and rich food
China
Cyclamen
Petroleum
Pulsatilla

Aversion to fish
Graphites

Aversion to fruit
China

Ignatia
Phosphorus
Pulsatilla

Aversion to garlic
Sabadilla

Aversion to meat
Calcarea
Calcarea sulph.
Carbon sulph.
China
Graphites
Muriatic ac.
Nux
Petroleum
Pulsatilla
Sepia
Silicea
Sulphur

Aversion to pork
Colchicum

**Aversion to meat while
    thinking of it**
Graphites

Aversion to milk
Ignatia
Lac defl.
Natrum carb.
Sepia
Staphisagria

Aversion to olives
Sulphur

Aversion to olive oil
Arsenicum

Aversion to salt and salty food
Graphites

Aversion to sweets
Causticum
Graphites

**Aversion to vegetables raw or
    in salads**
Helleborus

Desire for bitter food
Digitalis

Desire for bread and butter
Mercurius

Desire for cabbage
Cicuta

Desire for chocolate
Phosphorus

Desire for coffee
Nux
Selenium

Desire for cold food
Phosphorus
Pulsatilla
Veratrum

Desire for cucumbers
Antimonium

Desire for delicacies
China
Ipecac.
Tuberculinum

**Desire for eggs, especially
    hard-boiled**
Calcarea

Desire for starchy foods
Lachesis

Desire for fat
Arsenicum
Hepar sulph.
Nitric ac.
Nux
Sulphur

Desire for fat and sweet food
Sulphur

Desire for fruit
Phosphoric ac.
Veratrum

Desire for acidic fruit
Veratrum

Desire for herring
Nitric ac.

**Desire for highly seasoned
    spicy foods**
China
Phosphorus
Sulphur

Desire for hot food
Lycopodium

Desire for ice
Veratrum

Desire for ice cream
Phosphorus

**Desire for indigestible things
    like ashes, charcoal, paper,
    rags, tea grounds, etc.**
Alumina
Calcarea
Calcarea phos.

**Does not know what she
    wants, refuses food when
    offered it**
Bryonia
Ignatia
Ipecac.
Pulsatilla

**Desire for juicy refreshing
    things**
Phosphoric ac.

Desire for lemons
Arsenicum
Belladonna

Desire for lemonade
Belladonna

**Desire for lime in form of
    chalk and clay**
Alumina
Calcarea
Nitric ac.

Indistinct desires
Bryonia
Ignatia
Pulsatilla

Desire for meat
Magnesia carb.

Desire for pork
Crotalus

Desire for smoked meat
Causticum
Tuberculinum

Desire for milk
Rhus tox.
Sabadilla

Desire for olives
Lycopodium

Desire for olive oil
Arsenicum

Desire for oysters
Lachesis

Desire for pepper
Capsicum

Desire for raw food
Silicea
Sulphur

Desire for juicy things
Phosphoric ac.
Veratrum

Desire for salty things
Argentum nit.
Carbo veg.

Lac can.
Natrum mur.
Nitric ac.
Phosphorus
Veratrum

Desire for sand
Tarentula

Desire for smoked things
Calcarea phos.
Causticum

Desire for sour acidic things
Aconite
Arnica
Hepar sulph.
Sulphur
Veratrum

Desire for salt and sour
Carbo veg.
Natrum mur.
Phosphorus
Veratrum

Desire for sweet and sour
Sulphur

Desire for spices, condiments, highly seasoned pungent foods
China
Phosphorus
Sulphur

Desire for strange foods during pregnancy
Lyssin

Desire for vinegar
Hepar sulph.

Desire for sugar
Argentum nit.

Desire for sugar but can only digest it if she eats large amount
Staphisagria

Desire for sweets
Argentum nit.
Arsenicum
Cannabis ind.
China
China sulph.
Kali carb.
Lycopodium
Staphisagria
Sulphur

with headache
Calcarea

before periods
Sulphur

with salt
Argentum nit.

with sour foods
Sulphur

Desire for warm food
Arsenicum

Fatigue

Tiredness

Fatigue, or simple tiredness, is usually due to lack of sleep (see SLEEPING PROBLEMS), STRESS and overwork. It can also follow both emotional and physical trauma, such as after an operation, birth of a baby, or death of a loved one (see GRIEF). Fatigue can also be related to the amount and quality of food eaten, and its absorption (see WEIGHT PROBLEMS, p. 35), and is a feature of ANAEMIA, with paleness, difficulty in breathing and palpitations. It may be due to a specific nutritional deficiency, especially vitamin B1 and potassium.

Tiredness may be a result of metabolic or hormonal imbalance, such as PRE-MENSTRUAL SYNDROME (symptoms worse before periods and better almost as soon as period starts), MENOPAUSE (with hot flushes and irregular periods), HYPO-GLYCAEMIA (craving for sugar, sudden loss of energy, followed by adrenalin surges), diabetes (increase in thirst, increase in urination and loss of weight), HYPOTHYROIDISM (increase in weight for no reason, dry skin, hair falling out, intolerance of cold) (see also THYROID PROBLEMS), uraemia (lack of production of urine, vomiting and confusion), liver failure, (loss of weight, loss of appetite, vomiting and jaundice – yellowing of white of the eyes).

Fatigue may also be a feature of problems with the immune system, such as food intolerance, especially wheat (ALLERGY) or auto-immune disease, where the immune system attacks its own tissues.

Fatigue is a common side-effect of drugs, whether they are orthodox drugs or smoking, alcohol (see ALCOHOLISM), or caffeine, and can be a result of vitamin A overdosage.

Infections and infestations are commonly accompanied by fatigue, especially urinary tract infections (CYSTITIS), threadworm, CHRONIC FATIGUE SYNDROME (never well since an illness with tiredness and feeling unwell after over-exertion).

Fatigue is also one of the main symptoms of DEPRESSION.

Other causes of fatigue include chronic lung disease, e.g., asthma, heart disease, CANCER, neurological diseases, e.g., multiple sclerosis.

Symptoms that patients in our survey believe were caused by, or made worse by, tiredness included: heaviness in the head, and migraines, muscle tension and itchy scalp, dizziness, sore, painful eyes, anxiety, apprehension, apathy, lack of concentration, poor memory, weak voice, vaginal discharge, breast lumps, lack of sexual desire, back pain, fluid retention and increase in weight, itchy feet, eczema and intolerance of cold.

Self-help
First, see your GP for a thorough check-up to rule out physical causes. For simple fatigue a useful analogy is to imagine that the energy in your body is like a bank account, where you have a current and a deposit account (see CHRONIC FATIGUE SYNDROME). Lasting fatigue and tiredness may indicate that you have started to run your current off your deposit account, and that your deposit account is running low. To pull yourself out of fatigue you need to re-charge the deposit account. If tiredness is due to over-work and stress, have a holiday, if of course you can afford to. If you don't, and your health breaks down, that will be worse in the long run.

If the problem is due to over-tiredness try and increase the amount of sleep you get at night, by going to bed 15 minutes earlier every second or third night, until you have a refreshing night's sleep from which you can easily awake the next morning. A 15-minute nap after lunch is worth up to one hour's sleep at night, as it cuts the day into two halves. Try and cut back your energy output by a quarter, to allow 25 per cent of your available energy to go back into your deposit account. So if, for example, you find you get tired after walking for 4 miles, then next time walk only 3, and if you can study for 2 hours but then are tired, only study for 1 or 1½ hours. If you feel no better after a month see your GP again.

Homeopathic treatment
Constitutional treatment may be required.

Specific remedies to be taken twice daily for up to 7 days in the 6c potency.

Please remember to check your choice against the Remedy Pictures (p. 305).

Calcarea
Weakness in the morning; muscular and mental weakness, with perspiration; fatigue after pregnancy; anxiety; apprehension; lack of interest; depression; fear of death; dizziness; itchy scalp with headache; chronic headaches – worse before periods; stinging eyes; eczema in outer ear; sore tongue; hypothyroidism; distended stomach; cramping pains in abdomen; worms in bowels; irregular heavy periods; pain in the womb during period; burning discharge; weakness in voice; chronic bronchitis; swelling and tenderness of breasts pre-menstrually; stretching pains in back; pain in the neck and low back pain; trembling of the hand; varicose veins; cold hands and feet; tingling in hand, leg and foot; sleepiness in daytime; sleeplessness at night; eczema.

Generalities: Fatigue worse for cold – worse before periods; tendency to put on weight; feeling of extreme coldness inside; tendency to arthritis.

Pulsatilla
Fatigue in the morning, after childbirth, during pregnancy; brain fag; loss of interest; depression and irritability before periods; dizziness; one-sided headache; headaches before periods; decrease in appetite; cramping pains in abdomen; irritable bowel syndrome; constipation; chronic cystitis; irregular heavy periods; tenderness in vagina; pain in womb during periods; weakness in voice; chronic laryngitis; difficulty in breathing; lumpy breasts; pre-menstrual soreness in breasts; varicose veins; tingling in the foot; aching calves; rheumatic joint pains; tendency to inflamed skin.

Generalities: Tension in muscles – worse before periods; tendency to fluid retention and overweight – worse for eating bread; tendency to arthritis.

Lycopodium
Fatigue; weakness in morning; fatigue after childbirth and during pregnancy; muscular weakness; brain fag; sweating when fatigued; anxiety; difficulty in concentrating – worse for stress; poor memory; tearfulness; irritability before periods; dizziness; hair falling out; itchy scalp; headache before periods; painful eyes; chronic ear infections; sore tongue; hypothyroidism; distension of stomach; decreased appetite; craves sweets; cramping pains in abdomen; bloated abdomen before periods; constipation; irritable bowel syndrome; irregular periods; tendency to thrush; lack of libido; weak voice; difficulty in breathing; chronic bronchitis; varicose veins; numbness in forearm; tingling in hand; pain in right arm; sleepiness during the day.

Generalities: Worse in cold weather; worse before periods; tendency to weight problems – worse for eating bread; tendency to arthritis.

Sulphur

Fatigue generally; weakness in morning; weariness in evening; muscular weakness; fatigue worse for stress; heaviness in head; hair falling out; itchy scalp; drawing pains in head; headaches before periods; chronic ear infection; chronic sinusitis; bloated stomach; desire for sweets; itching around back passage; irritable bowel syndrome; chronic cystitis; irregular periods; tenderness in vagina; weakness in voice; chronic bronchitis; lower back pain; trembling in the hand; itchy foot; numbness in forearm; tingling in leg; sleepiness in daytime; tendency to inflammation of skin; eczema and dermatitis.

Generalities: Fatigue worse before periods; worse if hungry; tendency to overweight – worse for eating bread; tendency to arthritis.

Natrum mur.

Fatigue; weariness before periods and after eating; weakness in morning and evening; muscular weakness; fatigue worse for stress; indifference; depression – worse before periods; pre-menstrual irritability; dizziness; heaviness; hair falling out; itchy scalp; headache before periods; blurring of vision; burning pains in eyes; tendency to hypothyroidism; irritable bowel syndrome; tendency to thrush; loss of sexual desire; weakness in voice; trembling of hands; numbness in forearm.

Generalities: Muscular tension – worse before periods; general trembling before periods – worse for eating bread; tendency to arthritis.

Sepia

Weakness in morning and evening – better for physical exercise; fatigue during and after pregnancy; general muscular weakness; difficulty in concentrating – worse for stress; poor memory; indifference; depression; irritability before periods; hair falling out; headache from artificial light; sore tongue; tendency to hypothyroidism; worms in bowels; chronic cystitis; irregular periods; itchy vaginal discharge – worse after sexual intercourse; tendency to thrush; diminishing of sexual desire; low back pain; tingling in foot; sleepiness during the day.

Generalities: Muscular tension – worse for cold – worse before periods; tendency to arthritis – worse for eating bread.

Nux

Weakness in morning; fatigue after childbirth, and during pregnancy; brain exhaustion; difficulty in concentrating – worse for stress; indifference; great irritability – worse before periods; fear of death; dizziness; chronic vertigo; drawing pains in head; headache in morning; loss of appetite; cramping pain in abdomen; itching around back passage; irritable bowel syndrome; heavy irregular periods; pain in womb during periods; weakness in voice; chronic laryngitis; low back pain; trembling and tingling in hand.

Generalities: Muscular tension – worse for cold; tendency to fluid retention; extreme feeling of cold inside – worse after eating bread.

Phosphorus

Fatigue and weakness in morning; mental fatigue; difficulty in concentrating; apprehensive; poor memory; indifference; fear of death; dizziness and chronic vertigo; heaviness; hair falling out; chronic sinusitis; tendency to hypothyroidism; irritable bowel syndrome; heavy periods; weak voice; chronic laryngitis; difficulty in breathing; breast lumps; burning pains in back; low back pain; trembling of hand; tingling in hand and foot; sleepiness during the day.

Generalities: Tension in muscles – worse in cold conditions; tendency to overweight; feeling of extreme coldness inside.

Lachesis

Fatigue; weakness in morning and evening; fatigue after eating and during pregnancy; brain fag; difficulty in concentrating; poor memory; depression; heaviness; hair falling out; headaches before periods; chronic sinusitis; sore tongue; tendency to hypothyroidism; lack of appetite; bloated abdomen before periods; irritable bowel syndrome; irregular, heavy periods; chronic laryngitis; difficulty in breathing; breast lumps; tingling in hands; sleeplessness.

Generalities: Fatigue worse before periods.

Arsenicum

Weakness in morning; fatigue after eating; anxiety; poor memory; great fear of death; dizziness; drawing pains in head; desire for sweet things; irritable bowel syndrome; chronic cystitis; difficulty in breathing; chronic bronchitis; burning pains in back; pain in neck; cold hands and feet; sleeplessness; eczema.

Generalities: Fatigue worse for cold conditions; tendency to fluid retention and to put on weight; marked feeling of coldness inside.

Causticum

Weakness in evening; fatigue after childbirth, in pregnancy, after bereavement; anxiety; difficulty in concentrating; poor memory; depression; dizziness; pain in forehead; migraines; blurring of vision; stinging burning pains in eyes; hypothyroidism; decrease in appetite; diarrhoea;

irregular periods; lack of sexual desire; weakness in voice; chronic laryngitis; difficulty in breathing; dry cough – better for drinking cold drinks; shooting pains in the back; neckache; trembling hands; rheumatic pains in joints; pain in upper arm.

Generalities: Fatigue worse for cold, better in warm room; muscular pains; marked feeling of cold inside; tendency to arthritis; generally worse after eating bread.

Kali carb.
Fatigue after childbirth; brain fag; anxiety – worse for stress; hair falling out; headaches on one side; bloated stomach; irritable bowel syndrome; difficulty in breathing; numbness in forearm, tingling in hands, leg and foot; sleeplessness.

Generalities: Fatigue worse for cold – worse before periods – worse when hungry; tendency to put on weight; extreme feeling of coldness inside; tendency to arthritis.

Mercurius
Weakness in morning, and as result of infestation of worms; fatigue worse for stress; poor memory; drawing pains in head; recurrent vaginal thrush;

chronic laryngitis; sleeplessness; tendency to inflamed skin; dermatitis.

Generalities: Trembling with cold; arthritis.

Nitric ac.
Weakness in morning; muscular weakness; fatigue worse for stress; poor memory; fear of death; heaviness; hair falling out; painful eyes; sore tongue; irritable bowel syndrome; heavy irregular periods; vaginal discharge causing itching; tendency to thrush; chronic bronchitis; shooting pains in back; trembling hands; numbness in forearm; tingling in hand and foot; tendency to inflamed skin.

Generalities: Muscle tension – worse in cold conditions – worse before periods; feeling of extreme cold inside – generally worse after eating bread.

Carbo veg.
Fatigue worse in morning – worse during pregnancy; muscular weakness; brain fag; anxiety; difficulty in concentrating – worse for stress – indifference; heaviness; hair falling out; headaches before periods; sore tongue; bloated stomach; cramping pains in abdomen; diarrhoea; worms; heavy periods; weakness in voice; chronic laryngitis; difficulty in breathing; chronic bronchitis; varicose veins; cold hands and feet.

Remedy Finder for Fatigue

After injuries
Arnica
Conium
Hepar sulph.
Hypericum
Pulsatilla
Rhus tox.
Sulphuric ac.

Delirious with fatigue from over-exertion and studying
Lachesis

Muscular weakness and chilliness in menopause with fatigue
Calcarea

Persistently tired and exhausted womb in menopause with fatigue
Bellis

Heaviness in legs as if fatigued
Argentum nit.

Calcarea
Kreosotum
Magnesia mur.
Moschus
Murex
Natrum sulph.
Psorinum
Pulsatilla
Ruta
Sulphur

Swelling of joints from slightest fatigue
Actaea

Trembling of arms with fatigue from overwork
Cuprum
Plumbum

Tickling in arms and legs as if from fatigue
Natrum mur.

Pains in arms and legs as if from fatigue
Petroleum

Calf pains as if from fatigue
Sulphur

Drawing pains in foot as if from fatigue
Kali carb.

Sore legs after fatigue
Clematis

Trembling from fatigue
Plumbum

Fatigue worse in morning
Lachesis
Nux
Ruta
Sepia

Fatigue on waking
Bryonia
Calcarea
Carbo an.
Causticum
Conium
Lycopodium
Magnesia mur.
Natrum mur.

Nux
Thuja
Zinc

Sleepiness on waking up
Clematis
Cocculus
Graphites
Natrum mur.
Nux
Podophyllum
Sepia
Sulphur

Fatigue better in afternoons
Kali carb.

Fatigue in evening
Muriatic ac.
Sulphur

Especially in open air
Carbo veg.

Fatigue from climbing upstairs
Sulphur iod.

As if born tired
Onosmodium

After intercourse
Agaricus

From conversation
Ambra

After diarrhoea
Sulphur iod.

While eating
Kali carb.

After eating
Arsenicum
Baryta
Carbo an.
Lachesis
Natrum mur.
Nux mosch.
Rhus tox.

On slightest exertion
Baryta

Mental work tires her out
Aconite
Aurum
Conium
Graphites
Ignatia
Nat carb.
Nux
Selenium

Fatigue with vaginal discharge
Prunus

After vaginal discharge
Glonoinum

Before periods
Belladonna
Natrum mur.

During periods
Ammonium carb.
Causticum
Ignatia
Nitric ac.
Nux mosch.
Petroleum

Painful fatigue
Ruta

After playing piano
Anacardium

From reading
Aurum

From sexual excitement
Sarsaparilla

Whilst sitting down
Mercurius

More tired in morning than evening
Magnesia carb.

Unrefreshing sleep
Calcarea
Causticum
Kali carb.
Lachesis
Magnesia carb.
Magnesia mur.
Nitric ac.
Phosphorus
Tuberculinum

Fatigue with sleepiness
Antimonium

Fatigue with sleepiness when eating
Kali carb.

Worse for standing
Muriatic ac.

After talking
Alumina
Calcarea phos.

After a lot of talking
Calcarea

Better walking
Lac defl.
Muriatic ac.

Fatigue with acute illnesses
Anacardium
Carbo veg.
China
China ars.
Cocculus
Kali phos.
Phosphoric ac.
Phosphorus
Psorinum
Tarentula cub.

In acute illness with no fever
Arsenicum
Baptisia
Carbo veg.
China

Better in open air
Conium

Better for drinking alcohol
Cantharis

After childbirth
Graphites
Kali carb.
Pulsatilla
Sepia

Fatigue after miscarriage or termination of pregnancy
Ruta
Sepia

Worse for cold air
Agaricus
Allium
Arsenicum
Aurum
Badiaga
Baryta
Calcarea
Calcarea phos.
Camphora
Causticum
Cimicifuga
Cistus
Dulcamara
Hepar sulph.
Hypericum
Kali ars.
Kali carb.
Lycopodium
Magnesia phos.
Moschus
Nux mosch.
Nux

Psorinum
Ranunculus
Rhododendron
Rhus tox.
Rumex
Sabadilla
Sepia
Silicea
Strontium

Worse for cold wet weather
Ammonium carb.
Arsenicum
Badiaga
Calcarea
Calcarea phos.
Colchicum
Dulcamara
Medorrhinum
Natrum sulph.
Nux mosch.
Pyrogenium
Rhododendron
Rhus tox.
Silicea
Tuberculinum

From exposure to sun
Antimonium
Glonoinum
Natrum carb.
Natrum mur.
Pulsatilla

Worse in wet weather
Ammonium carb.
Arsenicum
Badiaga
Calcarea carb.
Dulcamara
Natrum sulph.
Nux mosch.
Pulsatilla
Rhododendron
Rhus tox.

Worse for cold winds
Belladonna
Hepar sulph.
Nux
Spongia

Worse in winter
Aurum
Fluoric ac.
Nux
Rhus tox.

Worse after being criticized or told off
Belladonna
Platina

From anger and anxiety
Aconite
Arsenicum
Ignatia
Nux

From anger and fright
Aconite
Ignatia

From anger and indignation
Colocynth
Staphisagria

From anger bottled up during grieving process
Ignatia
Staphisagria

Deterioration from anticipation
Argentum nit.
Calcarea
Graphites
Hyoscyamus
Lycopodium
Medorrhinum
Natrum mur.
Phosphorus
Plumbum
Psorinum
Pulsatilla
Silicea

After bad news
Calcarea
Gelsemium

After feeling unusually cheerful
Cannabis ind.
Coffea
Crocus
Hyoscyamus
Lachesis
Natrum carb.

From envy
Lachesis
Pulsatilla

From overexcitement
Aconite
Anacardium
Argentum nit.
Aurum
Belladonna
Causticum
Chamomilla

Coffea
Collinsonia
Graphites
Hepar sulph.
Hyoscyamus
Kali brom.
Kali iod.
Lac can.
Lachesis
Moschus
Natrum mur.
Nitric ac.
Nux
Opium
Phosphoric ac.
Phosphorus
Pulsatilla

From a feeling of being abandoned or forsaken
Aurum
Psorinum
Pulsatilla

After a fright
Aconite
Ignatia
Lycopodium
Natrum mur.
Opium
Phosphoric ac.
Phosphorus
Pulsatilla
Silicea

After grief
Aurum
Causticum
Cocculus
Ignatia
Lachesis
Natrum mur.
Phosphoric ac.
Staphisagria

From jealousy
Apis
Hyoscyamus
Nux
Phosphorus
Pulsatilla

From disappointment in love
Hyoscyamus
Ignatia
Natrum mur.
Phosphoric ac.

**After being deeply
 embarrassed**
Colocynth
Ignatia
Lycopodium
Natrum mur.

Palladium
Phosphoric ac.
Staphisagria

After being reproached
Ignatia

Opium
Staphisagria

Having been scorned
Bryonia
Chamomilla
Nux

Chronic Fatigue Syndrome

This is commonly called CFS, but is also known as Post Viral Syndrome, Post Viral Fatigue Syndrome, Icelandic Disease, Royal Free Disease, Fibromyalgia, Myalgic Encephalomyelitis (ME), or, in the media, 'Yuppie flu'.

This is possibly one of the most contentious syndromes in medicine at the moment. Controversy arises because there is no clear diagnostic test, and the symptoms can mimic a whole host of other diseases. The mere fact that it has been given so many names reflects how variable the condition is in different times and in different countries of the world: rather like trying to describe an iceberg from its appearance above the water.

In spite of the numerous theories as to causation and mechanisms underlying the disease, it can be best explained by simple analogy. Imagine that the energy in the body is like a bank account with a current and a deposit account. We believe that people who develop this condition have been running their current account off their deposit account for weeks, months or even years before the onset of the illness (see FATIGUE). There then comes a point when the deposit account is critically low, so that when the body next meets with infection, the current account ('the immune system') is overwhelmed. Because there are no reserves in the deposit account to back her up, the woman falls into chronic or sub-acute illness instead of fully recovering as she should. This results in some as yet not fully understood combination of immune system breakdown and metabolic imbalance.

Those who succumb to CFS usually have a history of recent viral infection of either the upper respiratory tract – such as a cold or flu – or of the gut, with diarrhoea and vomiting. Instead of a normal recovery the patient becomes dogged by long persistent fatigue, with other symptoms mentioned below. There is usually an accompanying low-grade fever which gradually subsides. The basic feature of the fatigue is that the recovery of muscle power is unduly prolonged. After moderate exercise from which the normal person would recover with a night's rest, the patient with CFS will take 3–4 days – after strenuous activity the period can be up to 2–3 weeks. If there is further expenditure in the recovery phase the effect is cumulative.

Symptoms

Currently 4 factors have to be met in order to diagnose Chronic Fatigue Syndrome:

1 Fatigue is the principal symptom, and has to be present for 50 per cent of the time, and have been present for more than 6 months (a Scottish specialist in this subject has recommended 3 months).
2 The condition must have a definite onset.
3 The fatigue must be severely disabling, affecting both mental and physical functioning.
4 Other symptoms will be present, including pains in muscles, weight fluctuation or sleep disturbance.

Other symptoms

These include: weakness, clumsiness, pins and needles, twitching muscles, headache, sensitivity to noise and light, palpitations, giddiness, gastrointestinal upset, recurrent sore throats, nausea, swelling of the lymph glands, cough, rashes, loss of appetite, recurrent fever, weight loss or weight gain and swelling of the fingers. Sensitivity in the temperature control system leads to overheating or marked chilliness. Alcohol also aggravates the condition, with additional aggravation before periods. Sore eyes and blurring of vision, muscle tension and vaginal discharge are additional problems.

Mental symptoms include poor memory and concentration, inability to speak properly, to understand speech or to express yourself, and confusion.

Emotional symptoms include: depression, anxiety, inability to handle stress, weepiness, irritability which is worse pre-menstrually and PANIC ATTACKS.

Many of the symptoms closely resemble those of HYPOGLYCAEMIA.

A full examination, and investigation where appropriate, is essential, but on examining patients there is usually little to find. Most look distressingly healthy, which does not help to get them sympathy for their disease. However, there may be signs of tenderness and swelling of the lymph glands in the neck, under the arms or in the groin, chronically inflamed throat and local muscle tenderness. CFS needs to be distinguished from other conditions, including infections such as TOXOPLASMOSIS, TUBERCULOSIS, brucellosis, AIDS, Epstein-Barr virus (responsible for GLANDULAR FEVER), pernicious anaemia and other ANAEMIAS, multiple sclerosis, DEPRESSION, hysteria and anxiety, epilepsy, and certain forms of CANCER, endocrine abnormalities such as Addison's disease, Cushing's syndrome and THYROID PROBLEMS, liver disease, chronic drug intoxication (DRUG ADDICTION), ALCOHOLISM and autoimmune diseases.

Possible causes of CFS

It is unlikely that there is one single cause for this syndrome – abnormalities in the immune system and metabolism can sometimes be detected (see below) but they are mostly thought to be a cause rather than an effect of the disease. Among the factors thought to drain the deposit account include: vitamin and mineral deficiencies, lack of rest, poor diet, FOOD ALLERGIES, candida (see THRUSH) infection, toxicity and pollution and geopathic stress, chronic carbon monoxide poisoning from faulty gas appliances, chronic intestinal parasite infestation particularly from giardiasis and *Entamoeba histolitica*. HYPERVENTILATING has also been included, and plays a part for many sufferers, as may magnesium deficiency.

The phenomenon known as geopathic stress causes problems in housing. It is known that natural radiations which rise up through the earth are distorted by weak electromagnetic fields, created by subterranean running water, rock and mineral deposits, fault lines and underground cavities. It is possible that these may in some circumstances be harmful to living organisms. If you feel that you have become unwell and cannot sleep since moving house or changing your bedroom, you may have been exposed to this or other magnetic phenomena. Try moving your bed or sleeping in a different room. (It has also been suggested that gypsies and other travelling people who rarely stay longer than 3 weeks in one spot, and who may have a feeling for places which are free of geopathic stress, do not suffer from cancer, despite bad living habits. If this information is true it certainly requires further investigation.)

Stress is a contributory factor in the lead up to the disease, and some 80 per cent of the time is the final straw which breaks the camel's back. It is possible that people who develop CFS are those who find it hard to accept themselves as they are, driving themselves too hard, obsessed with achievement, work and material advancement. According to new thinking in psychoneuroimmunology this causes a release of ACTH, which stimulates the adrenal glands. It also, unfortunately, inhibits the production of T-cell lymphocytes, which are vitally responsible for fighting off viruses. There has also been speculation that over-use of antibiotics has prevented the immune system from having a good fight, thereby weakening it. Immunizations may weaken the immune system in a similar way. Certainly the age onset of CFS appears to be getting lower, with children as young as 8 or even younger developing it.

Investigations

Various abnormalities have been found in patients with this condition, including those revealed by the VP1 (Virus Protein 1) test, which shows evidence of enteroviruses in the system. In the USA it is the Epstein-Barr virus (the virus which causes glandular fever) that is most commonly found. Virus proteins and nucleic acids may be found in muscle biopsy, and there may also be abnormalities in the complement of immunoglobulins, antibodies, and the numbers and activity of T-cells. Metabolically, HYPOGLYCAEMIA may be diagnosed by a 5-hour tolerance test, although this test does have its drawbacks. Great changes in carbon dioxide concentration may reveal evidence of HYPERVENTILATION. Red blood cell magnesium levels may also be low, although this test may be difficult to assess as different laboratories have slightly different methodologies, and give different results. Zinc deficiency may be detected on a sweat or taste test.

Treatment

As with everything else with this disease, there is considerable controversy about the treatment. The majority of authorities recommend rest, but some – mainly from the psychiatric world – advise exercise, and use the 'She will snap out of it' approach. The authors believe that this confusion arises because there are two phases to treatment and rehabilitation.

Phase 1

In this phase you must rest until you have 'bottomed out', as it were. Bottoming out is the time when you start to put energy back into the deposit account. It is entirely possible that the reason you have become ill with this condition is because you have not recognized that you have been over-riding the warning signals from your body. This means you will have to learn to recognize the danger signs again. If these are too subtle to pick up, then it is best to time your activities either by distance, or by the number of minutes you can do them for. In the early stages it may be necessary to cut down your energy output by up to 50 per cent of what it takes to make you tired. This may mean virtual bed rest for a period of days or even a couple of weeks. Otherwise, say if you walk 400 yards along a flat road one day and are ill and tired for the next day or two, you should try walking only 200 yards on the next occasion. If this is still too much, try 100 yards, and so on. Similarly, if you find that you can concentrate for only ½ hour, and it takes you a day or two to recover, then just study for 15 minutes. When you have reached the level where 50 per cent is getting into the deposit account you can increase your output to 75 per cent, which you should stay at until you get to Phase 2. Many sufferers appear to come to a stage – which is difficult to detect – after which it is as if the deposit account has risen to such a level that it can start to support the current account again. This means that if you do overdo things slightly, you don't go down so far or for so long.

It is at this point that a graduated scheme of exercise becomes important, because as psychiatrists have pointed out, there are harmful effects of disuse and inactivity on muscle, respiratory and heart function, not to mention the depression that comes with not being able to do what you want to do. There is also a secondary problem in that when you have suffered as a result of overdoing things, you tend to avoid the situations which brought them on in the first place; this can lead to the development of PHOBIAS.

Other treatment We will now go into further detail about the various other forms of treatment which are available once the principles of rest have been mastered. As we have indicated, other viruses may be present, although they are not the cause but the effect of the illness. In any case, there are no drugs capable of killing most of the viruses that are found in CFS. Treatment is therefore geared to strengthening the immune system by a variety of methods. The single most important method is of constitutional homeopathic treatment from an experienced homeopath. Remedies given later in this section are worth trying in the meantime.

Other measures are designed to stimulate the metabolism and detoxify it, and support the immune system. These include control of HYPO-GLYCAEMIA, HYPERVENTILATION, and candida (see THRUSH). Eat whole foods following the *twice-a-week rule*, including as much organically grown food as possible to eliminate chemicals, drugs and dietary toxins from the system. The COLON CLEANSE may be of benefit. Drink plenty of filtered or boiled water if you are in doubt about your water supply (up to 10 glasses a day are beneficial). The lymphatic system can be stimulated by exercising and stretching muscles gently with a graduated exercise programme, callisthenics or gentle yoga. We also highly recommend the Alexander Technique for CFS sufferers. Many patients appear to have problems in the spine and joints, particularly at the junction of the head and neck, which may also benefit from manipulation. When you sit down have your legs on a seat above the level of your bottom and stimulate the circulation by dry skin brushing. This is done for 2 minutes using a bristle (not nylon) bath brush with a flicking motion up to the chest, but do not brush the face or any areas where there are skin eruptions. It should be done before rather than after a bath. In the early stages cold applications, particularly to the upper right corner of the abdomen over the liver, may be beneficial. Apply for 1½ minutes hot then ½ minute cold, and repeat 5 times. Food allergies should be identified and eliminated if they are thought to be a problem or they can be treated by EPD (enzyme potentiated desensitization; see ALLERGIES). This is a method whereby a mixture of very dilute extracts of foods are combined with an enzyme which activates the immune system to respond to the foods. It is applied either by injection under the skin or by scratching the skin and applying a small plastic cup. This is usually repeated every 2 months to begin with, then every 3 months.

An anti-viral drug which shows promise in the treatment of CFS has been developed in the US.

Supplementation For details of doses see section on NUTRITIONAL SUPPLEMENTS. There are only 2 supplements which have been shown clinically to have any benefit in CFS:

1 A mixture of fish and plant oils, such as gammalinoleic acid and marine oils.
2 Magnesium, which may have to be given by injection.

Other recommended supplements include: multivitamins and minerals, vitamin D, vitamin B_5, iron, copper, selenium, beta carotene, vitamin E, vitamin C, and zinc. Some practitioners also use thymus extract. Orthodox medicines which have been used include anti-depressants, histamine 2 blockers – which act on the stomach – and ACE inhibitors (drugs used in hypertension). The latter 2 are based on an American theory which postulates that CFS is due to a lack of coordination between brain and gut. Vitamin B_6

is also used; here the problem is thought to be due to a deficiency in the enzyme which metabolizes it, therefore the supplements must be given as P5P (pyridoxal 5 phosphate).

An enormous amount of energy is needed to get well, and to decide what will achieve this. Obviously not all the measures described will be applicable to you. If it is possible to see a practitioner experienced in dealing with this condition we recommend it. The main things to do for yourself are to regulate the amount of energy you are using out of your current account, so that there is some saved in the deposit account. This may mean some hard decisions regarding the time that you spend at work and the quality of work that you do. Tiredness and poor concentration may make meetings with colleagues too exhausting. If you have the option, change the time that you work, and the type of work you do.

If you have anything more than a mild attack of this condition it may be necessary for you to work only half days. We have found that much benefit can be gained from working in the morning, coming home, having lunch, an afternoon nap, then getting up and doing some work at home. This way the day is broken into two halves, and you don't have to struggle on for a whole day at a time. In fact you should not have to struggle at all! It is very possible that it was struggling to fight the illness, by continuing to work long hours and taking strenuous exercise long after your body was telling you to stop, that brought CFS on in the first place. In first-class athletes, although exercise initially makes them feel better, there comes a point where the constant stress of having to keep fit and taking part in competition causes the immune system to break down (see STRESS and SLEEP PROBLEMS). In the case of the virus which attacked the North Sea seals, however, contrary to expectation the virus was found to be a common one; the seals' immune systems were no longer capable of fighting it properly, though, possibly due to pollution. Thus both the mental and physical stresses need to be removed. Indeed for many people CFS develops after they have been struggling in a situation which they should have got out of a long time ago, but could not take the decision to do so. In many cases once the decision has been taken to change the situation because of CFS, recovery starts to take place. If you have a long-standing conflict in your life try and resolve it now, no matter how painful this may initially be.

Phase 2

This phase of the recovery process begins when you have turned a corner; the deposit account climbs above the 60 per cent mark, and is now capable of supporting the current account. You should be starting to increase physical exercise, and feeling clearer mentally so that you can study or read for longer periods of time. We advise that at first you walk until you can do about 5 miles without suffering side effects, and then go on to swimming and cycling.

You should also now be willing to take up the challenge of going into situations in which you were previously ill – gradually become bolder and bolder. At this stage you do not need to be frightened of ordinary tiredness; this is a sign that your muscles have not been doing enough, rather than doing too much. Of course if it is associated with fever, swollen glands and the illness coming back, then you have overdone it and will have to be more careful. Even so, at this stage your recovery rate should be much quicker, and you should not go down so far. Remember that most people do recover from this illness, no matter how debilitating it is at first. However, it takes time and patience, and is probably one of the most frustrating diseases around; as you get better, you still have to be careful not to overdo things. You are constantly treading a tightrope between overdoing it and causing the symptoms to return on the one hand, and not doing enough and suffering from depression on the other.

Pregnancy and CFS

Many mothers and would-be mothers worry about whether they could cope with being pregnant, and whether CFS would affect the baby. There is no evidence that CFS is inherited. What is possible, of course, is that some of the factors that play a part in causing CFS could be passed on to the child – such as toxic overload, poor diet, tendency to allergies, chronic candida infection and stressful behaviour patterns. If you have taken any of the measures outlined above to get yourself well, however, it is much less likely that they will be passed on to your offspring. In general pregnancy does not seem to make the condition worse – in fact it sometimes appears to improve it. It is vitally important, though, that you consider how you are going to cope with a baby in case he or she is a poor sleeper. How are you going to get rest, particularly if you have other children? Back-up help is vital.

Healing

Whilst most recovery from CSF is a matter of hard slog, some women appear to benefit greatly from healing or bio-energy treatments. It is to be hoped that it might be possible to subject this to clinical trials, and have more people trained in the technique.

Homeopathic treatment

It is best to see an experienced homeopath for this condition for constitutional treatment. In the meantime see remedies below.

Specific remedies to be taken in the 30c potency twice a day for up to 2 weeks.

Please remember to check your choice against the Remedy Pictures (p. 305) where possible.

Natrum mur.

Swollen, painful neck glands; muscular pain; aching all over – worse for stress; difficulty in expressing herself; very weepy especially before periods; depression and irritability before periods; confusion; dizziness; itchy scalp and hair falling out; headache with fever; pain at back of the head going to the front; tired eyes; blurred vision; acidic stomach; burping; irritable bowel syndrome; thrush; fingers go to sleep.

Generalities: All symptoms can be worse before periods; weakness and weariness before periods; muscular tension.

Calcarea

Swelling of the glands in the groin and painful swollen neck glands; permanently cold; joint pains; weakness after the slightest exertion; poor memory; marked depression; great anxiety; very weepy; panic attacks; confusion; itchy scalp; pains from back of head to forehead; burning pains in side of head; bloated stomach; cramping pains in abdomen; thrush; fingers go to sleep; aching arms; sleeplessness.

Generalities: All symptoms can be worse before periods.

Arsenicum

Permanently cold; joint and muscle pains; aching and burning pains all over with stiffness – worse for stress; weakness from the slightest exertion; panic attacks; great anxiety; marked depression; poor memory; dizziness on the slightest exertion; headache with fever; migraines; sore, tired eyes; blurred vision; irritable bowel syndrome; fingers and toes asleep; aching arms; sleeplessness; breathlessness.

Generalities: Fainting in morning.

Belladonna

Swelling of glands in groin; swollen tender glands in the neck; muscle and joint pains; aching and burning pains all over – worse for stress; constant sore throat; confusion; great

anxiety; difficulty in concentrating; poor memory; difficulty in expressing herself; dizziness; headache with fever; pain in temples; migraine; burning pain in sides of head; sore eyes; burping; cramping pain in abdomen; thrush; sleeplessness.

Generalities: Weakness and weariness before periods.

Lycopodium

Swollen neck glands; joint and muscle pains; aching and stiffness all over – worse for stress; constant sore throat; poor memory; difficulty in expressing herself; difficulty in concentrating; marked anxiety; generally very weepy especially before periods; irritable and depressed before periods; dizziness; itchy scalp and hair falling out; pain in temples; sore, tired eyes; bloated stomach; burping; cramping pain in abdomen; irritable bowel syndrome with wind; fingers asleep; aching arms.

Generalities: All symptoms can be worse before periods.

Pulsatilla

Swollen glands in neck and groin; joint and muscle pains; aching all over – worse for stress; difficulty in expressing herself; very weepy and depressed especially before periods; dizziness – worse before periods; headache with fever; pain in temples; migraine; sore eyes; blurred vision; burping; cramping pains; irritable bowel syndrome with wind; thrush; breathlessness; fingers asleep; aching arms.

Generalities: Fatigue better for eating – worse before periods; muscular tension.

Lachesis

Swelling of glands in groin and neck – worse for stress; constant sore throat especially on left side; confusion; marked depression; poor memory and difficulty in expressing herself; difficulty in concentrating; dizziness before periods; hair falling out; headache with fever; pains go from back of head to forehead; sore eyes; irritable bowel syndrome; toes go to sleep; aching arms; sleeplessness.

Generalities: All symptoms can be worse before periods.

Nux

Permanently cold; joint pains; aching all over – worse for stress; confusion; irritability before periods; difficulty in concentrating and in expressing herself; dizziness; headache with fever; migraine; sore eyes; blurred vision; burping;

cramping pains in abdomen; wind, irritable bowel syndrome; thrush.

Generalities: Fainting in morning; muscular tension.

Mercurius

Swollen glands in groin, tender swollen glands in neck; joint and muscle pains; aching all over; constant sore throat; weakness after the slightest exertion; offensive sweat; intolerant of heat and cold; confusion; panic attacks; very weepy; poor memory; pains from back of head to forehead; sore eyes; burping; wind; thrush; toes go to sleep; aching arms; sleeplessness; dribbles on pillow at night.

Phosphorus

Swollen neck glands; permanently cold; joint pains – worse for stress; weakness after the slightest exertion; confused; panic attacks; weepy before periods; poor memory and difficult concentration; dizziness; hair falling out; burning pain in sides of head; tired eyes; burping; irritable bowel syndrome, wind.

Generalities: Fatigue better for eating, muscle tension.

Sepia

Swollen neck glands; stiff all over – worse for stress; weakness after the slightest exertion; numbness in throat; irritability before periods; marked weepiness; difficulty in concentrating; poor memory; difficulty in expressing herself; hair falling out; migraines; tired, sore eyes; acidic stomach; burping; thrush.

Generalities: Fatigue better for eating – worse before periods; muscular tension.

Causticum

Permanently cold; muscle and joint pains; stiff all over; weakness after slightest exertion; irritability before periods; great weepiness; marked anxiety and depression; difficulty in concentrating, poor memory; blurred vision; aching arms.

Generalities: Fatigue better for eating; great weakness after loss of a loved one.

Kali carb.

Swollen glands in neck and groin; permanently cold; joint pains; numbness in the throat; panic attacks; marked anxiety; difficulty in expressing herself; hair falling out; pain in temples; pain from back of head to forehead; migraine; blurred vision; bloated stomach; belching; irritable bowel syndrome; breathlessness; sleeplessness.

Generalities: All symptoms can be worse before periods.

Carbo veg.

Swollen, tender neck glands; aching and burning pains all over; confusion; marked anxiety; difficulty in concentrating; hair falling out; pain from back of head to forehead; sore eyes; bloated stomach, belching; cramping pains in abdomen; wind; thrush.

Generalities: Fainting in morning.

China

Joint pains; weakness after slightest exertion; great anxiety, marked depression; headache with fever; pain in temples; pain from back of head to forehead; migraines; over-acidic, bloated stomach; burping; wind; sleeplessness.

Generalities: Weakness before periods.

Remedy Finder for Chronic Fatigue Syndrome

Worse during heat of day
Selenium

Better for walking
Phosphoric ac.

Worse in morning
Arsenicum
Lachesis
Lycopodium
Phosphoric ac.
Sepia

Worse before lunch
Bryonia

Worse in afternoon
Sulphur

Worse in evening
Natrum mur.

Says she is well when very ill
Apis
Arnica

Restless limbs with fever
Arsenicum
China
Ferrum met.
Kali brom.
Lycopodium

Nux
Pulsatilla
Rhus tox.
Silicea
Stramonium
Tarentula
Zinc

Burning heat with fever
Aconite
Apis
Arsenicum
Belladonna
Gelsemium
Opium

Phosphorus
Pulsatilla
Tuberculinum

Sleepiness during fever
Mezereum
Opium
Palladium
Sambucus

Faintness during fever
Aconite
Arnica
Natrum mur.
Phosphorus
Sepia

Weakness with fever
Arsenicum
Baptisia
Bryonia
Ignatia
Natrum mur.
Nitric ac.
Phosphoric ac.
Phosphorus
Pulsatilla
Rhus tox.

Weakness from sweating
Bryonia
Camphor
Carbo an.
China
China sulph.
Ferrum met.
Iodum
Mercurius
Phosphorus
Psorinum
Sambucus
Sepia
Tuberculinum

Restlessness with fever
Arsenicum
Pulsatilla
Rhus tox.

Anxiety with fever
Aconite
Ambra
Arsenicum
Baryta
Ipecac.
Sepia

Falsely cheerful during fever
Aconite
Opium

Confusion with fever
Baptisia
Hyoscyamus

Delusions of animals
Arsenicum
Belladonna
Calcarea
Cimicifuga
Crotalus
Hyoscyamus
Opium
Stramonium

Visions of monsters
Belladonna
Stramonium

Despair with fever
Aconite
Arsenicum
Carbo veg.
Spongia

Despair of recovery
Aconite
Phosphoric ac.

Feverish cold
Aconite
Arsenicum
Belladonna
Bryonia
Hepar sulph.
Mercurius
Senega
Tarentula

Difficult breathing with fever
Apis
Cactus
Kali carb.
Lachesis
Sepia
Silicea
Tuberculinum

Snoring with fever
Opium

Nausea with fever
Natrum mur.

Pain in stomach eased during fever
Arsenicum
Bryonia
Nux

Vomiting with fever
Antimonium tart.
Eupatorium
Natrum mur.

Copious urine during fever
Stramonium

Copious urine with perspiration
Aconite
Dulcamara
Phosphorus
Rhus tox.

Giddiness with fever
Carbo an.
Cocculus
Kali carb.
Pulsatilla

Mental dullness with fever
Argentum nit.
Chamomilla
Ignatia
Pulsatilla

Excitement with fever
Apis
Ferrum
Petroleum
Rhus tox.
Sarsaparilla

Fever during heat
Arsenicum

Gesticulating during fever
Belladonna
Cocculus
Hyoscyamus
Stramonium
Tarentula

Impatience during fever
Ipecac.
Natrum mur.
Nux
Pulsatilla
Viola

Apathy during fever
Conium
Opium
Phosphoric ac.

Very busy with fever
Thuja

Irritability with fever
Arsenicum
Bryonia
Chamomilla
Ferrum
Natrum carb.
Natrum mur.
Nux

Psorinum
Rheum

Talkative during fever
Lachesis
Podophyllum
Tuberculinum

Moaning during fever
Arnica
Pulsatilla

Very quiet during fever
Bryonia
Gelsemium

Sad during fever
Aconite
Arsenicum
Natrum mur.

Emotionally sensitive during fever
Pulsatilla

Sighing with fever
Arnica
Chamomilla
Coffea
Ignatia

Stupefied with fever
Apis
Camphor
Sepia

Suicidal with fever
Arsenicum

Aversion to being touched
Antimonium carb.
Chamomilla
Kali carb.
Tarentula

Weeping during fever
Aconite
Belladonna
Pulsatilla
Spongia

Cold feeling during fever
Colchicum
Rhus tox.

Cold feet during fever
Arnica
Iris
Lachesis
Stramonium
Sulphur

Cold leg during fever
Stramonium

Eyes appear to sparkle
Belladonna
Camphora

Eyes appear glassy
Opium
Phosphoric ac.

Sore eyes during fever
Lycopodium
Valeriana

Pupils dilated in fever
Belladonna

Pain in head with fever
Apis
Arnica
Belladonna
China
Eupatorium
Natrum mur.
Silicea

Urine not passed during fever
Arnica
Arsenicum
Belladonna
Cantharis
Hyoscyamus
Opium
Plumbum
Secale

General chilliness
Antimonium tart.
Apis
Arnica
Arsenicum
Cantharis
Carbon sulph.
Carbo veg.
Cedrum
Chelidonium
China
Chininum sulph.
Eupatorium
Gelsemium
Helonius
Ignatia
Ipecac.
Ledum
Lycopodium
Mezereum
Natrum mur.
Nitric ac.
Nux
Nux mosch.
Pulsatilla
Rhus tox.
Sabadilla

Secale
Sepia
Staphisagria
Thuja
Veratrum
Veratrum vir.

Weakness with chilliness
China
Natrum mur.
Phosphorus

Mental dullness with shivering and chilliness
Capsicum
Chamomilla
Helleborus
Lachesis

Apathetic with chilliness
Opium
Phosphorus
Phosphoric ac.

Irritability with chilliness
Calcarea
Capsicum
Conium
Lycopodium
Platina
Rheum

Talkative during chilliness
Podophyllum

Moaning during chilliness
Eupatorium
Natrum mur.

Wants to be quiet when chilled
Bryonia
Kali carb.

Does not recognize relatives
Belladonna
Hyoscyamus

Restlessness with chilliness
Arsenicum

Sadness with chilliness
Aconite
Arsenicum
China
Glonoinum
Ignatia
Natrum mur.

Emotionally sensitive during chilly phase
Capsicum

Weeping with chilliness
Belladonna
Calcarea
Chamomilla
Lycopodium
Pulsatilla

Cold knees during chilly spell
Apis
Carbo veg.
Phosphorus

Difficulty in breathing with chilliness
Apis
Natrum mur.
Thuja

Hot head with cold extremities
Belladonna

Hot head during a cold
Arum

Cold ears during fever
Ipecac.
Lachesis

Hot ears
Calcarea

Noises in ear
Tuberculinum

Buzzing noises
Arsenicum

Chirping noises
Lycopodium
Natrum sulph.
Pulsatilla
Rhus tox.

Humming noises
Arsenicum
Nux

Roaring noises
Arsenicum
Nux

Cold nose
Camphora
Carbo veg.
Conium
Veratrum

Discoloured tongue

Black
Carbo veg.
China

Mercurius
Phosphorus

Blue
Antimonium tart.
Arsenicum
Digitalis

Brown
Ailanthus
Arsenicum
Baptisia
Bryonia
China ars.
Hyoscyamus
Kali phos.
Lachesis
Phosphorus
Plumbum
Rhus tox.
Secale

Dirty
China
Natrum sulph.

Pale
Mercurius

Red
Apis
Arsenicum
Belladonna
Mercurius
Nitric ac.
Phosphorus
Rhus tox.

Red tip
Argentum nit.
Arsenicum
Phytolacca
Rhus tox.
Rhus ven.
Sulphur

Yellow
Antimonium
Chelidonium
Mercurius
Nux mosch.
Rhus tox.
Spigelia

Cold face
Arsenicum
Carbo veg.
Cina
Platina
Veratrum

Pale face with fever
Arsenicum
Cina
Crocus
Hepar sulph.
Ipecac.
Lycopodium

Red face with fever
Belladonna
China
Petroleum
Sepia

Dryness of lips
Antimonium
Bryonia
Hyoscyamus
Nux mosch.
Pulsatilla
Rhus tox.
Sulphur
Veratrum

Hot face
Belladonna
Bryonia
Chamomilla
Cina
Graphites
Hepar sulph.
Nux
Opium
Pulsatilla
Stramonium
Tuberculinum

Pain in face
Aconite
Arsenicum
Aurum
Belladonna
Calcarea
Causticum
Cedrum
Colocynth
Gelsemium
Magnesia phos.
Natrum mur.
Nux
Phosphorus
Platina
Spigelia
Stannum
Staphisagria
Stramonium
Verbascum

Perspiration on face
Pulsatilla

Picking the lips
Aurum

Dry lips
Bryonia

Sensation of hair in throat
Kali bichrom.
Silicea
Sulphur

Painful neck glands
Belladonna
Calcarea
Capsicum
Carbo veg.
Mercurius
Natrum mur.
Silicea

Pain in neck glands

   with coughing
   Natrum mur.

   at night
   Mercurius
   Thuja

   turning the head
   Ignatia
   Kali carb.

Hard swollen neck glands
Baryta mur.
Calcarea
Conium
Iodum
Sarsaparilla
Silicea

Compression of chest
Bovista
Kali carb.

Pain in breast
Belladonna
Conium
Mercurius
Silicea

Palpitations
Arsenicum
Calcarea
Nitric ac.
Pulsatilla

Cough
Arsenicum
Calcarea
Conium
Ipecac.
Kali carb.
Natrum mur.
Nux
Phosphorus
Sabadilla

Coldness in abdomen
Zinc

Aching pains in abdomen
Antimonium
Arsenicum
Carbo veg.
Rhus tox.

Urge to urinate
Apis

Diarrhoea
Cina
Rhus tox.

Urine brown colour
Sepia
Veratrum

Periods suppressed
Belladonna
Conium
Cyclamen
Dulcamara
Ferrum iod.
Graphites
Kali carb.
Lachesis
Lycopodium
Pulsatilla
Senecio
Silicea
Sulphur
Veratrum

Never well after pneumonia
Kali carb.

   after meningitis
   Calcarea
   Silicea

   after influenza
   Abrotanum
   Cadmium met.
   Psorinum
   Tuberculinum
   Scutellaria

   after typhoid
   Carbo veg.
   Pyrogenium
   Sulphur

Pre-Menstrual Syndrome

This is a constellation of symptoms, both physical and emotional, which affect many women in the days leading up to a period, for anything from 2 to 14 days. It is only relatively recently that it has been recognized and accepted as a disorder with a physical cause. The term pre-menstrual syndrome (PMS) is more comprehensive than pre-menstrual tension, and is preferred by women as it has a less sexist, accusatory ring. The symptoms are relieved almost as soon as the period starts. It is a very common complaint, affecting 3 out of 4 women aged 30–40. This probably reflects the unnatural lifestyle led by many women in industrialized societies to-day, although pre-menstrual baboons in Kenya have been observed withdrawing from social contact and spending more time in the trees, feeding.

The social implications of PMS are considerable. There is an increased incidence of anti-social behaviour, accidents, illness and psychiatric crises in pre-menstrual women. Examples of this include poor standards of school work, with fewer passes and distinctions; schoolgirls receive more than the expected number of punishments, and are more forgetful and unpunctual. A 3–5 per cent increase in absenteeism from work occurs around the period time. Symptoms may be severe enough to cause a fear of crossing the road or driving, so the sufferer becomes isolated, preferring to stay close to home.

Behaviour of the sufferer that is different from the norm influences the lives of partners, children, neighbours and friends, etc. Aggressive behaviour towards the partner may lead to counter-violence. Children are very sensitive to their mother's emotional state, and may respond to inexplicable mood swings by psychosomatic symptoms e.g., a cough, runny nose, crying, vomiting (VOMITING IN BABIES), HEADACHES, etc. Thus, in addition to the unpleasant symptoms and feeling of not being in control that the sufferer experiences, she may also feel guilty about the effect she is having on those closest to her. This may account for the significant number of attempted suicides in the pre-menstrual phase. Sport may also be affected; pressure inside the eye may, for instance, reduce eyesight, affecting judgement. Women who are predisposed to aggression are also more likely to commit crimes of violence when they are in their pre-menstrual phase.

Causes and symptoms

The causes of PMS are many and varied. They include hereditary predisposition, emotional causes and dietary errors. It has been found that pre-menstrual syndrome patients consume 62 per cent more refined carbohydrate, 275 per cent more sugar, 79 per cent more dairy products, 78 per cent more sodium, 77 per cent less manganese, 53 per cent less iron and 52 per cent less zinc than symptom-free women. Metabolically it is possible to recognize 4 main sub-types of PMS, depending on the constellation of the symptoms experienced.

Type 1. PMS A: Symptoms are nervous tension, mood swings, anxiety and irritability (General Remedy Finder under ANGER). This is the most common type, affecting 65–75 per cent of PMS sufferers; it appears to be due to high oestrogen levels. These may arise because of VITAMIN B DEFICIENCY, which renders the liver unable to break down oestrogen for excretion. If CONSTIPATION is present the inert oestrogen can be reabsorbed in an active form. Excess oestrogen can affect mood and behaviour in several possible ways.

Firstly, by creating an imbalance in brain chemicals. Excess adrenaline and serotonin give rise to anxiety and irritability. Too little dopamine leads to a loss of calming effect.

Secondly, by blocking the VITAMIN B_6 METABOLISM which is necessary for dopamine synthesis. Up to 500 mg B_6 per day can be required before a satisfactory response is achieved. This should be done under the care of a nutritionally trained physician or dietician because of the danger of side-effects. Oestrogen/progesterone imbalances can increase B_6 requirements, so a woman may show a normal level of B_6 in the blood but in fact need a considerably higher level. Vitamin B_6 is also necessary for increasing the efficiency with which tissues make use of essential fatty acids. High saturated fatty acid levels in the diet will lead to poor metabolism of the essential fatty acids, which in addition to B_6 require supplies of magnesium, zinc, vitamin C, vitamin B$_3$ and chromium.

Deficiency of essential fatty acids may make women abnormally sensitive to ordinary levels of prolactin in the blood. Prolactin is a hormone produced by the pituitary gland which affects the amount of oestrogen and progesterone produced in the cycle. An excess of prolactin can affect breast tissue, making breasts enlarge and become swollen and tender (BREAST PROBLEMS). Few sufferers have abnormally high prolactin levels as such.

Thirdly, by affecting the body's regulatory system for maintaining normal blood sugar, resulting in recurrent HYPOGLYCAEMIA with associated mood changes.

Type 2. PMS H: Symptoms are of fluid retention (OEDEMA), weight gain (see WEIGHT PROBLEMS), breast heaviness and swelling (BREAST PROBLEMS) and abdominal bloating (ABDOMINAL DISTENSION). This affects 65–72 per cent of sufferers with PMS, and appears to be due to excess aldosterone production, which produces salt and water retention. A high salt intake on its own leads to increased fluid retention; the weight gain is likely to be more than 3 lb, and there may be swelling of the face, hands and ankles. PMS H is similar to PMS A in that the oestrogen level appears to be too high, resulting in excessive production of serotonin, in turn leading to over-secretion of aldosterone. As in PMS A there is also relative dopamine deficiency; dopamine normally suppresses aldosterone release.

Type 3. PMS C: Symptoms of Type 3 are sweet craving (General Remedy Finder) increased appetite, HEADACHE, PALPITATIONS, FATIGUE, dizziness and fainting. This affects 24–35 per cent of pre-menstrual women, and is due to decreased carbohydrate tolerance. The main mechanism here seems to be HYPOGLYCAEMIA. No clear explanation has emerged for this, although it seems that pre-menstrually there is increased sensitivity to insulin. Of course a high intake of refined carbohydrates and sugar is likely to lead to poor blood sugar control, resulting in mood changes. It also leads to decreased magnesium intake, which is involved with the production of progesterone, blood sugar control and essential fatty acid metabolism. Sugar is also likely to lead to water retention and bloating. High levels of coffee and tea interfere with nutrient absorption, and are associated with mood change, irritability (General Remedy Finder under ANGER), and insomnia (SLEEP PROBLEMS).

High intake of ALCOHOL may change the balance of vitamins and minerals and cause a reduction in the liver clearance of oestrogen, in addition to upsetting blood sugar control. In the absence of tea, coffee, sugar or alcohol, the body compensates for hypoglycaemia by producing more adrenalin; this increases the level of blood sugar by liberating stores of sugar from the liver. It also has the effect of causing anxiety, palpitations, sweating and shaking.

Type 4. PMS D: Symptoms are DEPRESSION, crying, confusion, forgetfulness, insomnia (see SLEEP PROBLEMS). This affects 23–35 per cent of women, and is more commonly found combined with PMS A, which occurs first and is followed by PMS D symptoms a few days before the onset of the period. It is characterized by high progesterone and low oestrogen. The low oestrogen may result in an increased breakdown of neurotransmitters. One theory is that LEAD POISONING, e.g., from exhaust fumes and factory outlets, blocks the action of oestrogen but not progesterone. If so, adequate intakes of VITAMIN B$_1$, MAGNESIUM, ZINC and IRON are important to decrease the absorption and deposition, and to increase excretion of the lead.

Additional symptoms

1 Skin disorders, increased tendency to ACNE. Skin becomes blotchy and dull with blemishes and whiteheads, and there may be a tendency to bruise. The skin is often more greasy.
2 Aches and pains due to: (a) increased pressure within the tissues as retained fluid starts to collect, pressing on the nerve endings; (b) increased state of tension of the muscle fibres, possibly due to actual pre-menstrual effect on the muscle fibre, though it may also be due to mental tension; (c) PAINFUL PERIODS caused by congestion of blood vessels in the pelvis and the genital regions – giving rise to a dull persistent pain in contrast to spasmodic period pains; (d) clumsiness (General Remedy Finder).

Other more unusual symptoms we have discovered in our patients are as follows: apathy, AGORAPHOBIA, PANIC ATTACKS, FRIGHT, PHOBIAS, aversion to company, suspicion, feeling of detachment, SUICIDAL TENDENCIES, swelling of upper eyelids, HAIR LOSS, sinusitis, sore throat, numbness of the throat, backache, swelling of the hip and lower back, cutting pain in the legs, itching irritation and burning in the vagina, vaginal discharge which may be yellow and offensive (see VAGINAL AND VULVAL PROBLEMS), aversion to intercourse, pain on intercourse (SEXUAL PROBLEMS), burning pain in bladder, increase in wind and alternate constipation and diarrhoea (IRRITABLE BOWEL SYNDROME), hot feet and a general feeling of being worse between 3–5 pm.

Other causes

There used to be a vogue for treating PMS as a progesterone deficiency state. This is, however, only the case for a small proportion of patients, and the vast majority of sufferers do not benefit from progesterone therapy. There is at least a 5–10 per cent incidence of side effects from its use, such as FATIGUE, lethargy, DEPRESSION, inertia, and HYPOGLYCAEMIA.

Prevention

As can be seen from reading through the causes and symptoms of PMS, the most important preventive measures to be taken include:

1 Regulation of blood sugar (HYPOGLYCAEMIA).
2 Reduction of salt intake.
3 Correction of nutritional deficiencies.
4 Prompt treatment of HORMONE IMBALANCES.

The best treatment for hormone imbalance is constitutional homeopathic treatment; it is also important to have optimum liver function, as the hormones are manufactured and destroyed by the liver.

Poor liver function may not always be reflected in a standard blood test, as a large proportion of the liver has to be knocked out before a test is abnormal. The diagnosis of sluggish liver rests on clinical evidence such as FATIGUE, malaise, digestive disturbance, ALLERGIES, pre-menstrual syndrome, CONSTIPATION.

One of the leading contributors to sluggish liver is likely to be reduction of bile fluid caused by:

1 Gallstones.
2 Alcohol.
3 Poor diet.
4 Stress.
5 Auto-intoxication from the bowel.
6 Steroids including the pill and oestrogens.
7 Pregnancy.
8 Other drugs and chemicals including environmental pollutants.
9 Hereditary disorders, e.g., Gilbert's syndrome.

Measures to protect liver:

1 Reduce ALCOHOL and saturated fat (see WEIGHT PROBLEMS) levels to decrease damage to the liver and slowing down of bile secretion. Increase fibre in your diet to promote bile secretion.
2 Increase antioxidants such as VITAMIN C, VITAMIN E, ZINC, SELENIUM to protect from free radical damage. (A free radical is a highly reactive molecule capable of destroying cellular structure unless effectively scavenged.) If you feel your liver is sluggish, do the LIVER DIET and COLON CLEANSE (see NUTRITIONAL SUPPLEMENTS AND SPECIAL DIETS).

Self-help

Avoid salted foods (do not cheat by adding salt at the table), junk food, fatty foods, and tea and coffee. The consumption of dairy products and refined carbohydrates, especially sugar, should be limited. Eat plenty of small, protein-rich snacks rather than large meals, but make sure most of the protein comes from vegetarian sources (pulses, nuts, whole grains, etc). Eat vegetables raw, and salads with sunflower oil dressing. Cut down on tobacco and try and eliminate smoking completely. If you are very overweight, try and lose some (see WEIGHT PROBLEMS).

Supplements

Below are supplements you may try yourself, but see general rules for supplements (p. 253).

1 Pyridoxine (vitamin B_6): dosage 50–200 mg a day. Higher doses than this may produce nerve damage.
2 Vitamin E: 150–300 units a day.
3 Evening primrose oil.
4 Multivitamins and minerals; the best one for this condition appears to be Optivite, which is available from most chemists and health shops: dosage 2 tablets 3 times a day.

With all supplements it is probably best to take them daily for the first month, then just in the 2 weeks pre-menstrually, or starting just before the expected onset of symptoms, unless advised otherwise by a nutritionally trained physician.

Other treatments

If changes in lifestyle, diet, supplementation and homeopathy do not work then see your GP, who will prescribe Vitamin B_6, or Evening Primrose Oil (see p. 252), and if they don't work, progesterone. Other possibilities include bromocriptine (which may help with breast tenderness), diuretics, Danazol. Where the emotional symptoms are the most trying psychotherapy may be helpful. For further information contact the Women's Nutritional Advisory Service (see Useful Addresses, p. 334).

Homeopathic treatment

The best course of action is homeopathic constitutional treatment, although the remedies listed below are well worth trying first.

Specific remedies to be taken every 12 hours for up to 3 days, starting 24 hours before pre-menstrual symptoms are due. All remedies to be taken in 30c potency.

Please remember to check your choice against the Remedy Pictures (p. 305) where possible.

Sepia

Irritability – worse for stress; depression; indifference; agoraphobia; weepiness; difficulty in concentrating; wanting to get away from everyone; emotionally flat; suicidal; fits of screaming; possible violence; anger; hair falling out; headaches in general; pressure on top of the head; chronic sinusitis; greasy facial skin; acne; hot flushes on face; sore throat with numbness; nausea; desire for sweets and salty things; tenderness, dragging, bearing down pains in lower abdomen; anal fissure; burning pain in bladder; burning pains in vagina; yellow, burning, offensive vaginal discharge; itching of vagina caused by discharge; discharge after intercourse with tendency to thrush – worse after childbirth; aversion to sexual intercourse or just reduced sex drive; prolapse of the womb; may have endometriosis; pain in vagina on intercourse, symptoms worse at menopause; sore nipples; palpitations.

Generalities: Muscular tension – worse between 3–5 pm; trembling; weakness and weariness in morning. Symptoms worse after periods.

Calcarea

Depression; indifference; agoraphobia; weepiness; irritability; panic attacks; suicidal; apprehension; fearful, especially in public places; dizziness; headache before periods; general tendency to headaches; pains in back of head; greasy facial skin; sore throat; desire for sweets, sugar and salt, and eggs; yellow, burning vaginal discharge causes itching; tendency to thrush; PMS worse since pregnancy; prolapse of womb; pain in womb during periods; swelling and tenderness of breasts before periods; backache; clumsiness; swollen ankles; swelling of hands; cutting pains in thigh; sleeplessness.

Generalities: Painful joints; tiredness and lack of energy; weakness with cold sweats; tendency to put on weight.

Lycopodium

Irritability – worse for stress; depression; lack of self-confidence; weepiness; difficulty in concentrating; wanting to be left alone; suspicious; mistrustful; feeling of being detached; violent behaviour; fearful in a crowd of people; weepy after periods; anger; hair falling out; headaches before periods; greasy facial skin; hot flushes on face; sore throat; nausea; desire for sweet things; desire for sugar; bloated abdomen; dull aching pains; bearing down pains in lower abdomen; irritable bowel syndrome; yellow vaginal discharge; aversion to sexual intercourse; may have endometriosis; tender nipples and breasts; backache, swelling of back; swollen fingers, hands, feet and ankles.

Generalities: Joint pains; general weakness; trembling; weakness in morning; weakness with sweating; tendency to put on weight.

Pulsatilla

Irritability – worse for stress; depression; indifference; lack of self-confidence; weepiness; bursts into tears for no reason; desire to be alone; suspicious; mistrusting; feeling of detachment; suicidal; indecisiveness; anxious about the future; fearful in public places; fearful in a crowd; dizziness; headaches before periods; swelling of upper eyelids; swelling of face; nausea; desire for sweets; bloated abdomen; dull aching pain and bearing down pains in lower abdomen; cramping pains – better for heat; irritable bowel syndrome; urgent need to pass water; burning pain; burning pains in vagina; burning yellow vaginal discharge, with tendency to thrush; PMS worse since pregnancy; prolapse of the womb; pain in womb during periods; periods irregular and may be scanty, symptoms worse at menopause; tender breasts; backache; hot feet; swollen fingers, ankles and feet.

Generalities: Joint pains; weakness; muscular tension; tendency to weight gain.

Sulphur

Weepiness; irritability; desire to be left alone; mistrustful; anxiety; violent; angry and apprehensive; hair falling out; headache before periods; drawing pains in head; swelling of upper eyelids; chronic sinusitis; greasy facial skin; hot flushes on face; sore throat; marked desire for sweets, sugar, and salt; dragging bearing down pain in lower abdomen; constipation; anal fissure; irritable bowel syndrome; urgent need to pass water; burning pains in vagina; yellow, burning offensive vaginal discharge which causes itching; aversion to intercourse or reduced sex drive; pain in vagina on intercourse, symptoms worse at menopause; painful nipples; clumsiness; hot feet; swelling of fingers and hands.

Generalities: Joint pains; PMS worse during convalescence from illness; tendency to put on weight.

Lachesis

Irritability; difficulty in concentrating; aversion to company; suspicious and mistrustful; detached feeling; suicidal; violent; indecisive; symptoms worse for stress; dizziness; hair falling out; headache before periods; sore throat worse on left side; bloated abdomen; tenderness in abdomen; constipation; anal fissure; irritable bowel syndrome; menopause; burning vaginal discharge; PMS worse since pregnancy; tender nipples; palpitations; backache; clumsiness; swollen ankles; aching pains in hips; swollen hands; sleeplessness.

Generalities: Symptoms better at beginning of period; weakness and weariness in morning – worse after periods are over.

Natrum mur.

Depression; indifference; lack of self-confidence; weepiness; definite aversion to company; detached feeling; anxiety; suicidal; violent; fearful in a crowd; symptoms worse for stress; hair falling out; headaches before periods; pressure on top of head; greasy facial skin; nausea; desires salty and sweet things; anal fissure; irritable bowel syndrome; burning pain in vagina; itching from vaginal discharge; tendency to thrush; aversion to intercourse or reduced sex drive; pain in vagina on intercourse; swollen tender breasts; palpitations.

Generalities: Weakness; muscular tension; trembling; weariness in morning; fluid retention.

Nux

Indifference; lack of self-confidence; agoraphobia; irritability; difficulty in concentrating; aversion to company; mistrustful; anxiety; suicidal; violent; fearful in public places; fearful in a crowd; anger, symptoms worse for stress; dizziness; drawing pains in head; pressure on top of head; chronic catarrh; acne on face; sore throat; nausea; desire for fatty foods, rich foods, alcohol; bearing down pain in lower abdomen; constipation; anal fissure; irritable bowel syndrome; frequent urgent need to pass water; yellow, offensive vaginal discharge, with tendency to thrush; PMS worse since pregnancy; pain in womb during periods, worse at menopause; tenderness of breasts; backache; clumsiness.

Generalities: Joint pains; muscular tension; weariness in the morning; generally worse after periods as well as before; chilliness.

Phosphorus

Worse for stress; indifference; panic attacks; difficult concentration; feeling of detachment; violent; apprehensive; weepiness after periods;

anger; dizziness; hair falling out; greasy facial skin; acne on face; nausea; desire for sweets, sugar, salt and salty things; dragging pain in abdomen; anal fissure; irritable bowel syndrome; urgent need to pass water; menopause; burning vaginal discharge; aversion to intercourse; clumsiness; swollen fingers, ankles, feet and hands; cramps in calves.

Generalities: Joint pains; weakness; PMS worse during convalescence from an acute illness; muscle tension; tendency to put on weight.

Graphites

Weepiness; irritability; difficulty in concentrating; anxiety; indecision; hair falling out; swollen face; hot flushes on face; constipation; anal fissure; burning pain in vagina; yellow vaginal discharge, with tendency to thrush; reduced sex drive, symptoms worse at menopause; tenderness in breasts and nipples; clumsiness; cutting pains in thigh; swelling of fingers, ankles and feet.

Generalities: Weakness; generally worse after periods; tendency to put on weight.

Kali carb.

Irritability; panic attacks; angry; tense; hair falling out; swollen upper eyelids, like a little bag or pouch; chronic sinusitis; swollen face; desires sweets, sugar; dull aching pain; gnawing pain in abdomen; constipation; irritable bowel syndrome; urgent need to pass water; reduced sex drive; pain in vagina on intercourse; symptoms worse at menopause; swollen, tender breasts; backache; sleeplessness.

Generalities: Joint pains; trembling; tendency to weight gain; exhaustion; symptoms worse around 3 am.

Silicea

Lack of self-confidence; difficulty in concentrating; hair falling out; pressure on top of head; greasy facial skin; acne on face; sore throat; cramping pains – better for warmth; constipation; anal fissure; offensive vaginal discharge; tender nipples; clumsiness; swollen feet.

Generalities: Joint pains; PMS symptoms worse during convalescence from acute illness; muscle tension.

Belladonna

Worse for stress; irritability; aversion to company; mistrustful; suicidal; violent; headache before periods; feeling of pressure on top of head; sore throat; dragging pains; burning in vagina; tendency to thrush; PMS worse since pregnancy; pain in womb during periods, symptoms worse at menopause; clumsiness; cutting pains in thigh; swollen hands; sleeplessness.

Generalities: Joint pains; weakness; weariness; tendency to weight gain.

Causticum

Depression; weepiness; irritability; difficulty in concentrating; suspicious and mistrustful; pessimistic; oversensitive; greasy facial skin; acne on face; sore throat; frequent urge to urinate or signs of cystitis; anal fissure; itching from vaginal discharge; PMS symptoms worse since pregnancy; aversion to sexual intercourse or reduced sex drive; tender nipples; backache; clumsiness; swollen feet.

Generalities: Joint pains; weakness.

Remedy Finder for Pre-Menstrual Syndrome

Abusive, insulting
Chamomilla

Anxiety in morning if period delayed
Natrum mur.

  before noon
  Ammonium carb.

  in evening
  Nitric ac.

Makes mountains out of molehills
Conium

Despair
Veratrum

Craving for alcohol
Selenium

Often frightened by trivial things
Calcarea

Impulsive need to run away
Lachesis

Becomes workaholic
Baryta
Calcarea
Calcarea phos.
Hyoscyamus
Ignatia
Lachesis
Magnesia carb.
Phosphorus
Sepia
Veratrum

Over-demonstrative
Veratrum

Lustful
Stramonium

Laughing inappropriately
Hyoscyamus
Nux mosch.

Nymphomania
Dulcamara
Phosphorus
Veratrum

Changeable mood
Chamomilla

Irritability before periods
Sepia

Cries with distress before periods
Graphites
Murex

Anxiety before periods
Cocculus
Graphites
Ignatia
Natrum mur.
Nitric ac.
Nux
Sulphur

Unusually cheerful and happy before periods
Aconite
Fluoric ac.
Hyoscyamus

Decreased ability to concentrate before periods
Calcarea

Confusion
Cimicifuga
Sepia

Over-excitement
Kreosotum
Lachesis
Lycopodium
Nux

Fear
Aconite

Easily frightened
Calcarea

Hysteria
Cimicifuga
Hyoscyamus
Ignatia
Magnesia mur.
Moschus
Platina

Irritability
Causticum
Chamomilla
Lycopodium
Natrum mur.
Nux
Pulsatilla
Sepia

Manic behaviour
Sepia

All mental symptoms worse pre-menstrually
Natrum mur.
Stannum

Discontented
Chamomilla
Lycopodium
Nux

Lovesick
Bromium

Lassitude
Belladonna

Giddiness and vertigo
Calcarea phos.
Caulophyllum
Conium
Lachesis
Pulsatilla

Veratrum
Zinc

Fullness in head
Aconite
Apis
Belladonna
Glonoinum
Kali carb.
Mercurius

Tension in skull
Hepar sulph.
Natrum carb.
Silicea

Itchy scalp
Magnesia mur.

Spotty scalp
Sepia

Hot head
Calcarea
Conium
Crotalus
Ignatia
Iodum
Lycopodium
Thuja

Heavy head
Cimicifuga
Crotalus
Ignatia

Throbbing in head
Belladonna
Borax
Crotalus
Glonoinum
Lachesis
Petroleum

Pulsating temples
Lachesis

Brain feels sensitive
Calcarea
Carbo veg.
Conium
Hyoscyamus
Natrum mur.
Phosphorus

Headache before and during periods
Belladonna
Cyclamen
Gelsemium
Glonoinum
Natrum mur.
Nux

Sanguinaria
Sepia
Sulphur
Ustaligo

Pain in forehead
Calcarea

Pain in temples
Lachesis

Boring pain in temples
Antimonium

Pressing pain
Natrum mur.

Pressing pain in forehead over eyes
Silicea

Shooting pains
Ferrum

Shooting pains in sides
Calcarea phos.

Heavy eyes
Natrum mur.

Whites of eyes full of dark vessels
Pulsatilla

Red eyes
Glonoinum

Red eyelids
Aurum

Staring eyes
Pulsatilla

Twitching eyelids
Natrum mur.

Noises in ear
Borax
Ferrum
Kreosotum

Tingling in ear
Ferrum

Bad hearing
Kreosotum

Cold in head before periods
Magnesia carb.

Cough and hoarseness
Graphites

Nosebleeds before periods
Baryta
Ipecac.
Lachesis
Natrum sulph.

Pulsatilla
Sulphur
Veratrum

Pain in nose – particularly the root
Conium

Bloated face
Graphites
Kali carb.
Mercurius
Pulsatilla

Blueness of face
Pulsatilla

Blue circles around eyes
Tuberculinum

Red flushes
Belladonna
Ferrum phos.
Sanguinaria

Skin eruptions around eyes
Magnesia mur.

Blotches on face
Magnesia mur.

Pimples
Magnesia mur.

Blisters on nose
Magnesia carb.

Hot face
Alumina
Lycopodium

Aching face
Stannum

Swollen face
Graphites
Kali carb.
Mercurius
Pulsatilla

Swollen cheeks
Phosphorus

Smelly breath
Sepia

Sore mouth
Phosphorus

Blood in saliva
Natrum mur.

Increase in saliva
Pulsatilla

Swollen gums
Baryta
Phosphorus

Bleeding mouth ulcers
Phosphorus

Blisters
Magnesia carb.

Toothache
Antimonium
Natrum mur.
Pulsatilla
Sulphur

Stinging pain in teeth
Sulphur

Tearing pains in throat
Arsenicum

Choking
Pulsatilla

Inflamed throat
Magnesia carb.

Burning pains in throat
Sulphur

Sore throat
Conium
Magnesia carb.

Tension in throat
Iodum

Ulcers
Magnesia carb.

Constricted feeling in stomach
Sulphur

Desire for sweets
Sulphur

Weak empty feeling in stomach
Ignatia

Ineffectual burping at night
Manganum

Burping in general
Kali carb.
Natrum mur.
Nux mosch.
Pulsatilla

Sour burps
Kali carb.

Sweetish burps
Natrum mur.

Watery burps
Manganum

Water comes into mouth
Nux mosch.
Pulsatilla

Heartburn
Sulphur

Fullness
Tarentula

Nausea – morning sickness
Ammonium mur.
Cocculus
Cyclamen
Ipecac.
Nux
Sepia

Nausea in general
Hyoscyamus
Ipecac.
Lycopodium
Natrum mur.
Pulsatilla

Pain in stomach before periods
Magnesia carb.

Stomach cramps
Belladonna
Pulsatilla
Sepia

Pressure
Nux mosch.

Thirsty for large quantities
Sulphur

Vomiting in morning
Ammonium mur.
Cocculus
Cyclamen
Ipecac.
Nux
Sepia

Vomiting any time
Calcarea
Cuprum
Kreosotum
Nux
Pulsatilla

Vomiting bitter tasting fluids
Caulophyllum

Sour vomiting
Calcarea
Pulsatilla

Contraction of abdomen
Natrum mur.

Bloat
Cocculus
Lachesis
Lycopodium
Pulsatilla
Zinc

Rash on abdomen
Apis

Rumbling in abdomen
Zinc

Hardness in abdomen
Manganum

Heaviness as from a stone
Pulsatilla

Dull aching pain in lower abdomen
Lachesis
Lycopodium
Natrum mur.
Sepia
Sulphur

Clawing pain
Belladonna

Abdominal cramps
Ammonium carb.
Belladonna
Calcarea phos.
Causticum
Chamomilla
Cocculus
Colocynth
Cuprum
Ignatia
Kali carb.
Lachesis
Magnesia phos.
Platina
Pulsatilla
Sepia

Cramping pains in belly button region
Kreosotum

Cutting pains
Chamomilla
Lilium

Pressing pains in lower abdomen
Platina
Sepia

Tender abdomen
Belladonna

Bryonia
Sepia

Sense of weakness in abdomen
Phosphorus

Constipation
Graphites
Kali carb.
Lachesis
Silicea

Diarrhoea
Ammonium carb.
Lachesis
Natrum sulph.
Silicea
Veratrum

Dragging feeling in rectum
Phosphorus

Haemorrhoids worse before periods
Aloe
Carbon sulph.
Carbo veg.
Collinsonia
Graphites
Ignatia
Lachesis
Pulsatilla

Itching in back passage
Graphites

Urge to urinate frequently
Alumina
Kali iod.
Pulsatilla
Sarsaparilla
Sulphur

Urge to urinate
Kali iod.
Pulsatilla
Sulphur

Painful urination
Sarsaparilla

Frequent urination – not urgent
Apis
Sarsaparilla

Cutting pain in urethra
Cantharis

Burning urine
Cantharis

Milky urine
Phosphoric ac.

Strong smelling urine
Mercurius

Scanty urine
Apis
Silicea

Mucus in urine
Lachesis

Whey-like urine
Phosphoric acid

Congestion in ovaries
Lac can.

Congestion of womb
China
Lachesis

Increase in sexual desire
Calcarea phos.
Phosphorus
Veratrum

Feeling as if ovaries enlarged
Silicea

Feeling as if womb enlarged
Sepia

Eruptions on vulva
Dulcamara

Spots of pus on vulva
Aurum mur.

Soreness of skin of vulva
Kali carb.
Sepia

Heat in vagina
Ignatia

Chilliness of vulva
Calcarea
Graphites
Kali carb.
Lilium
Mercurius
Sulphur

Itchy vagina
Graphites

Burning vaginal discharge
Graphites
Sepia
Silicea
Ustilago

Vaginal discharge like white of egg
Ustilago

Bland vaginal discharge before and after periods
Pulsatilla

Copious vaginal discharge
Lachesis
Nux

Jelly-like discharge before and after periods
Palladium

Vaginal discharge in general before periods
Bovista
Calcarea
Graphites
Kreosotum
Sepia

Thick discharge before and after periods
Zinc

Yellowy discharge
Natrum mur.
Pulsatilla
Sepia
Tarentula

Pain in ovaries
Apis
Belladonna
Cimicifuga
Colocynth
Lachesis
Lilium
Thuja
Zinc

Pain in womb during night before period starts
Calcarea

Pain in womb in general before periods
Calcarea
Calcarea phos.
Caulophyllum
Kali carb.
Pulsatilla
Sepia

Bearing down pains (dragging or labour-like)
Apis
Belladonna
Calcarea phos.
China

Cina
Conium
Kali carb.
Phosphorus
Platina
Sepia
Viburnum

Burning pains in genitalia
Sepia

Burning pain in labia
Calcarea

Burning pain in left ovary on movement
Thuja

Burning pain in womb
Natrum mur.

Burning pain in vagina
Ignatia
Sulphur

Cramping pains in womb
Calcarea phos.
Causticum
Chamomilla
Magnesia phos.
Viburnum

Pulling or drawing pains in ovaries
Colocynth

Pinching pain in womb
Alumina

Tender ovaries
Kali carb.
Lac can.

Tender womb
Bovista

Stinging pains in genitals
Zinc

Shooting pains in ovaries
Podophyllum

Shooting pains in womb
Borax

Tearing pains in womb
Natrum mur.

Sensitivity in genitals
Lachesis
Platina

Swelling of exterior genitals
Sepia

Swollen ovaries
Bromium

Difficulty in breathing
Cuprum
Natrum sulph.
Sulphur
Zinc

Cough in daytime
Graphites

Cough in bed in evening
Sulphur

Dry cough in daytime
Graphites

Dry cough in morning
Zinc

Dry cough in general
Sulphur
Zinc

Cough in general
Argentum nit.
Graphites
Sulphur

Coughing up blood
Zinc

Breasts icy cold
Medorrhinum

Swollen chest
Kali carb.

Constriction or tension in chest
Phosphorus

Fullness
Sulphur

Hardened lumps in breasts
Conium

Itchy armpits
Sanguinaria

Secretion of milk from breasts
Tuberculinum

Oppression of chest – heaviness in chest
Borax
Lachesis

Pain in chest on breathing
Pulsatilla

Pain in armpits
Calcarea

Pain in breasts in general
Calcarea

Conium
Kali mur.
Lac can.
Zinc

Sides of chest painful
Pulsatilla

Pain in heart region
Cactus
Lilium

Burning pain in chest
Zinc

Tenderness in chest before and during periods
Zinc

Sensitive tender breasts
Calcarea
Conium
Kali mur.
Lac can.
Pulsatilla
Tuberculinum

Swelling of breasts
Calcarea
Lac can.
Tuberculinum

Stitching pains in chest
Kali carb.

Stitching pains in side of chest
Pulsatilla

Palpitations
Cactus
Cuprum
Iodum
Lilium
Natrum mur.
Sepia
Spongia

Palpitations on waking
Alumina

Cramping in chest
Lachesis

Swelling of glands in armpit
Aurum

Weakness of chest with cough
Graphites

Eruptions on back of neck and between shoulder blades especially if itchy
Carbo veg.

Heaviness in lower back
Bovista

Backache
Berberis
Calcarea carb.
Causticum
Gelsemium
Hydrastis
Kali carb.
Kali nit.
Kreosotum
Lachesis
Lycopodium
Magnesia carb.
Nux
Nux mosch.
Podophyllum
Pulsatilla
Spongia
Ustilago
Viburnum

Drawing pains in neck
Natrum carb.

Tenderness in the tail
Spongia

Shooting pains in lower back
Natrum mur.

Perspiration on back
Nitric ac.

Pulsation in back
Nitric ac.

Neck tension
Natrum carb.

Cold arms
Manganum

Cold legs
Lycopodium

Clamminess of feet
Calcarea

Cold feet
Lycopodium
Nux mosch.

Contraction of thigh muscles
Chamomilla

Cramp in calves
Phosphorus

Tired heavy limbs
Lycopodium

Lameness of lower limbs
Nitric ac.

Numbness of thighs
Podophyllum

Numbness of feet
Hypericum

Cold sweats on limbs
Calcarea

Sweaty feet
Calcarea

Swollen feet
Lycopodium

Trembling limbs
Natrum mur.

Trembling legs
Kali carb.

Varicose veins worse
Ambra

Weakness of foot at night
Manganum

Painful joints
Caulophyllum

Pain in legs
Caulophyllum

Pain in hips
Cimicifuga

Pain in back of thigh
Magnesia mur.

Disturbed sleep
Alumina

Dreams about sex
Calcarea
Kali carb.

Anxiety dreams
Causticum

Many dreams
Alumina

Restless sleep
Kali carb.

Yawning with chilliness
Pulsatilla

Yawning with stretching
Pulsatilla

Chilliness at midnight
Lycopodium

Chilliness in general
Calcarea

Caulophyllum
Kali carb.
Lycopodium
Magnesia carb.
Pulsatilla
Sepia
Silicea

Heat before noon
Ammonium carb.

Heat at midnight
Lycopodium

Perspiration in morning
Natrum sulph.

Perspiration at night
Veratrum

Perspiration in general
Graphites
Hyoscyamus
Sulphur
Thuja
Veratrum

Cold skin
Silicea

Itchy herpes
Carbo veg.

Rashes
Dulcamara

Urticaria or nettle rash
Dulcamara
Kali carb.

Itchiness in general
Graphites
Silicea

Coldness of skin with feeling as if ants are running underneath it
Antimonium tart.

Hot flushes
Lachesis
Sanguinaria

Fainting
Lycopodium
Moschus
Muriatic ac.
Natrum mur.
Nux
Nux mosch.
Sepia
Thuja

Irregular pulse
Kali carb.

Shuddering pulse
Sepia

Trembling pulse
Natrum mur.

Weak pulse
Alumina
Ammonium carb.
Belladonna
China
Cocculus
Magnesia carb.

Natrum mur.
Veratrum

Weariness
Belladonna
Natrum mur.

Thrush (Candidiasis)

Candidiasis is caused by *Candida albicans*, a member of the yeast family. Under normal conditions it is harmless, but given optimal conditions it is capable of explosive growth, and can increase itself from 1 to 100 cells in 24 hours. These 100 cells can then produce 100 each in the next 24 hours, and so on. Apart from the bowel, it also likes the vagina and the skin. It has no helpful function, and is a pure parasite. The majority of infants will show a positive reaction by the age of 6 months if skin-tested for candida, showing that their immune system has been challenged to respond by producing immuno-globulins. It has been estimated that approximately 30 per cent of everybody in the world over 12 years – especially women – is suffering from yeast-related illnesses because of candida.

Studies have found a strong correlation between vaginal and intestinal cultures of candida, and it is thought that unrestricted spread of the organism may be the single most important predisposing factor in vulvo-vaginal candidiasis or thrush. It is interesting that there has been a 2-fold increase in the relative frequency and total incidence of vaginitis since approximately 1970, which corresponds to a decrease in incidence of gonorrhea and trichomonal vaginitis. The single most likely reason for this is the increased use of antibiotics, both therapeutically in humans, and as sub-therapeutic doses in animal feeds.

The role of antibiotics

Repeated courses of antibiotics given therapeutically, for instance for acne, cystitis or upper respiratory tract infections, disrupt the normal competition between separate members of the resident flora of the gut; in other words the normal balance of organisms in the bowel is upset. Candida is thus allowed to proliferate.

Sub-therapeutic amounts of antibiotics added to animal feeds, to promote rapid enhanced meat production, inevitably lead to acquired resistance by certain microbes in the gut to the antibiotics used. Increasing resistance of the salmonella population led in the 1960s and 70s to those antibiotics which were routinely used therapeutically being banned in the UK and EEC in animal feed. It was thought that the practice could lead to cross-resistance, i.e. certain microbes might acquire resistance to more than one antibiotic. In addition the stimulation of growth of yeasts was also inevitable.

Other predisposing factors

These include: an underlying inherited or acquired immune system deficiency, which may be due to a nutritional deficiency; increased demands on the immune system to combat environmental pollution; or damage to the immune system e.g., AIDS. Metabolic causes include diabetes mellitis (due to an increase in blood sugar), and raised vaginal alkalinity found in pregnancy, especially after multiple pregnancies. Drugs which exert an immuno-suppressive effect such as steroids (including hormone residues in meat), oral contraceptives (the Pill), and immuno-suppressive drugs (such as those used to treat cancer) can also contribute to candida. The progesterone component of the Pill appears to encourage candida growth, which is particularly noticeable in the second half of the menstrual cycle. Candidiasis can also follow the onset of allergies, and will resolve after the allergy has been treated.

Local predisposing causes include: underwear with non-cotton crotch, nylon tights (which promote the vulvo-vaginal warmth and moistness on which candida thrives), tight fitting jeans, vaginal deodorants, scented toilet tissues, etc. Sexual intercourse without enough lubrication can also predispose to it.

Symptoms

Symptoms spread throughout the body are many and varied, and include recurrent cystitis and recurrent 'thrush vaginitis' (vaginal soreness and itching with associated curdlike discharge which has a vinegar or yeastlike odour, and possible discomfort on intercourse). It is also associated with vulval itching. There may be oral thrush, painful irregular periods, pre-menstrual syndrome, endometriosis, low libido, and infertility. In the abdomen there may be indigestion, nausea, flatulence, bloating, diarrhoea, constipation or rectal itching. There is often a craving for sugar and refined carbohydrates or alcohol and yeasty food such as bread and cheese. These give a transient pick-up effect and then sudden energy loss (i.e., HYPOGLYCAEMIA).

The sufferer may have recurrent sore throat and nasal congestion, dizziness, fatigue, lethargy, blurring of vision and headaches. Mental effects include irritability, anxiety, depression, feelings of unreality, poor memory and hyperactivity.

There is a resulting wide range of both inhalational and food allergies. The skin complaints include acne, psoriasis, dermatitis, hives, athlete's foot and brittle, brown, discoloured nails. Aching, numbness and tingling of the muscles or aching pain and swelling in the joints is also possible. There is often a noticeable worsening of symptoms on damp days or in mouldy damp environments, i.e., damp earth or cellars. Finally, poor nutrient absorption and assimilation are likely. The above symptoms have been reported in classical attacks of candida.

In addition the women in our survey reported boils on the buttocks, deterioration of symptoms in the menopause, difficulty in concentration and in making decisions, swelling of the breasts, weight gain, bartholinitis, ulcers on the labia, facial hair, cracking of the skin on the labia, backache, burning pain in the eyes.

Diagnosis

Apart from oral and vaginal thrush which can be diagnosed from a swab, there is no definitive test for candidiasis. Diagnosis largely rests on history and symptoms and eventually on the success or otherwise of the treatment. There is, however, a test available in certain laboratories such as BioLab (see Useful Addresses, p. 336). In this, the Gut Fermentation Test, the patient fasts overnight and a blood alcohol level is taken. She is then given a loading dose of sugar (taken by mouth); the alcohol level is measured an hour later, along with short-branch fatty acids. If there has been a rise in alcohol level it will be because the sugar has been fermented into alcohol either by a fungus or a bacteria in the gut. By looking at the types of short-branch fatty acids present it is possible to tell whether the likely organism is bacterial or fungal.

Candida produces its effects by two routes. Firstly, there is a direct route initially by invasion of the gut and the vagina; candida is capable of spreading along the entire length of the gut. The presence of chronic vaginitis can often indicate wide-spread candidiasis. Secondly, there can be indirect effects caused by the spread of toxins through the bloodstream to other sites. In the gut candida can alter its form from a simple yeast organism to a 'mycelial fungal form', a network of root-like fibres called rhizoids. These can penetrate and damage the gut lining, allowing foreign food proteins to be absorbed into the bloodstream and to challenge the immune system so that multiple food allergy may result.

Toxic waste from candida infestations can also be absorbed into the bloodstream, producing a range of symptoms as above; some of the most disturbing may be those affecting the brain. Yeast toxin hypersensitivity can lead to anxiety, depression and impaired intellectual functioning. This is often not recognized as a candidal problem, and psychiatric referral is the result, which may be unsuccessful, and increase feelings of guilt, poor self-esteem and depression. In addition to the toxins produced by the candida organism itself, it can also affect the brain by way of the toxic substances manufactured from sugar and refined carbohydrates in the diet. The main substance implicated here is acetaldehyde, which is a normal by-product of metabolism, produced in small amounts and rendered harmless by the liver. If, however, there is excess production of this by candida and/or a lack of the appropriate liver enzymes which tend to be deficient in 5 per cent of the general population, the acetaldehyde will become bound strongly to human tissue. This may cause impaired neuro-transmission in the brain, resulting in anxiety, depression, defective memory and cloudy thinking.

Effects on the immune system

As an opportunist, candida is dependent on conditions which favour its steady growth. An immune system already undermined by other factors such as poor nutrition or exposure to environmental pollutants will be unable effectively to deter this relentless growth. Thus candida will in turn effectively weaken and disturb the immune system so that further damage may occur due to the invasion of viral agents such as Epstein-Barr virus, cytomegalovirus, herpes simplex and so on. Disturbance of the ongoing process of 'self recognition' by the immune system is likely to lead further to the possibility of a range of auto-immune diseases.

A note on the immune system

The main components of the immune system are:

1 B-lymphocytes: these produce proteins called immunoglobulins, which bind antigenic substances and render them harmless. An antigen is a substance which the body recognizes as being alien and therefore potentially harmful. An immunoglobulin is a particular kind of protein which coats the antigen; by being made harmless the antigens can then be digested by other cells.
2 T-lymphocytes; there are three types:
   a The killer cells; these attack and destroy substances with enzymes and hormones.
   b The helper cells; these help B cells to make the immunoglobulins.
   c The suppressor cells; these protect the body from the excesses of the body's defence system.

T-cell efficiency can be influenced to a useful extent by nutrition. It is largely the suppressors which are involved in fighting the candida challenge, partly because candida's adaptability allows it to produce disguising antigens which deter the immune system from recognizing it as foreign and harmful. In this way the immune system may eventually become non-responsive to the presence of *Candida albicans*. Candida toxins will then circulate virtually unchallenged, and candida will grow in a range of tissues either as a yeast or a mycelial fungus. This apparent tolerance of candida by the immune system can only be reversed in the long term by ending exposure of the body to yeast antigens and toxins. A high percentage of serum from symptomless people has been found to contain yeast toxin immunoglobulins. This indicates that the B-cell immune defences must be constantly counteracting candida toxin. When alive, yeasts are able to invade the immune system to a certain degree. When they are killed, proteins making up the yeast cell wall are absorbed through the lining of the intestine and can cause heightened allergy reactions, resulting in a phenomenon called 'Die off' or the 'Herxheimer reaction'. This may in fact signal a good response to treatment.

Allergic symptoms emerging as a result of weakness in the immune system may develop over a long period, or may proceed relatively quickly. This process seems to originate from the impaired production and function of the T-cell lymphocytes which can no longer effectively regulate B-cell immunoglobulin production. As a result the body cannot discriminate between harmless and potentially toxic agents.

Candida toxin tends to cause its effects by production of 'free radicals' (a kind of rogue molecule which can cause damage to cell membranes so that function is impaired). Thus, for example, the liver's detoxifying capability is likely to be impaired, so that the potentially toxic foreign substances are more likely to produce damage or reaction. It has been proposed, for instance, that increased sensitivity to mercury amalgam fillings may develop due to prior damage from candida toxins.

The candida syndrome appears to be more symptomatic in women, possibly due to its ability to upset the female hormone balance. It seems that candida can bind to adrenal steroids so that adrenal insufficiency may result. It can also be associated with ovarian and thyroid disorders, i.e. oophoritis (inflammation of the ovaries) and HYPOTHYROIDISM, due to thyroiditis or inflammation of the thyroid (see below and THYROID PROBLEMS). In the latter condition there may be no signs of thyroid swelling (goitre) and all thyroid function tests may be normal. It may, however, be suspected from a history of fatigue, depression, sensitivity to cold, constipation, and irregular periods and it responds well to anti-candidal treatment.

Similarly candidiasis can be associated with a range of auto-immune disorders apart from thyroiditis – the most commonly associated condition of candida – along with impairment of the immune system. Other conditions include rheumatoid arthritis. In such cases there may be a significant sequence of symptoms stretching right back to childhood including infant colic, childhood allergies, recurrent courses of antibiotics for respiratory tract infections, increased symptoms of allergy in adolescents, fatigue, PMS, irregular periods, pain on intercourse and endometriosis, depression and anxiety.

Treatment

N.B. All irritating or offensive discharges should be checked by a doctor for infection other than thrush before starting any self-help measures.

In the authors' opinion, constitutional homeopathic treatment is the single most effective treatment for deep-seated candida but it tends only to work to its best effect when combined with other measures as follows:

1 Anti-candida diet. This is essential for the long-term control of candida, because diet is one of the main precipitants of the condition.
2 Yeast growth must be eliminated in order to allow for strengthening of the immune system.

Optimal nourishment is required to rebuild and replace tissues damaged by candida infestation.

The two main principles are elimination of foods derived from or containing yeast or fungi, and a reduction of foods rich in refined carbohydrates. On average, the diet needs to be stuck to for at least 3 months, whereupon, if there is a clear improvement in symptoms, it should be possible to experiment gradually with the re-introduction of the forbidden foods. A recurrence of symptoms will indicate that the offending food must be eliminated for longer. (For further details see Yeast and Mould Free Diet in NUTRITIONAL SUPPLEMENTS AND SPECIAL DIETS section.)

Anti-candidal nutritional supplements

1 *Lactobacillus acidophilus* Culture of the bacteria normally found in the gut. It can be obtained as a powder, capsules or in live yoghurt, especially BA or Bio yoghurts. Conventional wisdom is that these supplements are a waste of time as they will be destroyed by the acid and other enzymes in the secretions of the gut, and would never reach the parts they are intended to. However, it may well be that in women with candida and other chronic illnesses, the acid and enzyme production is sufficiently impaired to allow a significant amount to get through and recolonize. It counters yeast growth by preventing mycelial extension, and is also capable of producing natural antibiotics which are effective against food-borne disease organisms.

2 *Olive oil* Two teaspoonsful 3 times a day helps to prevent mycelial extension.

3 *Biotin* One of the lesser-known B vitamins, this helps to prevent mycelial extension of fungi i.e., candida. It is found in meats, dairy products and whole grain cereals. It is possible to become deficient in biotin when on long-term antibiotics and by eating large amounts of raw egg, which contains a substance which counteracts biotin. (See also NUTRITIONAL SUPPLEMENTS section.)

4 *Garlic* Anti-bacterial and anti-fungal, due to its allicin content. Onions and cloves have similar properties. Garlic is best taken in the form of capsules.

5 *Caprylic acid* Coconut-derived fatty acid which has been found to help restore the normal balance of yeast to bacteria in the colon. It has strong anti-fungal effects and must be administered in a slow release form to have effect on the candida. It is sold under the brand name of Caprystatin. Clinical studies have shown the disappearance of candida from stool specimens within a few days. Caprystatin should be taken in increasing doses over several weeks, and then a maintenance dose taken for several months.

Immunity-enhancing nutritional supplements
see also NUTRITIONAL SUPPLEMENTS p. 252

1 Vitamin C 1–3 g a day.

2 Vitamin A best taken in the form of beta carotene 10,000 units a day.

3 Vitamin E 200–400 international units a day.

4 Vitamin B complex 1 capsule a day.

5 Calcium pantothenate (B_5) 500 mg a day (this is particularly advisable if allergic symptoms are present).

6 Folic acid 20–50 mcg a day (this is important for the correct differentiation of T-lymphocytes into suppressive and killer cells).

7 Selenium 100 mcg a day.

8 Zinc 20–25 mg a day (this should be taken at night).

9 Magnesium 250 mg a day.

10 Evening primrose oil 250 1–3 times a day (this is advisable since candida toxins can interfere with fatty acid production, in turn important for T-cell production).

N.B. All supplements must be labelled Yeast Free. As with all supplements, after one month leave them off at weekends unless advised not to by your homeopath or nutritionist.

Anti-candida drugs

1 *Nystatin* Doctor prescribable only. It is an anti-fungal antibiotic which kills or arrests the growth of a wide range of yeast and yeast-like fungi. It is lethal to yeast on contact, but yeast embedded in the gut wall might be relatively unaffected. Nystatin is available as a powder – which is probably the most effective – as tablets or drops for candida in the gut, or as a suspension for babies. It is also available as creams, ointments and powder for surface areas. Although virtually non-toxic, and cheap, some patients may become dependent on it and weaning can be difficult. It also tastes like potting compost! Along with other anti-candida drugs it can only deal with the short-term situation. The bowel must be adjusted by diet and lactobacilli, and the immune system must be strengthened. The average length of a course is 3 months. The maintenance dosage is ¼-½ teaspoonful 4 times a day but the dosage is fairly individual. It is not absorbed through the gut wall.

2 *Amphotericin (Fungilin)* Doctor prescribable only, this drug is more widely used in Europe than the UK. It acts in a similar way to Nystatin, but is absorbed and can be highly toxic, causing kidney damage. It should be used very selectively.

3 *Diflucan (Fluconazole)* Doctor prescribable only, this is a highly effective anti-fungal which is absorbed and can deal with candida anywhere in the body. As with all the other anti-candidal drugs, however, the candida will quickly come

back unless the bowel flora has been adjusted and the immune system strengthened. For this reason the authors do not recommend it except at the end of a course of more natural anti-candidal measures. It can be given in a single high dose or a lesser dose over a period of days. Fluconazole is a relatively new drug, but as a similar drug caused liver damage when given over a long period of time, fluconazole should also be used cautiously.

Anti-candida immunotherapy

If a candida-syndrome patient does not respond well to the measures above it may be advisable to attempt to influence the immune system's reactivity directly with regard to candida, particularly if there is an associated multiple allergy syndrome. This can be done in two ways.

1 *Neutralizing dose immunotherapy* A highly complex therapy, which takes advanced training and experience for success.

This treatment is not advised for the patient acutely overloaded with candida, and so would tend not to be used as a first-line treatment. In any case, for lasting symptom relief the diet and supplements are essential. Neither should it be used in the presence of auto-immune disorders such as rheumatoid arthritis because of the likelihood of aggravation.

2 *EPD (Enzyme Potentiated Desensitization)* An injected desensitization technique relatively lacking in side-effects, since it uses extremely small doses of allergens compared with traditional forms of skin testing and desensitization. Each injection must be associated with a strict low food allergen diet for 24 hours before and after. Allergy relief is likely to occur in 80 per cent of patients.

Self-help

Apart from the doctor-prescribed pessaries and creams such as Nystatin and Canesten there are various effective measures which may be applied. In the second half of the menstrual cycle – for instance, when candida is encouraged by hormonal changes – or in circumstances where repeated sexual intercourse may cause both candida and cystitis (see CYSTITIS), try the following measures:

1 Yoghurt douches: one pot natural live yoghurt to 1.75 litres (3 pints) boiled cooled water, douche 3 times a day or use acidophilus powder, ½ teaspoonful to 8 oz water.
2 Douches of vinegar or lemon juice.
3 Acigel, available in any chemist.
4 Extract of garlic douche using odourless form, i.e., kyolic.

5 Always remember to treat your partner as well. A man may carry thrush under the foreskin, as a result of transfer from a partner with vaginal thrush; he may be unaware of this and may also re-infect his partner. He may notice burning, itching, redness and irritation around the head of the penis shortly after intercourse, but it is generally self-limiting. It may represent a hypersensitivity reaction to candida toxin or antigen.

Detoxification

Many people suffering from this syndrome have poorly functioning organs of elimination. When cellular waste products accumulate in the bloodstream the individual feels ill in herself and cannot effectively absorb the nutrients provided by the candida control diet and nutrition supplements. The main detoxification organ is the liver. In addition to the usual metabolic waste, the liver also helps to remove from the body environmental pollutants and other toxins. Any toxins in the bowel may be removed using the colon cleansing regime (see COLON CLEANSING). Coffee enemas help to cleanse the colon, as coffee makes a good solvent for encrusted waste in the wall of the large bowel. They also seem to stimulate the functioning of the liver and gall bladder which helps to eliminate toxic wastes.

Orthodox Viewpoint

The concept of candida infection affecting other systems of the body apart from the bowel and vagina is a contentious one, and most orthodox doctors do not believe in its power to do so. This is understandable, as there is no reliable test for candida outside the vagina, mouth and possibly bowel. Indirect confirmation of the hypothesis, however, comes from work being done in infants. This shows that in the early days of life at least they have a leaky bowel, allowing larger fragments of protein than would normally be absorbed to get into the bloodstream and set up an antigen-antibody response. As you will have seen, it is thought that candida may work in a similar fashion. Certainly we have noted an improvement in patients who do follow an anti-candida regime where indicated.

Homeopathic treatment

Constitutional treatment is recommended.

Specific remedies to be taken in the 6c potency 6 times a day for up to 5 days.

Please remember to check your choice against the Remedy Pictures (p. 305) where possible.

Calcarea

Marked vaginal itching associated with cervical erosion; discharge is yellow, or milky, with itching of vagina before periods; thrush worse before and after periods; burning discharge with inflammation of the vulva – worse on becoming warm – worse during pregnancy; depression; anxiety; dizziness; chronic headache – worse before periods; burning pains; appetite increased; dull, aching pain in abdomen; frequent urination; itching worse after passing urine; heavy periods; chronic vaginitis; vaginal warts; swollen tender breasts pre-menstrually; backache; stiff neck; dry skin.

Generalities: Symptoms worse before periods; weakness; tendency to put on weight.

Sepia

Very offensive discharges with marked vaginal and vulval itching; soreness and burning in vagina; cervical erosion possible; ulcers on labia; vaginal discharge after sexual intercourse; very irritating, burning or smarting yellow discharge – worse before and after periods; vulval inflammation – worse for stress – worse during pregnancy; weepiness before periods; difficulty in concentrating; depression; chronic headache; anal fissure; distended abdomen; urgent need to urinate; chronic vaginitis; sharp, stinging pains in womb – worse in menopause; backache; itchy skin.

Generalities: Weariness – worse between 3–5 pm – worse on walking.

Sulphur

Very offensive discharge causing marked itching; vaginal soreness – worse for stress; itchiness in vulva; yellow or white discharge; itchy vagina before periods; vaginal discharge after periods; burning or stinging discharge; burning pain in vagina; pain in vagina during intercourse; pain and discharge worse in the week before the period; chronic headache – worse before periods; burning pains in eyes; appetite increased; irritable bowel syndrome; offensive wind; itching around the back passage; cramping pains in abdomen; pinching sensation around navel; frequent urination with urge to urinate; pain in urethra after urination; general thickening of skin of vulva from itching – worse in menopause; backache; pain in neck radiating to shoulder; swollen fingers; dry and itchy skin.

Generalities: Tendency to put on weight; thrush worse during convalescence from another acute illness; weariness.

Graphites

Vaginal soreness; thrush worse pre-menstrually; ulcers on the labia; very irritating discharge; itching in vagina pre-menstrually; vaginal discharge after periods; burning pain in vagina; chronic thickening of skin of vulva from scratching; difficulty with concentration; indecisiveness; depression; appetite increased; dull aching pain in abdomen; anal fissure; frequent urination; menopause; backache, especially in neck; swollen fingers; dry itchy skin.

Generalities: Tendency to put on weight; weariness – worse after periods.

Pulsatilla

Vaginal soreness associated with possible cervical erosion; very irritating burning discharge – worse in pregnancy; burning smarting pain in vagina; discharge after periods; watery, cloudy discharge – worse before and after periods – worse lying down; weepiness before periods; indecisiveness; dizziness; chronic headache – worse before periods; burning pains in eyes; appetite increased; bloated abdomen pre-menstrually; irritable bowel syndrome; offensive wind; frequent urination; urgent need to urinate; chronic cystitis; pain in urethra after urinating; heavy periods – worse at menopause; chronic vaginitis; tender breasts; backache; swollen fingers; itchy skin.

Generalities: Weariness.

Lycopodium

Thrush – worse for stress; very irritating vaginal discharge – worse after periods, with itching; chronic thickening of the skin of vulva from scratching; weepiness before and after periods; difficulty in concentrating; anxiety; dizziness; headaches pre-menstrually; appetite increased; bloated abdomen pre-menstrually; dull aching pain in abdomen; irritable bowel syndrome; itching around back passage; frequent urination; chronic cystitis; genital warts; backache; neck stiffness; swollen fingers; dry and itchy skin.

Generalities: Worse before periods; tendency to put on weight; weariness – worse before periods.

Carbo veg.

Very offensive itchy, greenish, burning discharge – worse from becoming hot, associated with possible cervical erosion, itching of vulva, with cracks; worse in pregnancy; discharge during and after periods; difficulty in concentrating; depression; anxiety; headache pre-menstrually; burning pains; dull, aching pain in abdomen; offensive wind; itchy skin.

Generalities: Weakness.

Mercurius
Very irritating, stringy offensive discharge with marked itching and burning soreness of vagina; possible cervical erosion – worse for stress; itching in vagina before periods; burning discharge; inflammation of vulva; chronic headache; dull aching pain in abdomen; frequent urination; chronic vaginitis; genital warts; tender breasts; swollen fingers; itchy skin.

Generalities: Weariness; chills alternating with sweats.

Natrum mur.
Marked vaginal itching – worse becoming warm – worse for stress; burning pain in vagina; vaginal pain during intercourse; weepiness before periods; dizziness; chronic headache – worse before periods; burning pains in eyes; increased appetite; irritable bowel syndrome; offensive wind; urgent need to urinate; backache; itchy skin.

Generalities: Weariness – worse before periods.

Nitric ac.
Very offensive irritating, stringy, greenish or pinkish discharge – worse after periods; marked vaginal itching, and burning soreness; possible cervical erosion, worse for stress; ulcers and cracks on labia; inflammation of vulva; chronic headache; irritable bowel syndrome; offensive wind; anal fissure; heavy periods; genital warts; neck stiffness; swollen fingers.

Arsenicum
Possible cervical erosion; ulcers on labia; very irritating offensive, yellow burning vaginal discharge; chronic thickening of skin of vulva due to scratching; depression; anxiety; chronic headaches; burning pains in eyes; increase in appetite; dull aching pains in abdomen; irritable bowel syndrome; offensive wind; pain in the neck; swollen fingers; dry and itchy skin.

Generalities: Weakness; tendency to put on weight.

Kreosotum
Very offensive itchy, milky or yellow, irritating discharge, smelly like rye bread; vaginal soreness and burning; possible cervical erosion – worse pre-menstrually, preceded by flushed face and pains in small of the back – worse after periods; pain in vagina during intercourse; inflamed vulva with chronic thickening of the skin due to scratching; headache pre-menstrually; bloated abdomen after periods; heavy periods; chronic vaginitis.

Generalities: Great weakness – worse after periods.

Lachesis
Burning discharge – worse during pregnancy; difficulty in concentrating; indecisiveness; depression; chronic headache – worse before periods; bloated abdomen pre-menstrually; irritable bowel syndrome; offensive wind; frequent urination; heavy periods – worse at menopause; neck stiffness.

Generalities: Weariness – symptoms worse before and after periods.

Nux
Very offensive discharge – worse on becoming warm – worse for stress – worse during pregnancy; difficulty in concentrating; dizziness; chronic headache; increased appetite; irritable bowel syndrome; itching around back passage; frequent urination; urgency of urination; pain in urethra after urination; heavy periods; backache; neck stiffness.

Generalities: Weariness – symptoms worse after periods.

Kali carb.
Vaginal soreness; itching in vagina worse before periods; pain in vagina during intercourse – worse becoming warm – worse for stress; depression and anxiety; burning pain in eyes; dull aching pain in abdomen; irritable bowel syndrome; urge to urinate; swollen breasts pre-menstrually; backache; neck stiffness; dry skin.

Generalities: Tendency to put on weight – worse before periods; weariness – worse in afternoon.

Other remedies to consider
- Frequent, copious, straw-coloured discharge which causes vulva to itch and smart and stiffens underwear, itchiness relieved by washing in cold water, discharge worse before and after period *Alumina 6c*
- Discharge transparent like egg white and highly irritant, scalded feeling on inside of thighs *Borax 6c*
- Yellowish, burning discharge *Carbo an. 6c*

Remedy Finder for Thrush

Possible cervical erosion
Apis
Arsenicum
Belladonna
Cantharis
Lac can.
Lachesis
Lycopodium
Pulsatilla
Sabina
Secale
Terebinth

With dryness of vagina
Aconite
Arsenicum
Belladonna
Berberis
Ferrum

Graphites
Lycopodium
Natrum mur.
Sepia

Intense itching in vagina
Caladium
Kreosotum
Lilium

Creamy vaginal discharge
Calcarea phos.
Natrum phos.
Pulsatilla
Secale

Burning pains in vagina
Belladonna
Berberis
Calcarea phos.

Cantharis
Chamomilla
Chelidonium
Graphites
Kali bichrom.
Kreosotum
Mercurius
Natrum mur.
Nitric ac.
Petroleum
Pulsatilla
Sulphur
Thuja

Burning pain in vagina during intercourse
Kreosotum
Lycopodium
Sulphur

Cystitis

Cystitis principally affects women because the female urethra is short and easily invaded by bacteria and other microbes present in the vagina, bowel and vulva area (in men cystitis is usually associated with PROSTATE PROBLEMS, bladder tumours, or congenital abnormality of the bladder and urethra).

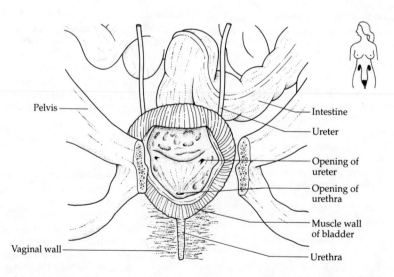

Pelvis

Intestine

Ureter

Opening of ureter

Opening of urethra

Muscle wall of bladder

Vaginal wall

Urethra

The anatomy of the bladder

The location of the urethra

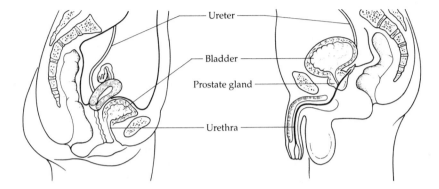

An attack of acute cystitis is so painful that the woman can be quite incapacitated, with all the inconvenience this causes. Repeated attacks are also likely to make the sufferer less than enthusiastic about sex – especially if this is a trigger – which can result in considerable strain on a relationship.

The term cystitis is often used rather loosely to describe 3 different conditions that have similar symptoms. These symptoms are a frequent urge to urinate, urine which smells strongly, stings or scalds as it is passed and may have blood in it, sometimes accompanied by a dull ache in the lower abdomen.

1 Cystitis proper is inflammation of the bladder due to infections, usually by E. coli bacteria transferred from the bowel.

2 Urethral syndrome is chronic irritation of the bladder and urethra usually from causes other than infection. Antibiotics, certain contraceptives, hormone imbalances caused by STRESS or fear, poor diet, food allergy, poor hygiene, clothing, urination patterns, intercourse and bruising of the urethra during intercourse have all been cited as possible causes.

3 Urethritis is inflammation of the urethra, occasionally due to infection, particularly by chlamydia and possibly also candida (see THRUSH and non-specific urethritis in SEXUALLY TRANSMITTED DISEASES). It is more often due to bruising during intercourse, lasting for 2–3 days at most, and is common in women who have just started having intercourse. Infective cystitis is distinguished from the other two by its severity and the presence of infection in a sample of urine. Some dipsticks can now predict urine infections quite accurately.

A Gallup poll was conducted in 1986 to find out women's awareness of urinary tract infection. It revealed the following:

1 50 per cent of adult women have had a urinary tract infection.

2 A large number of women do not know what causes urinary tract infections or what the symptoms are. The survey also showed that a large proportion of women still need educating about self-help measures.

3 Some 10 per cent of women experienced side-effects, most commonly nausea or rashes from the antibiotics given for urinary tract infections.

Patterns of infection

There are 3 common patterns of infection:

1 Isolated episodes which clear spontaneously or rapidly on treatment.

2 Relapsing urinary tract infection, where the treatment results in disappearance of symptoms and an apparent cure. However, not all the bacteria in the bladder are eliminated, and infection is likely to recur in a few days as the remaining bacteria multiply. This may happen if antibiotic courses are cut short.

3 True re-infection, which happens in approximately 80 per cent of women who develop cystitis frequently. The bacteria responsible are eliminated, but as a result of a susceptible urinary tract, re-infection by the same or a different organism can still occur weeks or months later.

Such recurrent urinary tract infections can be a significant problem for some women, and they should be investigated. Approximately 55 per cent of infections will involve the upper urinary tract, including the kidneys, with a possibility of renal failure. Failure of a correctly selected antibiotic to treat the infection may be due to bacterial resistance or to not taking the antibiotic properly.

Complications of cystitis may include the following:

1 Cystitis cystica, characterized by small, bacteria-filled cysts or swellings in the bladder lining. The symptoms are those of simple cystitis and can recur over months or years.

2 Acute pyelonephritis, an acute infection of both kidneys, symptoms of which may include chills accompanied by high fever, pain in lower back radiating to the groin, with nausea and shaking.

3 Chronic pyelonephritis. If the urinary tract infections continue for a number of years, kidney damage may result. This is rare nowadays, but if untreated can result in renal failure. Also, infections of the kidneys over a long time interfere with the manufacture and release of particular substances in the kidney which maintain normal blood pressure. This can lead to salt and water retention, with an increase in the volume of the blood and raised blood pressure. In pregnancy hormone changes can cause a general relaxation in muscle tone in the urinary tract, resulting in the retention of urine in the bladder or urethra. If this leads to a urinary tract infection it can cause an increased risk of premature labour.

Predisposing factors

The most commonly offending organism in about 85 per cent of cases is E. coli, a normally harmless inhabitant of the bowel. When E. coli gains access to the bladder it begins to act as a hostile organism. Under normal conditions the immune system responds by employing white cells (lymphocytes) to destroy the invaders. Some women, however, appear to have a particularly hospitable urinary tract lining, allowing the bacteria to adhere and multiply. This may be associated with a deficiency of glycosaminoglycan (GAG). Protection must involve a free flow of large quantities of urine, avoidance of retention of urine, complete emptying of the bladder, and optimum immune function.

The E. coli bacteria can come from the anal or vulval area due to faulty hygiene, particularly wiping back to front after passing a stool.

The main danger time after sexual intercourse is generally 36 hours. If sex is the predisposing factor drink plenty of fluids during this time, and add 1 teaspoon bicarbonate to the occasional drink. Cystitis may be triggered by sexual intercourse or masturbation due to pressure on the urethra, which pushes the bacteria into the bladder. In addition, contraceptive diaphragms may cause pressure on the bladder. Although a snug-fitting cap acts efficiently as a contraceptive barrier it may also tend to diminish the flow of urine from the bladder. In addition it can affect the bacterial balance in the vagina; one study showed an increased count of E. coli colonies in diaphragm users. If a diaphragm is the problem, check with your doctor to see if the next size smaller is possible.

Tight-fitting clothing, e.g., body suits, tight jeans, etc., provide a warm, moist, hospitable environment for E. coli and candida. After swimming, change out of your swimsuit as soon as possible, pass urine and wash off salt or chlorine.

Finally, 50 per cent of hospital-acquired infections are urinary tract infections due to catheterization (where a small tube is passed through the urethra into the bladder to drain it because the patient is incapable of draining it herself, or is incontinent).

Other predisposing factors

The presence of vaginal candidiasis (see THRUSH) provides a good breeding ground for E. coli, and depletes the natural vaginal secretions. This is encouraged by antibiotics, therefore potentially prolonging or causing recurrence of cystitis. Always take acidophilus after antibiotics (see PRO-BIOTICS p. 260).

Uncircumcised male partners may find it difficult to clean under the foreskin, which can harbour a range of bacteria which are then introduced into the vagina and urethra on intercourse. Vaginal dryness can also lead to possible bruising and cracking of the vaginal lining, allowing bacteria to breed more quickly – KY jelly may help this. Having intercourse with a full bladder or bowel can also lead to increased vaginal trauma, as can certain coital positions e.g., missionary position and hand petting.

Causes in the urinary tract itself include congenital deformities, especially reflux up the ureter due to a faulty valve in the upper-bladder opening, which allows urine to be retained in the ureter, leading to kidney infection and damage.

Metabolic causes include diabetes, in which there is excess sugar in the blood stream, and consequently in the urine, providing ready sustenance for E. coli and candida. Kidney stones result in restricted urine flow and tendency to infection. Diverticulae, or pouches in the bladder lining, can allow stagnation of small amounts of urine, leading to infection. Stress can also create problems by causing the ovaries to malfunction, which then affects vaginal secretions. These secretions can either be too little or too much, either of which can lead to increased tendency to harbour infection. Finally, iron deficiency anaemia due to persistent heavy periods leads to deficiency in resistance to infection.

Symptoms

1 A constant desire to urinate.
2 A feeling of trying to force urine out of urethra with a drawing sensation.
3 Incomplete emptying or poor stream sensation, just passing a trickle of urine.
4 Pain or burning sensation in urethra during urination.
5 Desire to pass urine at night.
6 Cloudy urine which can be reddish due to presence of blood, or actual blood stains.
7 Fever, nausea and vomiting.

Similar conditions

These include: ENDOMETRIOSIS, where implants of uterine wall may be found in the bladder, leading to irritation and infection; urge or STRESS INCONTINENCE due to weakening of the muscles following childbirth (here the symptoms would frequently be apparent following the menopause, when changes in hormone levels affect tissue tone); overflow incontinence when there is leaking of small amounts of urine because the bladder is too full (this can occur transiently when the bladder is over-distended after surgery or childbirth, or during a first attack of herpes, which can affect the bladder's nerve supply).

Cystitis can also occur secondary to more permanent damage as in multiple sclerosis, after spinal cord injuries or as a complication of diabetes, etc. Incontinence can be a feature of cystitis if left largely untreated after recurrent episodes. This is due to persistent irritation of the urethra lining and bladder outlet valve by urine rendered acidic by infection.

N.B. Women with incontinence for the first time should be investigated for urinary tract infection; if infection or prolapse is absent then further investigation is necessary. Various SEXUALLY TRANSMITTED DISEASES (p. 109), including gonorrhea and genital herpes (see relevant section), also resemble cystitis.

FIBROIDS, depending on their size and position, may sometimes cause bladder pressure sufficient to trigger cystitis-like symptoms. Vulvo-vaginal candida can often predispose to and co-exist with cystitis. In some women, thrush may only exist in the urethra or bladder, but not the vagina or bowel. This needs to be treated with the appropriate sugar- and mould-free diet and homeopathy. If severe, it may need drug treatment e.g., Diflucan (see THRUSH). Itching and burning of the vulva and vaginal discharge may be associated with burning on urination.

Self-help There is a lot you can do for yourself in an acute attack of cystitis. To reduce acidity of urine – responsible for the stinging and scalding – and to flush infected urine out of the bladder as quickly as possible, drink 0.25 litre (½ pint) cold water, barley water, or water with bicarbonate of soda in it every 20 minutes. Don't overdo the bicarbonate – 1 teaspoon per hour for up to 3 hours only is the maximum you should take; if you have a heart condition, stick to plain water or barley water. Curling up with a hot water bottle or ice pack clasped to the lower abdomen also offers relief.

There are also a number of preventive measures you can take, whether you suffer from cystitis, urethral syndrome, or urethritis.

Urinary habits Never suppress the urge to urinate; try to develop the habit of emptying the bladder every 4 hours, and do it twice each time to make sure the bladder is completely empty.

Fluid intake and diet Increase fluid intake to 3 litres (5 pints) per day, or until urine is a normal colour. Tea, coffee, and alcohol are not a good idea, except perhaps twice a week. The more alkaline your urine the better; a daily bowl of vegetable broth, or a teaspoon of bicarbonate of soda taken in water twice a day, or a daily glass of Effercitrate, obtainable from the chemist, will achieve this. Alkaline urine turns pink litmus paper blue, so buy some litmus from the chemist and test it. If thrush in the urethra or bladder is the problem, do not alkalinize your diet too much, as this will encourage growth.

Foods Known to aggravate cystitis and related conditions are asparagus, spinach, raw carrots, potatoes, tomatoes, citrus fruits and strawberries, red meat, milk and ice cream, grapes (especially red or grape juice), condiments, junk food in general, chlorinated water. Alcohol, which is acidic and dehydrates, should be avoided, especially red wine. Long drinks such as beer are less problematic than shorts unless there is thrush in the urethra, in which case avoid both. Liqueurs and hard spirits should be avoided. If wine or champagne prove irresistible, drink water or squash before and after, or dilute the drink with mineral water. Aduki beans are said to be beneficial, and cranberry juice is found to be effective in diminishing the ability of the bacteria to adhere to the bladder lining. Most of the cranberry juice on the market contains excessive sugar, so try to find one that doesn't. Sugar and caffeine should be avoided wherever possible.

Hygiene In her invaluable book on cystitis (see Books for Further Reading, p. 341), Angela Kilmartin recommends the following cleansing routine after every bowel movement:

1 Wipe bottom from front to back with soft white toilet paper.
2 Wash hands.
3 Soap hands with non-perfumed soap and wash anal area (not vaginal area) with fingers.
4 Rinse hands.
5 Fill a small bottle with warm water, sit back on lavatory, and pour water down past urethral opening and vagina, using free hand to wash out nooks and crannies.
6 When all traces of soap have been washed away, pat dry with a soft towel kept only for that purpose.

This method uses only hands, unscented soap, and the flow of clean warm water to clean anal and vulval area; using flannels, cloths, or cotton wool is not recommended – they only harbour germs. Nor are bidets or squatting in the bath and douching with the shower – that way germs may spread or be forced up the urethra. Nor are vaginal deodorants, vaginal douches, medicated creams, bath oils, bath salts, bubble baths, talcum powder, or antiseptics like Dettol – all of which can irritate the skin. If possible, tampons should be avoided too.

Sexual intercourse If possible have a drink of water and empty the bladder before intercourse. Be as relaxed as possible and spin out time spent in foreplay. Use KY jelly as a lubricant, and don't be afraid to experiment with different positions to see if these relieve pressure on bladder or urethra. After intercourse, empty bladder and wash away semen using the bottle-of-warm-water technique described above. The man should wash his hands and penis before intercourse. Since long fingernails harbour germs, both partners should keep nails short.

Clothing Swap nylon underwear for cotton, and nylon tights for those with a cotton gusset, and change them every day. Wash them in pure soap – never with biological washing powders or bleach – and rinse thoroughly.

Other preventives include garlic, which has anti-microbial activity against many disease organisms, including those associated with urinary tract infections, including E. coli, proteus, klebsiella, etc. Golden seal (Hydrastis) is one of the most effective of the herbal anti-microbials, and has long been used by herbalists in infections. It should be taken in a tincture of 1 : 5 dilution, 1 teaspoonful 3 times daily, and works best in an alkaline urine. Also Uva ursi when available as a herbal tincture, or the herb itself. Herbal preparations containing acacia gum, e.g., colonite, can be extremely effective.

Immune enhancement May be helped by taking buffered vitamin C, but avoid sustained high doses of a gram or more for long periods of time as this may lead to kidney stones. (Also be aware of vitamin B high potency complexes which can irritate the bladder if taken without sufficient water.) Vitamin A and zinc may be of benefit (see NUTRITIONAL SUPPLEMENTS).

Yoga If the infection spreads up to the kidneys in addition to other treatments, try this yoga technique. Sit with your back against the wall, bring your feet together in front of you, and now try and get both feet back as close into the crotch as possible. This will help relieve the pain.

Homeopathic treatment

The homeopathic approach to recurrent attacks is constitutional, although the remedies given below will relieve symptoms in an isolated flare up.

Please remember to check your choice against the Remedy Pictures (p. 305) where possible.

Specific remedies to be taken every ½ hour for up to 10 doses in the 30c potency.

Pulsatilla
Acute or chronic cystitis; frequent urination; burning or aching pain in bladder – worse while urinating, on walking, after exposure to cold conditions; chills after urinating; stricture; pain; constant pain in urethra – worse after urinating; dull aching in lower abdomen caused by delay in passing water; vaginal discharge, either non-irritating white copious vaginal discharge or thrush.

Generalities: Symptoms worse before periods; fluid retention; joint pains.

Sulphur
Acute or chronic cystitis – worse in diabetics; leaking of urine if passing of urine is delayed; frequent urination; urge to urinate at night; pain in bladder from getting cold; chills after urination; constant pain in urethra – worse after urination; bloated abdomen; copious bland vaginal discharge; thrush; worse for stress.

Generalities: Symptoms worse before period.

Sepia
Acute or chronic cystitis; urine leaks if urination delayed; aching, burning, or shooting pain in bladder – worse in evening – worse after urination; chills after urinating; cystitis worse in pregnancy; pain in urethra after urinating;

sensation of few drops of urine having been passed; aching dull pain in lower abdomen if urination is delayed; copious white vaginal discharge, thrush; worse for stress.

Generalities: Symptoms worse before periods.

Calcarea

Frequent urination; acute cystitis; pain in bladder during urination – worse in diabetics; chills after urinating; bloated abdomen; copious white vaginal discharge; thrush; feeling anxious.

Generalities: Weakness – worse before periods.

Lycopodium

Chronic cystitis – worse in diabetics; frequent cystitis; burning pain in bladder after urination; urge to urinate at night; bladder feels as if it does not empty properly; constant pain in urethra; feels anxious – worse for stress; bloated abdomen; ovarian cysts.

Generalities: Symptoms worse before periods.

Arsenicum

Acute or chronic cystitis – worse in diabetics; burning pains in bladder; bladder feels as if not emptying properly; feeling anxious; restless; bloated abdomen; copious white vaginal discharge; thrush.

Generalities: Weakness; fluid retention; chilly.

Nux

Pain in bladder before urinating; frequent and painful urging with little result; aching bladder; acute cystitis; bladder feels as if it does not empty properly; cystitis worse in pregnancy; pain in urethra after urination; symptoms worse for stress; bloated abdomen; white vaginal discharge.

Generalities: Fluid retention; joint pains.

Mercurius

Frequent urination; acute cystitis; symptoms worse for stress; bloated abdomen; copious bland white vaginal discharge; thrush.

Generalities: Fluid retention.

Causticum

Frequent urge to urinate – worse for coughing and sneezing; acute cystitis; cystitis worse for getting cold; bladder feels as if it is not emptying properly, but obeying urge rewarded after 15 minutes by involuntary passage of urine; pain after urinating; itching around opening of urethra; cystitis worse in pregnancy; feeling anxious; copious vaginal discharge; thrush.

Generalities: Weakness.

Belladonna

Acute cystitis; bladder feels as if it does not empty properly; cystitis worse in pregnancy; bladder sensitive to jarring; urine bright red and with little clots of blood; burning sensation in urethra; feeling anxious; white vaginal discharge.

Generalities: Fluid retention.

Conium

Acute cystitis; pain in bladder on walking; bladder feels as if it is not emptying properly; symptoms worse for stress, feeling anxious; copious white vaginal discharge.

Generalities: Weakness.

Cantharis

Acute or chronic cystitis; frequent urination; burning cutting pain in bladder with non-stop urgent need to urinate; bladder does not empty properly; pain too severe to ignore; ache in small of back – worse in afternoon; merest trickle of urine with blood in it; stricture of urethra; constant pain in urethra – worse after urination.

Apis

Acute cystitis; frequent urination; burning, sharp, stinging pain in bladder – worse after urination; frequent urgency to urinate; urine scant, hot and bloody; bloated abdomen; copious white vaginal discharge; thrush.

Generalities: Symptoms worse for heat – better for cold.

Other remedies to consider

- Attack comes on after getting damp and cold after exertion, especially in autumn, urine bloody and frequent *Dulcamara 6c*
- Pains come on as urination ceases, urine thick and milky-looking, urgency and pressure to pass urine, feeling thirsty *Sarsaparilla 6c*
- Frequency and burning sensation as urine is passed, with pain in small of back, blood in urine, drowsiness, tingling in ears, tongue red and shiny, rest makes symptoms worse but walking in open air alleviates them *Terebinth 6c*
- Attack comes on after sexual intercourse or after catheterization for an operation, urethra feels as if a drop of urine is continuously trickling along it, burning sensation almost constant, even when not passing water *Staphisagria 6c*
- Stream of urine slow and intermittent *Clematis 6c*
- Pain worse at start of urination, no urine passed despite intense and urgent straining,

muscles at base of bladder in spasm, cold makes symptoms worse *Camphora 6c*
- High fever, excruciating pain in bladder area, bladder swollen and hard, feeling extremely restless, great sense of hurry *Tarentula 6c*
- Urine slimy, with fine mucus in it, burning, radiating pains which get worse during and after passing urine, and during rest *Berberis 6c*

Remedy Finder for Cystitis

Chronic cystitis
Arsenicum
Benzoic ac.
Cannabis sat.
Cantharis
Dulcamara
Eupatorium
Hydrastis
Kali mur.
Mercurius corr.
Pulsatilla
Sabal
Sepia
Sulphur
Terebinth
Tuberculinum

Pressing pain in bladder
Lycopodium

Mucous discharge
Benzoic ac.
Colocynth
Dulcamara
Lycopodium
Nux
Pulsatilla
Sulphur

Acute cystitis
Aconite
Apis
Belladonna
Cantharis
Equisetum
Lachesis
Lycopodium
Pulsatilla
Sarsaparilla
Sepia
Terebinth

Tenesmus (painful straining)
Arsenicum
Cantharis
Digitalis
Lilium
Mercurius
Nux
Pareira
Plumbum
Prunus

Pulsatilla
Terebinth
Thuja

Urgent need to urinate
Apis
Argentum nit.
Belladonna
Berberis
Bryonia
Camphor
Cannabis ind.
Cannabis sat.
Cantharis
Causticum
Chimaphila
Kali carb.
Lilium
Mercurius corr.
Natrum mur.
Nux
Phosphoric ac.
Pulsatilla
Sabina
Sarsaparilla
Sepia
Staphisagria
Thuja

Frequent urination
Ammonium carb.
Apis
Argentum
Argentum nit.
Baryta
Calcarea
Calcarea ars.
Cantharis
Castoreum
Causticum
Euphrasia
Gelsemium
Graphites
Ignatia
Lachesis
Lactic ac.
Lycopodium
Mercurius
Mercurius corr.
Nux
Pulsatilla

Staphisagria
Sulphur

Pain in bladder if desire to pass urine postponed
Lactic ac.
Pulsatilla
Sulphuric ac.

Painful urge to urinate
Nux
Phytolacca

Pain in bladder before urinating
Fluoric ac.
Lilium
Nux
Phytolacca

Pain at beginning of urination
Cantharis
Clematis
Mercurius

Pain in bladder during urination
Phytolacca
Pulsatilla

Pain in bladder better as soon as she starts to pass water
Prunus

Pain in bladder as soon as few drops of urine pass
Cantharis
Causticum

Pain in bladder extending up to kidneys
Aesculus
Cantharis

Pain in bladder extending to thighs
Pulsatilla

Pain in neck of bladder
Belladonna
Berberis
Calcarea phos.
Cannabis sat.
Cantharis
Ferrum phos.

Nux
Zinc

when attempting to urinate
Copaiva

at beginning of urination
Clematis

at close of urination
Cannabis sat.
Pulsatilla
Sarsaparilla

with urge to urinate
Calcarea phos.

before urinating
Lilium
Nux

after urinating
Apis
Pulsatilla

while walking
Ignatia

Aching pain in bladder before urinating
Fluoric ac.
Nux

after urinating
Cantharis
Fluoric ac.

Burning pain in bladder before urinating
Apis
Berberis
Cantharis
Capsicum
Fluoric ac.

during urination
Cantharis
Terebinth

after urination
Berberis
Fluoric ac.
Lycopodium

Burning in bladder better for walking in open air
Terebinth

Burning in neck of bladder
Berberis
Cantharis
Chamomilla
Nux
Prunus
Pulsatilla

Staphisagria

during urinating
Cantharis
Nux

after urinating
Apis
Pulsatilla
Sarsaparilla

extending through to urethra
Cantharis

Constriction pain in bladder neck
Lycopodium
Mezereum

Constricting pain generally
Berberis
Ledum
Mezereum
Sarsaparilla

Cutting pains in bladder
Terebinth

Cutting pain in bladder neck which may extend to urethra
Cantharis

Dragging pain in bladder
Cantharis
Chelidonium
Lycopodium

Pinching pain
Berberis

Pressure in bladder
Aconite
Apis
Lilium
Nux
Sepia

Pressing pain in bladder before urinating
China
Kali sulph.
Nux
Pulsatilla
Sepia

during urinating
Camphor
Chimaphila
Hepar sulph.
Lachesis
Natrum mur.
Nux
Silicea

after urinating
Calcarea phos.
Camphor
Digitalis
Equisetum

Pressing pain in neck of bladder
Cantharis
Nux

Pressing pain in neck of bladder before urinating
Nux
Phytolacca
Pulsatilla

Smarting in neck of bladder
Cantharis

extending to the meatus
Chimaphila

Tender bladder
Cantharis
Equisetum
Terebinth

Tenderness in neck of bladder
Calcarea phos.
Carbo veg.
Nux
Pulsatilla

Tenderness in neck of bladder after urinating
Calcarea phos.

Spasmodic pain in neck of bladder
Berberis
Cantharis
Caulophyllum
Chelidonium

Stabbing pains in bladder
Chelidonium

Stinging in bladder
Berberis
Chelidonium
Clematis
Conium
Kali carb.
Lilium
Lycopodium
Natrum mur.
Sulphur

Stinging pains in bladder with ineffectual urging
Guaiacum

before urinating
Lilium
Mancinella

on beginning to urinate
Mancinella

during urinating
Natrum mur.

Stinging in neck of bladder
Belladonna
Calcarea phos.
Cantharis
Carbon sulph.
Chamomilla
Guaiacum
Lilium
Lycopodium
Opium
Pulsatilla
Thuja

**Stinging in neck of bladder
   before urinating**
Cantharis

   when not urinating
   Chamomilla

Cramping pains in kidney
Causticum
Chelidonium
Nitric ac.

**Pains in ureters
   right-sided**
   Lycopodium
   Nux
   Sarsaparilla

   left-sided
   Berberis
   Lycopodium
   Pareira

**Pain starting in kidney going
   down to bladder**
Berberis

Blood in urine
Apis
Argentum nit.
Arnica
Arsenicum
Bothrops
Cactus
Calcarea
Cannabis sat.
Cantharis
Coccus
Crotalus
Hamamelis
Ipecac.
Mercurius corr.
Millefolium
Phosphorus
Pulsatilla
Secale
Squilla
Terebinth

Offensive smelling urine
Apis
Arnica
Baptisia
Benzoic ac.
Calcarea
Carbo veg.
Dulcamara
Nitric ac.
Sepia
Sulphur
Viola

Urine smelling of ammonia
Iodum
Moschus

Putrid smelling urine
Calcarea

Scanty urine
Arsenicum
Cantharis
Carbon sulph.
Causticum
Conium

Digitalis
Equisetum
Graphites
Gratiola
Kali nit.
Lac can.
Lactic ac.
Lilium
Mercurius
Mercurius corr.
Mercurius dulc.
Natrum sulph.
Nitric ac.
Nux
Opium
Plumbum
Ruta
Sarsaparilla
Selenium
Sepia
Staphisagria
Sulphur
Terebinth

Bloody sediment
Cantharis
Chimaphila
Phosphoric ac.
Pulsatilla
Sepia

Mucous sediment
Benzoic ac.
Berberis
Chimaphila
Equisetum
Mercurius corr.
Natrum mur.
Pareira
Pulsatilla
Sarsaparilla
Sepia

Pus sediment
Arnica
Cantharis
Clematis
Uva ursi

Note: **Any pain in the kidneys or ureters, or blood in the urine,
should be reported to your GP 12 .**

Menstrual Problems

Endometriosis

This is a condition in which fragments of the lining of the uterus (endometrium) are found in abnormal sites such as the pelvic peritoneum, the ovaries, the bladder or the bowel. As they are still under the influence of progesterone and oestrogen they engorge with blood every month, irritating and scarring the surrounding tissues. The condition is most common in childless women between the ages of 30–40. It is rarely seen in girls under 20, but if it is found in adolescents it is then accompanied by severely PAINFUL PERIODS. The cause is not known, although oestrogens are certainly involved; selenium deficiency and the use of tampons have also been suggested.

Symptoms

HEAVY PERIODS, dragging period pains which tend to get worse towards the end of the period, INFERTILITY and perhaps PAINFUL INTERCOURSE. Between 15 and 30 per cent of infertile women have endometriosis. Of those women already suffering from endometriosis, up to 40 per cent may be infertile.

Other symptoms reported in our survey included: burning pain in bladder on urinating, irritability and weepiness before periods, breast swelling before periods, backache before periods, apathy, calf cramps, DEPRESSION, nausea before periods, swollen fingers, dizziness, pain in shoulders, URTICARIA, weight gain (see WEIGHT PROBLEMS) and fluid retention (see OEDEMA). Sometimes endometriosis does not cause any symptoms.

Diagnosis

Endometriosis is diagnosed during laparoscopy, when a small telescope is passed into the abdomen, through a tiny cut in the navel, allowing the small particles of tissue to be seen.

Treatment

Orthodox treatment may include the use of the oral contraceptive pill, or of danazol, which inhibits ovulation and gives the body time to re-absorb the dispersed fragments of the endometrium. The particles can also be burnt out with a laser or removed surgically. Hysterectomy may be advised if severe pain has been experienced, if the ovaries are scarred and the woman does not want any more children.

Self-help

If you have a craving for sweet foods and refined carbohydrates read HYPOGLYCAEMIA, and if relevant try the BLOOD SUGAR LEVELLING DIET for one month. Also take OPTIVITE 2 tablets 3 times a day.

Homeopathic treatment

Constitutional treatment is recommended. In the meantime take the following remedies for pain.

Specific remedies to be taken in the 30c potency for up to 10 doses.

Please remember to check your choice against the Remedy Pictures (p. 305) where possible.

Pulsatilla
Pain in womb during periods; cramping pains in abdomen before and during periods; dull aching in abdomen before periods; dragging pain in abdomen; irritable and weepy before periods; indifferent; depressed; dizziness before and after periods; nausea before periods; may vomit with pain; bloated abdomen before periods; heavy periods; swollen breasts; backache before periods.

Generalities: Weight gain.

Calcarea
Dull aching pain in left groin; pain in womb during periods; dull aching pain in iliac region; burning pain in abdomen; dull aching pain in abdomen before periods, and at the beginning of periods; indifference, depression; heavy periods; painful swollen breasts at all times – worse before periods; backache before periods; urticaria.

Generalities: Weight gain.

Lachesis
Pain in left ovary – worse before periods; cramping or cutting lower abdominal pain before periods; depression; dizziness before periods; bloated abdomen before periods; heavy periods; swollen breasts; backache before periods.

Belladonna

Pain in coccyx during periods; pain in uterus during periods; cramping abdominal pains before and during periods; pain in ovaries before periods; shooting pain in lower abdomen; pain in womb – worse for motion; aching dragging pain – worse for lying down; bright red flow; heavy periods; heavy swollen breasts; skin hot and flushed.

Generalities: Fluid retention; weight gain.

Kali carb.

Pain in coccyx during periods; cramping abdominal pain before and during periods; shooting or dull aching pain in lower abdomen before or at the beginning of periods; pain at beginning of periods; bloated abdomen before periods; swollen painful breasts pre-menstrually; backache before periods.

Generalities: Fluid retention; weight gain.

Lycopodium

Shooting pain in iliac region; pain in lower abdomen before periods; irritable and weepy before periods; depression; nausea before periods; bloated abdomen before periods; burning on urinating; backache before periods; swelling of the fingers.

Generalities: Weight gain.

Phosphorus

Pain in left ovary; dull aching pain in iliac region; burning pain in abdomen; pain in lower abdomen before periods; weepy before periods; indifference; dizziness before periods; burning pain in bladder on urinating; heavy periods; painful swollen breasts; cramps in calves before periods; swelling of fingers.

Generalities: Weight gain.

Sepia

Dull aching pain in left groin extending to the back; pain in womb during periods; cramping pain in abdomen during periods; pain in vagina with intercourse; cramping abdominal pain before periods; burning pain in abdomen; pain in lower abdomen before periods; dragging pain in abdomen; irritability before periods; indifference; depression; pain in vagina on intercourse.

Generalities: Fluid retention.

Sulphur

Dull aching pain in left groin extending to the back; cramping pain during periods; pain in lower abdomen before periods; dragging abdominal pain; depression; pain in vagina on intercourse; painful swollen breasts; swollen fingers; urticaria.

Generalities: Weight gain.

Platina

Pain in left ovary; cramping pain in abdomen before and during periods; dull aching pain in iliac region; indifference; depression; heavy periods; pain in vagina on intercourse; pain in ovaries and womb after intercourse.

Generalities: Fluid retention.

Nux

Pain in womb during periods; cramping abdominal pain during periods; burning abdominal pain; stitching pain in lower abdomen; dragging pains; periods arrive early, prolonged; irritability before periods; indifference; burning pains on urinating; heavy periods; painful breasts pre-menstrually; backache pre-menstrually.

Generalities: Chilliness; exhaustion.

Causticum

Pain in coccyx during periods; cramping abdominal pain before and during periods; dull aching pain in left iliac region; dull aching abdominal pain – worse lying on right side – before periods, at beginning of periods and after intercourse; burning abdominal pain; shooting pains in lower abdomen; irritable before periods; depression; backache before periods; urticaria.

Generalities: Weight gain.

Chamomilla

Severe cramping abdominal pains before and during periods; shooting pains in iliac region; cutting pains in abdomen before periods; dull aching abdominal pain before periods; irritability before periods; depression; anger with periods; restlessness; burning pain on urinating; painful swollen breasts.

Conium

Cramping abdominal pain during periods; burning abdominal pain; shooting pains in left iliac region – worse during periods; pain in womb – worse for motion; indifference; dizziness before and after periods; swollen, painful breasts generally – worse before periods.

Mercurius

Pain in coccyx during periods; pain in left ovary; shooting pains in iliac region; dull aching abdominal pain – worse for lying on right side; pain in lower abdomen before periods; depression; painful swollen breasts; swollen fingers.

For further remedies see PAINFUL PERIODS.

Remedy Finder for Endometriosis

(See also remedies in 'Painful Periods', p. 101)

Abdominal pain before periods
Lachesis
Lycopodium
Natrum mur.
Sepia
Sulphur

during periods
Calcarea
Pulsatilla
Sepia
Sulphur

Pain in coccyx during periods
Causticum
Cicuta
Cistus

Pain in ovaries after intercourse
Apis
Platina
Staphisagria

before periods
Apis
Belladonna
Colocynth
Lachesis
Zinc

during periods
Apis
Belladonna
Lachesis

Palladium
Phosphorus
Platina
Thuja

Pain in womb during intercourse
Ferrum phos.
Hepar sulph.

extending to lower back
Calcarea phos.

Pain in vagina during intercourse
Argentum nit.
Natrum mur.
Sepia

Infertility
Aurum
Borax
Natrum carb.
Natrum mur.
Sepia

Spasm of vagina (vaginismus)
Plumbum

Constipation before periods
Graphites
Kali carb.
Lachesis
Silicea

Constipation during periods
Ammonium carb.
Apis

Aurum
Graphites
Kali carb.
Natrum mur.
Natrum sulph.
Nux
Platina
Sepia
Silicea

Pain in back passage before periods
Ignatia
Petroleum

during periods
Aloe

Pain in back passage during passing of stool
Aloe
Ignatia
Mercurius
Muriatic ac.
Nitric ac.
Sulphur

after passing stool
Arsenicum
Calcarea
Colchicum
Collinsonia
Graphites
Lycopodium
Nitric ac.
Podophyllum
Silicea
Sulphur

Heavy periods (menorrhagia)

Defined as profuse bleeding ('flooding'), which quickly leaks through sanitary protection; discharge of large clots of blood, or bleeding which continues for more than 7 days. The average amount of blood loss during a normal period is less than 60 ml. A woman with menorrhagia may lose more than 90 ml. It may be caused by HORMONE IMBALANCE, FIBROIDS or ENDOMETRIOSIS and PELVIC INFECTION. In a minority of women IUDs increase monthly flow. Consistently heavy periods can lead to iron deficiency ANAEMIA. If periods are getting heavier and heavier see your GP. If you may be pregnant and your period is heavier than usual, you may have had a MIS-CARRIAGE; appropriate action is 12. If associated with pain in the lower abdomen, it may be an ECTOPIC PREGNANCY ②.

Heavy periods caused by hormone imbalance are conventionally treated by prescribing oral contraceptives or drugs to lessen the bleeding; in other cases antibiotics, laser therapy or surgery may be appropriate; iron tablets may also be given. An exploratory operation called Dilatation and Curettage (D & C) may be necessary to find the cause of the bleeding; this involves scraping the womb. If a D & C fails to cure the problem a HYSTERECTOMY is conventionally recommended. Indeed some 18,000 women are referred for hysterectomy for heavy or painful periods in the UK each year.

Other symptoms

Some of the following symptoms may represent manifestations of hormonal imbalances, including: ACNE, itchy vagina, unusual VAGINAL DISCHARGE, PAINFUL PERIODS, nausea and vomiting, DEPRESSION, FAINTNESS, weight gain (see WEIGHT), anxiety, perspiration, irritability, apathy, painful, swollen breasts (see BREAST PROBLEMS) before periods, CONSTIPATION, clumsiness (see General Remedy Finder), difficulty in concentrating and backache.

Treatment

A new technique called transcervical resection of the endometrium (TCRE) is available, in which the lining of the womb is cauterized (cut and sealed with an electrical loop or with a laser) under general anaesthetic. This appears to be 90 per cent effective, and as it is less traumatic and indeed much cheaper, may replace some hysterectomies in due course.

Self-help

The following measures should be tried:
1 Cut out tea, coffee and alcohol.
2 Reduce consumption of milk and dairy foods.
3 Eat lots of raw vegetables.
4 Increase intake of CALCIUM, ZINC, IRON, VITAMIN A, VITAMIN B$_6$ and bioflavonoids.
5 Take 30 minutes of moderate exercise a day, but avoid overstraining yourself.
6 Take several short cold baths in between periods.
If these measures fail try the LIVER DIET for one month.

Homeopathic treatment

Constitutional treatment is recommended; in the meantime see below.

Specific remedies to be taken in the 30c potency every 8 hours for up to 10 doses.

Please remember to check your choice against the Remedy Pictures (p. 305) where possible.

Calcarea

Heavy white discharge with periods; PMS; cramping pain in womb before periods; at onset of and during periods; bright red flow; irregular periods; irritability; indifference; anxiety; depression; headaches before periods; head feels congested; blind boils on face; pale face; nausea with the periods; itchy vaginal discharge; fibroids; swollen tender breasts before periods; painless swollen breasts during periods; backache in small of back during periods; clumsiness; clammy, sticky sweats – worse before periods.

Generalities: Tendency to weight gain; chilliness.

Pulsatilla

PMS; pain in womb before and during periods; vomiting during periods; clots; cramping pain in womb during periods; irregular periods; indifference; irritability before periods; depression; headache before periods; acne on face with irregular periods; nausea with periods; cramping pain in abdomen – worse for walking and before periods; vaginal discharge; may have endometriosis; tender breasts before periods; swollen breasts during periods; backache during periods.

Generalities: Worse for warmth.

Lycopodium

PMS; bright red flow; irregular periods; difficulty in concentrating; irritability in general – worse before periods; anxiety; depression; headache before periods; blind boils; nausea with periods; bloated abdomen before periods; may have endometriosis; pain in womb before periods; fibroids; backache during periods; clammy, sticky sweats.

Generalities: Symptoms worse for cold.

Sepia

PMS; pain in womb before periods; cramping abdominal pain during periods; fainting with periods; irregular periods; difficulty in concentrating; indifference; irritability before periods; depression; zig-zags before eyes; acne on face; cramping pain in abdomen before periods; copious itchy vaginal discharge; may have endometriosis; sweating during periods.

Generalities: Symptoms worse for cold; worse at beginning of periods.

Kali carb.

PMS; pain in womb before periods and at onset of periods; cramping pains in womb during periods; thin watery flow without clots; irritability; anxiety; fear of dying; blind boils; nausea with periods; cramping pain in abdomen – worse before periods; copious vaginal discharge, may have fibroids; swollen breasts pre-menstrually and during periods; backache during periods; sweaty during periods.

Generalities: Cold extremities; feet worse for warmth – worse at onset of periods; exhaustion.

Nux

Pain in womb during periods; cramping abdominal pain during periods; vomiting with periods; faintness with periods; cramping in womb during periods; irregular periods; difficulty in concentrating; indifference; irritability before periods; acne on face; nausea with periods; clumsiness; clammy, sticky sweats.

Generalities: Symptoms worse for cold.

Lachesis
PMS; pain in womb at onset of periods; fainting during periods; clotting; irregular periods; difficulty in concentrating; depression; headache before periods; bloated abdomen before periods; cramping pain in abdomen before periods; may have endometriosis, fibroids; backache during periods; clumsiness.

Generalities: Symptoms worse for warmth; generally worse at beginning of periods.

Belladonna
Pain in womb during periods; cramping abdominal pain during periods; clotting; cramping pain in womb during periods; bright red flow; irregular periods; irritable; anxiety; headache before periods; throbbing head; face hot and flushed; cramping pain in abdomen – worse for walking; backache during periods; clumsiness; sweating before and during periods.

Sulphur
PMS; cramping pain in abdomen during periods; vomiting during periods; irregular periods; depression; headache before periods; copious vaginal discharge; pain in womb before periods; backache during periods; clumsiness; sweaty before and during periods.

Generalities: Symptoms worse for warmth.

Natrum mur.
PMS; cramping abdominal pain during periods; indifference; irritability before periods; depression; headaches before periods; zig-zags before eyes; copious vaginal discharge.

Generalities: Symptoms worse for warmth.

Phosphorus
Vomiting during periods; bright red flow; difficulty in concentrating; indifference; acne on face; cramping pains – worse for walking; may have fibroids; backache during periods; clumsiness; clammy, sticky perspiration – worse before and during periods.

Generalities: Symptoms worse for cold.

Chamomilla
Cramping abdominal pain during periods; vomiting during periods; clotting; cramping pains in womb during periods; bright red flow; irritability – worse before periods; depression; swollen breasts during periods; clammy and sticky.

Cocculus
Cramping abdominal pain during periods; cramping pains in womb during periods; irregular periods; cramping pains in abdomen before periods; bloated abdomen before periods; clumsiness.

Other remedies to consider
- Intermittent bleeding, dark clots of blood, abdominal cramp, headache, giddiness, faintness, face very pale *China 30c*
- Blood dark or red, with or without clots in it, labour-like pains in small of back, emotional upsets increase blood loss, difficulty controlling weight *Sabina 30c*
- Profuse bleeding, blood bright red, nausea *Ipecac. 30c*
- Flooding, blood dark and watery, face pale, occasional flushes, walking around seems to improve things *Ferrum 30c*
- Clots of blackish blood, sensation of movement inside uterus, feeling weak, sick, and worried *Crocus 30c*
- Profuse bleeding, with abdominal cramps and nausea, especially in first day or two of period, pain and bleeding worse at night *Borax 30c*

Remedy Finder for Heavy Periods

Anxiety
Cannabis ind.

Despair
Cocculus

Obstinacy
Nux

Toothache
Ferrum sulph.

Burning urine
Ferrum

When heavy periods occur associated with termination or miscarriage
Plumbum

Burning vaginal discharge and chronic menorrhagia
Iodum

Sleeplessness
Cannabis ind.

Yawning
Apis

Headache and chilliness
Chininum sulph.

Anaemia
Calcarea
Cannabis ind.
Cyclamen
Ferrum
Graphites
Hydrastis

Kali carb.
Natrum mur.
Pulsatilla

Anxiety at night after periods
Sepia

Anxiety during night
Sabina

Odd behaviour after periods
Sepia

Nausea
Ipecac.

Heaviness in abdomen
Apis

Aching dull pain in lower stomach
Magnesia carb.

Stinging pain in abdomen
Apis

Labour-like pains
Caulophyllum

Chamomilla
Cimicifuga

Difficulty in breathing
Fluoric ac.

Restless sleep during periods
Sabina

Restless sleep after periods
Sepia

Fainting
China

Irregular periods

Menstruation is said to be irregular if there is a variation from the normal pattern. Periods can become widely variable in the amount of time between the first day of each period, the number of days for which the woman bleeds, or the amount of blood lost. If the periods have stopped altogether see AMENORRHOEA.

Infrequent periods

Infrequent periods (oligomenorrhoea) are of normal duration but occur less frequently than every 26–28 days. They are very common as the menopause approaches, although for a few women infrequent periods are the norm due to their particular hormone cycle. The only problem is that this reduces the chances of getting pregnant. If INFERTILITY is due to irregular egg production, hormone injections or fertility drugs may be prescribed. Homeopathic treatment is constitutional – see remedies below.

Causes of breakthrough or abnormal bleeding

Always consult your GP. Spotting of blood between periods can be due to stress, travel, or may be a side-effect of interuterine devices, certain oral contraceptives, and other drugs. A profuse discharge of watery blood between periods, possibly made worse by intercourse, suggests cervical erosion (see CERVICAL PROBLEMS) or cancer (see CANCER OF THE CERVIX, CANCER OF THE UTERUS); early diagnosis is important, so see your GP as soon as possible. Cancer is also a possibility if bleeding restarts more than 6 months after the MENOPAUSE.

If you are pregnant, bleeding accompanied by pain in the lower abdomen may signal an ECTOPIC PREGNANCY or impending MISCARRIAGE; prompt medical attention is vital so ②. In an ectopic pregnancy (most often associated with IUD failure, or with infection or abnormality of the

Fallopian tubes) the embryo starts to develop outside the womb, causing severe pain and internal bleeding; the risk of shock setting in is very real.

Most irregular periods are due to a disturbance in the balance of oestrogen and progesterone hormones (see diagram, The Menstrual Cycle, p. 33). These imbalances may also be the reason why women in our survey reported other symptoms along with their irregular periods, although some may be coincidental.

Associated symptoms

These include: painful breasts before periods, acne, dizziness, faintness, pain in lower limbs, numbness in legs, clumsiness, headache, watery eyes, abdominal distension, weariness, weakness of memory, allergy to bread, weeping, sweating in the armpit, dry skin, cold feeling in the body, sensation as if water splashing about in body, hot head, stiff neck, irritability before periods, palpitations, weight gain, growth of hair on chin, sleeplessness, leakage of milk from the breast when not pregnant or suckling, aggravation from tea, loss of appetite, nausea, constipation, etc.

Homeopathic treatment

The best course of action is constitutional treatment from an experienced homeopath. In the meantime see remedies below.

Specific remedies to be taken in the 30c potency once weekly for up to 4 doses.

Please remember to check your choice against the Remedy Pictures (p. 305) where possible.

Lycopodium

Weepiness and irritability before periods; pressure on head in company; headache before periods; watery eyes; appetite diminished; abdomen bloated pre-menstrually; flatulence;

painful breasts pre-menstrually; chronic mastitis; pain in left breast; milk leaking from breast in non-pregnant woman; dry skin.

Generalities: Weariness on waking; fainting before periods; tendency to put on weight; fatigue.

Pulsatilla

Irregular periods – worse at puberty; heavy periods; pain in womb before periods; clots; weepiness and irritability before periods; migraine; headache before periods; watering eyes; acne on face; nausea; bloated abdomen pre-menstrually; cramping pain in left side; painful breasts before periods; chronic mastitis; milk leaking from breast in non-pregnant woman; backache before periods.

Generalities: Body feels heavy; weariness on getting up – worse for eating bread; tendency to put on weight; general fatigue.

Calcarea

Periods heavy; pain in womb before periods; periods too early and frequent; tendency to fall to the right; watering eyes; acne on face; flatulence; painful breasts before periods; clumsiness; sleeplessness; dry skin.

Generalities: Body feels heavy; weariness on waking; tendency to put on weight.

Lachesis

Heavy periods; periods become irregular after death of loved one; tendency to fall forward; pressure on head while walking; poor appetite; bloated abdomen before periods; chronic mastitis; pain in left breast; clumsiness; sleeplessness.

Generalities: Fatigue.

Natrum mur.

Heavy periods; periods too frequent and too early; irritability before periods; irregular periods started after death of loved one; weepiness before periods; forgets what she is about to do; tendency to fall forward; migraine; watering eyes; zig-zags in front of eyes; acne on face; nausea; cramping pain in left side; painful breasts before periods.

Generalities: Body feels heavy; weariness on waking; sensation of cold water splashing on organs; fainting before periods; fatigue.

Nux

Heavy periods; periods too frequent and too early; irritability before and during periods; irregular periods started after death of loved one;

tendency to fall forward; acne on forehead; poor appetite; nausea; cramping pain in left side; painful breasts before periods; clumsiness.

Generalities: Body feels heavy; weariness on waking; faintness before periods; fatigue – worse after drinking tea.

Belladonna

Heavy periods; periods too frequent; clots; hot head with cold face; pressure on head while walking; watering eyes; acne on face; nausea; chronic mastitis; milk from breast in non-pregnant woman; clumsiness; sleeplessness; dry skin.

Generalities: Sensation of cold water splashing in inner organs; tendency to gain weight.

Phosphorus

Heavy periods; periods too early; irregular periods following death of loved one; weepiness before periods; forgets what she is about to do; watering eyes; bloated abdomen not relieved by passing wind; chronic mastitis; milk leaking from breast in non-pregnant woman; clumsiness.

Generalities: Body feels heavy; tendency to put on weight; fatigue.

Sulphur

Long and variable intervals between periods; cramping abdominal pain better for bending double; irritable during periods; forgets what she is about to do; tendency to fall forward; pain at top of head; watering eyes; acne on forehead; flatulence; cramping pain in left side; sweaty armpits; clumsiness; dry skin.

Generalities: Body feels heavy; tendency to put on weight; fatigue.

Sepia

Pain in womb before periods; abdominal cramping pain better for bending double; irritability before periods; zig-zags in front of eyes; acne on forehead; nausea; sweaty armpits.

Generalities: Body feels heavy; fainting before periods; fatigue worse after drinking tea.

Bryonia

Periods too early; tendency to fall forward; pressure in head while walking; sore eyes; nausea; cramping pain in left side; painful breasts before periods; sweaty armpits; chronic mastitis; sleeplessness; dry skin.

Generalities: Weariness on waking; intolerance of bread which aggravates symptoms.

Causticum

Irregular periods; irritability before periods; irregular periods started after loss of loved one; tendency to fall to the right, and to fall forward; acne on forehead; appetite poor; clumsiness; feels fatigued on waking.

Silicea

Irregular periods; tendency to fall to the right and to fall forward; acne on forehead; flatulence; sweaty armpits; chronic mastitis; clumsiness; dry skin.

Generalities: Body feels heavy; fatigue.

Remedy Finder for Irregular Periods

Acne associated with irregular periods
Cimicifuga
Graphites
Pulsatilla
Sanguinaria

Bleeding between periods (see BREAKTHROUGH BLEEDING)
Belladonna
Bovista
Calcarea

Causticum
Chamomilla
Cocculus
Coffea
Elaps

Periods irregular in time and amount
Cimicifuga
Coccus
Ignatia
Nux mosch.

Platina

Vaginal discharge before periods
Sepia

Periods at long and variable intervals
Sulphur

Periods irregular at puberty
Pulsatilla

Painful periods (dysmenorrhea)

Most women experience some discomfort during the first 2–3 days of a period, which is quite normal. Depending on the individual, the 'discomfort' may be a dull ache in the lower back or abdomen, or cramping pains severe enough to cause nausea and vomiting. STRESS and ANXIETY can make the pain considerably worse. Most teenage girls and young women suffer from painful periods, known as primary dysmenorrhea.

The problem usually begins 2–3 years after the periods start, once ovulation is established, and tends to disappear between the ages of 25 and 30 or following childbirth.

Causes and primary symptoms

These may be due to an excess production of – or sensitivity to – prostaglandins, hormones that cause the muscles of the uterus to contract. If the periods suddenly become painful after several years of relative freedom from pain (secondary dysmenorrhea) there is usually an underlying cause. This may be FIBROIDS (for prolonged or heavy periods see UTERUS PROBLEMS), ENDOMETRIOSIS (pain worse towards end of period), or PELVIC INFECTION (earlier heavy periods, mild fever, smelly vaginal discharge). If any of these conditions is suspected see your GP. Interuterine devices or coming off the Pill can also make periods more painful.

Other symptoms

Some of these may be coincidental, some may be due to other obscure effects of hormone imbalance. These include: weakness and weariness, irritability, itching of the scalp, depression, headache, dizziness, suspiciousness, trembling before periods, weepiness, pain in breast before periods, mental dullness, over-sensitivity to noise during periods, fainting during periods, weight gain, acne, aggravation from warm or cold conditions, excessive perspiration – which could be sticky or clammy – migraines, apathy, anger and diarrhoea.

Self-help

A general approach to the whole body is the best way of trying to sort out period problems. The diet should include as much raw fruit and vegetables as possible. Try the LIVER DIET for one month, and if you weigh more than you should, try to do something about it. You may take extra VITAMIN E, VITAMIN C, VITAMIN B COMPLEX, MAGNESIUM, CALCIUM, ZINC and EVENING PRIMROSE OIL. Step up the amount of exercise you are taking, and in the week before your period have a long hot bath every other night. In between periods take the occasional short cold bath. Osteopathic or chiropractic manipulation or physiotherapy sometimes achieves excellent results. Slantboard exercises, which gently shift the contents of the abdomen, can also be beneficial. Many women recommend orgasm as a cure for painful periods, and as one woman said 'Right, I'll go out and buy one today'!

Homeopathic treatment

Where there is no obvious organic cause for the painful periods, homeopathy offers constitutional treatment. The specific remedies below, however, are effective relievers of pain and tension. These should be tried with preference to over-the-counter analgesics.

Specific remedies to be taken in the 30c potency every hour for up to 10 doses as soon as period pains come on.

Please remember to check your choice against the Remedy Pictures (p. 305) where possible.

Pulsatilla

Cramping; abdominal and womb pains before periods – better for warmth; vomiting or nausea with pain in womb during periods; cramping abdominal pain during period – worse for walking; tenderness of abdomen; tearing pain in womb; cutting pains in abdomen – better for motion; depression; irritability before periods; suspicious and mistrustful; weepiness before and during periods; dullness; indifference; dizziness before periods; headache pre-menstrually; migraine with periods; bloated abdomen before periods; diarrhoea during periods; heavy periods; may have endometriosis; heavy periods with clots, alternatively period may be scanty; breasts tender pre-menstrually; backache during periods.

Generalities: PMS; worse for warmth.

Sepia

Cramping pains in abdomen pre-menstrually – better for bending double; pain in womb before periods; tearing pains in womb with periods – better for lying on right side; depression; irritability before periods; indifference; bad-tempered before periods; migraines, especially right-sided; acne on face; pain in vagina with intercourse; may have endometriosis; sweating during periods.

Generalities: Weakness with periods; PMS with trembling before periods; fainting with pain and before periods; cold aggravates.

Calcarea

Pain in womb before and at beginning of periods, with nausea, becoming cutting with period; sadness; dullness; indifference; headache before periods; migraines especially right-sided during periods; heavy periods which are bright red; breasts painful pre-menstrually, with swelling and tenderness; backache; clammy and sticky.

Generalities: PMS; tendency to put on weight – worse for cold.

Nux

Cramping pain and tenderness in abdomen – better for bending double; nausea and vomiting with pain; irritability before and during periods; anxiety before periods; indifference; migraines; acne on face; heavy periods; prolonged periods that arrive early; constipation during periods; clammy.

Generalities: Weakness and exhaustion during periods; fainting with pain during and before periods – worse for cold.

Lycopodium

Pain in womb before periods; nausea with periods; depression, irritability and weepiness before periods; suspicious and mistrustful; sluggish brain; headache before periods; migraines during periods; bloated abdomen before periods; may have endometriosis; backache during periods; clammy and sticky.

Generalities: PMS; trembling before periods – worse for cold; fainting pre-menstrually.

Belladonna

Cramping abdominal pain worse just before periods – worse for walking; tender abdomen during periods with tearing aching or dragging pains in womb – worse for lying down; sluggish brain; headache before periods; right-sided migraine with periods; heavy periods with clotting; bright red gushing – worse for slightest motion; skin hot and flushed.

Lachesis

Pain in womb at beginning of periods – better after flow established; tearing pains in abdomen during periods; dizziness before periods; headache before periods; bloated abdomen before periods; heavy periods, may have endometriosis; backache.

Generalities: Weakness during periods; PMS; fainting with pain – worse for warmth.

Sulphur

Pain in womb before periods; cramping pains in abdomen especially low down – better for bending double; vomiting with pain; cutting pains in abdomen – better wrapping up warmly; anxiety before periods; irritability during periods;

depression; suspicious and mistrustful; headache before periods; pain in vagina on intercourse; backache; sweaty before periods.

Generalities: Weakness during periods; PMS – worse for warmth.

Kali carb.

Cramping pains in lower abdomen before periods; pain in womb before and at beginning of period; cramping or cutting pains in womb during period; nausea with periods; pain in vagina during intercourse; breasts swelling before periods; backache.

Generalities: Weakness and weariness during periods; PMS; trembling before periods – worse for cold.

Natrum mur.

Cramping pain in lower abdomen – worse with periods – extending to the back; depression, anxiety, irritability and weepiness before periods; weepy during periods with indifference and sluggish brain; headache before periods; pain in vagina on intercourse.

Generalities: PMS; trembling and fainting before periods – worse for warmth.

Cocculus

Cramping lower abdominal pains before and during periods, with tenderness of the abdomen; cutting pain in womb; anxiety before periods; weepiness during periods; bloated abdomen before periods.

Generalities: Weakness during periods.

Phosphorus

Vomiting with pain; cramping pain in abdomen – worse for walking; weepiness before periods, with indifference and sluggish brain; acne on face; diarrhoea during periods; heavy periods, bright red and gushing – worse for slightest movement; clammy and sticky.

Generalities: Weakness during periods – worse for cold.

Causticum

Cramping pain before and during periods; pain in womb at beginning of periods; cutting and tearing pains in womb during periods with tearing pains in abdomen; depression; irritability before periods; suspicious and mistrustful; acne on face; diarrhoea during periods; backache; sweating during periods.

Generalities: Weakness and weariness during periods – worse for cold.

Chamomilla

Severe cramping abdominal pain before and during periods; vomiting with pain; irritability before periods; depressed and bad-tempered during periods; restless; heavy periods with clots.

Graphites

Cramping or tearing lower abdominal pain during periods – worse for walking; with nausea; backache.

Generalities: Weakness during periods; tendency to put on weight – worse for cold.

Other remedies to consider

- Pain comes in spasms, soothed by heat, pressure, and movement, membranes present in blood flow *Magnesia phos. 30c*
- Periods late and scanty, pain extends into thighs *Viburnum 30c*
- Periods late and scanty, sharp pains which are soothed by heat, uterus feels heavy *Gelsemium 30c*
- Strong contractions of uterus, rather like labour pains, headaches in days leading up to periods *Cimicifuga 30c*
- Pain extends down into thighs, nausea, muffled buzzing in ears *Borax 30c*

Remedy Finder for Painful Periods

Desire for coffee
Lachesis

Piles
Collinsonia

Wind
Viburnum

Painful urination
Nux mosch.

Senecio
Veratrum vir.

Increase in sexual desire
Cannabis ind.

As a result of anger
Chamomilla

After termination or miscarriage
Senecio

Pain in abdomen
Calcarea
Calcarea phos.
Carbon sulph.
Cimicifuga
Graphites
Nux
Pulsatilla
Ratanhia
Sabina

Sepia
Sulphur
Viburnum

Pain better for heat
Arsenicum

Bearing down pain in womb
Belladonna
Lilium
Pulsatilla
Sepia

Burning pains in womb
Calcarea phos.

Cramping pains in womb
Caulophyllum
Chamomilla
Nux
Sabina
Ustilago

Cutting pains
Cocculus

Labour-like pains
Chamomilla

Pain in womb better for bending double
Aconite
Cimicifuga
Colocynth
Nux

Pain in womb during period
Belladonna
Cactus
Calcarea
Nux
Pulsatilla

   at beginning of period
   Calcarea
   Crotalus
   Lachesis

   better for bending back
   Lac can.

   better for bending double
   Colocynth
   Kali carb.
   Opium
   Pulsatilla

Has to bend double
Colocynth
Pulsatilla

Blotches all over body
Dulcamara

Chilliness
Kali carb.
Veratrum

Worse at menopause
Psorium

Worse for catching cold
Aconite

Cold feeling all over
Veratrum

After colic
Kali carb.

After evening meal
Phytolacca

Better after discharge of clots
Viburnum

Worse for emotions
Chamomilla

Belching
Viburnum

From excitement
Calcarea

Better for pressing feet against some support
Medorrhinum

Worse for getting feet wet
Phosphorus
Pulsatilla
Rhus tox.

Flatulence
Viburnum

Greater the flow the more pain
Cimicifuga

Smaller the flow the greater the pain
Lachesis

Pain better for flow
Magnesia phos.
Moschus
Zinc

After fright
Aconite

Irregular painful periods since first period
Pulsatilla

Horrible pain with crying and weeping
Cactus
Coffea
Cuprum

Infantile behaviour
Calcarea phos.

Jerks
Platina

Irregular painful periods
Belladonna
Calcarea
Caulophyllum
Cimicifuga
Cyclamen
Natrum mur.
Nux
Pulsatilla
Senecio
Sepia

When periods painful every two weeks
Bovista
Calcarea
Phosphorus

Prolapse of womb
Veratrum vir.

Painful periods at puberty
Phytolacca
Pulsatilla

Sexual desire
Chamomilla

Screaming with pain
Platina

Spasmodic pains
Belladonna
Caulophyllum
Cimicifuga
Gelsemium
Magnesia phos.
Nux
Pulsatilla
Viburnum

Infertility
Phytolacca

Frequent urination
Medorrhinum

Worse for walking
Sabina

Better for warmth
Arsenicum

Magnesia phos.
Nux mosch.
Sabina

Better for washing
Kali carb.

Worse after getting wet
Zinc

Pain in left breast while coughing
Causticum

With aching pain in heart
Crotalus

Retraction of nipples
Sarsaparilla

Frightful dreams
Cyclamen

Sleeplessness
Cocculus

Cold sweats
Sarsaparilla
Veratrum

Sexual and Relationship Problems

Problems of sexual identity and problems arising from chromosomal anomalies lie outside the scope of this book and are, more properly, the province of the psychotherapist and psychosexual counsellor. However, constitutional homeopathic prescribing can help to relieve tension and anxiety where these are part of the picture.

Erection, orgasm, and ejaculation are reflexes, but there is nothing automatic about them. They can be helped or hindered by thoughts and emotions. They can be helped by trust, relaxation, and fantasy. They can be hindered by guilt, sexual taboos, and fear of inadequacy even when all the right sensual stimuli are there, even when all the nerves, blood vessels, glands, and hormones involved in sexual response are perfectly normal. Female orgasm is a less reliable response than male orgasm, during intercourse that is; during masturbation both sexes' capacity for orgasm is about equal.

Sexual anatomy and the techniques of sexual intercourse are described at length in many books, but as anyone who has been in a long-term sexual relationship knows, sexual intercourse is a great deal more than the art of applying the right techniques to the right erogenous zones. Indeed, sexual intercourse is only one aspect of sexuality. To concentrate on it to the exclusion of dress, humour, flirting, seduction, affection, and so on is like insisting that music begins and ends with Beethoven and Haydn.

There is no reason why sexual drive and sexual function should not continue into our 80s or even 90s, with, as one wag put it, this important proviso: those who enjoy the party tend to leave last! Intercourse does make demands on the heart, but if you can climb two flights of stairs without suffering from palpitations or getting painfully out of breath, you should be quite safe.

Penis size has very little to do with female satisfaction, primarily because it is the outer third of the vagina which is the most sensitive.

Much has been written about the mismatch of the male and female 'sexual response cycle' as a source of sexual dissatisfaction; both are described in terms of an excitation phase, a plateau phase, orgasm, a resolution phase, and a refractory phase. The most common complaint is that she climaxes too slowly, he too fast – however, anthropologists have pointed out that this may be a cultural rather than a physiological phenomenon. What does seem to be a physiological phenomenon, however, is that quite a few women over the age of 25 reach orgasm more than once in a love-making session. Few men do. Foreplay is a way of prolonging the man's excitement and plateau phase and bringing the woman to plateau phase or even orgasm before penetration. Women are not responsible for men's orgasms; both sexes are responsible for their own.

What a woman expects during sexual intercourse and what actually happens may be rather different. This is often a cause of problems. For example, orgasm is not always dramatic or obvious – some women moan or cry out, others are silent; nor is it experienced the same way on every occasion. Synchronized climaxes happen a lot in novels but not in the real world – psychologists would say that 'coming' together is an intermittent reward that serves to strengthen rather than diminish sex drive. Techniques that please one person may not excite someone else – we are all different in our capacity for pleasure.

What a woman wants from intercourse may be unreasonable – this too can be a source of conflict. Love-making seldom solves problems in other areas of life, nor does it always shut them out. Quite the reverse, in fact. Job worries, money problems, identity problems, depression, boredom, fatigue, and so on have a habit of getting into bed with us.

Sexual education begins with the way in which we treat our children. Hitting or beating a child, or denying physical affection, may make it very difficult for that child to have loving sexual relationships; her sexuality may be tinged with sadism or masochism. Many films and advertisements on television subtly suggest that sex equals power and possession, that sex is not real sex unless it is violent and exploitative. In the authors' view, parents should do everything possible to combat this distortion.

Like every other part of the body the genitals are susceptible to infection, especially to sexually transmitted infection. There are specific homeopathic remedies for such ailments, but in these days of global travel and high mobility the giving of antibiotics for some of these conditions is, the authors feel, justifiable on medical and social grounds. However, a susceptibility to sexually transmitted infections indicates an underlying miasm which constitutional treatment can help to dispel.

Many of the sexually transmitted diseases will become less frequent as a result of people practising safer sex (see below) as part of AIDS prevention. Indeed the level of gonorrhea in the homosexual community has been used to monitor the degree of safer sex being practised. When asked, many women said men were their greatest problem regarding sex, so we have included an A–Z of men's problems at the end of this chapter.

Safer sex

When AIDS was contained within the homosexual and drug-taking population there seemed to be little need for the majority of heterosexual women to feel threatened by it. Now, however, as the number of cases of HIV infection and AIDS in the UK continues to rise, new cases among heterosexual women are rising most rapidly. The HIV virus is found mostly in blood and other body fluids such as semen and vaginal secretions. Penetrative sexual intercourse involves mixing these body fluids, and therefore presents a risk of transmission. The sexual practice which puts women most at risk is unprotected anal intercourse, but it is also important to realize that most women infected become so through vaginal intercourse. Any infection present already in the vagina, such as herpes or syphilis, increases the risk, whereas the use of condoms reduces it, especially in conjunction with spermicides which kill viruses.

Medium risk activities include oral-anal and other oral-genital contact; the risk is increased if there is any inflammation or ulcerative condition in either partner. This risk will be reduced by using condoms, rubber mouth shields and by avoiding ejaculation into any orifice. If an infected woman is menstruating at the time of intercourse the potential risk to her partner will be significantly increased. Similarly any practice involving urinating into the mouth or anus conveys a medium risk.

Lower risk practices are those such as mutual masturbation, body rubbing and using (non-shared) sex toys. Spermicides seem to kill the virus to some degree, so always use them with barrier contraceptives where possible.

No-risk activities include touching, dry kissing, embracing, sharing utensils or drinking from the same cup or glass. The HIV virus cannot be caught from one-use disposable needles used in blood tests, injections or in acupuncture and tattooing; make sure your practitioner is using them. It cannot be caught from toilet seats, contrary to popular misconception.

The effect that AIDS has had on sexual behaviour, or at least on attitudes to sexual behaviour, can best be illustrated by the change in viewpoint of Dr Alex Comfort's book *The Joy of Sex*. Group sex is out and kissing is in. Tenderness, touching and being together are as much 'real sex' as vaginal intercourse. Comfort goes on to caution that the only sane assumption in planning sexual behaviour is that any new partner, however innocent or attractive, may endanger your life.

For further details about how safer sex can be practised the authors recommend the series of booklets produced by the Terrence Higgins Trust (see Useful Addresses, p. 335). These include a booklet on safer sex for women and one for lesbian couples, both of which give useful contact addresses, helpline telephone numbers and suppliers of recommended products. We have also included the address and client services telephone number for Positively Women, an organization specifically for women and AIDS.

Relationship problems

It appears that we choose our partners largely unconsciously. They appear to fit in with our subconscious projections, probably based on our experience of our parents' marriage. The first stumbling block for a relationship could therefore be that the roles our parents gave us were not suitable to form a basis for a healthy relationship. Before we can form a genuine relationship with another person we have to separate ourselves from our parents. Having overcome that hurdle, any change in circumstances between a couple can give rise to problems. The most obvious one is the birth of the first child, where the woman gives up a satisfying and lucrative career and starts making demands on her partner. He, in turn, may respond by getting more and more involved in work to shut off the demands. When the youngest child first goes to school a mother who has not worked outside the home, and has given up everything to look after children, may feel that she has been left behind and has lost touch with her partner. Either then or later, when the children have left home, she may decide to go out to work. On finding that raising children has made her very good at organizing, for example, she may start a successful new career, just at a time when her partner's is beginning to peak. This may lead to change, which in turn can cause more problems.

Other changes involve the death of parents and retirement, and losses such as infertility, miscarriage or death of a child. All these changes require adaptation in a relationship, and any of them can either be overcome by honesty about feelings, or can lead to a breakdown in communication due to an inability to express feelings and share problems. If you do develop a problem in your marriage the first port of call should be your own GP; if you feel you would rather seek other advice try Relate (see Useful Addresses p. 336). Whatever happens, don't take your problems as a couple out on the children, or this may lead to them making the same mistakes in their adult life. In the authors' experience the happiest marriages are those where couples are capable of standing on their own but have an open and caring relationship with each other. As Khalil Gibran wrote in *The Prophet*: 'Give your heart but not into each other's keeping, for only the hand of life can contain your hearts. And stand together, yet not too near together for the pillars of the temple stand apart and the oak tree and the cyprus grow not in each other's shadow.' In any relationship there are four elements – physical, emotional, intellectual and spiritual. It is rare to find a perfect match for all these elements, and each relationship will have its strong and weak points. We hope that the following A–Z of both women's and men's sexual problems will help solve any worries and difficulties you may have, whether or not you are in an ongoing relationship.

Women's sexual problems

Anxiety about intercourse

Can be due to lack of knowledge, fear of AIDS, herpes, and other SEXUALLY TRANSMITTED DIS-EASES, lack of physical affection in childhood, or parental strictures against exploring genitals or masturbating. Escaping into drugs or alcohol generally makes problem worse. Where anxiety is bound up with general insecurity or difficulty forming intimate relationships, constitutional homeopathic treatment is recommended; in the meantime, the remedies below may be helpful.

Specific remedies to be taken every 12 hours for up to 5 days:

- Woman who is very emotional, cries and blushes easily, hates being in hot stuffy rooms *Pulsatilla 30c*
- Phobias and irrational thoughts, obsessive fear of 'catching something' *Argentum nit. 30c*
- Difficulties caused by grief or disappointment in a previous relationship *Ignatia 30c*

Excessive desire for sex

Rarely has a physical cause but may be aggravated by certain drugs; not a problem unless compulsion to have intercourse (see OBSESSIONS AND COMPULSIONS) becomes a burden to person concerned or makes unreasonable demands on a partner. Constitutional homeopathic treatment may be necessary, but the remedies below should be tried first; if urge to have sex does not become more controllable within 3 weeks, see your GP.

Specific remedies to be taken every 12 hours for up to 5 days:

- Woman who has enormous sexual appetite, despises men, suffers from depression *Platina 30c*
- Woman who behaves in a highly emotional way, makes obscene remarks, strips off and exposes genitals, suffers from paranoia *Hyoscyamus 30c*
- Woman who is always seeking excitement and has inflated sense of her own importance *Gratiola 30c*

Specific remedies for partners exhausted by sexual demands, to be taken every 4 hours for up to 3 days:

- Apathy, lethargy, indifference *Phosphoric ac. 30c*
- Physical exhaustion, chilliness, oversensitivity *China 30c*

Incest

Incest is the name given to intercourse between relatives such as parent / son / daughter / brother/ sister / uncle / aunt / nephew / niece / grandparent / grandchild. This is not just a taboo based on emotional reasoning; it probably reflects the fact that in-breeding gives rise to a higher number of congenital malformations. It is thought that up to 10 per cent of women have had sexual contact with a male relative. This is often associated with child abuse, and is becoming more frequently reported due to telephone helplines and greater awareness amongst medical and social services. The victim suffers considerable feelings of anxiety, guilt and depression, which may take years to recover from. The authors would urge anyone who finds herself in this situation to report it to a responsible person either within or outside the family as soon as it occurs, even if it means ignoring threats made by the perpetrator. Homeopathic treatment is given below. If necessary see your homeopath.

Specific remedy to be taken 4 times a day for up to 1 week:

- For trauma relating to the aftermath of incest *Staphisagria 30c*

Lack of desire for sex

The root cause is usually psychological – STRESS, DEPRESSION, fear of getting pregnant, performance anxiety (see LACK OF ORGASM), and frequently boredom – rather than hormonal or physical. Labels such as 'frigidity' are old-fashioned and extremely unhelpful. There is no 'normal' level of desire for sex (libido) in men or women, although in both sexes it is the 'male' hormone testosterone which sustains it; testosterone levels can be depressed by poor liver or kidney function, pituitary problems, fatigue, pain, illness, depression, and stress, and also by tranquillizers, opiates, drugs used to treat high blood pressure, appetite suppressants, and alcohol.

For some women libido goes right down before a period (see PRE-MENSTRUAL SYNDROME); temporary loss of interest in sex is perfectly natural after childbirth or gynaecological surgery; in some women oral contraceptives and hormone replacement therapy have a lowering effect on sex drive. In general, if sex is pleasurable before the MENOPAUSE it will continue to be pleasurable after it; indeed, for some women, cessation of fertility and relief from some of the pressures of home-making are a boost to libido. If sex drive falters after the menopause or after HYSTERECTOMY and this causes relationship problems, your GP may prescribe testosterone.

Treatment of underlying conditions mentioned above is obvious first step to restoring libido. Where cause is mainly psychological, sex therapy can be very helpful. Homeopathic approach is constitutional, provided there are no physical problems, but the remedies below should be tried first.

Specific remedies to be taken every 12 hours for up to 5 days:

- General weakness, especially after prolonged or frequent intercourse *Agnus 30c*
- Irritability, feeling chilly, exhausted and indifferent to sex, energy revives after brisk exercise *Sepia 30c*
- Loss of libido associated with grief or repressed emotions *Natrum mur. 30c*
- Loss of libido following periods, vagina feels raw and sore *Causticum 30c*
- Formation of allergies *Apis 30c*
- Lumps in breasts *Conium 30c*
- Weepiness and depression *Pulsatilla 30c*
- Apathy and indifference *Phosphoric ac. 30c*

Lack of orgasm

Orgasm during intercourse is a much more reliable response in men than in women; as anthropologists have pointed out, this may be related to the fact that until a few decades ago, in the UK at least, women were not supposed to enjoy sex to the extent of having orgasms; now that they are, not having orgasms can create the kind of performance anxiety which causes ERECTION PROBLEMS and EJACULATION PROBLEMS in men. Even if the right sensory information goes to the brain, orgasm can be blocked by anxiety, anger, guilt, mistrust, or determination not to lose control. In isolated cases, lack of orgasm is caused not by psychological blocks but by drugs or damage to vital nerve pathways.

For the majority of women, the clitoris is the primary focus of sensations which lead to orgasm, with the vagina and labia important but secondary; on most occasions the clitoris is not sufficiently stimulated by thrusting movements of the penis in the vagina to trigger off orgasm; only 30 per cent of women are regularly orgasmic through vaginal stimulation alone.

If lack or infrequency of orgasm, your own or your partner's, worries you or is beginning to cause problems, try the self-help methods below; constitutional homeopathic treatment might also help, although the remedies listed below or under ERECTION PROBLEMS should be tried first. If situation does not improve, and your GP has ruled out physical causes, you might consider sex therapy.

Specific remedies for women, to be taken every 12 hours for up to 5 days:

- Inability to let go of emotions *Natrum mur. 30c*

- Fatigue and lack of energy *Agnus 30c*
- Difficulty follows grief or painful end to a love affair *Ignatia 30c*

Self-help
Try to de-emphasize orgasm by making other phases of response cycle more pleasurable. Tell or show your partner where your most sensitive areas are and what you find most exciting, and allow yourself to fantasize – fantasies can take the brakes off! Read *Becoming Orgasmic*, a sexual growth programme (see Further Reading, p. 00)

Masturbation worries
May be justified if masturbation is causing problems within a marriage or within a valued relationship, or if self-stimulation is compulsive (see OBSESSIONS AND COMPULSIONS), associated with extremely sadistic fantasies, or a symptom of inability to socialize. Worries about masturbation sapping health, leading to homosexuality, retarding development of adult sexual relationships, or undermining ability to have orgasm during intercourse are unfounded. Studies have shown that women who continue to masturbate once they are in a sexual relationship are less likely to seek help for sexual problems than women who don't; for some couples, mutual or self-masturbation is part of intercourse or sex play. However, if the urge to masturbate is causing anxiety, see your GP and ask about sex counselling or psychotherapy. Constitutional homeopathic treatment can help to defuse anxiety and tension; in the meantime the remedies below may be helpful.

Specific remedies to be taken every 12 hours for up to 5 days:

- Sinking feeling in stomach, untidiness, being oblivious to what other people think of appearance or behaviour *Sulphur 30c*
- Irritability, resentment, bottled up emotions, masturbating to get your own back on the world *Staphisagria 30c*
- Obesity, feeling sweaty and chilly by turns, masturbating to release tension or relieve boredom *Calcarea 30c*
- Increasing isolation and withdrawal, feeling worn out after masturbation or intercourse, constipation *Natrum mur. 30c*
- Masturbation followed by great weakness *Phosphoric ac. 30c*
- Masturbation associated with increase in sexual appetite *Calcarea phos. 30c*

Painful intercourse (dyspareunia)
In women intercourse may be painful due to vaginal or vulval infections, which cause unusual discharge or itchiness (see VAGINAL AND VULVAL PROBLEMS), CYSTITIS (frequent urge to urinate), or VAGINISMUS (spasm of muscles at entrance to vagina); pain on deep penetration or in certain positions may be a symptom of endometriosis or retroversion of the uterus (see UTERUS PROBLEMS), or of cervical erosion (see CERVICAL PROBLEMS). Dryness of vagina can cause discomfort and soreness for both partners; vaginal secretions tend to become scantier after MENOPAUSE, but sometimes lack of lubrication is due to ANXIETY ABOUT INTERCOURSE, or too perfunctory foreplay; KY jelly usually helps. Resuming intercourse too soon after having a baby can be painful, as can intercourse for the first time ever.

For orthodox and homeopathic treatment, see causative conditions mentioned above. If none of the homeopathic remedies given seems to meet the case, try one of the remedies below; if there is no improvement within 3 weeks, see your GP or homeopath.

Specific remedies to be taken every 4 hours for up to 2 weeks:

- Vulva and vagina feel very sensitive, pain in ovary during intercourse, 'honeymoon' cystitis *Staphisagria 6c*
- Vagina very sensitive, severe pain in left ovary after intercourse, vulval warts *Thuja 6c*
- Vulva and vagina feel itchy and twitchy, burning sensation in uterus and ovaries after intercourse, increased desire for sex *Platina 6c*
- Dry vagina, constipation, emotional upset *Natrum mur. 6c*
- Heavy, dragging sensation in lower abdomen, intercourse causes pains which shoot up through vagina and uterus to navel *Sepia 6c*

Rape
There has been a considerable increase in the number of rape cases reported in recent years. Whether this means a greater incidence or a better understanding and attitude on the part of the police and society in general, women are now more willing to report it. However, it is still thought to be under-reported due to shame, fear of being disbelieved or rejected, or of the publicity and emotional trauma of a trial, or of being assaulted by the rapist. Rape mostly occurs between people who know each other and is not always accompanied by additional violence. Rape is not provoked by the victim, and is now thought to be a crime of violence rather than a sexual event, with a need for the man to dominate the woman. Men who commit rape are usually angry and have a hostile attitude to women, and are frequently drunk.

Physical injuries as a result of rape include swelling of the labia, bruising of the vaginal walls or cervix and occasionally tearing of the anus or perineum (the skin between the genitals and the anus). There may also be evidence of beating or attempts to choke. Psychological effects are usually severe, including anxiety and depression. Some victims may develop a variety of Post Traumatic Stress Disorder (PTSD), more commonly known from the field of military combat as shell shock. PTSD may also be found in survivors and relatives of those killed in disasters, and in those who have been kidnapped or held hostage for a significant period. Symptoms include disturbed sleep and concentration, recurring dreams and memories, guilt, apathy, irritability, sense of isolation and depression.

If you are raped and decide that you will report it, either on your own account or to prevent it happening to someone else, you will have to undergo a physical examination by a doctor. If the doctor is a man, a woman will be present as well. The doctor will take samples from you and examine you. If as a result of the rape you become pregnant you may consider TERMINATION. You will also be tested for any SEXUALLY TRANSMITTED DISEASES. Get in touch with a Rape Crisis Counselling Service, details of which can be obtained from your doctor, local social work department, or Citizens' Advice Bureau. You may need expert help from a homeopath.

Specific remedies to be taken 4 times a day for up to a week:

- For significant bruising *Arnica 6c*
- For trauma relating to aftermath of rape *Staphisagria 30c*

Vaginismus

Unusual condition in which muscles around entrance to vagina go into spasm, making intercourse, vaginal examination, or use of tampons painful or impossible; spasm may be accompanied by arching of back and drawing together of thighs. If problem has a physical basis, your GP will probably refer you to a gynaecologist; if psychological, sex therapy may be the answer. Constitutional homeopathic treatment may also be beneficial, but the remedies below should be tried first.

Specific remedies to be taken every 12 hours for up to 5 days:

- Extreme sensitivity of vulva and vagina, constipation *Plumbum 30c*
- Extreme sensitivity of vulva and vagina, made worse by sitting, irritable bladder *Staphisagria 30c*

- Where spasms are a hysterical reaction to grief or a broken love affair *Ignatia 30c*
- Vagina feels burning hot and as heavy as lead, sensation made more unpleasant by slightest jarring *Belladonna 30c*
- Extreme sensitivity of vulva accompanied by pleasurable itching, general restlessness and insomnia, attention-seeking behaviour *Coffea 30c*
- Painful periods, copious early flow of dark blood which ceases on lying down, heart condition *Cactus 30c*

Sexually transmitted diseases see SAFER SEX

Diseases whose main means of transfer is through sexual intercourse. Fear of AIDS and herpes (see below) is changing attitudes to casual sex. It pays to be choosy about who you have sex with, especially if you or your partner have other partners. Be fastidious about genital hygiene and do not ignore unusual discharges, itches, bumps, or sores in the genital area. If you think you have an infection, *do not pass it on*; tell your partner (or other sexual contacts) so that they can tell any sexual contacts they have had. Go and see your GP or local STD clinic, refrain from intercourse until you are symptom-free and make sure that your partner gets treated as well.

If you trust a person enough to want to go to bed with them, have the courage to ask, perhaps with a half smile, 'Do you have anything I could catch?' If you cannot bring yourself to do this, at least check that your intended partner has no obvious signs of infection; the best place to do this, and the most fun, is in the bath or shower. Risk of infection can also be reduced by using a condom, whether this is necessary from the contraceptive point of view or not.

AIDS (Acquired Immune Deficiency Syndrome)

Human immunodeficiency virus, HIV for short, is responsible for a spectrum of conditions of which AIDS is only a part. These are: HIV positive (virus present in blood but no noticeable symptoms); PGL or persistent generalized lymphadenopathy (lymph glands remain swollen and sometimes painful for at least 3 months following HIV infection); ARC or AIDS-related complex (a range of relatively mild signs and symptoms including seborrhoeic dermatitis, malaise, fever, night sweats, profound fatigue, recrudescent acne, cold sores around mouth, shingles, weight loss, diarrhoea); and AIDS (symptoms include fever, malaise, HEADACHE, breathlessness, dry COUGH, ORAL THRUSH, abdominal tenderness, DIARRHOEA, swollen lymph glands, a subcutaneous form of CANCER called Kaposi's sarcoma, rapid weight loss, cerebral abscess, fits, encephalitis, meningitis, pneumonia (including *Pneumocystus carinii*), DEPRESSION, PSYCHOTIC ILLNESS, dementia, personality changes).

HIV causes its devastating effects by going straight to the heart of the immune system and knocking out the T4 helper cells, which are vital for recognizing infecting organisms. They are also required to direct the activities of other elements in the immune system (see note on Immune System in CHRONIC FATIGUE SYNDROME). HIV may also cause changes in the gastro-intestinal tract, leading to malabsorption of one or several nutrients essential for immune function and absorption of microbes and microbe products not normally admitted into the bloodstream.

Recently there has been speculation that AIDS may be related to syphilis (see below); AIDS symptoms are similar to those of advanced syphilis, and blood tests in patients with AIDS are often positive for syphilis. There has been no further evidence brought forward to corroborate this, however.

HIV is transmitted from person to person through blood and blood products, and through any bodily secretion. Groups most at risk are homosexual men and drug users who share needles; it is through drug use and bisexual behaviour, and through heterosexual relation-ships with people from countries where AIDS is endemic, that AIDS is slowly spreading into the heterosexual population. Where blood has not been properly screened and heat-treated, people receiving transfusions, organ transplants, or Factor VIII injections for haemophilia are at risk.

Pregnancy and AIDS. If a woman has symptoms of AIDS there is a substantial risk not only that the baby will be infected, but that the pregnancy will cause a more rapid deterioration in her disease. If she is HIV positive but has no symp-toms, the risk of infecting the baby could be as low as 2 per cent. This figure may be higher if she actually becomes symptomatic, or is re-infected whilst pregnant, or around conception. If you are HIV positive and desperately want to have a baby, the best currently available advice is: recognize when you are most likely to conceive, (see INFERTILITY). At other times avoid inter-course, or use strict barrier methods of contra-ception.

Breastfeeding and AIDS. Current thinking is that there is a definite risk of transmitting the virus from mother to baby through breast milk. Regrettably, therefore, advice from experts and the government is not to breastfeed, at least in the UK, where safe alternatives are available.

Drug addiction and AIDS. In many cities AIDS is endemic amongst the drug community. The main source of infection is infected needles. Nowadays you should be able to get hold of a supply of sterile works, but if you can't, then follow the instructions below (you should note that this will not protect you from Hepatitis B).

About 30 per cent of people diagnosed as HIV positive develop AIDS within 7 years; the percentage of HIV positives who develop ARC within the same timescale is about the same; other people with the virus develop PGL or remain symptom-free. *Everyone* who has the virus can transmit it to others through activities which involve exchanging blood or body fluids; for most people, this means sexual activity, with some forms of sex being safer than others (see self-help measures below).

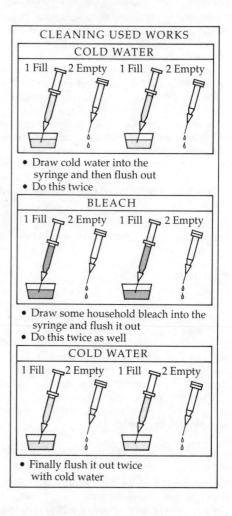

The user's guide to safer drug use

If you think you have been exposed to HIV or if you develop any of the symptoms mentioned above, see your GP and ask for a blood test. If the test is positive, the most constructive approach is holistic; accept treatment (usually antibiotics) offered by your GP, adopt immunity-boosting habits, implement the self-help measures described below, and seek constitutional treatment from an experienced homeopath.

Recently, doubt has been cast on the role of HIV in AIDS. It is held by some that general lifestyle factors and previous medical conditions such as repeated infections and street drugs may be more important in the causation of AIDS than HIV itself. This would confirm that the holistic approach to AIDS outlined above is the most important one.

Self-help

Always use a condom during vaginal or anal sex and read the information on safer sex on p. 105. If possible, avoid surgery, blood products, and injections in developing countries or countries where AIDS is endemic. Never share razors, toothbrushes, or other articles which may have blood on them, burn sanitary towels or if this is not possible put them in a double bag, flush tampons down the lavatory, always cover wounds, and after accidents carefully wipe all blood off skin and furniture, then clean furniture with diluted bleach (1 part bleach to 10 parts water) using a disposable cloth, and carefully dispose of all swabs and dressings.

If a child is HIV positive, warn him or her against blood-mixing rituals, ear-piercing, tattooing, and giving blood in science classes. He or she should also be trained to take the precautions outlined above. The sharing of toys, and of pens and pencils which have been chewed or sucked, should be kept to a minimum. Various organizations offer information and support to people with AIDS and to those diagnosed as HIV positive (see Useful Addresses, p. 335).

Gonorrhea ('clap')

Bacterial infection spread by oral, vaginal, or anal intercourse with person who is incubating infection or already has symptoms; condition is related to promiscuity and affects twice as many men as women; incubation period is 3–5 days, followed by discomfort when urinating and increasingly thick and copious discharge of pus from tip of penis; occasionally, however, the man may have no symptoms; in women, there may be no obvious symptoms or unusual discharge from vagina. If rectum is infected, there may be a feeling of wetness inside rectum or pus in faeces; after oral intercourse, throat may feel sore. Un-checked, infection can spread, causing rashes and joint problems, pelvic infection, or stricture of the urethra (see PENIS PROBLEMS).

If gonorrhea is suspected, see your GP or visit your local STD clinic immediately; if diagnosis is positive, take penicillin or other antibiotics offered, refrain from intercourse until you are symptom-free, then seek constitutional homeopathic treatment in order to boost resistance to further infection. There are specific remedies for treating gonorrhea, but these should be taken only under guidance of an *experienced homeopath*.

Herpes (herpes genitalis)

Caused by same type of virus which causes cold sores around mouth; transmitted by oral–genital or genital–genital contact with someone who is incubating virus or who already has symptoms; virus incubates for about 10 days, then causes itchiness and crop of small blisters on penis or vulva; these quickly become moist and ulcerated, glands in groin become swollen and tender, and slight fever develops; symptoms usually clear up within 2 weeks, but for 50 per cent of sufferers, the virus goes to ground in a bundle of nerve cells at base of spine and causes further attacks, milder and less and less frequent, whenever health is below par. Herpes can be fatal to babies, so if infection is active at time of birth, baby will have to be delivered by caesarian section. If herpes is suspected, see your GP or visit your local STD clinic – an anti-viral ointment will probably be prescribed – and refrain from intercourse until ulcers heal. Alternatively, you can treat yourself, using the self-help measures and homeopathic remedies below. Constitutional homeopathic treatment may help to prevent recurrence.

Specific remedies to be taken 4 times daily for up to 14 days:

- Bad ulcers which bleed, especially at night, whole genital area very tender and painful *Sempervivum 6c*
- Skin of genitals very dry, lesions hot and puffy, with pearl-like blisters *Natrum mur. 6c*
- Genitals burn and itch, discomfort aggravated by cold or damp, general restlessness *Rhus tox. 6c*
- Genitals burn and sting, skin cracked, with red, itchy rash *Capsicum 6c*

Self-help

Avoid intercourse during an attack or if you feel tingling or tenderness which heralds an attack. Always wash your hands with soap and water after touching ulcers, and expose ulcers to air as much as possible. Ulcers can be bathed in

Hypericum and Calendula solution (5 drops of mother tincture of each to 0.25 litre [½ pint] boiled cooled water) 4 times a day, or Calendula ointment can be applied. Frequent warm baths with salt added to the water are soothing and speed healing.

Non-specific urethritis (NSU)

Infection and inflammation of urethra due, in 45 per cent of cases, to organisms called CHLAMYDIA, which are half-way between a virus and a bacterium; in other cases cause of infection cannot be pinpointed. Three-quarters of sufferers are men. Infection is usually, though not invariably, spread through sexual contact and may take 1–5 weeks to incubate. In men, first sign is tingling sensation at tip of penis, especially after urinating first thing in morning; this is followed by clear discharge from penis, scanty at first, then thicker and heavier. In women, there may be no symptoms at all, or slightly increased discharge from vagina.

If infection is suspected, see your GP or visit your local STD clinic at once; take antibiotics prescribed, and do not have intercourse until course of antibiotics is finished and you are symptom-free; your partner should take antibiotics too, even if he or she has no symptoms. Constitutional homeopathic treatment is recommended after antibiotics.

Pubic lice ('crabs')

Crab-shaped species of louse about 2 mm (¹⁄₁₀ in) long which lives in pubic hair and in hairs around anus, sucking blood and causing itching, especially at night. Adults move from one body to another during sexual contact, but symptoms of infestation may take several weeks to appear because eggs (nits) laid by adults take a week or two to hatch. If pubic lice are suspected, see your GP or visit your local STD clinic; a special cream or ointment will be prescribed to kill the lice, and you may be advised to shave pubic hair to get rid of nits, which cannot be removed by normal washing.

Reiter's syndrome

A combination of CONJUNCTIVITIS, joint pains (see OSTEOARTHRITIS, rheumatoid arthritis), and acute urethritis (see CYSTITIS) or DIARRHOEA; probably due to an infection-triggered change in immune system; may be acute or chronic, and in majority of cases is sexually transmitted. Orthodox treatment consists of antibiotics in acute stage, and non-specific anti-inflammatory drugs. If the homeopathic remedy given below does not produce some improvement within 2 weeks, constitutional treatment should be sought. For self-help measures, see conditions mentioned above.

Specific remedy to be taken every 4 hours for up to 2 weeks:

• *Sulphur 6c*

Syphilis

Bacterial infection transmitted during oral, anal, or vaginal intercourse. Though once a killer, the disease is now very rare and is almost always cured before it reaches serious stage; two-thirds of sufferers are men, usually homosexual; blood tests in AIDS patients are also positive for syphilis. Incubation period is 9–90 days; first stage, highly infectious, is a painless sore or chancre on penis, anus, or vulva which disappears in a few weeks; second stage, also highly infectious and lasting for only a few weeks, is a non-itchy rash all over body, including palms of hands and soles of feet, accompanied by swollen lymph glands and moist warts around anus or under arms. Disease then becomes latent, but may re-emerge years later to attack heart valves and walls of arteries supplying brain and vital organs.

Any sores on penis, vulva, or around anus should be promptly investigated by your GP or local STD clinic; it is essential that antibiotics are taken, and that all sexual contacts are traced and treated; intercourse should be refrained from until course of antibiotics is finished and symptoms have disappeared. Afterwards, constitutional homeopathic treatment is recommended.

Men's sexual problems

As men play such an important part in women's lives, we felt that some information about men's special health problems might be of use. As far as the sexual difficulties men encounter is concerned read *Men and Sex* by Bernard Zilbergeld, which deals with the subject excellently (see Books for Further Reading, p. 341.)

Reproductive organs

The testicles manufacture sperm and also produce the male sex hormone testosterone. They lie outside the body, the left usually lower than the right, because sperm production requires slightly cooler conditions than those which reign inside the body. Normally, both testicles descend into the scrotum, the pouch of skin behind the penis, shortly before birth. At puberty they enlarge and begin to produce sperm.

Each testicle consists of an almond-shaped testis, where sperm are manufactured at the rate of 10,000–30,000 million a month, and a much coiled tube called the epididymis, inside which the sperm mature for about 3 weeks. In all it takes 60–72 days for a sperm to develop fully.

From the epididymis, sperm move into the vasa deferentia and seminal vesicles for storage; in the seminal vesicles a sugar-rich fluid is added to provide the sperm with energy. If mature sperm are not ejaculated, they disintegrate and are reabsorbed into the body, but if psychological conditions are right and orgasm occurs, the seminal vesicles and prostate gland contract powerfully, expelling about 3 ml (half a teaspoonful) of semen into the urethra and out of the end of the penis; this is ejaculation. Once in the female reproductive tract, sperm have a maximum life of 3 days. It is not possible to urinate and ejaculate at the same time because the reflexes which cause the bladder to empty automatically shut off entry of semen into the urethra.

The prostate gland is bulb-shaped and completely encircles the urethra at the point where it leaves the bladder. Its role is to add acids, trace elements, and enzymes to seminal fluid at the moment of ejaculation. These activate the sperm and also give semen its distinct smell. For reasons which are not known, the prostate tends to enlarge and stiffen with age, narrowing the exit from the bladder; this obliges the bladder muscles to work harder to expel urine, and can make urination slow and painful.

The penis relies, for its hydraulic power, on three cylinders, two hollow and one spongy. These are arranged protectively around the urethra and only fill with blood during sexual arousal. Erection is maintained by strands of muscle at the base of the penis which slow the rate at which blood drains back into general circulation. The head of the penis is most sensitive to touch, the shaft to pressure.

Infections are the commonest kind of disorder, for although the male urethra is relatively long and less prone to invasion than the female, it has direct communication with the testes, epididymis, and prostate. This means that kidney, bladder, or urethral infections can spread to the organs concerned with reproduction.

Ejaculation problems

Rarely due to any physical disorder, although spinal cord injury, urethral stricture (see PENIS PROBLEMS), or surgical removal of prostate gland or testis may interfere with the ejaculatory mechanism. Ejaculation can occur without orgasm, and if refractory period (time between one climax and the next) is short, orgasm can occur without ejaculation; capacity for repeated ejaculation decreases rapidly after puberty – only 5 per cent of 40-year-olds are capable of ejaculating more than once during a love-making session. Ejaculation during dreams, 'wet dreams', is quite normal.

There is nothing abnormal about 'premature' ejaculation – climaxing before or as soon as penis enters vagina – but it does suggest anxiety, however caused, lack of concern for partner's satisfaction, and perhaps ignorance of female sexual response and of techniques for delaying orgasm. If it happens regularly, it can lead to profound sexual dissatisfaction for both partners; woman begins to feel used, cheated, angry – all of which may depress her desire for sex (see LACK OF DESIRE FOR SEX); man begins to feel self-conscious, dreads climaxing too soon, and may become so anxious about his sexual performance that even erection becomes difficult (see ERECTION PROBLEMS). Rapid orgasm and ejaculation is common at beginning of many relationships; as trust and affection increase and anxiety wears off, timing of orgasm is easier to control. In isolated cases, urethritis (see PENIS PROBLEMS), prostatitis (see PROSTATE PROBLEMS), or a nervous disorder may make it difficult to delay orgasm and ejaculation, but if early ejaculation is causing problems and has no physical basis, try the self-help measures below; if you still feel you need expert help, ask your GP about sex therapy; it may be necessary for you *and* your partner to attend sessions since problem is seldom one-sided. Constitutional homeopathic treatment is strongly recommended; in the meantime, the remedies below are useful dissolvers of anxiety and tension.

Specific remedies to be taken every 12 hours for up to 5 days:

- Feeling short-tempered and impatient, craving excitement, use of drugs such as cocaine *Nux 30c*
- Increased desire for sex accompanied by lack of self-confidence and expectation of failure *Lycopodium 30c*

Self-help
Relax before you make love, and don't make love when you are tired or in a hurry. When orgasm is near, you or your partner should firmly squeeze the penis just below glans; this will not affect erection, but will delay orgasm and ejaculation.

Erection problems
Physical causes include injury or surgery to spinal cord or genitals, chronic illnesses such as diabetes, various nervous disorders, many groups of drugs (tranquillizers, diuretics, anti-depressants, barbiturates, drugs for high blood

pressure and stomach ulcers, recreational drugs such as alcohol, marijuana, cocaine), fatigue, and sometimes lack of appropriate stimulation. It used to be thought that in 90 per cent of cases the inability to have or sustain an erection was due to psychological factors. The current view is that the majority of cases may in fact be due to physical causes. Having said that, STRESS, a state of general mental and emotional turmoil induced by pressures of modern living, or anxiety about intercourse can easily inhibit erectile response. Most men have erectile difficulties at some time in their lives, often with women they feel strongly about, but a single failure or even occasional failure does not spell 'impotence'. However, if fear of failure becomes a self-fulfilling prophecy, try the self-help measures and homeopathic remedies below; constitutional homeopathic treatment is strongly recommended where stress and anxiety are the culprits. If you go to see your GP, you may be offered testosterone or anti-anxiety drugs, injections of papaverine or prostaglandin. Sex therapy is also an option.

Specific remedies to be taken every 12 hours for up to 5 days:

- Surge of desire, anticipation of failure, penis cold and small *Lycopodium 30c*
- Erection not firm enough for penetration, general weakness, penis cold and small, especially if intercourse has been very frequent or if erectile difficulties have come on recently *Agnus 30c*
- Following bruising injury to penis *Arnica 30c*
- Following injury which has bruised spinal cord *Hypericum 30c*
- Erection does not last, great surge of sexual feelings after long abstinence, legs feel cold and cramped *Conium 30c*
- Erectile difficulties associated with dribbles of semen during sleep, increased desire for sex, erotic fantasies *Selenium 30c*
- Erection occurs when half asleep but disappears on waking up; even when sexually excited penis remains flaccid *Caladium 30c*

Self-help
Try making love in different places and at different times, and try out different forms of foreplay; forget intercourse for a while and concentrate on giving and receiving pleasure with all your senses and with every part of your body except your genitals.

Excessive desire for sex
Rarely has a physical cause but may be aggravated by certain drugs; not a problem unless compulsion to have intercourse (see OBSESSIONS AND COMPULSIONS) becomes a burden to the person concerned or makes unreasonable demands on a partner. Constitutional homeopathic treatment may be necessary, but the remedies below should be tried first; if urge to have sex does not become more controllable within 3 weeks, see your GP.

Specific remedies for men, to be taken every 12 hours for up to 5 days:

- Intense desire to have intercourse, ejaculation during erotic dreams *Phosphorus 30c*
- Local irritation of penis *Camphora 30c*
- Profuse ejaculation of semen, great exhaustion, absence of erotic dreams *Picric ac. 30c*
- Man very easily aroused, especially after alcohol or cocaine *Nux 30c*

Specific remedies for partners exhausted by sexual demands, to be taken every 4 hours for up to 3 days:

- Apathy, lethargy, indifference *Phosphoric ac. 30c*
- Physical exhaustion, chilliness, over-sensitivity *China 30c*

Lack of desire for sex
Root cause is usually psychological – STRESS, DEPRESSION, fear of getting pregnant, performance anxiety (see ERECTION PROBLEMS, EJACULATION PROBLEMS, LACK OF ORGASM), and frequently boredom – rather than hormonal or physical. A label such as 'impotence' is old-fashioned and extremely unhelpful. There is no 'normal' level of desire for sex (libido) in men or women, although in both sexes it is the 'male' hormone testosterone which sustains it; testosterone levels can be depressed by poor liver or kidney function, pituitary problems, fatigue, pain, illness, depression, and stress, and also by tranquillizers, opiates, drugs used to treat high blood pressure, appetite suppressants, and alcohol.

In men testosterone production, and therefore libido, slowly declines with age; this leads to less urgency for coitus, slower erection, and delayed orgasm, all of which can add to sexual enjoyment rather than detract from it. In both sexes the ability to be mentally aroused lasts longest.

Treatment of underlying conditions mentioned above is the obvious first step to restoring libido. Where the cause is mainly psychological, sex therapy can be very helpful. Homeopathic approach is constitutional, provided there are no physical problems, but the remedies below should be tried first.

Specific remedies for men, to be taken every 12 hours for up to 5 days:

- Loss of sex drive or positive aversion to sex, premature ejaculation or no ejaculation, especially if herpes is diagnosed *Graphites 30c*
- Premature ejaculation or inability to have an erection *Lycopodium 30c*
- Irritability, self-criticism and extreme sensitivity to real or fancied criticism from others, despair, thoughts of death *Nitric ac. 30c*
- Formation of allergies *Apis 30c*
- Apathy and indifference *Phosphoric ac. 30c*

Phimosis see PENIS PROBLEMS

Painful intercourse

In men a burning sensation when ejaculating or urinating, and perhaps unusual discharge from penis, suggests urethritis (see PENIS PROBLEMS) or prostatitis (see PROSTATE PROBLEMS); pain during intercourse may be balanitis (see PENIS PROBLEMS) or herpes (see SEXUALLY TRANSMITTED DISEASES), especially if head of penis is red, itchy, sore, or blistered. Soreness or itchiness around head of penis after intercourse suggests sensitivity to spermicidal creams or vaginal secretions; problem is easily solved by using a sheath; if the rubber of the sheath causes an allergic reaction, switch to a non-allergenic brand. Occasionally the tip of the penis may be irritated by friction against trailing threads of the partner's IUD; this can be solved by asking your GP to shorten the threads. Erection and intercourse can also be painful if the foreskin is too tight (see PHIMOSIS); if the foreskin has recently been removed, intercourse may be painful for several months until the glans becomes less sensitive.

For orthodox and homeopathic treatment, see causative conditions mentioned above.

Non-specific urethritis see SEXUALLY
TRANSMITTED DISEASES

Penis problems

Balanitis

Swelling and soreness of foreskin or head of penis, often caused by friction against damp underwear, or by irritants in sheaths and contraceptive creams; can also be caused by the herpes virus (see SEXUALLY TRANSMITTED DISEASES). Complaint is most common in men who suffer from diabetes mellitus, since sugar in urine encourages microbes to flourish. If homeopathic remedy and self-help measures mentioned below do not clear problem up, see your GP; an antibiotic cream will probably be prescribed, but if inflammation keeps recurring, making it difficult or painful to draw back foreskin, your GP may recommend circumcision.

Specific remedy to be taken every 4 hours for up to 5 days:

- *Mercurius 6c*

Self-help In addition to taking the remedy above, bathe foreskin and head of penis with Hypericum and Calendula solution (5 drops of mother tincture of each to 0.25 litre [½ pint] boiled cooled water) every 4 hours. Always keep penis clean and dry, and wash well under foreskin.

Blood in sperm (haemospermia)

Pink, red, or brown streaks in semen due to rupture of small veins in urethra during erection; quite common, but harmless, and usually clears up within a day or two; however, if blood appears in urine, see your GP as soon as possible.

Injury

Usually the testicles rather than the penis bear the brunt of blows to the groin. The most common injury to the penis is getting it caught in a trouser zip; if this happens, cut the zip free of trousers and go to the nearest hospital casualty department; in the meantime, bathe the wound with Hypericum and Calendula solution (5 drops of mother tincture of each to 0.25 litre [½ pint] boiled cooled water); attempting to undo the zip, especially if you are not circumcised, may make matters worse.

Painful penis

If pain accompanies erection, the cause may be that the foreskin is too tight or PRIAPISM (erection occurring in absence of sexual excitement); if pain is felt during intercourse, partner's vagina may be too dry; after intercourse, inflammation or soreness may be due to chemicals in sheath, cap, spermicidal creams, etc. Redness or swelling of the head of the penis may be BALANITIS. Painful open sores are likely to be due to herpes (see SEXUALLY TRANSMITTED DISEASES); lumps or bumps caused by penile warts (see below) or syphilis (see SEXUALLY TRANSMITTED DISEASES) are generally painless.

Penile warts (condylomata)

Like warts elsewhere on body, virally caused and moderately contagious; not necessarily contracted through sexual intercourse, although susceptible individuals easily become re-infected if a partner has genital warts. Since wart-like growths can be the first sign of cancer of the penis or of syphilis (see SEXUALLY TRANSMITTED DISEASES), ask your GP for diagnosis as soon as possible.

Conventionally treated by very careful application of specially prescribed wart paint; over-the-counter preparations should be avoided. Homeopathic treatment is constitutional, but while treatment is being sought one of the remedies below should be tried. Your partner should also be examined and treated if necessary.

Specific remedies to be taken 4 times daily for up to 14 days:

- Remedy of first resort *Thuja 6c*
- If Thuja produces no improvement, and if foreskin is swollen and warts bleed *Cinnabar 6c*
- Warts accompanied by inability to obtain erection, or by great increase in sexual desire and premature ejaculation *Lycopodium 6c*

Phimosis
Foreskin which is too tight to draw back from head of penis; may not be diagnosed until first erection, which causes considerable pain, although the condition is usually diagnosed much earlier; showing a child, from age of 3 or so onwards, how to gently draw back the foreskin to wash underneath it may help to prevent problem. Condition may require surgical removal of foreskin, but in meantime one of the remedies below might help.

Specific remedies to be given 3 times daily for up to 14 days:

- Itching and irritation under foreskin, ejaculation during sleep *Mercurius 6c*
- Painful erections, foreskin swollen, with itchy pimples on it *Jacaranda 6c*

Self-help If foreskin itches, bathe it and head of penis with Hypericum and Calendula solution (5 drops of mother tincture of each to 0.25 litre [½ pint] warm water).

Priapism
Rare and painful condition in which penis erects and stays erect even though individual is not sexually aroused; cause is sudden, inexplicable obstruction of outflow of blood from penis, or injury to nerves in spinal cord. A priapismic erection lasting for longer than 3 or 4 hours can do lasting damage to spongy tissues of penis, making further erection impossible, so appropriate action is ②. Surgery may be needed to assist excess blood in penis to drain back into general circulation. In meantime, give one of the homeopathic remedies below.

Specific remedies to be given every 15 minutes for up to 10 doses:

- General feebleness and impotence *Kali brom. 6c*
- Erection usually painful *Cantharis 6c*
- Generally sluggish venous system, individual may have piles or varicose veins *Carbo veg. 6c*

Self-help A 3-week course of vitamin E is strongly recommended; take 100 units a day to begin with, increasing intake to 600 units a day. If suffering from high blood pressure, see your GP first as vitamin E can temporarily raise blood pressure.

Thrush
Fungal infection mainly found in women but occasionally in men if genital hygiene is poor or sexual partner is infected; yeast grows under foreskin of penis, causing itching and inflammation. Conventional treatment consists of antifungal cream (see also THRUSH).

Specific remedy to be taken 4 times daily for up to 14 days:

- *Mercurius 6c*

Self-help Bathe penis in Hypericum and Calendula solution (5 drops of mother tincture of each to 0.25 litre [½ pint] boiled cooled water) 4 times a day for up to 15 days, then apply Calendula ointment.

Trichomoniasis
Caused by trichomonas organism which lurks under the foreskin of the penis, causing soreness and inflammation; condition is far more common in women than in men, and may be the result of poor genital hygiene or intercourse with an infected partner. Conventionally treated with drugs such as Metronidazole. See THRUSH for homeopathic treatment.

Urethral stricture
Rare condition in which the urethra becomes narrowed by scar tissue as the result of injury or infection, making urination and ejaculation painful or impossible; shrinkage of urethra may also force the penis into a bent position. Occasionally, urethra may narrow as result of nervous spasm. If homeopathic remedies below do not improve matters, see your GP; the urethra may have to be stretched under local anaesthetic, or scar tissue may have to be incised or replaced with a graft.

Specific remedies to be taken twice daily for up to 1 month in chronic cases:

- Stricture due to scarring *Silicea 6c*

- Sore, burning sensation when passing water *Cantharis 6c*
- Discharge of pus *Mercurius 6c*
- Nervous spasm and discharge of pus *Camphora 6c*

Specific remedy to be taken every hour for up to 10 doses in acute cases:

- Painful spasms during urination, tingling or smarting sensation when not urinating *Aconite 30c*

Self-help Bathe the penis in cold water twice a day – easiest way to do this is in the shower. Avoid spicy foods, and take a 3-week course of vitamin E, gradually increasing dosage from 100 units to 600 units a day but see note under priapism in PENIS PROBLEMS.

Urethritis
Inflammation of urethra, often caused by infection transmitted during sexual intercourse; symptoms are a burning sensation when urinating or ejaculating, and a thick yellowish discharge from tip of penis. See CYSTITIS and SEXUALLY TRANSMITTED DISEASES (gonorrhea and non-specific urethritis) for conventional and homeopathic treatment and self-help measures. Intercourse should be refrained from until symptoms disappear; repeated infection can cause urethral stricture (see above).

Priapism see PENIS PROBLEMS

Prostate problems

Enlarged prostate
Extremely common in men over 45, although cause is not known; symptomless until tissues become sufficiently stiff and enlarged to interfere with expulsion of urine from bladder; at this point sufferer may find it difficult to start stream of urine, especially in mornings, despite urgent signals from bladder, and may have to get up several times in night; the stream of urine is also weak, and there may be blood in it; some sufferers complain of a dragging sensation between the legs. Symptoms clear up of their own accord in 1 in 3 of mild cases; however, if the condition persists and is not treated, possible complications include CYSTITIS (bladder infection), acute pyelonephritis (kidney infection), retention of urine (bladder expands to hold more urine, less and less urine passed), and eventually kidney failure. A localized lump rather than general enlargement suggests the possibility of cancer of prostate; to rule out cancer, a biopsy is necessary.

Excess prostate tissue can be removed surgically by making an incision in the abdomen or by passing very slender instruments through the urethra; most prostatectomy operations completely relieve urinary difficulties, but ability to obtain an erection and ejaculate sperm is sometimes lost.

Specific remedies to be taken 4 times daily for up to 21 days:

- Difficult or painful urination, with spasms of bladder or urethra *Sabal 6c*
- Where person is senile, urinates frequently at night, complains of pressure on rectum and smarting sensation at neck of bladder *Ferrum pic. 6c*
- Frequent urge to urinate, slow stream of urine, person thin, underweight, prematurely impotent *Baryta 6c*
- Frequent, urgent desire to pass urine *Thuja 6c*
- Loss of potency, shrunken testes, prostate gland feels hard, though hardness may not be due to cancer *Iodum 6c*
- Impotence because erection is lost on penetration, or lack of desire for sex, or pain on intercourse *Argentum nit. 6c*

Self-help Many sufferers find that Lecithin and calcium and magnesium tablets help – both are obtainable from chemists and healthfood shops. Correct dosages are 2 or 3 dessertspoons of Lecithin per day, and one calcium and magnesium tablet 3 times a day for 1 month. Evening primrose oil can also be beneficial.

Prostatitis
Inflammation of the prostate, usually due to infection spreading from elsewhere in the urinary tract; an acute attack causes fever, pain and tenderness around base of penis, and difficulty passing urine; if left untreated, the prostate may fill with pus and burst, releasing pus into urethra and causing further infection. The condition is most common in elderly men with enlarged prostates (see above), and tends to recur; a mild attack may clear up of its own accord. Conventionally treated by antibiotics; in resistant cases, pus may need to be drained surgically. Homeopathic treatment is constitutional, but in an acute attack the remedies below may help; if there is no improvement within 24 hours, see your GP.

Specific remedies to be taken every 2 hours for up to 10 doses:

- Where prostate is enlarged and area around prostate feels cold, or where ejaculation is impossible or intercourse is painful *Sabal 6c*

- Burning sensation at neck of bladder, frequent urge to pass urine *Thuja 6c*
- Thick yellow discharge from penis, urgent need to pass urine, lying on back makes matters worse *Pulsatilla 6c*

Self-help If condition is mild but recurrent, extra zinc and two daily 10–15 ml doses of cold-pressed linseed oil may be beneficial.

Testicle and scrotum problems

It is very important to detect problems early by regular examination of testicles, preferably in a hot bath so that scrotal muscles are relaxed; the testes themselves should feel smooth through skin of scrotum; the epididymis should feel cord-like, with no noticeable bumps or lumps; any nodules, areas of tenderness, or swelling should be reported to your GP.

Enlarged or painful testicle

A painless lump in one testicle is most likely to be an epididymal cyst (see below); in rare cases, it may be cancer of the testicle. A painful swelling in one testicle, followed by pain and swelling of scrotum, suggests torsion or epididymitis (see below); both conditions require prompt medical attention, so ②. A blow to the testicles can cause severe pain; if pain does not wear off within an hour or so, or if the scrotum is obviously bruised and swollen, ②; surgery may be necessary to prevent internal bleeding causing permanent damage to testes; in meantime, give Arnica 30c every 5 minutes for up to 10 doses.

Epididymal cysts

These are benign, painless, fluid-filled swellings which develop in one or more of the many tubes leading from testis to seminal vesicle; quite common in men over 40, and can occur in one or both testicles; since the epididymis lies behind the testis, swelling is usually located in the upper rear part of testicle. Surgery is seldom necessary or advised, as it can result in partial sterility. Constitutional homeopathic treatment is recommended, but the remedies below should be tried first.

Specific remedies to be taken 4 times daily for up to 7 days:

- Remedy of first resort *Apis 30c*
- If Apis does not reduce swelling *Graphites 6c*

Epididymitis

Bacterial infection of epididymis, usually as result of urinary tract infection; results in a hot, tender, painful swelling at back of one testicle. Conventionally treated with antibiotics; however, the remedies given below should be tried first. If there is no improvement within 12 hours, see your GP.

Specific remedies to be taken every hour for up to 10 doses:

- Testicle extremely hot, red, swollen, tender, and sensitive to slightest jarring *Belladonna 30c*
- Infection onsets very suddenly, dramatic swelling of testicle, pains in scrotum and lower abdomen *Pulsatilla 6c*
- Fever, restlessness, infection comes on after exposure to cold dry winds *Aconite 30c*
- Testicle hot, swollen, and aching as if someone had kicked it, pains shooting up towards bladder *Hamamelis 6c*

Hydrocele

Excess fluid in double-layered sheath around testis, causing soft, painless swelling; in most cases, the cause is not known, though occasionally the condition is precipitated by injury; most common in older men. Condition is usually kept under observation rather than treated, but if swelling is large, GP may recommend drawing off excess fluid under local anaesthetic; if this does not prevent recurrence, surgery may be necessary. If the homeopathic remedies below produce no improvement within a month or so, see your homeopath.

Specific remedies to be taken 3 times daily for up to 3 weeks:

- Swelling follows injury *Arnica 30c*
- If Arnica does not help *Bryonia 30c*
- Testicle tends to ache in thundery weather *Rhododendron 6c*

Torsion of the testicle

Occurs when one of testicles twists out of its natural position, pinching veins and blocking outflow of blood; the result is sharp pain, sometimes sharp enough to cause nausea and vomiting, and swelling. The condition is rare, but can happen at any time, even in sleep; in susceptible individuals, double-layered sheath enclosing testis is not as close-fitting as it should be. The twist often undoes itself spontaneously, but if it doesn't, ② as arteries as well as veins may become blocked. While waiting for medical help, take *Aconite 30c* every 5 minutes for up to 10 doses. Standard treatment is surgical exploration as this is the only sure way to prevent torsion recurring.

Varicocele

Abnormal distension of veins draining one of the testicles, analogous to VARICOSE VEINS in legs;

symptoms are swelling, which disappears when lying down, and a dragging pain, especially in hot weather or after exercise; problem is most common in adolescence; in rare cases, increase in local heat can interfere with fertility. The pain and dragging sensation can be relieved by supporting testicles with a jock strap; surgery to remove or bypass distended veins is not always successful.

Specific remedies to be taken 2 times daily for up to 21 days:

• Person pale and anaemic, pain made worse by pressure but relieved by cold applications *Ferrum phos. 6c*
• Pain radiates up from testicle into lower abdomen, person also suffers from piles *Hamamelis 6c*
• Heat and lying on painless side make pain in testicle worse, cold applications relieve pain *Pulsatilla 6c*

Urethral stricture see PENIS PROBLEMS

Urethritis see PENIS PROBLEMS

Varicocele see TESTICLE AND SCROTUM PROBLEMS

Fertility and Pregnancy

Anyone searching for evidence of miracles need look no further than the process of conception. Every month, as each ripe egg is released from its ovary and enters the Fallopian tube, the mucus at the entrance to the womb becomes less sticky. If intercourse takes place, millions of vigorously swimming sperm make their way through the mucus, into the womb, and into the Fallopian tubes. Here they congregate around the egg, causing it to spin round with the movement of their beating tails. Eventually one sperm penetrates the egg, the nuclei of sperm and egg fuse, and the process of cell division begins. The fused nuclei split into 2 cells, then 4, then 8, then 16, all containing the 46 individual packages of information or chromosomes which will create a new and totally unique human being.

7 days after fertilization the ball of cells embeds itself in the wall of the uterus. At 20 days the placenta begins to form, at 30 days the spinal cord, at 6 weeks the heart, and by 13 weeks all the body organs are formed. At 5 months the baby can be felt to move. At 6 months the lungs become functional and the nostrils open. At 7 months the baby turns into the head down position ready for birth.

A full-time pregnancy usually lasts 38 weeks, counting from the moment of conception to the

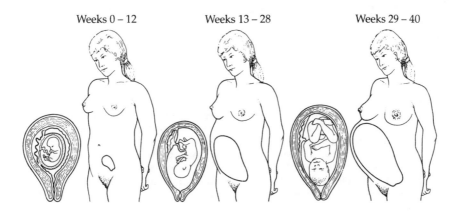

Weeks 0 – 12   Weeks 13 – 28   Weeks 29 – 40

The stages of pregnancy

time the baby is born. Conception usually takes place halfway between periods if your cycle is 28 days and regular. However, since many women's periods are not exactly 28 days, pregnancy is usually measured as being 40 weeks from the first day of the last period. Common pointers to pregnancy are missing a period, more than usually tender or swollen breasts and darker nipples, nausea, tiredness, a frequent urge to pass urine, and sometimes loss of appetite or cravings for unusual foods. To confirm your pregnancy you should have a pregnancy test. This can be done by your GP, a family planning clinic, or a pregnancy testing service. If you use a home pregnancy testing kit from the chemist, read the instructions very carefully, and if you are still in doubt see your chemist or GP.

Your chances of having twins are about 1 : 80! Identical twins develop from the same egg and share the same placenta; non-identical twins develop from different eggs and have a placenta each. Only three pairs of twins in every ten are identical. Triplets are much rarer, only occurring in 1 : 6,400 pregnancies. According to recent evidence, efforts to determine the sex of a baby by having intercourse at a particular time during ovulation or by altering the acid-alkaline balance of the vagina do not work.

Once you have established that you are pregnant, do go for regular antenatal check-ups, even it it means frustrating waits in hospital antenatal clinics or in your GP's waiting room. Normally your GP will share your antenatal care with a midwife and a hospital consultant. If you want to have your baby at home, write to the Supervisor of Midwives at your local Maternity Unit, stating you intend having a home birth and asking her to provide you with a midwife.

Antenatal care is important since it allows you to find out at an early stage if there are any problems. Ultrasound (a sound picture of the baby in the womb) is thought to be harmless to mother and baby and can be used to monitor the size, shape and position of the baby at any stage of pregnancy. Amniocentesis (taking a sample of the amniotic fluid around your baby) is usually carried out between 16 and 18 weeks, but only if a previous baby has been abnormal or there is a family history of congenital problems, or if the mother is over 35. An earlier test, chorion villous biopsy, can be done at 10 weeks in some centres. Conditions such as spina bifida or Down's syndrome can be detected in this way. However, the procedure does involve a slight risk of miscarriage. You should also consider carefully what your attitude would be if your baby was found to be abnormal. Would you want to terminate the pregnancy or not?

In brief, some of the dos and don'ts of pregnancy are as follows:

1 Treat your developing baby as a person – moderate exercise, swimming and walking in the fresh air, are very good, but avoid anything which involves repeated compression of the spine, such as horse-riding or trampolining.
2 Try to keep 25 per cent of your energy in reserve.
3 Go to antenatal classes. They will teach you what to expect and how to breathe in order to cope with pain during labour.
4 As your tummy expands avoid tight-fitting clothes.
5 Get as much sleep as you can, and avoid late nights wherever possible.
6 If you faint easily or have a tendency to bleed, do not sit in a hot bath for longer than 10 minutes or so.
7 If you have had a threatened miscarriage, or there are complications in your pregnancy, or you suffer from travel sickness, avoid travelling any great distance. Most airlines prefer women not to fly after 32 weeks. If you must fly, check with the airline first.
8 If your work is very strenuous or stressful, try and stop before the time when maternity benefit can be claimed.
9 It is important that pregnant women should reheat cooked, chilled meals and ready-to-eat poultry until they are piping hot rather than eating them cold.
10 Avoid smoking at all.

The old idea that an expectant mother needs to 'eat for two' has been comprehensively demolished in recent years. Everything depends on the efficiency of the mother's metabolism. Increase consumption of iron and calcium foods and also ensure a modest increase in protein intake, preferably in the form of oily fish, nuts, seeds, pulses and wholegrains. The latter, with generous helpings of raw vegetables and fruit, will help to guard against constipation. Tea, coffee, and alcohol should be avoided in the first 14 weeks, and if you have problems with HYPOGLYCAEMIA make sure that your diet is pretty strict, especially for the first trimester.

As for sex during pregnancy, there are no rules really, except to say that if you do not feel like it your partner should respect your wishes. Intercourse during the first 16 weeks should be avoided if you have had a threatened miscarriage or previous miscarriages; it is also unwise if there is still occasional vaginal bleeding, or if you are excessively nervous and worried about the effects of intercourse on your pregnancy. In the later months of pregnancy, deep penetration should be avoided. There are women who feel that orgasms in the later stages of pregnancy make labour less painful.

Homeopathic remedies during pregnancy During the first three months of pregnancy, the most vulnerable time, you should AVOID ALL MEDICATION if you possibly can. This includes, especially in the first 14 weeks, stopping smoking and drinking alcohol and any 'street' or over-the-counter drugs. If you are on medication consult your doctor about giving it up. The main drugs to avoid are aspirin and other non-steroidal anti-inflammatories, which can cause foetal heart problems and delay the onset of labour because of their inhibition of prostaglandin production. Under other circumstances this may be a good thing (see MISCARRIAGE). Aspirin and ibuprofen may lead to increased blood loss during delivery; therefore do not take in last 3 months. Of the antibiotics only penicillin and cephalosporins are considered safe. Other antibiotics and anti-fungals, apart from Nystatin, should be avoided if at all possible. Magnesium trisilicate is too high in sodium, as is Gaviscon. Avoid over-the-counter medicines containing codeine either as a painkiller or cough linctus, as they can cause constipation. Neither should you take herbs, vitamin and mineral supplements. You should even avoid homeopathic remedies unless they are really necessary. There is no evidence that homeopathic remedies cause any problems during pregnancy, but to be on the safe side they should not be taken in potencies less than 6c except for tissue salts. It is probably best to avoid low potency Apis altogether and take 30c if you need to.

There are many schools of thought among homeopaths as to the most appropriate treatment f or pregnancy. There are homeopaths who only treat if there are symptoms to treat; others recommend a 'miasmatic clear-out', giving nosodes for all the diseases or weaknesses which appear in the family history; others favour a systemic clear-out using Sulphur, Calcium carb., Lycopodium, and tissue salts; others favour constitutional treatment for both the mother and the father; others give Caulophyllum in the last stages of pregnancy to stimulate the womb.

In fact pregnancy is a very good time to treat someone because constitutional features tend to declare themselves very strongly due to the general mobilization of the Vital Force. Also by treating the mother's symptoms the baby can be treated as well. Indeed some of the mother's symptoms are the baby's. Our treatment approach depends on the length of time we have known the parents and the family, the family's medical history, the health of the mother during pregnancy, and sometimes the health of the father too. Where possible we advise pre-conceptual constitutional treatment for both parents.

For minor complaints during pregnancy, homeopathic remedies should be tried first. If you feel very unwell, see your GP before taking anything.

Abdominal pain in pregnancy

Griping, pinching sensations in the lower abdomen, most common during the first trimester of pregnancy, and sometimes described as 'colic'. If pain persists for more than 3 hours, especially if it is associated with vaginal bleeding, an ECTOPIC PREGNANCY should be suspected; appropriate action is ②.

Specific remedies to be taken ½-hourly for up to 6 doses:

- Griping sensation behind navel, bowels full of trapped wind, symptoms brought on by anger *Chamomilla 6c*
- Constipation, ineffectual straining to pass stools *Nux 6c*
- Bowels feel as if they are being clutched by a hand, hot, bloated feeling, discomfort made worse by jarring *Belladonna 30c*
- Bowels feel as if they are being pinched between two stones, pain relieved by bending double or pressing hand hard against abdomen *Colocynth 6c*

Abortion see TERMINATION OF PREGNANCY

Anaemia during pregnancy see also ANAEMIA
pp. 217–18

Ideally, of course, anaemia should be corrected before conception. However, iron deficiency anaemia and folic acid deficiency anaemia can develop quite quickly during pregnancy; symptoms are pallor, fingernails which look unhealthily white, tiredness, weakness, fainting, breathlessness, even palpitations. Vitamin B_{12} deficiency anaemia, which mainly affects vegetarians, is of more insidious onset; in addition to the symptoms above there may be abdominal pain, weight loss, yellowing of the skin, and tingling in hands or feet. The main dangers of anaemia are to the mother rather than the foetus; low iron and haemoglobin levels can predispose her to post-natal infections and POSTNATAL DEPRESSION.

The forms of anaemia mentioned above usually respond to dietary change or nutritional supplements (see PART 4). Green leafy vegetables contain plenty of folic acid. Vitamin B_{12} is a constituent of animal products and of brewer's yeast.

Iron can be taken in the form of iron tablets, with extra vitamin C or tissue salts Ferrum phos. and Calcarea phos. to aid absorption and assimilation. It is not necessary, or advisable, to take iron supplements during pregnancy if you are not anaemic.

Antepartum haemorrhage
Bleeding from the vagina any time after the 28th week of pregnancy; before then, bleeding is classified as a threatened MISCARRIAGE. Sometimes due to a burst varicose vein in the vagina or damage to the cervix; more seriously, blood loss may be due to PLACENTA PRAEVIA, in which part of the placenta becomes detached from the wall of the womb (placental abruption), preventing an adequate flow of nutrients to the foetus and slowing foetal growth; in severe cases, this can be fatal to mother and foetus.

Any bleeding after the 28th week requires prompt investigation; the best course is (2), or (999) if bleeding is very heavy. You will probably be admitted to hospital; if you have lost too much blood, the situation may be stabilized by a blood transfusion, or it may be necessary to induce labour or deliver the baby by Caesarean.

Specific remedies to be taken every 5–10 minutes for up to 6 doses until help arrives:

- Sudden onset of bleeding, fear for baby's life *Aconite 30c*
- Bleeding brought on by injury *Arnica 30c*
- If Arnica does not stop bleeding *Bryonia 30c*
- Blood bright red and hot *Belladonna 30c*
- Bleeding profuse and continuous, feeling sick *Ipecac. 30c*
- Blood partially clotted, slightest movement seems to increase blood loss, shooting pains in vagina *Sabina 30c*
- Blood loss temporarily stopped, feeling exhausted and very much on edge *China 30c*

Backache during pregnancy
Lower back pain is common in pregnancy as extra weight accumulates forward of the spine and as the ligaments of the pelvis begin to stretch in preparation for birth. Extra care should be taken when bending, lifting, or twisting; when standing and walking, the baby's weight should not be allowed to pull the pelvis too far forward; when side-lying, a pillow buttress for the abdomen takes some of the strain off the lower back.

Specific remedies to be taken 4 times daily for up to 7 days:

- Back feels weak and tired, dragging pains in middle and lower back *Kali carb. 6c*

- Hard, tense feeling in lower abdomen, head feels hot *Belladonna 6c*
- Hard, tense feeling in lower abdomen, feeling hot all over, symptoms worse in stuffy rooms *Pulsatilla 6c*
- Hard, tense feeling in lower abdomen, feeling chilly *Nux 6c*

Specific remedy to be taken 2-hourly for up to 10 doses:

- Backache due to injury or strain *Arnica 30c*, followed by *Rhus tox. 6c* every 6–8 hours for up to 7 days if backache persists.

Self-help
If you are prone to backache even when you are not pregnant, take tissue salts Calcarea fluor. and Calcarea phos. 3 times daily for 5 days out of 7 during pregnancy.

Bleeding see MISCARRIAGE, ANTE-PARTUM HAEMORRHAGE

Breast discomfort during pregnancy
Distension of the breasts during the first few months of pregnancy is quite normal, and due to hormone changes; in the last 2 or 3 months, feelings of fullness and discomfort are due to incoming milk. However, if discomfort is accompanied by fever and tender glands under the armpits, MASTITIS should be suspected, in which case 12.

Specific remedies to be taken 4-hourly for up to 5 days:

- Mild discomfort caused by enlargement *Conium 6c*
- Breasts feel hard and tense *Bryonia 6c*
- Breasts feel hard and tense, with red streaking of skin *Belladonna 6c*

Breech and other mal-presentations
Before 36 weeks it is sometimes possible to turn a baby in the womb – that is, turn the head down and the buttocks up, or turn the body so that the baby is facing the mother's buttocks – by giving three doses of Pulsatilla 30c at 12-hour intervals. If the mal-presentation persists, the baby may have to be delivered by forceps or Caesarean.

Cardiovascular problems during pregnancy
Pregnancy puts extra strain on the heart and circulatory system. It is not uncommon, for example, for heart murmurs to develop during pregnancy; these represent slight alterations in blood flow through the heart and are usually not serious, but your GP will probably want

to investigate. If you have an existing heart problem, rest as much as possible during pregnancy, don't smoke, learn some form of relaxation or meditation and see dietary suggestions for HIGH BLOOD PRESSURE. If you have a congenital heart defect, see your GP; he or she will probably send you to see a specialist. If one of your heart valves is damaged antibiotics may be prescribed to prevent infection, which could prove fatal, but if you are unable or unwilling to take antibiotics, take 3 doses of Silicea 6c for 5 days out of 7 throughout pregnancy. To relieve the strain which delivery puts on the heart, you may need an episiotomy (an incision in the vulva so that the baby's head slips out more easily).

High blood pressure

This can be due to general anxiety; constitutional homeopathic treatment, rest, relaxation, and the diet suggestions given below will almost certainly help. If high blood pressure is accompanied by headaches, blurred vision, nausea, vomiting, intolerance of light, and swollen ankles, the chances are that you are developing PRE-ECLAMPTIC TOXAEMIA so ②.

Self-help Change to a diet low in animal protein and high in raw vegetables and fruit. Cut down on your salt intake.

Palpitations

These are not uncommon during pregnancy; they are a sign that the heart is having to work harder to pump an increased volume of blood.

Specific remedies to be taken every 2 hours for up to 10 doses:

- Palpitations onset suddenly after a shock of some sort, fear of dying *Aconite 30c*
- Palpitations brought on by heat or rich, fatty food, general weakness *Pulsatilla 6c*
- Palpitations worse at night, especially when lying on left side *Lycopodium 6c*
- Heartbeats seem to shake whole body, constricted feeling in chest, heat and sympathy make discomfort worse *Natrum mur. 6c*

Swollen ankles

These are most common in the 6th and 7th month of pregnancy, tend to occur in women who take too little exercise and whose lymphatic drainage is poor; rest and walking usually improve matters. More seriously, puffy ankles can be a sign of HIGH BLOOD PRESSURE or developing PRE-ECLAMPTIC TOXAEMIA. Provided your GP rules out the latter, constitutional homeopathic treatment would be beneficial.

Swollen or inflamed vulva

This has similar causes to swollen ankles.

Specific remedies to be taken 4 times daily for up to 7 days:

- Bearing down sensation as if contents of womb are about to escape through vagina, sensation makes you cross your legs *Sepia 6c*
- Itchy, raw, scalding sensation after passing water, soothed by washing *Mercurius 6c*
- Vulval swelling associated with constipation, ineffectual straining to pass stools and always feeling there is more to come, urge to urinate *Nux 6c*
- Vulva and vagina excessively tender and itchy, but too sensitive to scratch *Coffea 6c*
- Swelling due to venereal disease *Thuja 6c*

Varicose veins

These are usually aggravated rather than caused by pregnancy, as the weight of the uterus begins to bear down on the veins of the pelvis. Usually one leg is more affected than the other; exercise tends to make distended veins more painful, and in severe cases they may burst. Get as much rest as possible, with legs raised above hip level, and avoid constricting clothing.

Specific remedies to be taken every 4 hours for up to 2 weeks:

- Remedy of first resort *Pulsatilla 6c*
- If Pulsatilla does not work, and skin is marbled, with knotted, painful veins *Carbo veg. 6c*
- One foot hot, the other cold *Lycopodium 6c*

Cervical incompetence

Weakness of the cervix which causes it to open up at some time after the 12th week of pregnancy and cause MISCARRIAGE; weakness may be due to damage caused by previous deliveries or by D & Cs (stretching of the cervix in order to remove a foetus, fibroids, or cysts from the uterus). Standard treatment is a minor operation in which a suture is put around the cervix, like a purse string, and tightened; it is removed at 38 weeks, unless labour begins earlier.

Constipation during pregnancy

see also CONSTIPATION p. 224

The hormone which maintains pregnancy, progesterone, decreases the tone of the bowel muscles, and the growing foetus also presses on the large intestine; the net result is delayed transit of faeces. If constipation does not respond to the homeopathic remedies or self-help measures below see your GP. On no account take laxatives – they may cause MISCARRIAGE or premature labour.

Specific remedies to be taken 4 times daily for up to 14 days:

- Dull headache, feeling of fullness in rectum, frequent but unsuccessful straining to pass stools *Nux 6c*
- Hard, knobbly stools, never emptying bowels properly, piles or inflammation around anus *Sulphur 6c*
- Hard, dry, burnt-looking stools, especially during morning, discomfort made worse by movement and cold drinks, thirst for large quantities of fluid at infrequent intervals *Bryonia 6c*
- Large, hard stools, rectum feels as if there is a hard ball inside it, pains which shoot up rectum *Sepia 6c*
- No desire to pass stools unless rectum is full, even soft stools are difficult to pass *Alumina 6c*
- Hard, small stools, passed with difficulty, never emptying bowels properly, ineffectual straining, passing a lot of wind *Lycopodium 6c*

Self-help
Drink more, increase the amount of fibre in your diet. Try taking oranges and prunes, take more exercise and never suppress the urge to pass stools. If these measures fail, try taking psyllium husks or linseeds, once a day to begin with, then three times a day; the correct dose is 1 teaspoon husks (1 dessertspoon linseeds) stirred into a cup of water and drunk immediately, followed by 2 more cups of water. Most healthfood shops stock both psyllium husks and linseeds.

Contraception
We feel that this book is not the place for a full discussion of contraception. Contraceptive requirements vary considerably from couple to couple, and we recommend that you discuss them with a suitably trained person such as your GP or Family Planning Clinic before coming to a decision. Unfortunately there is no such thing as a homeopathic contraceptive which would be completely free from side-effects! We would also like to point out that breastfeeding, which has a mildly contraceptive effect, is not reliable enough on its own to be used as a method of contraception.

Cramp during pregnancy
Cramp in the calves is common during pregnancy, and very exhausting if it occurs at night as well as during the day.

Specific remedies to be taken every 4 hours for up to 7 days:

- Cramp worst in calves, but relieved by warmth and walking *Veratrum 6c*
- Cramp in calves and soles of feet, numbness or pins and needles in arms and hands, rest relieves discomfort, cold makes it worse *Nux 6c*
- Cramp mainly affects left leg but wears off when pressure is applied *Colocynth 6c*
- Legs feel cold and numb, but better for cold applications *Ledum 6c*

Self-help
If cramp is persistent take Magnesia phos. tissue salts as well as one of the remedies above. You might also consider calcium or magnesium supplements.

Cravings and aversions during pregnancy
Strong food likes and dislikes during the first 3–4 months of pregnancy are very common, but not compulsory! If health is good, there is nothing to worry about. However, if cravings or aversions persist, try one of the remedies listed in the Remedy Finder for WEIGHT PROBLEMS. The remedy you choose should be taken in 6c potency 3 times daily for up to 6 days.

Diabetes during pregnancy
Can declare itself during pregnancy, especially if previous babies have weighed 4 kg (9 lb) or more at birth. If urine tests during regular antenatal check-ups reveal high levels of glucose, you will be given a glucose-tolerance test; if this is positive, your GP will prescribe dietary and/or insulin treatment as necessary. Constitutional homeopathic treatment is also recommended.

Pre-existing or not, diabetes during pregnancy requires careful management since risks to mother and baby are twice as high as normal; risk of neonatal death is also much higher. If diabetes is severe, you may need to spend the last 10 weeks of pregnancy in hospital; induction or a Caesarean may be recommended at 36 weeks.

Self-help
Control of diabetes takes considerable self-discipline, especially where diet is concerned. Your GP may give you a detailed diet sheet, but if not, follow the BLOOD SUGAR LEVELLING DIET on p. 265.

Diarrhoea during pregnancy
see also DIARRHOEA p. 225

The danger of diarrhoea during pregnancy is that it may trigger off a MISCARRIAGE. If 3 or more successive bowel movements are very loose and watery, ②. In the meantime, select a remedy from the list below.

Specific remedies to be taken every hour for up to 10 doses:

- Cramping pains in abdomen, yellow-green stools which look like chopped egg *Chamomilla 6c*
- Cramping pains in abdomen, stools yellow-green and watery, slimy tongue and bitter taste in mouth, no thirst, symptoms worse at night *Pulsatilla 6c*
- Diarrhoea follows over-chilling after exertion *Dulcamara 6c*
- Diarrhoea makes you rush to the lavatory first thing in morning, no abdominal pain *Sulphur 6c*

Ectopic pregnancy

This occurs in the first three months. Development of foetus in one of the Fallopian tubes or in the abdominal cavity rather than in the uterus; symptoms are persistent abdominal pain and bleeding, as placenta burrows into surrounding tissues to establish foetal blood supply; cause may be some abnormality of the Fallopian tubes due to previous operations or infections, or the presence of an IUD. If there is bleeding and abdominal pain lasting for more than 3 hours, ②; you will be sent to hospital, and may need an operation to remove the developing pregnancy, and possibly the tube as well. If the other tube is in good shape, you stand a good chance of becoming pregnant again, and in the normal way.

Specific remedies to be taken ½-hourly for up to 10 doses if ectopic pregnancy is suspected:

- Feeling very worried and afraid *Aconite 30c*
- Abdominal pain accompanied by bleeding *Arnica 30c*

Emotional disturbance during pregnancy

Pregnancy is an emotional time for many women; moods fluctuate very rapidly; joy, fear, anger, and so on seem to be more intense than usual. Hormone changes are partly responsible, but cognitive processes are also involved. In the authors' experience, very strong emotions in the mother affect the baby, so if you find your emotions distressing, take one of the remedies below.

Specific remedies to be taken every 12 hours for up to 3 days:

- Fear/apprehension – fear of dying, pale face, palpitations, fainting fits *Aconite 30c*
- Fear/apprehension – feeling of anguish, trembling, breathlessness, face dark and flushed *Opium 30c*
- Fear/apprehension – diarrhoea, feeling chilly all the time *Veratrum 30c*
- Fear/apprehension – face red and hot *Belladonna 30c*
- Grief – feeling sad, constricted feeling in chest, lump in throat, headache *Ignatia 30c*
- Grief – indifference to people and surroundings, lack of energy *Phosphoric ac. 30c*
- Anger – breathlessness, fidgeting, diarrhoea, bilious attacks *Chamomilla 30c*
- Anger – irritability, being over-critical *Nux 30c*
- Anger – wanting to be left alone, worrying about money *Bryonia 30c*
- Joy – inability to sleep, going 'over the top' *Coffea 30c*

Excessive salivation during pregnancy

Profuse salivation during first trimester of pregnancy, distressing because one wants to spit all the time; most sufferers cope by carrying a large box of tissues around with them; the remedies below are also recommended.

Specific remedies to be taken 4 times daily for up to 7 days:

- Profuse salivation, dribbling on to pillow at night, sweet, metallic taste in mouth *Mercurius 6c*
- Excessive salivation accompanied by nausea, aversion to food, tongue looks white or yellow *Pulsatilla 6c*
- Symptoms as for Pulsatilla, but tongue clean *Ipecac. 6c*
- Too much saliva, feeling weak, chilly, restless, and worried *Arsenicum 6c*
- Too much saliva, forehead cold and sweaty, feeling weak and apathetic *Veratrum 6c*

Fainting during pregnancy

Can occur for no obvious reason, or may be due to extra circulatory load, blood loss, poor diet, previous illness, or wearing clothes which are too tight around the waist.

Specific remedies to be taken every 12 hours for up to 3 days:

- Fainting associated with sadness or grief *Ignatia 30c*
- Fainting associated with irritability *Chamomilla 30c* or *Nux 30c*
- Fainting due to general overloading of cardio-vascular system, fear and apprehension *Aconite 30c*
- Fainting due to heat *Belladonna 30c*

- Faints brought on by movement *Bryonia 30c*
- Fainting due to illness or blood loss *China 30c*

False pains

In the last few months of pregnancy the muscles of the uterus start to tone up and contract at infrequent intervals in preparation for labour (see pp. 134–8); there is no cause for alarm unless contractions are prolonged or increasing in frequency, or unless there is a discharge of blood or fluid from the vagina.

Specific remedies to be taken every hour for up to 10 doses in the following order, if false pains are more than just a nuisance:

- *Pulsatilla 6c, Coffea 6c, Nux 6c, Secale 6c, Caulophyllum 6c*

Fluid retention during pregnancy

see CARDIOVASCULAR PROBLEMS DURING PREGNANCY

Foetal growth problems

If you fail to gain weight, or start losing weight, or if the baby stops moving, ② – all of these symptoms suggest that the placenta is not functioning properly. Possible causes include PRE-ECLAMPTIC TOXAEMIA, ANTE-PARTUM HAEMORRHAGE, high blood pressure (see CARDIO-VASCULAR PROBLEMS), diabetes, smoking, and drugs.

Haemorrhoids during pregnancy

see PILES DURING PREGNANCY

Heartburn during pregnancy

Affects nearly 50 per cent of all women. The pregnancy-maintaining hormone progesterone causes the muscles which close the entrance to the stomach to slacken; this allows stomach acid to splash up into the oesophagus, causing a burning sensation. Upward pressure of the womb on the stomach in later pregnancy aggravates reflux problems.

Specific remedies to be taken 4 times daily for up to 7 days:

- Burning sensation behind breastbone, great thirst, drinking causes shuddering and marked flatulence *Capsicum 6c*
- Sight or smell of food causes nausea, cold feeling in pit of stomach, craving for fizzy drinks *Colchicum 6c*
- Craving for ice-cold drinks which are vomited up as soon as they become warm in stomach, craving for salt *Phosphorus 6c*

- Heartburn worse around 11 am, gnawing sensation in stomach, craving for sweets, marked thirst but little appetite, drinking milk makes heartburn worse *Sulphur 6c*

Self-help

Eat small meals at frequent intervals; this will go a long way towards easing discomfort. If you suffer from heartburn at night raise the head of your bed by a few inches; this is not recommended, however, if you have swollen ankles.

High blood pressure during pregnancy

see CARDIOVASCULAR PROBLEMS DURING PREGNANCY

Hydramnios

An excessive amount of fluid (amniotic fluid) around the baby during later months of pregnancy; more common in mothers who are carrying twins or who have diabetes or PRE-ECLAMPTIC TOXAEMIA; may be symptomless or accompanied by increasing breathlessness, indigestion, a dull ache in the abdomen, and swelling of the legs, thighs, and face; sometimes symptoms onset suddenly, with nausea, in which case there is a risk of premature labour. Appropriate action is ②; in the meantime, rest and take one of the remedies below.

Specific remedies to be taken every 15 minutes for up to 6 doses if symptoms onset suddenly:

- Fear and apprehension *Aconite 30c*
- Face hot and flushed *Belladonna 30c*

Specific remedies to be taken 4 times daily for up to 7 days if symptoms are of more gradual onset:

- Increased breathlessness, puffy legs and face *Arsenicum 6c*
- If symptoms include constipation or frequent urination or vomiting *Nux 6c*
- Symptoms come on after loss of fluid or blood *China 6c*
- If none of the above remedies seems appropriate *Sulphur 6c*

Indigestion during pregnancy

see also HEARTBURN DURING PREGNANCY

Often a feature of late pregnancy, when the digestive tract and its veins and arteries become compressed by the expanding uterus; breathing may also be affected (see RESPIRATORY CHANGES DURING PREGNANCY).

Specific remedies to be taken 15 minutes before meals for up to 3 days:

- Remedy of first resort *Nux 6c*

- If Nux does not prevent indigestion, and main problem is bloating and flatulence *China 6c*
- If fatty foods are the problem, with vomiting and lack of thirst, and stuffy rooms make indigestion worse *Pulsatilla 6c*

Infertility

If you have been having regular, unprotected intercourse for 12 months and have not become pregnant, you or your partner may be infertile. Infertility is quite common – one in eight couples, researchers say, although a recent GP survey put the figure rather lower, at 3.3 per cent of 35-year-olds – and in most cases can be traced to a specific problem in the woman or the man. Oddly enough, coming off oral contraceptives – which appears to lead to AMENORRHOEA in most women – can give a rebound fertility in some. The 12-month rule for infertility is dated from coming off the Pill.

Female infertility may be due to damage to the uterus (from infection or fibroids), to retroversion of the uterus (see UTERUS PROBLEMS), or to the presence of a wall or septum in the uterus, a congenital defect; mucus produced by the cervix may be too viscous for the sperm to penetrate or it may contain antibodies which kill the sperm; one or both Fallopian tubes may be blocked, as the result of gonorrhea (see SEXUALLY TRANS-MITTED DISEASES), ENDOMETRIOSIS or tuberculosis; one or both ovaries may be affected by OVARIAN CYSTS or endometriosis, and fail to produce the necessary hormones; or chronic ill health, STRESS or emotional trauma may depress production of follicle stimulating hormone by the hypothalamus and so prevent eggs maturing in the ovaries (see HORMONE IMBALANCES). Investigation will be by physical examination initially, at which time a full medical history will be taken; you may also be asked to keep a temperature chart – a slight rise in temperature in mid-cycle indicates that ovulation is occurring. If ovulation is not the problem, the next step is to take a sample of semen from your cervix shortly after intercourse to see what effect your cervical mucus has on the sperm. If this is not the problem you will be given blood tests to check hormone levels, followed by X-rays and a small operation to see if your Fallopian tubes and ovaries are normal.

Specific remedies to be taken every 12 hours for up to 7 days while waiting for constitutional treatment:

- Breasts tender, with areas of hard swelling, desire for sex suppressed for some reason *Conium 30c*

- Tenderness in lower abdomen over right ovary, dry vagina *Lycopodium 30c*
- Previous miscarriages before 12 weeks *Sabina 30c*
- Irregular periods, womb feels as if it is about to drop out of vagina, feeling chilly, weepy, and irritable, aversion to sex *Sepia 30c*

If a pituitary problem has been diagnosed, take Agnus 6c up to 3 times daily for 3 weeks out of 4 (if your periods are regular, stop during the week of your period).

Male infertility may be due to a low sperm count (causes include mumps, too much heat around testicles, varicocele, steroids, drugs, alcohol, excessive smoking, lead or carbon-monoxide poisoning, and X-rays), or sperm may be deformed or unable to swim vigorously; testicles or vasa deferentia may be damaged by gonorrhea or syphilis; stress, overwork, tiredness, and psychological factors can cause ERECTION PROBLEMS and EJACULATION PROBLEMS.

Diagnosis is by physical examination and history taking; a sample of semen will be needed to check sperm numbers and quality; if no sperm are found, a testicular biopsy (analysis of a small sample of tissue from the testes) may be necessary.

Specific remedies to be taken every 12 hours for up to 7 days while waiting for constitutional treatment:

- Ineffectual erection, lack of energy, absent-mindedness *Agnus 30c*
- Inability to sustain erection, cramp and coldness in legs *Conium 30c*
- Increased desire for sex but intercourse spoiled by anticipation of failure, general insecurity *Lycopodium 30c*
- Dragging sensation in genitals, no desire for sex *Sepia 30c*

Self-help

If infertility is due to a low sperm count, try to abstain from intercourse in the week leading up to ovulation; this will allow sperm numbers to build up, increasing the chances of conception. The ovulation method can also be used to pinpoint the time of ovulation, maximizing the chances of success. Ask your GP for advice on this and on predictor tests.

Orthodox treatment of infertility is by drugs – to ensure ovulation, increase sperm production, boost certain hormones and suppress others. There are also various implantation techniques. Occasionally, such drugs result in multiple pregnancy. Some abnormalities can be corrected by surgery. Otherwise, the options are artificial insemination or test-tube fertilization, both of which require careful thought, and considerable effort and commitment.

Before embarking on orthodox treatment, the authors advise nutritional therapy (see Pre-conceptual care, p. 129) and constitutional homeo-pathic treatment.

Listeria in pregnancy

Pregnant women should avoid eating certain types of soft cheese, according to government advice, because of the presence in it of listeria. This can cause miscarriage, stillbirth or death soon after birth. These cheeses are likely to be soft, ripened cheeses such as Brie, Camembert and blue vein. They can be made from pasteur-ized or non-pasteurized milk from a cow or goat. Hard cheeses do not present the same problem.

Mature mothers

With the increase in the number of women who choose to establish themselves in a career before starting a family there are inevitably questions about whether it is as safe for a woman in her 30s or 40s to become pregnant and be a mother as it is for a younger woman. There are usually no additional medical problems for mature women, although the older you become the less able you may be to keep up with an energetic offspring. However, you bring a greater experience of life which they can benefit from. The main problem is whether the baby is more likely to be born deformed. A recent reassuring Canadian study looked at 1½ million live births and found that apart from certain well-known conditions such as Down's syndrome, the majority of congenital abnormalities are no more common in children of mature mothers. In some conditions the risks are actually reduced. If you are worried you should ask your GP or obstetrician to have any pre-natal diagnostic tests done that may be appropriate. Otherwise this report is very reassuring.

Miscarriage

The main causes of miscarriage – defined as losing a baby before 28 weeks – are foetal abnormality, structural problems in the uterus, CERVICAL INCOMPETENCE, HORMONE IMBALANCES, and falls; however, miscarriage as the result of a fall is rare – the baby is well protected inside the womb. Losing a baby after 28 weeks is, technically speaking, a stillbirth if the baby is dead; a premature baby is a live baby born after 28 weeks but before term.

A miscarriage is inevitable if the foetus dies in the womb; this is technically a *missed miscarriage* if there are no symptoms – and MORNING SICKNESS

and fullness in the breasts disappear and at your next check-up your GP will find that your uterus has not increased in size. Usually, however, there are obvious signs – discharge of blood and solid matter from the vagina – and crampy pains in the lower abdomen and back; if part of the foetus is retained in the uterus – this is an *incomplete miscarriage* – pain and bleeding may persist for several days. Scanty brown or bloody discharge at around the time when periods are due is not uncommon; this is a *threatened miscarriage*, but in most cases the baby is not lost and the pregnancy proceeds normally. The pain from a miscarriage, no matter at what stage it occurs, can be just as severe as full labour pains.

Any vaginal bleeding during pregnancy is potentially serious, so best course is [12]. If bleed-ing is associated with abdominal pain, (2) and give one of the remedies listed under ECTOPIC PREGNANCY. If you pass any solid matter, keep it for the doctor to see. In the meantime, rest. Since it is usually necessary to remove the remains of the foetus and placenta from the uterus under general anaesthetic in order to prevent infection and anaemia, don't eat or drink while waiting to see your GP.

It is possible that repeated miscarriages are caused by tiny clots in the placenta due to an imbalance between two substances that dilate blood vessels. It has been suggested that a low dose of aspirin every day may help prevent mis-carriage in women with this type of problem. A miscarriage, especially if late, can be just as traumatic as losing any other relative. We would encourage you to grieve fully for the baby rather than just try to pretend it hasn't happened (see GRIEF).

We further suggest that you ask to see the child – or a photograph of her – in order to focus your grief, particularly if she is malformed. It is usually far better to see the worst rather than to be left imagining. Have constitutional homeopathic treatment afterwards.

Specific remedies to be taken every hour for up to 10 doses while waiting to see your GP:

- Bleeding and pain after a blow, a fall, or a particularly violent movement *Arnica 30c*
- Feeling feverish, restless, thirsty, and very worried, dry skin *Aconite 30c*
- Steady loss of bright red blood, cramping pains in abdomen, weakness, nausea *Ipecac. 30c*
- Appearance of dark, coagulated blood towards end of third month or at times when periods would normally occur, tearing pain between lower back and vagina, nausea and vomiting, diarrhoea *Sabina 30c*

- Face hot and dry, distended abdomen, bearing down sensation in vagina *Belladonna 30c*
- Feeling very nervous and agitated, unable to sleep, vulva and vagina extremely sensitive *Coffea 30c*
- Intermittent bleeding which is more profuse each time it occurs, blood dark and coagulated, cramping pains *Pulsatilla 30c*
- Profuse discharge of thick, blackish blood, feeling weak, exhausted, and afraid of dying *Secale 30c*
- Missed miscarriage, no symptoms *Sepia 30c* followed by *Coffea 30c*

Morning sickness

Many women, especially first-time mothers, experience nausea and vomiting in the second and third month of pregnancy, and not just in the mornings; symptoms usually wear off by 14–16 weeks, although a few women go on to develop 'hyperemesis', severe vomiting which causes fluid and chemical imbalances and may require hospital treatment.

As a first resort, try the self-help measures below; if these do not help, try one of the homeopathic remedies given below or see your homeopath. If you are vomiting most of your meals, see your GP; anti-vomiting drugs are available, although there is increasing reluctance to prescribe them.

Specific remedies to be taken 2-hourly for up to 3 days:

- Nausea worse in morning, vomiting small amounts of food with mucus in them *Nux 6c*
- Non-stop nausea, everything vomited up, liquids and solids *Ipecac. 6c*
- Nausea in evening, wearing off at night *Pulsatilla 6c*
- Nausea a few hours after eating, suddenly vomiting everything *Ferrum 6c*
- Vomit full of milky mucus, especially if temperament is melancholy, irritable, and weepy *Sepia 6c*
- Breasts hard and swollen *Conium 6c*
- Heartburn, keeping nausea at bay by constant eating, getting up at night to eat, aversion to meat and fat, cabbage aggravates symptoms *Petroleum 6c*
- Diarrhoea, burning sensation in abdomen, feeling restless and exhausted *Arsenicum 6c*
- Aversion to bread, fat, and slippery foods, craving for salt, feeling very thirsty *Natrum mur. 6c*
- If none of the above remedies seems appropriate *Sulphur 6c*

Self-help
Eat small, frequent meals, avoiding greasy foods, and get plenty of rest. If you feel sick in the mornings, a dry biscuit before you get up might help. Using fresh ginger in cooking can also help. An acupressure device called a Seaband, worn around the wrist, may also be effective (obtainable from your chemist or direct from Seaband UK, Church Walk, Hinckley, Leics.).

Oedema during pregnancy

see CARDIOVASCULAR PROBLEMS DURING PREGNANCY

Piles during pregnancy see also PILES

Varicose veins in the rectum and around the anus are related to constipation and pressure of the uterus on the veins of the pelvis (see CONSTIPATION and CARDIOVASCULAR PROBLEMS DURING PREGNANCY).

Specific remedies to be taken 4 times daily for up to 7 days:

- Remedy of first resort *Pulsatilla 6c*
- If Pulsatilla does not work, and if piles are aggravated by drinking wine or coffee and you are constipation-prone, even when not pregnant *Nux 6c*
- Burning, fiery pains in rectum, soothed by heat *Arsenicum 6c*
- Distended veins look bluish, burning pains after passing stools *Carbo veg. 6c*
- Anal fissures with cutting pains *Chamomilla 6c*

Placenta praevia

Condition in which placenta is attached to the wall of the uterus close to the cervical canal rather than higher up; in this position, it can more easily become detached or damaged, causing bleeding (see ANTE-PARTUM HAEMORRHAGE), but no pain; if bleeding is severe, a blood transfusion and an emergency Caesarean section may be necessary. However, as the uterus grows, the placenta is usually pulled upwards, decreasing risk of complications.

Pre-conceptual care

You owe your baby the best start in life so when you begin to think about pregnancy (ideally 3–6 months before conception) make sure you and your partner are in good health and physically fit. It is a matter of common sense that a healthy baby will only come from healthy sperm and an egg which when fertilized grows in the womb of a healthy mother.

Stop smoking and drinking alcohol and taking

'street' drugs, and read the introduction to this chapter.

Foresight gives warnings about the following drugs:

1 *Marijuana* – upsets the menstrual cycle, although it is possible to become tolerant to it. May induce chromosome damage and behaviour effects if large quantities are smoked. Prolonged or arrested labour may also occur. A heavy use (5–18 joints a week for 6 months) is noted to cause a marked lowering of blood testosterone, low sperm count, greater than average impotency and diminished libido. Sperm mobility is affected, and there is an increase in the number of abnormal sperm.

2 *Cocaine* – abuse in humans significantly reduces the weight of the foetus. Poor placental separation increases the still-birth rate. Cocaine is associated with a higher malformation rate. Babies also suffer mild withdrawal symptoms.

3 *Opiates* – include opium, morphine, codeine. May lead to increased infertility, and cause atrophy of the male accessory sex organs and decreased testosterone production. In women there are many complications during pregnancy – greater risk of stillbirth, prematurity, growth deficiency and general abnormalities, respiratory distress syndrome, lower birth weight and small size for age. There is an increase in perinatal mortality, and maybe long-term effects on growth and behaviour.

4 *Alcohol* – it is now well known that there is a Foetal Alcohol Syndrome (FAS) although a safe level of alcohol in pregnancy is difficult to set. We advise that no alcohol in the pre-conception phase and first 14 weeks of pregnancy is the safest policy. The most dangerous periods are from day 14–18, and from ovulation to the end of the cycle. In its classic form FAS babies are of low birth weight with facial abnormalities including a low nose bridge, no upper lip, small chin and fat face. There is also mental retardation in varying degrees, and heart and dental defects, amongst others.

Stop taking oral contraceptives or have any IUD removed 3 months before you intend to become pregnant, using natural family planning and barrier methods or cap during the fertile period in the meantime. Read 'Nutrition' (p. 247) and ensure that your diet is wholesome and nutritious, with adequate vitamin and mineral intake. If possible, have as much of your food organically grown as is practical, and if there is any doubt about your water supply use a water filter or boiled water. Try to avoid exposure to PESTICIDES. Most vitamins and minerals are necessary for the formation of a healthy baby. Vitamins A, C, E and B complex, zinc, iodine and selenium are essential for fertility (see NUTRITIONAL SUPPLEMENTS).

If either you or your partner have any long-standing health problems it would be best to have constitutional homeopathic treatment. If you have back trouble see a physiotherapist, osteopath or chiropractor before conceiving. If you suffered from phenylketonuria (PKU) as a child, then you should do the PKU diet for 2 months before conception. If there is a history of hereditary diseases such as cystic fibrosis, sickle cell anaemia, thalassaemia or inborn errors of metabolism in your immediate family, it would be wise to have genetic counselling or screening before going ahead.

In addition, if you have had a miscarriage, or are having problems with fertility, consult Foresight (see Useful Addresses, p. 334). Read the Foresight book *Planning for a Healthy Baby* (see Further Reading).

Avoiding specific problems

For the information contained below we are grateful to Foresight, who will supply further information on request. We have not given all the conditions for which nutritional deficiency has been proposed as a cause, but list below some examples. If you have had a baby with a congenital abnormality we recommend that you contact Foresight and go and see one of their doctors. You should be aware that the evidence for the nutritional cause of certain abnormalities is not 100 per cent; there may well be other reasons for it, so do not feel guilty on reading this section if you have a child with any of the abnormalities described. Please just take it in the spirit in which it is intended, i.e. that it is one thing you can do for yourself that may help to lessen the risks of this happening again. It should not do you any harm, providing that if you do take supplements, after one month of taking them all the time, take them only 5 days out of every 7, unless a doctor instructs you otherwise. It is probably best to avoid supplements in the first 3 months of pregnancy unless a physician directs you to take them.

Specific conditions in which nutritional deficiency or toxic levels may play a part

1 Cleft lip and palate – deficiency of vitamins B_2, B_3, B_5 and folic acid.

2 Diaphragmatic hernia – deficiency of vitamin A and folic acid; zinc.

3 Down's syndrome – increase in lead, cadmium, aluminium, copper and decrease in selenium.

4 Eye defects and malformations – vitamin A and B_5, folic acid, iron, zinc and chromium deficiencies.

5 Cataracts – deficiency of B_2 and selenium.

6 Squint – deficiency of vitamin E.

7 Hearing loss – deficiency of manganese.

8 Heart defects – deficiencies of vitamin A, B_5, E; biotin, manganese, zinc and nickel.

9 Kidney defects – deficiency of vitamin B_2, B_5 and E; folic acid, choline, essential fatty acids, zinc and nickel.

10 Liver defects – deficiencies of biotin, vitamin B_2, choline and nickel.

11 Jaundice (of the baby) – deficiency of vitamin B_2, E, biotin, choline, essential fatty acids, selenium, nickel and zinc and increase in toxic metals.

12 Club foot and limb reduction deformities – deficiencies in vitamin B_2, B_3, B_5 and E, folic acid, manganese, iron and zinc.

13 Underdevelopment of the lung – deficiencies of vitamin E and folic acid.

14 Urogenital problems such as undescended testicles and deformed penis – deficiency of vitamin A, B_5, folic acid and zinc.

Hazards of parents' occupation

As far as risks at work for the future of unborn babies is concerned, Foresight quotes a number of occupations where rates of deformity, still-births and perinatal infant mortality appear to be higher than the average. If you are in a high-risk occupation in your pre-conceptual time we suggest you contact Foresight, or have a consultation with one of their doctors, to try and lessen the risks where possible.

Foresight can also recommend a specialized doctor in your area who can conduct a medical examination and any further tests such as hair mineral analysis, blood tests, and test for specific infections such as toxoplasmosis and chlamydia. Screening for cytomegalovirus, which may affect 1 : 1,500 children, causing severe retardation and deformities, with some mothers being affected prior to pregnancy, appears not to be worthwhile. Some 60 per cent of the population are carriers, but screening gives no reliable indication of which babies are at risk.

Having a healthy baby should never be put in jeopardy. Remember that relaxation and exercises are vital. In neural tube defects such as spina bifida, folic acid has been proved to be essential to prevent the condition. A daily 5 mg supplement is now recommended by the government.

Pre-eclamptic toxaemia (PET)

A complication of late pregnancy, associated with raised blood pressure (see CARDIOVASCULAR PROBLEMS). In mild cases, there may be no obvious symptoms apart from raised sphygmomanometer readings. In severe cases, symptoms are head-

aches, blurred vision, intolerance of light, nausea and vomiting, and swollen ankles due to fluid retention; protein may appear in urine. If blood pressure is not brought under control, the symptoms of eclampsia – convulsions, drowsiness, unconsciousness – develop, threatening the life of mother and baby.

Eclampsia is now rare, thanks to better antenatal care, but PET is quite common, especially in first pregnancies. PET is routinely treated by drugs to lower blood pressure; in some cases it may be necessary to induce the baby early.

If convulsions develop or if other symptoms are severe, (999) and give one of the emergency remedies below. The other remedies given below are interim palliatives only – *they are no substitute for expert medical care.*

Specific remedies to be taken every 5 minutes for up to 10 doses while waiting for help:

- Face hot, dry, and flushed, staring eyes, congestive headache *Belladonna 30c*
- Severe symptoms accompanied by great fear *Aconite 30c*
- Severe symptoms aggravated by grief *Ignatia 30c*
- Severe symptoms aggravated by fright *Opium 30c*

Specific remedies to be taken 3 times daily for up to 3 days:

- Stinging pain in legs, aggravated by heat *Apis 30c*
- Feeling chilly, exhausted, and anxious *Arsenicum 30c*

Self-help

The most sensible thing you can do is cut down on salt, and rest as much as possible.

Respiratory changes during pregnancy

Respiratory symptoms such as shortness of breath and coughing are not uncommon in the last months of pregnancy, especially if the baby is large and the mother small. Diaphragm and rib movements which pull and push air into and out of the lungs are, to some extent, hampered by upward pressure of the uterus; the lungs also become congested because of pressure on veins and arteries, making gaseous exchange less efficient. Digestion is often affected too, for similar reasons (see INDIGESTION DURING PREGNANCY).

If coughing is severe, (2); in the meantime take Aconite 30c every 5 minutes for up to 10 doses, especially if fear is the overwhelming emotion. If you are short of breath even when at rest, 12 .

Coughing
Specific remedies to be taken 4 times daily for up to 7 days:

- Coughing after meals, shortness of breath *Nux 6c*
- Frequent, dry, exhausting cough which gets worse at night, salty taste in mouth *Sepia 6c*
- Cough accompanied by nausea and vomiting *Ipecac. 6c*
- Cough accompanied by involuntary passing of urine, alleviated by drinking cold water *Causticum 6c*

Shortness of breath
Specific remedies to be taken every 5 minutes for up to 10 doses as soon as symptoms come on:

- With palpitations, fainting, fear *Aconite 30c*
- With weakness, swollen ankles, face pale and anguished looking, feeling chilly and restless *Arsenicum 6c*
- With nausea, fainting *Ipecac. 6c*

Rhesus incompatibility

Rhesus factor is one of several factors used to type blood; a mother who is Rh− (Rhesus negative) will make antibodies against her own baby if the baby's blood (and the father's) is Rh+ (Rhesus positive) and mixes with hers during pregnancy; if this happens, the mother's antibodies will start to destroy the baby's red blood cells, and the baby will be born jaundiced (see NEONATAL JAUNDICE). Risks to second or third Rh+ babies are higher, the mother's immune system having been primed by the first.

However, stillbirths and neonatal problems due to Rhesus incompatibility are now rare, thanks to maternal blood tests during pregnancy and to the practice of giving Anti-D serum injections to Rh− mothers of Rh+ babies immediately after delivery (or after MISCARRIAGE, ANTE-PARTUM HAEMORRHAGE, or TERMINATION OF PREGNANCY, which can also result in a mixing of foetal and maternal blood); because Anti-D serum kills Rh+ red blood cells, full-scale antibody production is forestalled.

Rubella (German measles) during pregnancy

Can cause congenital defects if contracted during the first trimester of pregnancy; can be prevented by immunization at age of 13, though immunization is not necessary if you have already had the disease and therefore have immunity to it; immunity can be confirmed by a blood test, a wise precaution since many viruses produce symptoms similar to those of German measles. Conception should be avoided for 3 months after immunization.

If you become pregnant and have not had German measles/been immunized, take Rubella nosode 30c immediately, 3 doses at 12-hour intervals to begin with, then 1 dose every 3 weeks until you are past the 12th week of pregnancy.

If you contract German measles during early pregnancy, you may wish to consider a TERMINATION OF PREGNANCY; you should discuss this with your GP.

Skin changes during pregnancy

These are caused by raised hormone levels; if neither of the remedies below seems suitable, see remedies given under ACNE and CHLOASMA.

Specific remedies to be taken 4 times daily for up to 7 days:

- Brown/dirty yellow freckling over bridge of nose *Sepia 6c*
- Skin dry, itchy, hot, and scurfy, made worse by washing *Sulphur 6c*

Sleep problems during pregnancy see also
SLEEP PROBLEMS pp. 237–8

Anxiety about pregnancy and birth, heartburn, the urge to urinate, general discomfort, the baby kicking . . . all of these can break sleep during pregnancy; then worrying about not sleeping makes sleeping more difficult, and so a vicious circle is set up.

Specific remedies to be taken before going to bed for up to 5 nights and hourly if still awake:

- Over-excitement, mental over-stimulation, excessive joy *Coffea 30c*
- Feeling you will never get to sleep again, especially after some form of grief *Ignatia 30c*
- Feeling very afraid *Aconite 30c*

Self-help
If you cannot get comfortable in bed, tuck a pillow under your abdomen, into the small of your back, between your knees, or wherever you feel you need support. If you still cannot sleep, don't be tempted to take sleeping pills, especially in the first 16 weeks of pregnancy; get up and read a book or do housework, and make up for lost sleep later, enlisting your partner's help if necessary.

Termination of pregnancy

As the law now stands, termination is illegal unless 2 doctors agree that it is necessary for one of the following reasons: the baby is abnormal; there is a risk to the physical or mental health of the baby; the health of the mother or of other children may be jeopardized if the pregnancy continues.

According to the Human Fertilization and Embryology Act of 1990 there is a 24-weeks time limit for terminations performed on the grounds of risk. There is also a new ground for termination – grave permanent injury to the physical or mental health of the pregnant woman. This allows termination to be carried out without time limit where there is risk to the life of the pregnant woman or substantial risk that the child, if born, would suffer such physical or mental abnormalities as to be seriously handicapped.

If pregnancy is unwanted and bringing up a child yourself is totally unfeasible, you have two choices: termination or adoption. Adoption preserves life; on the other hand, pregnancy and labour are not without risks, the baby has to be given up shortly after birth, and you may come to regret that you took no part in his or her growing up. Termination also has its pros and cons; it is less risky than carrying a baby to term, although there is a slight risk of CERVICAL INCOMPETENCE in subsequent pregnancies; guilt, sometimes severe, is a common reaction.

The decision to terminate a pregnancy is often made purely from the head and under time pressure. At the time it may seem quite logical, when you feel that you would not be able to care for the baby properly, or you would have to give up your career or in some other way lose your independence. It may be that in days, weeks, months or even years to come you will suffer reaction from the heart. If this does happen admit to yourself that you may have made a mistake, and forgive yourself – for truly you are only human. You may then grieve for yourself and the loss of your potential baby as you should (see GRIEF).

If your GP is not sympathetic to termination, the British Pregnancy Advisory Service, Family Planning Association, Brook Advisory Centre, or National Council for One-Parent Families (addresses pp. 333–8) will give you all the advice and information you need.

Termination in the first 3 months of pregnancy involves a D & C (dilatation and curettage, or suction removal of the contents of the womb); this is a 15-minute procedure done under general anaesthetic and seldom involves a hospital stay of more than 12 hours. Early terminations can sometimes be carried out using hormones inserted vaginally.

Specific remedies to be taken every 4 hours for up to 3 days after operation:

- Feeling very upset, with lump in throat and tight feeling around chest *Ignatia 30c*
- Where symptoms are more physical – i.e. abdominal pain, cystitis *Staphisagria 30c*

Toothache during pregnancy
The best preventive is good dental care and adequate calcium before conception and during pregnancy.

Specific remedy to be taken as required for up to 10 doses:

- *Sepia 6c*

Urinary problems during pregnancy
These are usually caused by pressure on the bladder, urethra, and pelvic floor muscles, and can be aggravated by tight jeans, non-cotton underwear, bubble baths, etc.

Cystitis causes a burning sensation on passing water and a frequent urge to urinate. If none of the remedies given below seems appropriate, more remedies – and self-help measures – are given under CYSTITIS.

Specific remedies to be taken up to 2-hourly daily for up to 3 days:

- At first sign of discomfort, especially if weather is cold and windy and you are feverish, restless, and apprehensive *Aconite 30c*
- Slightest tension causes leakage of urine, scalding sensation during and after urination, lack of thirst, heat and lying down make discomfort worse *Pulsatilla 6c*
- Bladder and urethra feel itchy and irritable, dribbles of urine passed frequently and with some difficulty *Nux 6c*
- Urge to pass urine most frequent at night, burning and soreness after passing urine, urgency, urine copious and almost colourless *Sulphur 6c*
- Passing copious amount of cloudy urine at frequent intervals, burning sensation, urge to pass urine most frequent at night *Phosphoric ac. 6c*
- A bad attack of cystitis, with constant burning and urgency *Catharis 30c*

Incontinence of urine during pregnancy is due to extra strain on the muscles which close the sphincter from the bladder. See STRESS INCONTINENCE for more information.

Specific remedies to be taken 4 times daily for up to 14 days:

- Remedy of first resort *Pulsatilla 6c*
- Bearing down sensation as if contents of womb are about to fall out of vagina *Sepia 6c*
- Incontinence made worse by coughing *Causticum 6c*

Retention of urine is not uncommon in later pregnancy, and tends to come on gradually; urine flow becomes scantier, with intermittent pain in the bladder area; scanty flow can also contribute to cystitis (above). If pain becomes severe and urination impossible, ②; your GP will pass a small tube called a catheter into the bladder to drain off the urine. The remedies given below are only suitable in the early stages of retention, when urination starts to become difficult.

Specific remedies to be taken ½-hourly for up to 10 doses:

• Remedy of first resort *Nux 30c*
• If Nux does not bring relief *Pulsatilla 30c*

Varicose veins during pregnancy
see CARDIOVASCULAR PROBLEMS DURING PREGNANCY

Childbirth and Postnatal Problems

The process of labour

More and more women today feel that birth should not be a high-tech affair unless there are definite reasons for it. Hospitals are notoriously unrelaxed, noisy, insensitive places in which to give birth, although they have their merits. One of the authors saw a mother in her second pregnancy nearly die because the womb inverted as the placenta was delivered; this is very rare and could not possibly have been foreseen, but the mother would certainly have died if she had been at home. On the other hand, although it may be an ordeal, a calm and controlled birth leaves the mother much less traumatized; it is much more rewarding, and appears to be safer for the baby, than a high-tech birth. There is less likelihood of postnatal depression, and it may increase the baby's ability to cope with stress.

Barring unforeseen complications, if a woman is calm, relaxed and undisturbed then her hormones will function normally, enabling her to deliver the baby spontaneously without any need for interference.

Labour requires the total integration of the woman's body, mind and spirit for all the natural physiological functions to work properly. If this delicate balance is upset, and any one level becomes distressed, there is a strong likelihood of complications in the delivery. The labour can stop, become inefficient and prolonged, or the woman may lose control and panic, so needing medical assistance. As we have pointed out before, routine obstetric technology is life-saving, but in itself can create problems not already present in a labour.

Increasingly obstetricians and midwives are coming to rely on modern medical techniques for assessing the progression of labour. There is a danger that they are losing touch with the natural ways of helping and sustaining a woman

through her labour. In an ideal world the solution would be to make hospitals homelier and more responsive to women's real needs. In special birthing units mothers could be attended by their own midwife, give birth in a way that suits them rather than in a hospital, and have members of their family present at the birth if they wish. Back-up emergency help would be available within minutes.

If complications are expected, it is best to have the baby in hospital.

If you have strong views on specific procedures or specific drugs, approach your consultant at some point during the antenatal period and make your wishes clear. This is also the time to ask if there is any objection to using homeopathic remedies; these would not interfere with any drugs you may be given. The National Childbirth Trust (p. 335) offer 'birth plans' as part of their classes.

What homeopathy can do in labour
Remedies can bring about a profound change in the course of labour, during times when the mother is unable to maintain total involvement with the job that her body is trying to perform; she may be resisting, getting frightened, so that labour is not progressing and is exhausting her. Homeopathic treatment has a remarkable power to put a woman 'back in the process' so that labour can proceed as it should.

Homeopathy can help in particular conditions such as raised blood pressure, induction, turning a breech baby, postnatally etc.

Homeopathy can also be used to help with pain relief.

Finally, remember that labour is very like running a marathon, and the older we are the harder it becomes. There is a strong correlation between fear, tension, trying too hard and pain. Midwives tend to have terrible labours and doctors and homeopaths seem to fare little better! So whilst you should make all the arrangements you can, and try to do everything the right way and have everything on hand you might need, once the process begins just relax, let go, trust mother nature and surrender.

Onset of labour

It is impossible to predict exactly when labour will begin, except to say that it will usually be within three weeks before or after the expected date of delivery. In the last week or so of pregnancy the baby's head slides down into the pelvis – this relieves pressure on the diaphragm and stomach but increases pressure on the bladder and rectum; the whole vulval area becomes moister. The signals that labour is about to begin include the following:

1 The show – a fairly large amount of clear, thick, flecked or blood-stained mucus. (This is the mucus plug from your cervix.) Labour is likely to begin within the next 24–28 hours, but could be delayed for up to 7 days.
2 Waters break – may or may not happen before the onset of labour. If you lose a lot of water – a flood and not just a mugful – then labour must begin within the next 24–48 hours or there is a danger of infection reaching the baby (see INDUCTION).
3 Regular painful contractions – you may have had episodes of strong fairly regular contractions towards the end of pregnancy (see FALSE PAINS), but when labour really begins the pain reaches a strong level. At this point anyone else who is with you may notice a mild note of apprehension in your voice instead of the rather jovial excitement of previous reportings!

First stage

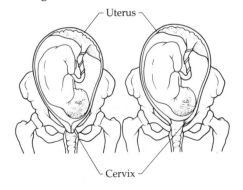

Uterus

Cervix

In the first stage of labour the uterine muscles are pulling open the cervix to dilate it from 0–10 cm in diameter. It is also pulled upwards, so the uterus, cervix and vagina form a single tube or birth canal. You will be given a vaginal examination during the first stage of labour to assess how close you are to giving birth. In the very early stages the cervix is thin (or effaced) but not yet dilated. At 2 cm it is still early. At 6–7 cm things are going to progress quite rapidly, especially if it is not your first baby. In the first stage of labour, in some hospitals, you may be given an enema to empty your bowels, and will be encouraged to pass urine. The old-fashioned habit of shaving pubic hair is not now considered necessary to prevent infection.

The first stage of labour lasts on average 12 hours in a first pregnancy, and 6 hours in the second. There are no hard and fast rules – sometimes the first stage takes up to 24 hours, and sometimes, apparently, only a few minutes. The waters can break at any time during the first stage, and labour tends to intensify after this happens. This is potentially the most painful part of giving birth and is a time when homeopathy can most help (see LABOUR PAINS). As labour proceeds, the pulse will become harder and faster, and your mouth may feel dry; restlessness, nausea, and sometimes vomiting are quite common, especially at transition, where things may come to a halt before the second stage begins.

Transition

The first 2 stages overlap. The rhythm changes, and it may seem to you that everything is going wrong; you may feel tearful. The cervix is very nearly fully dilated, the intensity of the pain has lessened and there is a pause, a lull. The baby's head has to rotate and flex into the right position to come down the birth canal; otherwise the head will become stuck in the pelvis and have no room to get out. There is a time when you feel that you do not want to go on. Unless anything goes wrong, however, you are over the worst. The contractions become confusing, and they begin to change as the urge to push starts. Your midwife will instruct you to resist these tentative urges to push until there are signs that the baby's head has definitely entered the birth canal, the main sign being pouting of the rectum during each contraction.

Transition may last anything from a few seconds to 3 hours. Until your midwife tells you that you are ready, resist the urge to bear down; the cervix would be damaged if you pushed before it had completely opened around the baby's head. During the contraction you need to blow out with short puffs as if blowing out a candle that is about 3 feet away. It is impossible to push while panting like this. If there is an anterior lip of the cervix which is not shifting it may be helpful if you go into the knee/chest position lying with bottom up and head down. If you are lying on your side or leaning forward it is a great help if someone can lightly separate your buttocks during the contraction, helping everything to relax.

Once the rectum starts to pout this is the signal that the first stage is done. The urge to push comes from pressure of the baby on the rectum sending signals to the brain that something must be pushed out!

Second stage

The baby's head is now clear of the cervix and is ready to come down. You must throw yourself into the very powerful urge to push with each contraction: finally you may expel the pain from your body. Although each contraction is not so intensely painful, you may find this the most difficult stage. The baby's head feels like a melon coming down; it can seem an impossible task to get it out, but it can also be a very satisfying experience.

This stage usually lasts an hour or so in a first pregnancy, and about half an hour in subsequent ones, although it may be anything from 3 minutes to 2 hours. If it is much over 2 hours the baby may begin to register distress.

Midwives often do not give reminders about positions, and it can transform a second stage to find a position that suits you. Use gravity, and positions where you are leaning forward, as this will reduce the likelihood of tearing. Positions include kneeling on all fours with arms round your partner's waist, squatting with support under each arm, standing with support while squeezing someone's hand tight. On all fours with a horizontal back will slow down a second stage if it is happening too fast. Upright will encourage as fast a second stage as possible. If it is your first baby, remember it will feel as if you are pushing the baby out through your bottom rather than your vagina. Imagine that the huge bulge that is coming down is going out! This will help the muscles of the pelvic floor to thin out as the head comes down; otherwise there is a tendency for them to tense against the head which again increases the likelihood of tearing. You may also find it helpful to visualize the perineum opening. Everything is now stretched to the absolute limit in the perineum as the head crowns. The midwife or other helper will control it so that it slips through the vagina without

stretching too much, causing splitting. If there is a fear that the vagina will be badly torn you may need an episiotomy. However, with good control and gentle massage of the vaginal skin this is not often necessary.

Once the head emerges the shoulders and body soon follow. The baby can then be delivered on to your tummy. Breathing is started by clearing the baby's airways of mucus, and tipping his or her head down. You may then suckle. The baby may or may not whimper a little and may start to guzzle right away, or she may want to look around for a bit. The cord will not be clamped until it has stopped pulsating unless it is round the baby's neck. Sucking the breast will stimulate hormones which will make the placenta separate from the uterus, although this should happen anyway. Eye contact between mother and baby has also been shown to stimulate the third stage.

If there is any reason why you cannot hold your baby right away, for instance if you need stitches, make sure the father holds her. Even if he is initially a little nervous of the newborn, he will be very glad afterwards. The first half hour is considered by many to be the most sensitive period for bonding between newborn and parents, and it is lovely for all three to have this opportunity.

Third stage

Within 5–15 minutes of the baby being born the uterus will have contractions which separate the placenta from the wall of the womb and expel it. If it hasn't been delivered in half an hour or so there is a danger of the womb shrinking round it. Should this happen it may have to be removed surgically (see RETAINED PLACENTA). To prevent haemorrhage after birth, most obstetricians give an injection of Syntometrine as soon as the baby's head has appeared; this induces immediate contraction of the uterus. It is certainly necessary for anyone who has had an epidural or other anaesthetic which reduces the ability of the uterus to contract spontaneously. It should also be used if there is excessive bleeding, or if the mother and baby are separated at birth. (It is interesting to note that Syntometrine is derived from the same source as the homeopathic remedy Secale.) If there is no excessive bleeding there is no need to hurry the process, and it can be quite a pleasurable experience to expel the placenta spontaneously. For this reason it is unnecessary for the midwife to pull on the cord to speed up the process. This is a good time to have a quiet cuddle and suckle the baby.

Bleeding, however, indicates that the placenta has not come away intact. In the rare event that there is a tear in the uterine wall, and it is not contracting down fast enough, then

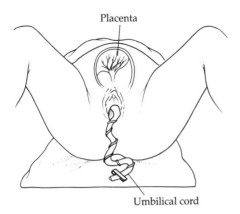

Placenta

Umbilical cord

a woman can haemorrhage, losing blood very quickly. If you are at home the Flying Squad must be called immediately ⑨⑨⑨ (see POST-PARTUM HAEMORRHAGE).

Baby check
Usually after birth the midwife or doctor will check to see if your baby is all right; a more thorough check will be done later. This will include looking in the baby's mouth, at the genitals, the back passage, fingers and toes, back and navel. Hips and feet will also be examined.

After the birth
Once baby has been settled you will be washed or you can have a shower if you are able. Bathing the vaginal area with Arnica solution (10 drops of mother tincture to 0.25 litre [½ pint] warm water) will take away some of the soreness and promote healing. If you have had an EPISIOTOMY or a lot of small tears use Calendula solution in the same dilution. After that you should be allowed to sleep, or at least be very quiet and tranquil. At this time well-meaning visitors and telephone calls can be very exhausting.

Advice for your partner/companion
Once labour begins and you are asked to be present take a few minutes to soak up the atmosphere. If the woman is still up and about and busy between her contractions then that is fine. If she is finding the contractions difficult but seems to be in a world of her own, re-laxed, focused inwards and involved in her own rhythm, this is also fine. If, however, she is finding contractions difficult, has not settled into a rhythm and is not relaxed, then she is resisting, and you can help a great deal. There is a danger that she will lose energy in this state, and the labour will not proceed well. The uterus becomes inefficient, and even though contractions are forceful and painful the uterus does not work properly to dilate the cervix. To help her find her rhythm:

1 Stop any chit-chat in the room. Provide a balanced, calm atmosphere. Act as an inter-mediary between her and other people, hospital staff, etc.

2 Help her relax, gently encourage her to try alternative positions for greater comfort and effectiveness. Some women find moving about relaxes them; some need to sit still and gently rock; some need to sit motionless; some need to lean forwards; some need to lie on one side (with the top leg supported by several pillows). Any pressure on an area in pain is excruciating; lying on her back is almost impossible. An upright position is preferable, as then gravity helps, but by far the most important thing is that she is relaxed. If she is sitting, it is a good idea to get her a ring to sit on so that there is no upward pressure. This becomes particularly important when the cervix is 5 cm dilated.

3 Use key words as reminders, such as 'go with it', 'relax', 'open up', 'breathe', 'loose lips', 'don't resist'.

4 Breathe with her through a contraction – follow the subtle changes in her breathing pattern. Encourage her to go with the different rhythms her body suggests.

5 Gently massage any area which is tense. Some women relax best in the face of pain if they are moving around; others need to become like a limp lettuce leaf.

6 Frequently tell her how well she is doing. This is powerful magic, however transparent.

7 Keep all interactions to a minimum. Ask only questions requiring a 'yes/no', 'good/bad' answer.

Remember, always give loads of encouragement. It works tremendously well, and takes away some of the pain. As the second stage proceeds and the baby's head appears, give lots of feedback.

Massage in labour
In the first stage if the mother is in her own world and managing then do not intervene. If she is seeking help then massage is invaluable as a support. Massage the feet and legs to speed up labour, and help the mother settle into herself. Use effleurage or butterfly stroking. If the most distress is in the front, this is because the con-tracting womb is causing undue tension in the tummy muscles. Effleurage desensitizes the skin, enabling the muscles below to relax. Aroma-therapy oils can be beneficial, but avoid those which antidote homeopathic remedies (see p. 195 for list).

Technique

Rhythmic *light* movement with the fingertips (any pressure causes distress). Massage the area of pain in the tummy as soon as it starts for most effective results. Massage continuously throughout a contraction, either with both hands going up the midline and then out to side and then down in line with the nipples, or from side to side with one hand. The woman may be able and wish to do this herself, or get you to do it.

Massage for backache labour

1 Pressure on the base of the spine. Slow rhythmic pushes in with the heel of one or both hands during contractions.
2 Heavy pressure on coccyx. Like pushing a rolling pin up and down with all your strength. (In a true backache labour a woman may feel her back is going to fly off at 100mph, because the pressure of the baby's head on her back is so great.)
3 Knead the sacro-iliac joint (the joint between the spine and pelvis) with your thumbs and knuckles, and maybe with a follow-on outwards motion.
4 Butterfly massage. Tapping with the fingertips disperses underlying tension.

Aching thighs

This may occur towards the end of the first stage. The return of blood from the legs is sluggish because of the pressure in the pelvis. Try and get the knees higher than the pelvis in order to use gravity. Using the palms of both hands, massage with firm pressure upwards from knees to trunk, running them lightly back to knees. It may be needed for a few contractions.

Massage any area that is tense or aches, and as a general tonic massage the feet.

Acupuncturists and many primitive cultures believe in 'mother roasting'. If the woman becomes very cold after giving birth, it is done immediately, otherwise after a day or two. This can be done by the father using moxibustion. Also take Arnica 30c 4 times a day for up to 3 days to reduce pain and bruising and to ward off infection.

You will probably not feel very hungry for a day or two. Thin vegetable soup is good on the first day, with salads and fruit on the second, and a return to your normal diet on the third. Tea, coffee, chamomile tea, and wine are best avoided. The most important nutrients in the weeks after birth are iron (to make up for lost blood), protein (to aid healing), and calcium (if you are breastfeeding). To get back into shape, cut down on starchy foods.

A mixture of blood, fluid, and mucus is discharged from the womb in the days immediately following delivery. After-pains are common at this time, and tend to be worse if labour has been relatively easy. It is quite normal to feel very weary and stiff. Some women also find themselves perspiring a lot. Within 12–15 days the womb returns to its normal size. After an episiotomy or a tear, the vulva and vagina will take several weeks to heal.

Periods usually restart 6–8 weeks after delivery, but may not reappear for several months, especially if you are breastfeeding. If you are worried, see your GP.

Breastfeeding

Breast milk contains, in ideal proportions, everything your baby needs – not only carbohydrates, proteins, fats, vitamins, and minerals, but also antibodies against many infections, including those which cause diarrhoea. In Western countries breastfeeding tends to prevent obesity; in many Third World countries it prevents the opposite marasmus or wasting diseases. There is mounting evidence too that breastfeeding for the first 4–6 months helps to prevent allergy-formation, especially if there is a family history of allergy. Cot deaths, constipation, intestinal obstruction, hypocalcaemic convulsions and tooth decay also occur less frequently in breastfed babies than in bottle-fed. Child abuse is also less common, probably because of the strong emotional bond which grows out of the physical contact between mother and baby. From the mother's point of view the breast is much cheaper than the bottle and always handy. Lactation also helps to balance her hormone secretions.

Formula milk contains additives such as pH adjusters, anti-oxidants, carag[een, hydroxy-propyl starch, emulsifiers, and thickening agents. Though some constituents – zinc for example – are in the same proportion as those found in breast milk, they are less well absorbed.

Breastfeeding should not be undertaken if the mother is suffering from:

1 Severe disease such as Crohn's, or renal failure.
2 An infection such as tuberculosis, septicaemia or breast abscess, or AIDS/HIV infection (see AIDS).
3 Persistent inverted nipples which do not come out.
4 Psychotic illness.
5 Is on certain drugs such as lithium, cytotoxic and immunosuppressors (used in cancer particularly), radioactive drugs, ergot alkaloids (used in treatment of migraine).

Breastfeeding should also be avoided for infants who are acutely ill unless it is expressed and given by tube, if they have an inborn error of metabolism, or a cleft palate. However, it can be continued if there is jaundice. Finally, remember that just because a baby cries after feeding it does not necessarily mean he or she is still hungry; it may be because he or she has wind, is thirsty, wants company, is not hungry but still wants to suck, or needs a new nappy. Try comforting and other measures first. The only true guide as to whether the baby is getting enough food is whether it is growing and putting on weight and developing normally.

The quantities required by an infant on average are 150 ml of fluid per kilo of body weight per day (2½ oz per 1 lb per day), although in babies up to one month old it can be up to 200 ml per kilo daily. The energy requirement is between 100–120 kcals per kilo (1 fluid oz is about 30 ml). Most proprietary cans of milk formula provide the equivalent of about 25 kcals per fl. oz.

Try to breastfeed in the first 24 hours if you can, as this is the most sensitive time for your baby. At first your milk (colostrum) will be very watery, but rich in protective antibodies.

As your baby sucks on the pigmented area around the nipple, messages go to your pituitary gland telling it to produce oxytocin, a hormone which stimulates the glands in your breasts to produce milk. Proper milk comes in on the second or third day, at which time you may experience sudden chills or notice that blood and fluid loss becomes scantier.

Feed on demand if you can, otherwise your milk production may drop or cease altogether. Breastfeeding is not considered to be a totally reliable form of contraception although it is pretty good unless more than 6 hours between feeds (see CONTRACEPTION). Combined oral contraceptives should be avoided, as they interfere with the volume and composition of breast milk.

If you cannot breastfeed, don't feel guilty or despairing about it, but have a really good try first. Not everyone takes to breastfeeding like a duck to water. There is a knack to it, so don't be afraid to ask your nurse or midwife what to do or contact the La Leche League (see Useful Addresses, p. 335). If the bottle turns out to be best, you can always kick your partner out of bed in the middle of the night to feed junior! If using bottles remember that they must be sterilized properly. Continue to sterilize bottles until the baby has reached the stage of putting objects into her mouth. Return to routine sterilizing if there is an outbreak of infection in the family. The steam method is best; the new Avent Steam Sterilizer, which is fully automatic and only takes 45 minutes, is ideal as it is safe and relatively cheap. Boiling is hazardous, difficult and having boiling water near young infants can be dangerous. Chemical sterilization is convenient, can be done anywhere and is also cheap. Mistakes that occur are generally due to using stale solution, or in the wrong concentration.

Problems in labour and after the birth

Breastfeeding problems

Failure to breastfeed

Very full breasts are difficult for the baby to suck; if this is the case, expressing some milk before feeding will solve the problem. Sometimes the milk is too watery or it may have a salty or bitter taste which the baby does not like; this can be due to emotional problems in the mother, or maternal malnutrition, or the mother may be taking salty or strongly spiced foods, strong tea, chamomile tea, or drugs, which give an odd taste to her milk. Sometimes the mother needs to be nurtured by another female figure (her own mother, for example) before she can produce enough milk. Difficulties may also increase with successive babies. The La Leche League (see Useful Addresses, p. 335) give the following advice:

1 Wear breast shields during pregnancy to help draw out flat or inverted nipples.
2 Begin breastfeeding as soon as possible after birth of the baby, preferably on delivery table as this exploits the baby's strong need to suck.
3 Give feeds as often as the baby wants them.
4 In the rare instance of the baby refusing to suck do not give a bottle – instead give milk on a spoon.
5 Breast pumps are useful for mother if she has to return to work, but avoid plastic bulb pumps as these can bruise the breast tissue.
6 Freeze milk at −18°C in a proper domestic freezer; if frozen in the freezer compartment of a fridge it can only be kept for 24–48 hours.
7 Expect 6–8 wet nappies each day.
8 If you wish to wean the baby before she wants to, do it very gradually and gently.

Constitutional homeopathic treatment can sometimes help, but in the meantime one of the remedies below should be tried.

Baby refusing milk or vomiting

Specific remedies to be taken 4 times daily for up to 3 days:

- Poor quality milk, mother large and prone to chills and sweats *Calcarea 30c*

- If downward movements while nursing cause baby to scream *Borax 30c*
- If baby is thin, with a large, sweaty head, and vomits after feeds *Silicea 30c*
- Sudden excessive milk production in a young, healthy mother *Aconite 30c*
- Breasts hard and swollen *Bryonia 30c*
- Overproduction of milk, mother young, timid, and weepy *Pulsatilla 30c*

Engorgement

If the baby refuses to feed or if you decide to stop breastfeeding the breasts can become painfully distended with milk. Expressing milk provides immediate relief, but one of the remedies below should also be taken.

Specific remedies to be taken every 4 hours until engorgement passes:

- Feeling weepy and sensitive to cold, hating to be in stuffy rooms *Pulsatilla 30c*
- Extreme sensitivity to cold, cold sweats, tendency to be overweight *Calcarea 30c*

Exhaustion from breastfeeding

This is an unusual reaction, but can occur because of the fluid loss which breastfeeding entails. In addition to the remedy below you could try expressing some milk so that your partner can give one of the night feeds.

Specific remedy to be taken every 4 hours for up to 10 doses:

- *China 30c*

Hardness of the breasts

Specific remedies to be taken every hour for up to 10 doses:

- Suspected breast abscess or mastitis *Bryonia 30c*
- Suspected breast abscess or mastitis, with red streaks on skin *Belladonna 30c*
- If neither Bryonia nor Belladonna help *Calcarea 30c*

Loss of milk

Specific remedies to be taken 4 times daily for up to 3 days:

- Remedy of first resort if milk production stops *Agnus 6c*
- If Agnus fails and milk stops after exposure to cold, breasts swollen, sore, and sensitive *Dulcamara 6c*
- If Dulcamara fails *Pulsatilla 6c*
- If due to grief *Ignatia 6c*
- If due to anger *Chamomilla 6c*

- If due to shock or fright *Aconite 30c*
- If due to jealousy *Hyoscyamus 6c*
- If due to extreme joy *Coffea 6c*

Sore or cracked nipples

After each feed bathe the nipples with Arnica solution (10 drops mother tincture to 0.25 litre [½ pint] boiled cooled water), then dry them thoroughly and apply Calendula cream (from chemist or health food shop). One of the remedies below should also be taken.

Specific remedies to be taken every 4 hours for up to 6 doses:

- Nipples inflamed and very tender to the touch *Chamomilla 6c*
- Sore nipples, especially if associated with grief *Ignatia 6c*
- Sore nipples, especially if mother is timid and weepy *Pulsatilla 6c*
- Pain and soreness made worse by exposure to cold *Aconite 6c*
- Cracked nipples which cause smarting, burning pain *Sulphur 6c*
- Nipples cracked and sore, with blisters on them *Graphites 6c*
- Cracked nipples associated with plentiful milk production and distended breasts, although milk is poor and baby dislikes it *Calcarea 6c*
- Ulcerated nipples *Silicea 6c*

Delayed periods after childbirth

Periods usually restart within 6–8 weeks of birth, but may be delayed for several months if you are breastfeeding on demand. Orthodox treatment is to give drugs to stimulate ovulation or recommend a D & C to make sure that none of the products of conception remain in the womb. Before such measures are taken, try one or other of the remedies below.

Specific remedies to be taken every 12 hours for up to 7 days:

- Lack of thirst, weepiness, feeling worse in hot, stuffy surroundings *Pulsatilla 30c*
- Feeling chilly, tired, depressed, irritable, and turned off by sex, constipated *Sepia 30c*

Emergency childbirth

If labour comes on suddenly and proceeds very fast (see description of labour, pp. 134–8), and there is no time to get the mother to hospital, you must be prepared to deliver the baby yourself. Don't panic – birth is a natural event and in most cases proceeds perfectly normally with only minimum assistance from those in attendance.

Make sure the room is warm, and put fresh

sheets on the bed, with a large plastic sheet underneath to keep the mattress clean. Up to 0.5 litre (1 pint) of blood and fluids will be lost during the birth; this is quite normal. Boil a pair of scissors and a length of string to sterilize them. Wash your hands thoroughly, taking care to scrub under your fingernails.

The baby's head will appear first, followed by the shoulders. As soon as the shoulders are out, support the head, but do not pull on it or the umbilical cord. Once the body and legs have emerged, gently wipe the mucus away from the nose and mouth and tip the baby's head downwards. This should start the baby breathing, but if it doesn't do so within 1 minute, begin artificial respiration and dial ⑨⑨⑨.

Once the cord stops pulsating, tie it with the sterilized string in two places, one about 10 cm (4 in) away from the baby's tummy and the other about 20 cm (8 in) away; then cut the cord between the pieces of string with the sterilized scissors. Swaddle the baby in a clean sheet and give him or her to the mother to hold.

Within about 30 minutes of the birth, the placenta should appear; gently massage the mother's stomach to assist delivery of the placenta, but do not pull on the cord. If bleeding continues after delivery of the placenta, ⑨⑨⑨, give reassurance, and massage the mother's stomach every few minutes until help arrives.

Once the placenta has been delivered and the baby has settled, encourage the mother to take a shower, and bathe the whole vulval area with Arnica solution (10 drops of mother tincture to 0.25 litre [½ pint] warm water). If there are large tears in vulva or near back passage, suturing will be necessary. For remedies see under LABOUR PAINS and PROLONGED LABOUR.

Episiotomy

If during the second stage of labour there is a fear that the vagina will be badly torn – which can even affect the bowel if it is very severe – you may need an episiotomy. This is an incision of the skin of the vagina, done under local anaesthetic. After the delivery this will be stitched up by a doctor or midwife. Remember to take Arnica 30c four times a day until you begin to feel comfortable. Bathe the area in a solution of Calendula, 10 drops of mother tincture to 0.25 litre (½ pint) warm water.

High blood pressure

see also PRE-ECLAMPTIC TOXAEMIA

Blood pressure should not be allowed to rise during labour if possible, as this may be a sign that the mother is not going with the flow. Read Advice to Partner/Companion for help with relaxation, massage etc. It is also claimed that immersing the mother in a warm bath will help to bring down the blood pressure.

Specific remedies to be given every 15 minutes for up to 7 doses:

- With red or livid face, dilated pupils, jerking and violent pulsations of the carotid artery (in the neck) *Belladonna 30c*
- When associated with very weak and irregular pains, woman weak, feverish and thirsty, with moist genitals *Caulophyllum 30c*
- Where there is violent vomiting, clenching of the fingers *Cuprum 30c*
- Where blood pressure has been high towards end of pregnancy, pulse is full, hard and quick, head and chest feel full of blood *Veratrum vir. 30c*

Induction

see POST-MATURITY

If the baby is more than 2 weeks overdue there is a possibility that it may cease to be sufficiently well nourished by the placenta. As hospital induction can create a rather overpowering labour which is difficult for the mother to deal with, we recommend the following:

Specific remedy to be taken 3 times a day after the expected date of delivery:

- *Caulophyllum 30c*

If you have been overdue in a previous pregnancy we recommend that you start Caulophyllum 30c in the following dosage: from 36–38 weeks once a week; from 38–40 weeks once a week; 40+weeks one dose 3 times a day.

Labour pains

Psychoprophylactic techniques, especially breathing techniques, learnt at antenatal classes help many women to control pain during labour. In hospital, pain control options include nitrous oxide gas and air, a local anaesthetic if forceps delivery is necessary, or an epidural (injection of anaesthetic into the space around the lower part of the spinal cord). The danger with an epidural is that the mother may not be able to push properly, so the baby may have to be delivered by forceps; the mother may also have a violent headache afterwards and low blood pressure. The drug pethidine is sometimes given, but not immediately before birth as it can cause respiratory distress in the baby and make the mother very spaced out.

Hypnotherapy and acupuncture deserve wider use in labour – for information, contact addresses on p. 336–7 – but they are not widely available yet. Homeopathic remedies are more widely accepted. Those most commonly used are listed below, but there are many others; if possible, consult your homeopath beforehand.

Specific remedies to be given every 5 minutes for up to 10 doses:

• Labour proceeding normally but contractions so violent they are almost unbearable, woman cries out with pain, and is nervous and restless between contractions *Coffea 30c*
• Pains accompanied by frequent urge to pass water or stool, woman very irritable and impatient *Nux 30c*
• Woman in great anguish, talking incoherently, limbs twitching, eyes staring *Belladonna 30c*
• Sensation of constant pressure in womb, constant bearing down sensation, forcing pains, mother very distressed *Secale 30c*
• Mother very restless, chilly, and tearful, labour very slow *Pulsatilla 30c*
• Pains so severe that she can hardly bear them, just wants to get away from herself and the pain, cross, unreasonable, fretful, does not want anyone near her, spiteful, cries out sharply, cannot be satisfied by anything done for her *Chamomilla 30c*
• Labour pains on the left side, weeps with pain and with extreme sensitivity of her vagina and vulva *Platina 30c*

• *Backache labour:* take every 5 minutes for up to 10 doses:
• Contractions so violent they are almost unbearable, woman cries out with pain and is nervous and restless between contractions *Coffea 30c*
• Distressing sore aching pain in back, spasmodic labour pains, woman becomes tired and fretful towards the end of labour *Causticum 30c*
• Drawing pains in back and thighs accompanied by frequent urge to pass water or stool even in first stage, woman very irritable and impatient *Nux 30c*
• Pain relieved by pressure *Kali carb. 30c*

Specific remedies to be taken after an epidural:

• *Arnica 30c* ½-hourly for up to 7 doses, followed by *Hypericum 6c* every 4 hours for up to 5 days

Mal-presentation

Normally babies emerge from the birth canal with their face pointing towards the mother's back; mal-presentation occurs when the baby faces forwards or fails to turn into the head-down position in the last few weeks of pregnancy. The face-forward or occipito-posterior position usually causes prolonged labour and severe back-

ache – 'backache labour'; the buttocks-down or 'breech' position can make delivery extremely difficult since the buttocks do not enlarge the birth canal sufficiently for the head to follow easily. In these and other forms of mal-presentation the baby may have to be delivered by Caesarean.

If you have discomfort then ask your doctor if the baby is in the wrong position. The doctor may review your scan for evidence of a very short cord, or cord round the neck etc.

Specific remedy to be given hourly for up to 3 doses:

• *Pulsatilla 30c*

Nausea and vomiting in labour

Specific remedies to be taken every 2 hours for up to 7 doses:

• Os of the cervix thick and rigid, not dilating properly, accompanied by great feeling of sickness and difficulty in breathing, especially in women who have history of pelvic inflammation *Antimonium tart. 30c*
• Nausea and vomiting, with fainting due to spasmodic pains in womb; vomiting may be of bile *Cocculus 30c*
• Constant nausea, especially with sharp cutting pains at the umbilicus extending down to the womb *Ipecac. 30c*
• Nausea with need for cool air, so doors and windows must be open, lacks thirst, weepy *Pulsatilla 30c*

Post-delivery problems

After-pains

These are a sign that the womb is contracting back to its normal size; discomfort tends to be worse if labour has been relatively easy. If the remedies below produce no improvement within 24 hours, contact your GP or midwife; if you begin to run a temperature, [12].

Specific remedies to be taken every 2 hours for up to 10 doses:

• Sharp pains, especially if woman is oversensitive and has lost a lot of sleep *Coffea 6c*
• Pains associated with frequent urge to pass water or stool *Nux 6c*
• Pains made worse by drinking coffee *Chamomilla 6c*
• If part of placenta has been retained *Pulsatilla 6c*

Appetite changes

Strange cravings or difficulty controlling appetite in the weeks immediately after delivery are due to hormone changes, as pregnancy ends and lactation begins.

Specific remedies to be taken every 12 hours for up to 3 days:

- Craving for salt and salty foods *Natrum mur. 30c*
- Craving for sweets and sugary foods *Lycopodium 30c*
- Indigestion after fatty foods *Pulsatilla 30c*

If you are having difficulty losing weight, increase the amount of exercise you take, and reduce your salt, fat, and carbohydrate intake. Constitutional homeopathic treatment is recommended, but in the meantime one of the remedies below may help.

Specific remedies to be taken 4 times a day for up to 7 days:

- Insatiable appetite, feeling hotter than usual, diarrhoea first thing in morning *Sulphur 6c*
- Not losing weight, constipation, feeling chilly, irritable, and apathetic *Sepia 6c*
- Fluid retention and a craving for salt *Natrum mur. 6c*
- Not losing weight, especially if woman tends to be pale, chilly, sweaty, and clumsy *Calcarea 6c*

Constipation
Specific remedies to be taken every 4 hours for up to 10 doses:

- Ineffectual straining to pass stool *Nux 6c*
- Stools hard, brown/black, and burnt-looking *Bryonia 6c*
- Feeling chilly, exhausted, and irritable as well as constipated *Sepia 6c*

Discharge from uterus (lochia)
Following delivery of the placenta, a quantity of blood, fluids and mucus is discharged from the womb, pure blood at first, and then a milky mixture of mucus and fluid. If discharge is very scanty or very copious, see your midwife; in the meantime try one of the remedies below.

Specific remedies to be taken every hour for up to 10 doses:

- Scanty discharge, red in colour, made even scantier by strong emotions or exposure to cold *Aconite 30c*
- Scanty discharge, diarrhoea, abdominal pain, headache or toothache *Chamomilla 30c*
- Scanty discharge, distended abdomen *Colocynth 30c*
- Scanty discharge, delirious behaviour *Belladonna 30c*

- Scanty discharge, desire for sex *Platina 30c*
- Copious bloody discharge *Secale 30c*
- If no response to Secale and whole vulval area is extremely sensitive *Platina 30c*
- Discharge very slow *Calcarea 30c*
- Discharge very slow, woman feels worn out *China 30c*
- Excessive discharge after over-exertion *Arnica 30c*
- Profuse discharge made worse by chamomile tea *Coffea 30c*
- Profuse discharge made worse by coffee and alcohol *Nux 30c*
- Profuse milky discharge *Pulsatilla 30c*
- Profuse milky discharge which then becomes bloody *Calcarea 30c*
- Bearing down sensation in womb, milky discharge which becomes streaked with pus, or feeling generally chilly, with cold, clammy extremities *Sepia 30c*
- Sweating, increased saliva, offensive-smelling discharge, sensitivity to heat and cold *Mercurius 30c*
- Excessive milky discharge with putrid smell *Carbo an. 30c*

Exhaustion
The effort of giving birth leaves most women extremely tired and stiff and very drained emotionally; this is perfectly normal. Rest and quiet are the best healers. However, one of the remedies below may be helpful; if there is no improvement within 3 days, and there are no complications, consult your homeopath.

Specific remedies to be taken 4 times daily for up to 3 days:

- Exhaustion follows profuse sweating or loss of blood *China 30c*
- Exhaustion accompanied by profuse sweating *Carbo veg. 30c*
- Exhaustion accompanied by hair loss *Calcarea 30c*
- Distended abdomen, bearing down pains *Sepia 30c*
- Distended abdomen, spasmodic abdominal pain *Colocynth 30c*

Incontinence
Bladder control may temporarily be lost as the result of trauma to the muscles of the pelvic floor. Stopping and starting the flow of urine several times as you pass water will help to tighten these muscles (see also Pelvic Floor Exercises under MENOPAUSE). If, despite these exercises and taking the remedy below, there is no improvement within 3 days, see your homeopath.

Specific remedy to be taken 4 times daily for up to 3 days:

- *Belladonna 30c*

Injury to vulva or vagina

Overstretching, tears, or incisions and stitches in this area should be bathed three or four times a day with Arnica solution (10 drops of mother tincture to 0.25 litre [½ pint] warm water) to aid healing.

Piles

These are the result of extreme pressure on the pelvic veins. If the remedy below produces no improvement within 3 days, see your homeopath.

Specific remedy to be taken every 4 hours for up to 3 days:

- *Pulsatilla 6c*

Post-maturity

The risks of stillbirth and brain damage rise significantly after 40 weeks in utero; if the placenta starts to fail, the baby may die from lack of oxygen; lack of oxygen can also cause brain damage. Since the baby's head is also larger and harder than normal, labour is often more difficult, making forceps delivery or Caesarean section more likely. The baby may need to be induced (see INDUCTION).

Postnatal depression see also DEPRESSION

Many women feel 'down' after giving birth, and for many reasons – hormonal changes, tiredness (possibly due to a drop in blood sugar levels), previous episodes of postnatal depression, strains within the marriage or relationship, anxiety about coping with a new baby, financial problems, the sudden realization that life has changed for good. . . In a few women such feelings, initially a natural response to a new situation, last for much longer than a few weeks and seriously undermine their ability to cope. Symptoms include tiredness, an increase or decrease in appetite, feeling that one is a failure, feeling very aggressive towards the baby when he or she cries and guilty afterwards, withdrawing from family, friends, and all forms of social contact, and not least feeling that everything is unreal, that the whole world is made of cardboard. If the depression is associated with coldness, changes in hair growth, increase in weight and general sluggishness it may be that the thyroid gland has been affected (see THYROID PROBLEMS).

A few women completely lose touch with reality, in which case their behaviour can be said to be psychotic (see PSYCHOTIC ILLNESS) rather than depressed; if this happens ② and give Aconite 30c ½-hourly until help arrives. Otherwise, select a remedy from the list below; if there is no improvement within a week or so, seek constitutional treatment from an experienced homeopath or see your GP.

Specific remedies to be taken 4 times daily for up to 3 days:

- Not interested in anything, sex least of all, feeling tired, irritable, and chilly, constipated, yellow-brown discoloration across bridge of nose, morale very good during pregnancy but very low afterwards *Sepia 30c*
- Talking excitedly and incoherently, face red and flushed, eyes staring *Belladonna 30c*
- Persistent obscene thoughts, unusual talkativeness and suspicion, inappropriate laughter, breaking off encounters abruptly and running away *Hyoscyamus 30c*
- Depression brought on by grief *Ignatia 30c*
- Feeling very weepy, not at all thirsty, and worse for heat *Pulsatilla 30c*
- Woman withdrawn, irritable, full of guilt and resentment, refuses to be consoled or comforted, says she just wants to be left alone *Natrum mur. 30c*

Self-help

Mild postnatal depression can be helped by getting more sleep, and by getting out of the house away from the baby. Don't bottle up your feelings; talk things over with a confidante. Taking extra zinc and trying the BLOOD SUGAR LEVELLING DIET for a month or so might also help.

Post-partum haemorrhage

In hospital the drug Syntometrine (derived from the same source as secale) is given to staunch bleeding after delivery. If you are not in hospital, ⑨⑨⑨ and take one of the remedies below.

Specific remedies to be taken every 5 minutes for up to 6 doses:

- Remedy of first resort *Secale 30c*
- Blood dark and clotted, labour pains continue *Pulsatilla 30c*
- Profuse bleeding, backache which feels like period pain, tingling sensation in vagina, body feels as if it is getting larger *Crocus 30c*
- Exhaustion from blood loss during labour *China 30c*
- Continuous, profuse bleeding, bright red blood, nausea and vomiting, feeling cold and clammy, gasping for breath *Ipecac. 30c*

- Dark clots of blood lost intermittently, haemorrhage associated with outburst of anger *Chamomilla 30c*
- Bright red blood which clots easily, pulse hard and full, face burning hot *Ferrum 30c*
- Slightest movement causes bleeding, blood mixed with fluid, blood dark and clotted as well as bright red *Sabina 30c*
- Profuse bleeding with intermittent after-pains, blood hot and bright red, feeling of pressure in abdomen *Belladonna 30c*

Premature birth

Birth before 37 weeks can be caused by conditions such as PRE-ECLAMPTIC TOXAEMIA, PLACENTA PRAEVIA, ante-partum haemorrhage, and high blood pressure during pregnancy (see CARDIOVASCULAR PROBLEMS IN PREGNANCY), but in many cases the cause is not known. Premature babies are at risk of respiratory distress syndrome and NEONATAL JAUNDICE due to the immaturity of their lungs and liver; nevertheless even babies of 26 weeks can be viable, given intensive care. If labour begins several weeks before you expect it, ⑨⑨⑨; in some cases, drugs are given to relax the uterus and prevent labour. If the delivery goes ahead, take Aconite 30c 4 times daily for up to 7 days afterwards

Prolonged labour

Specific remedies to be given every 15 minutes for up to 7 doses:

- Mother exhausted, muscles of uterus no longer able to push, death of baby suspected *Secale 30c*
- Severe backache, muscles of uterus exhausted, mother of strong constitution, or if death of baby is suspected *Pulsatilla 30c*
- Pain stops suddenly due to emotional upset, face red, hot, and puffy *Opium 30c*
- Mother delirious *Hyoscyamus 30c*
- Pulse thin and rigid, labour slow and tedious, feels on and off pressure on sacrum *Belladonna 30c*
- First stage prolonged because the os of the cervix is round, hard, thick, rigid and undilated *Gelsemium 30c*
- Long feeble, ineffectual labour in woman who tends to suffer from nervous exhaustion at best of times *Kali phos. 30c*
- Pains feeble, then stop altogether, and woman very sad and foreboding *Natrum mur. 30c*
- Labour does not progress despite intense pains accompanied by frequent urge to pass water or stool in woman who is very impatient and irritable *Nux 30c*

Puerperal fever

This is caused by infection of the genital tract shortly after birth, although any fever within 2 weeks of childbirth is dangerous since it can cause INFERTILITY or septicaemia. Puerperal fever is now rare thanks to improved hygiene during delivery and of course antibiotics. However, if you begin to run a temperature, ⑫, inform your midwife and take one of the remedies below.

Specific remedies to be taken every hour for up to 10 doses:

- Sudden rise in temperature, skin hot and dry, pain in uterus, vivid thoughts about dying *Aconite 30c*
- Sudden onset of fever, face hot and red, eyes staring, delirium, distended abdomen, great thirst, bowels feel as if they are being clutched by a giant hand *Belladonna 30c*
- Profuse sweating, great sensitivity to heat and cold, offensive-smelling discharge from vagina, increase in saliva, mucus or blood in stools, symptoms worse at night *Mercurius 30c*
- Vaginal discharge suddenly stops, constipation, nausea and vomiting, irritability *Nux 30c*
- Womb feels very sore, slightest movement aggravates soreness, irritability, feeling very apprehensive and pessimistic about the future *Bryonia 30c*

Retained placenta

Normally the placenta is shed within about half an hour of birth, or sooner if the drug Syntometrine is given; if retained for more than an hour, it may have to be removed by hand under general anaesthetic. The homeopathic remedies below aid contraction of the womb and expulsion of the placenta.

Specific remedies to be given every 5 minutes for up to 10 doses:

- Intermittent bleeding, retention of urine, lower abdomen hot, red, sore, and painful to the touch, especially if woman is of a mild, tearful disposition *Pulsatilla 30c*
- Bearing down sensation continues, pains strong and continuous but ineffectual, muscles of uterus no longer able to contract, woman throws bedclothes off and craves fresh air *Secale 30c*
- Vagina feels dry and hot, profuse bleeding, woman red in face, moaning, very distressed, and sensitive to slightest jarring *Belladonna 30c*
- Vulva and vagina extremely sensitive, severe cramping pains in abdomen, constant ooze of dark blood *Platina 30c*

Self-help
Try suckling the baby to stimulate your hormones. If this does not work, try squatting to help gravity remove the placenta.

Sex after childbirth

Intercourse should not be resumed until the vagina has healed; this takes at least 10 days, and several weeks after a tear or an episiotomy. However, many couples prefer to wait for at least 6 weeks, when a full postnatal check-up is routinely done. The vagina will be very sensitive at first, and possibly dry, in which case a lubricant such as KY jelly should be used. Pelvic floor exercises will help to tone up the muscles around the vagina; when you pass water, try to stop and restart the flow of urine several times. Many factors can cause loss of libido at this time – pain, lack of sleep, emotional exhaustion, anxiety, fear of another pregnancy. . . It is possible to become pregnant again even before your periods restart, so some form of contraception will be necessary for a few months even if you are planning to have another baby; breastfeeding cannot be relied on to prevent ovulation.

The remedies listed below are helpful in that they boost energy levels generally. However, if loss of libido persists for more than a few months, constitutional homeopathic treatment should be sought; if the problem lies in the relationship between you and your partner, sexual counselling might be more helpful (see Useful Addresses, p. 333–8).

Specific remedies to be taken every 12 hours for up to 2 weeks:

- Feeling very battered, bruised, and low in energy *Arnica 30c*
- Feeling exhausted after loss of blood, sweat, or other body fluids *China 30c*
- Feeling emotionally fragile and weepy, especially in stuffy rooms *Pulsatilla 30c*
- Aversion to sex, chilliness, irritability, depression *Sepia 30c*

Stretch-marks (striae)

The best treatment for these is vitamin E (100 units a day for 5 days a week) for up to 3 months; you could also try Calc. fluor. tissue salts, 3 tablets 3 times a day for 5 days a week for up to 3 months. These measures should be started after the 14th week of pregnancy.

Special Problems in Infants

There can be little doubt that breastfeeding gives a baby the best possible start in life. However, milk is not 'let down' immediately a baby is born. For 3 days or so after birth the breasts secrete a clear, yellowish fluid called colostrum, which gives the baby valuable antibodies and hormones. The baby's sucking causes extra large amounts of a hormone called oxytocin to be released from the pituitary; this stimulates milk production and also helps the walls of the uterus to contract.

The balance of minerals, vitamins, and proteins in cow's milk is not ideal for babies. It contains many times more sodium, potassium, magnesium, calcium, and phosphorus than the baby needs, 3 times as much protein, which overtaxes acid secretion in the baby's stomach, resulting in indigestion and a proliferation of harmful bacteria, and only a third of the vitamin C and a tenth of the vitamin D.

At birth the head is very large compared with the body – about a quarter of body length is head. This is because the brain develops well in advance of the body. At birth the brain weighs about a quarter of its adult weight, at 6 months about 50 per cent, and at 12 months about 60 per cent. By contrast, birth weight is only 5 per cent of young adult weight, although this doubles within 6 months and triples within 12. Head circumference is measured 3–4 days after birth and serves as a baseline for growth and for detecting any abnormalities.

The pace of brain development is most easy to observe in the way a baby looks at things. In the first few weeks, a baby sees and reacts to objects about 20 cm (8 in) away from the face. By the age of 3 months the eyes are sufficiently coordinated to be able to track slowly moving objects, provided they are no more than 30 cm (12 in) away. At 4 months full accommodation or focusing occurs. At 6 months objects are watched with great attention until they disappear from sight and are then 'forgotten'; the realization that people and things continue to exist when the eye can no longer see them comes much later. At 12 months a baby recognizes familiar people as soon as they come within a range of 6 m (20 ft).

Even newborn babies 'corner' their eyes towards certain sounds. In tests babies have shown themselves to be far more sensitive to the human voice than to pure tones and household noises; in other words they possess an innate ability to distinguish speech sounds from other sounds, an ability fundamental to language acquisition. The first recognizable syllables, usually produced towards the end of the first year, are preceded by burbling and babbling as the pitches and rhythms of speech are tried out. Other tests have shown that even very young babies have a good memory for smells – they recognize mum by her smell.

Chart for detecting hearing problems

'Can your baby hear you?'
Here is a checklist of some of the general signs you can look for in your baby's first year:

Shortly after birth
Your baby should be startled by a sudden loud noise such as a hand clap or a door slamming and should blink or open his eyes widely to such sounds.   Y/N

By one month
Your baby should be beginning to notice sudden prolonged sounds like the noise of a vacuum cleaner and he should pause and listen to them when they begin.   Y/N

By 4 months
He should quieten or smile to the sound of your voice even when he cannot see you. He may also turn his head or eyes towards you if you come up from behind and speak to him from the side. Y/N

By 7 months
He should turn immediately to your voice across the room or to very quiet noises made on each side if he is not too occupied with other things.   Y/N

By 9 months
He should listen attentively to familiar sounds and search for very quiet sounds made out of sight. He should also show pleasure in babbling loudly and tunefully.   Y/N

By 12 months
He should show some response to his own name and to other familiar words. He may also respond when you say 'no' and 'bye bye' even when he cannot see any accompanying gesture.   Y/N

Your health visitor will perform a routine hearing screening test on your baby between 6 and 8 months of age. She will be able to help and advise you at any time before or after this test if you are concerned about your baby and his development. If you suspect that your baby is not hearing normally, either because you cannot answer yes to the items above or for some other reason, then seek advice from your health visitor.

Physical development is most obvious between 16 and 28 weeks, when the neck and trunk muscles develop, allowing the baby to sit up and look around and take experimental swipes at nearby objects. By 40 weeks most babies are experienced crawlers, eager for horizons beyond the cot and the pram. Shortly afterwards there are wobbly attempts to stand, though unsupported standing is not usually achieved until about a year old.

The things to watch out for particularly in infants are fever and dehydration. Temperature quickly rises in response to infection, hot weather, too many blankets, and so on, and measures to reduce it should be taken very swiftly (see FEVER). To take a baby's temperature, put the bulb of the thermometer under the armpit for 3 minutes. Persistent diarrhoea or vomiting can easily cause dehydration; usually the cause of diarrhoea is premature introduction of solids or too much sugar in feeds.

Daily immersion in soap and water is not essential for a baby. The essential areas to clean thoroughly are eyes, face, hands, and bottom, the traditional 'topping and tailing' method.

Granules are the most convenient way of giving homeopathic remedies to babies; they quickly dissolve on the tongue and cannot be spat out as easily as pilules. Alternatively, crush a pilule between two clean spoons, dissolve it in a little warm water, and drop it on to the tongue with a dropper.

Asphyxia of the newborn
The failure of a newborn baby to breathe, more common in small-for-dates babies, overdue babies, and babies whose mothers have received pethidine in labour. The baby doesn't move or cry, and turns blue; after 5 minutes of not breathing brain damage is likely, and after 10 minutes the baby will die. If the baby has been delivered at home ⑨⑨⑨. Hold him or her upside down and massage the back. If this fails start mouth to mouth resuscitation, removing any fluid or mucus from the baby's mouth first; once the baby is breathing, give one of the emergency homeopathic remedies below.

If mouth-to-mouth resuscitation does not work, artificial respiration may be necessary (a tube is inserted through the baby's mouth and into the lungs, and attached to a respirator); in meantime, give Carbo veg. 30c in the dosage specified below.

Specific remedies to be given every 2 minutes until baby loses blue tinge and is breathing and crying normally:

- Baby collapsed, limp, cold, nearly dead *Carbo veg. 30c*
- Baby cold, blue, gasping for breath, failing pulse *Laurocerasus 6c*

Birthmarks
Caused by local pigmentation of skin or by an accumulation of tiny blood vessels (NAEVI) close to surface of skin.

Pigmented spots, also known as 'café au lait' spots because they are coffee-coloured, are usually permanent; they are much larger than ordinary moles, irregular in shape, and may have hairs growing out of them.

There are 3 types of naevi: *capillary naevi*, which are flat pink or pink-brown spots – these usually fade within 18 months; *strawberry naevi*, which are strawberry-red, raised, about 2.5 cm (1 in) across, and grow rapidly at first, then slow down and grow with the child – most fade after 3 years; and *port wine stains*, mulberry-coloured, slightly raised, and often extensive patches on face or limbs – these generally persist into adult life. Disfiguring or unsightly birthmarks can be treated by cosmetic surgery or disguised with skin-coloured creams.

If a strawberry naevus bleeds, apply pressure and give Phosphorus 6c every 5 minutes until bleeding stops, then give 3 doses of Phosphorus 30c at 12-hour intervals. For a strawberry naevus which does not bleed, give 3 doses of Thuja 30c at 12-hour intervals and apply Thuja mother tincture every day for 3 weeks. If these measures do not help, see your homeopath.

Bronchiolitis
Viral infection which causes swelling of the membranes lining the smaller airways (bronchioles) in the lungs. Usually occurs in children under 18 months old, often after COLDS, and is most dangerous in children under 6 months old. If, within 2–3 days of starting a cold, the child begins to wheeze, has difficulty breathing, looks blue around lips, and refuses food, ② as there may be a danger of heart failure or pneumonia.

Specific remedies to be taken every 10 minutes for up to 10 doses until help arrives:

- Child hoarse, wheezy, blue in face, exhaled breath feels cold, attack comes on in evening *Carbo veg. 30c*

- Child exhausted with trying to breathe, too weak to cough up loose phlegm, nostrils sucked in with effort of breathing, vomiting *Antimonium tart. 30c*

Circumcision
Surgical removal of foreskin of penis; usually an elective procedure but occasionally necessary in cases of balanitis, phimosis (see PENIS PROBLEMS), or repeated swelling of foreskin when urine is passed. Do not attempt to pull back the foreskin until the child is at least 3 years old, as it may tear and lead to phimosis. As soon as the child can comfortably move it back, he should be taught to wash underneath it in the bath. If there is any irritation, apply Hypericum and Calendula solution (5 drops of mother tincture of each in 0.25 litre [½ pint] warm water).

Colds
Quite common in young babies, but not harmful unless they interfere with feeding, or spread to throat, lungs, ears, or brain. See below for suitable homeopathic remedies. Decongestant nose drops (1% saline solution or 0.5% ephedrine, both obtainable from chemist) can be given just before feeding or sleeping if a stuffy nose is causing problems, but always in strict accordance with instructions on bottle and never for more than a day at a time as they can damage sensitive lining of nose. Homeopathic remedies should always be tried first.

Specific remedies to be taken every 2 hours for up to 4 doses:

- Cold comes on suddenly, especially after exposure to cold, dry wind, sneezing, burning throat, restlessness, symptoms worse at night *Aconite 30c*
- Cold comes on suddenly, with a high temperature, skin dry, hot, and burning, light hurts eyes, sore throat worse on right side, tickly cough, person very thirsty *Belladonna 30c*
- Baby more than usually irritable, feels cold, nose runs during day but becomes blocked at night *Nux 6c*
- Sweating, excessive salivation, sneezing, catarrh thick and yellowish-green, bad breath *Mercurius 6c*
- Baby not at all thirsty but wants lots of attention *Pulsatilla 6c*

Colic
Sharp tummy pain which causes baby to pull legs up, scream, and go red in face; may be a reaction to dairy products, wheat, cabbage, citrus fruit in mother's diet, or mother's tension and anxiety; in

a bottle-fed baby it may be due to air-swallowing because hole in teat is too small. Most common form of colic is *3-month colic*, typically coming on in evening and lasting anything from a few minutes to several hours; burping or laying baby over knee or shoulder usually has little effect. If baby turns very pale and limp, or vomits, or has DIARRHOEA, a more serious condition should be suspected; to be on safe side, 12.

Specific remedies to be given every 5 minutes for up to 10 doses:

- Symptoms relieved by firm pressure on stomach *Colocynth 6c*
- Symptoms relieved by warmth and gentle pressure *Magnesia phos. 6c*
- Baby very irritable, screams at slightest movement *Bryonia 30c*
- Baby impossible to please, but seems to improve when carried around *Chamomilla 6c*
- Where mother is breastfeeding and grieving or emotionally upset *Ignatia 6c*

Self-help
If mother's exhaustion is affecting baby, try to arrange for someone else to do the household chores for a day or two and encourage her to remain in bed. Resting will encourage milk production, and drinking more fluids will encourage a better milk supply in evenings and at night. If mother is irritable from lack of sleep, give Nux 30c every 8 hours for up to 5 days.

Constipation
Baby is said to be constipated if she passes infrequent hard stools which are causing considerable pain, discomfort or straining. If stools are soft they are not constipated. If constipation has been present since birth see your GP, as it may be Hirschsprung's disease, intestinal atresia or intestinal stenosis. First try giving extra fluids and Nux 6c 1 to 6 times a day for up to 36 hours; if there is no improvement see your GP.

Cot death (Sudden Infant Death Syndrome – SIDS)
Happens to 13–15 in every 10,000 babies, usually between age of 6 weeks and 4 months; girl babies, first babies, breastfed babies, and babies born into fairly affluent families do not succumb as often as boy babies, second, third, and fourth babies, bottle-fed babies, and babies born into poorer families. Suffocation by pillows, blankets, etc. is very rarely the cause. However, there does seem to be a link between SIDS and various respiratory problems – FEEDING PROBLEMS which are respiratory in origin, ASPHYXIA OF THE NEWBORN (when baby fails to breathe at birth), cyanotic attacks (breathing difficulties which cause skin to turn blue), and minor respiratory tract infections, especially those occurring in winter. One cot death in 4 is attributed to a combination of factors, including brain malfunction, respiratory tract abnormalities, and sudden severe infection. In other cases, death may occur because nervous control of breathing is jeopardized by larynx descending into throat – this happens when infant is about 3 months old; atmospheric pollution (carbon monoxide, lead, organo-phosphate pesticides) at this critical age is known to affect nervous control of breathing.

Other speculative causes include a particular type of microorganism when it is associated with a certain type of mattress, ALLERGY to cow's milk, botulism (a particularly severe form of food poisoning), hyperthermia from being in an overheated room, hyperthyroidism (see THYROID PROBLEMS) and a deficiency of biotin, vitamin E, selenium, or potassium.

The World Health Organization, in its attempt to reduce incidence of SIDS worldwide, recommends that women should not get pregnant too young, that number of pregnancies should be limited, with 2–3 years between pregnancies, that mothers should not smoke or take drugs, and that babies should be breastfed for 4–6 months.

The Foundation for the Study of Infant Deaths recommend now that infants should only be placed on their backs. If they are put on their sides they should be three-quarters on their backs with the arm of the side they are lying on out in front to prevent them from rolling face downwards. There is now evidence that babies who sleep on their fronts are 9 times more likely to become victims of cot death than those who lie on their backs. The reason for not placing babies on their backs in the past was that doctors believed they could choke on inhaled milk, but apparently this does not happen. Further advice includes paying careful attention to controlling your baby's body temperature, so that she does not become too hot or too cold. Taking your baby into bed with you is dangerous if you are under the influence of drugs or alcohol. You should take care that baby does not overheat. Mothers are also advised not to smoke during pregnancy, and not to allow anyone to smoke near the baby.

Crying and screaming
A baby's way of communicating hunger, thirst, discomfort, pain, loneliness, boredom, anxiety. . . If the cause of crying is not understood, parents become angry and worried and their feelings communicate themselves to the baby, who reacts by crying more – the classic vicious circle. If you

cannot work out why your baby is crying, talk to your GP or health visitor.

Generally speaking, the more lustily a baby bawls, the more healthy he or she is; a healthy newborn baby may spend many of its waking hours crying, but by age of 6 months a lot of waking time is spent gurgling and playing. So if crying is feeble or infrequent, especially in a newborn baby, or if a 6-month-old baby does nothing but cry when he or she is awake, something may be wrong. Other danger signs are FEVER, runny nose, cough, DIARRHOEA, VOMITING, and SLOW WEIGHT GAIN. An unusually high-pitched cry, coupled with vomiting, a bulging fontanelle (soft spot on top of head where bones of skull meet), and intolerance of light, may be a sign of brain infection, possibly MENINGITIS; appropriate action is (999).

Most frequent cause of crying is hunger; if your baby stops crying when fed, increase frequency of feeds; if she starts crying less than 2 hours after being fed, increase size of feeds. FEEDING PROBLEMS can also cause crying. If a few sips of water between feeds relieve crying, the cause may be thirst.

Babies also cry because of COLIC (screaming attacks in evening, especially around age of 3 months), TEETHING (usually from 6 months onwards), or NAPPY RASH, or because nappy pins are sticking in, or bath water is too hot, or fingers get caught in shawls, or because they get worried by too much noise, very bright lights, too much laughter, too much hugging, too much tickling. . . Crying when passing water is quite normal; if observed closely, it can be seen that a baby usually cries just before passing water, which helps to raise pressure in bladder and so expel urine. Excessive crying may also be an early sign of hyperactivity.

If a baby stops crying when picked up, he or she may simply be feeling bored or excluded; even if you cannot give your undivided attention, place the cot where he or she can watch what you are doing. Babies are very accurate sensors of tension in the family, especially of tension and tiredness in the mother; crying then becomes a way of expressing emotional discomfort and asking for reassurance.

Self-help

Only a parent who has had to care for a constantly crying baby knows how exhausting it is. For the sake of her health and sanity, the mother should try to rest while the baby is sleeping, even if that means letting the housework slide. She also deserves an evening out and a good night's sleep at least once a week; if she is breastfeeding, milk can be expressed beforehand and left in a bottle. For suggestions about how to get a good night's sleep for both self and baby, see SLEEP PROBLEMS. Parents who feel ragged from loss of sleep might also benefit from constitutional homeopathic treatment.

A crying baby often responds to rhythmic sounds (a tape recording of mother's heartbeat, for example), or to being rocked. Sucking a dummy or a thumb also has a soothing effect; dummies should be changed every week or so as they quickly become germ-ridden.

Only a very thin line separates parents who manage to cope with a continually crying baby and those who don't. If you have ever battered your baby, or feel that you might, seek help immediately, and don't be afraid to do so; talk to your GP, health visitor, or the Social Work Department of the NSPCC (address on p. 335). CRY-SIS (address on p. 334) also offers support. If you have good reason to believe that someone is battering his or her baby, tell one of the agencies mentioned above; you will be helping both baby and parent in the long run. A word of caution, however; some cases of 'baby battering' have been found to be due to mineral deficiencies, which produce X-ray images very similar to those seen in genuine cases. This should not deter you from reporting as above.

Dehydration

see GASTROENTERITIS, DIARRHOEA, VOMITING

Diarrhoea

Potentially serious in very young babies as it quickly leads to dehydration. Diarrhoea is one of the symptoms of GASTROENTERITIS (fever of 38°C [100°F] or more, with or without VOMITING, lack of enthusiasm for feeds, torpor); if gastro-enteritis is suspected, or if stools are mixed with blood, or if diarrhoea persists for longer than 12 hours, call your GP. In meantime, give frequent sips of water to prevent dehydration and select a remedy from the list below.

Occasionally diarrhoea in infants is caused by too much sugar (too little water added to fruit juices or too much sugar added to fruit purées, for example); some drugs are also given in a very sugary base. Gripe water can also cause diarrhoea. Liquid stools in a baby who has just been weaned usually indicate that he or she is still unable to cope with solids; wait 2–3 weeks, then reintroduce them.Occasionally diarrhoea is due to too early reintroduction of milk after an attack of GASTROENTERITIS.

Specific remedies to be given every hour for up to 10 doses:

- Diarrhoea comes on after exposure to cold wind *Aconite 30c*

- Diarrhoea brought on by food which has gone off slightly, or diarrhoea which gets worse when baby is given cold food or drinks, with baby exhausted, breathless, and emaciated *Arsenicum 6c*
- Diarrhoea associated with teething, greenish stools, baby irritable and difficult to please *Chamomilla 6c*
- Diarrhoea associated with colic *Colocynth 6c*
- Diarrhoea caused by over-feeding *Nux 6c*
- Baby passes watery stools after eating or drinking, and even during washing *Podophyllum 6c*
- Diarrhoea caused by sour fruit or by drinking cold drinks when overheated, slightest movement makes diarrhoea worse *Bryonia 30c*

Eye inflammation

Usually a combination of a mild infection and blocked tear ducts; if tear ducts cannot be unblocked by gently massaging skin on either side of nose, a paediatrician will use a probe to open them. Wipe eyes every 4 hours with Hypericum and Calendula solution (5 drops of mother tincture of each in 0.25 l [½ pint] boiled cooled water) and give Argentum nit. 6c every 2 hours for up to 10 doses. If inflammation persists, see your GP; an eye swab may have to be taken. In rare cases, eyes may be inflamed because of gonorrhea (see SEXUALLY TRANSMITTED DISEASES) during pregnancy.

Failure to thrive

see SLOW WEIGHT GAIN, FEEDING PROBLEMS

Febrile convulsions

Fits brought on by FEVER. There is no evidence that febrile convulsions cause permanent brain damage, but if they recur without fever, constitutional treatment should be sought. In an acute attack (999) if homeopathic remedies fail to take effect within 2 minutes. It may be necessary for your GP to give a tranquillizer by rectum to stop convulsions. If child loses consciousness, put him or her in recovery position.

Specific remedies to be given every minute for up to 3 doses or until fit subsides:

- First signs of fit *Aconite 30c*
- Fit accompanies gastroenteritis *Aethusa 6c*
- Fit preceded by staring eyes and excited, incoherent behaviour *Belladonna 30c*
- Child very pale, has sunken fontanelle *Zinc sulph. 6c*

Self-help see FEVER for care of feverish child.

Feeding problems

Modern wisdom is that babies should be fed on demand and allowed to feed until satisfied. Breastfeeding may need to be every 2 hours at first (see pp. 138–9 for pros and cons of breastfeeding and bottle-feeding). Time to introduce solids is when a baby's hunger increases, causing more frequent waking at night.

Government recommendation is that infants should not be started on mixed feeding until they are around 4 months old, to prevent allergy and possible overweight. However, they also recommend that solids should be introduced no later than 6 months, because if the infant is fed primarily on milk there is a risk of iron deficiency, rickets and anaemia, particularly amongst Asians. Adequate milk intake should be continued as solids are being introduced.

Consult your GP or health visitor if your baby loses interest in food or stops gaining weight (see SLOW WEIGHT GAIN). Regurgitation of small amounts of food is quite normal, but this should happen less and less once solids are introduced. However, if the baby actually vomits (brings up large amounts of half-digested food), and this happens several times within 24 hours, or if VOMITING is accompanied by FEVER or DIARRHOEA, 12. Possible causes include a digestive tract abnormality, GASTROENTERITIS, lactose intolerance, and INTUSSUSCEPTION; see VOMITING for further information.

Breastfed babies

Baby should be put to the breast as soon as possible, and certainly within 24 hours of birth, and then fed on demand, if possible, until age of 4 to 6 months. If breasts are too full for the baby to suck comfortably, some milk should be expressed before feeding. If milk is too watery, salty, or bitter, the baby will probably cry and draw away from the breast. Self-help measures and homeopathic remedies for distended breasts, sore nipples, loss of milk, unpleasant-tasting milk, etc. appear under BREASTFEEDING PROBLEMS on p. 139.

Bottle-fed babies

Carefully follow mixing instructions on container. Feed which is too dilute will result in small, firm, dark green stools; feed which is not sufficiently diluted will make the baby thirsty because salt content is high for its volume; in both cases baby is likely to express discomfort by crying. If the baby nods off while feeding, wake him or her up. Observe careful sterilization of bottles procedure (p. 139).

Weaning

Best policy is to introduce solids one by one at first, just in case there are any intolerances. Best foods to wean on are rice, potatoes, vegetables (especially carrots and greens), fruit, avocados, and fish or lean meat, all well puréed of course. Avoid wheat, nuts, corn, and mushrooms, which are not digested well, and keep dairy products to a minimum. If any food produces wind or other upsets, note it down and wait for a month or two before reintroducing it. If there is a family history of food intolerance, delay introduction of wheat and dairy products until age of 12 months.

Fever

Generally a sign that body is marshalling its resources to fight and destroy infection; however, in very young babies, whose temperature regulation mechanism may not be mature, temperature quickly rises in response to hot weather, hot rooms, or too many clothes or blankets.

Automatically reaching for aspirin, paracetamol, etc. when a baby has a temperature is not necessary; aspirin should not be given to young children because of risk of Reye's syndrome, a rare but fatal disease which seems to be linked to taking of aspirin. In most cases the homeopathic remedies listed below effectively bring temperature down; sometimes simply undressing the baby or giving tepid sponge-downs brings temperature back to normal. Junior paracetamol should only be given if fever rises above 39°C (102°F) and homeopathic remedies are not working, if the baby is prone to FEBRILE CONVULSIONS (fits which come on when temperature rises above normal – see p. 151), or if fever is preventing baby from sleeping. Give extra fluids.

If, despite all efforts, the baby's temperature remains above 39°C (102°F) for more than 2 hours, call your GP. Also, if your baby has a history of febrile convulsions, call your GP as soon as fever develops. If baby goes into convulsions, or if skin develops bluish tinge, (999).

Conditions such as croup and stridor (crowing intakes of breath), acute bronchitis and bronchiolitis (rapid breathing, gasping for breath), pneumonia (dry cough, wheezing, rapid breathing), and MENINGITIS (unusual drowsiness or irritability, unusual high-pitched cry) are accompanied by fever, and require prompt medical attention; appropriate action is ②. Fever can also be an indication of GASTROENTERITIS (diarrhoea, perhaps vomiting as well) or of one of the childhood fevers; appropriate action is 12. Middle ear infection (sudden waking, crying, pulling at affected ear) and throat infections (refusing solids) can also be accompanied by fever; keep infant under close observation, and if there is no improvement within 24 hours, see your GP.

Specific remedies to be given every hour for up to 10 doses as soon as fever comes on:

- Sudden rise in temperature after exposure to cold dry wind, baby restless, shivery, and thirsty *Aconite 30c*
- Sudden onset, baby very thirsty, with burning hot skin and staring eyes, unusual noises and movements *Belladonna 30c*
- Baby very restless and thirsty for small drinks at frequent intervals, symptoms worse between midnight and 2 am *Arsenicum 6c*
- Slightest movement causes baby to cry out, large quantities of fluid gulped down *Bryonia 30c*

Self-help

Tepid sponging is a very effective method of bringing temperature down. Spread a clean towel on the floor in a warm room, undress the child, and lay her on the towel; sponge face, arms and legs, and front of body with tepid water, then pat dry with a second towel; turn the baby over, wet-sponge arms, legs, and back, and pat dry. Repeat this procedure, front and back, 6 times. If temperature has not come down within 2 hours, repeat the process. Give the baby as much to drink (dilute, unsweetened apple juice, for example) as he or she seems to want.

Sometimes, simply undressing the baby and giving frequent small drinks does the trick.

If fever is not due to overheating nor accompanied by any other obvious symptoms, a low-level infection may be the cause. If this is the case, give Ferrum phos. (see Tissue Salts, p. 24) every 30 minutes for up to 4 doses, then every 2 hours for up to 4 doses. If there is no improvement within 48 hours, see your GP.

Gastroenteritis

Potentially serious in very young babies since inflammation of stomach and small intestine causes DIARRHOEA and VOMITING, and therefore dehydration; stools are green and watery, baby develops slight FEVER, tends to feed poorly, and becomes miserable and tetchy. Signs of dehydration are a dry mouth, sunken eyes and fontanelle (spot on top of head where cranial bones meet), and irritability. Condition is less common among breastfed babies who are, to some extent, protected against bacteria and viruses by antibodies in mother's milk; bottle-fed babies not only miss out on this protection but are also exposed to germs harboured by bottles, teats, and other feeding utensils.

If remedies below do not produce some improvement within 12 hours, or if signs of dehydration develop, call your GP.

Specific remedies to be given every 1–2 hours (depending on severity) for up to 10 doses:

- Milk makes symptoms worse, stools green and watery, baby limp and passive, upper lip looks very pale *Aethusa 6c*
- Baby cold, weak, restless, and obviously miserable *Arsenicum 6c*
- Symptoms come on in cold wet weather, or after catching a chill, stools greenish-yellow and slimy *Dulcamara 6c*
- Colicky stomach pain, with legs drawn up, gentle pressure seems to relieve pain *Colocynth 6c*
- Copious vomiting and diarrhoea *Nux 6c*
- Baby chilly, apathetic, and makes a fuss if touched, stools yellow and frothy, a lot of wind *China 6c*
- Baby very thirsty for cold water, which is vomited up as soon as it becomes warm in stomach *Phosphorus 6c*
- Diarrhoea, with undigested food in stools; baby seems better after passing stools but shows no obvious pain on doing so *Phosphoric ac. 6c*

Self-help
If you are bottle-feeding, make sure all utensils are sterilized each time you use them; avoid touching teats once they have been sterilized, and never put them in your mouth. Stop feeding for 24 hours, and give water with a little glucose and salt in it (1 teaspoon glucose and ½ teaspoon salt to 0.5 litre [1 pint] boiled cooled water) instead; on the second day give quarter-strength feed, the next day half-strength, and the next day three-quarters-strength; on the fifth day, go back to normal strength, but feed a little and often rather than a lot all at once.

If you are breastfeeding, give extra spoonfuls of boiled cooled water (made up as above) between feeds.

These measures should produce some improvement within 24 hours, but if they don't, call your GP.

Intussusception
Condition in which small intestine telescopes into large intestine, causing violent ABDOMINAL PAIN and screaming. Usually occurs around 6 months of age and is more common in boys than girls. In intervals between pain, child is limp and pale, and may vomit. Stools may be red and jelly-like. If intussusception is suspected ② and

give nothing by mouth, except homeopathic remedies; if intestine cannot be manipulated back into place, an operation may be necessary.

Specific remedies to be given every 15 minutes while waiting for help to arrive:

- First choice: colon seen as a lump during colic *Belladonna 30c*
- Pain relieved by bending child double *Colocynth 6c*
- Pain not relieved by bending child double *Nux 6c*
- Child restless and passing red, jelly-like stools *Rhus tox. 6c*

Jaundice
see NEONATAL JAUNDICE

Meningitis
Potentially more serious in infants and toddlers than in older children and adults as there is a slight risk of brain damage if condition is not detected and treated in early stages. First symptom is FEVER of 39°C (102°F) or more; early signs of head pain are unusual irritability or quietness, and turning eyes away from light; infant may also hold neck rigid or arched back despite attempts to push head forward; other symptoms may be VOMITING and convulsions (see FEBRILE CONVULSIONS), an unusual high-pitched cry, and a purplish rash on trunk; in very young babies, fontanelle (meeting point of skull bones on top of head) may bulge due to pressure of cerebrospinal fluid around brain.

If meningitis is suspected, ⑨⑨⑨; baby may need antibiotics and intravenous drip. Chances of complete recovery, with no residual mental handicap, are good.

Specific remedies to be given every 5 minutes until help arrives:

- Symptoms onset after head injury *Arnica 30c*
- Baby restless, panicky, thirsty, skin feels very dry *Aconite 30c*
- Baby very hot, making unusual noises and movements, pupils wide and staring *Belladonna 30c*
- Baby obviously in great pain, unusually quiet, unable to look into light *Bryonia 30c*

Nappy rash
Usually caused by ammoniacal reaction between urine and faeces, or by irritating chemicals in faeces; not thoroughly rinsing soap or detergent out of nappies is another possible cause. Baby's buttocks, thighs, and genitals become sore, red, spotty, and weepy in areas touched by soiled

nappies; in boys, foreskin may become inflamed, making urination painful; rash may become secondarily infected with candida fungus if baby has been given antibiotics or if breast milk has antibiotics in it, or if mother has oral THRUSH or genital thrush (see VAGINAL AND VULVAL PROBLEMS).

If homeopathic remedies listed below produce no improvement, see your homeopath.

Specific remedies to be given 4 times daily for up to 5 days:

- Rash dry, red, and scaly *Sulphur 6c*
- Skin itchy, with little blisters *Rhus tox. 6c*
- Nappy area very moist and sweaty, baby produces more saliva than usual *Mercurius 6c*
- Rash area raw and bleeding *Medorrhinum 6c*
- Nappy rash in a fat baby who suffers from copious head sweats at night *Calcarea 6c*

Self-help
Simplest and most effective treatment is to allow the baby to spend as much time out of nappies as possible, provided room is warm and dry; rash almost always clears up when exposed to air. After washing rash area with warm water only (no soap), pat dry with sterile cotton wool, and apply Calendula ointment. If you are using washable nappies, be extra careful about rinsing out all soap or detergent; if rash persists, try disposable nappies, and if one brand doesn't seem to help, try another. At all events, change nappies more frequently. Excluding cow's milk and dairy products along with food colourings may also be beneficial. See ALLERGY and talk to your GP or health visitor if prolonged avoidance becomes necessary.

Neonatal jaundice
Many babies, especially babies born before term, develop a yellowish tinge within 2–3 days of birth due to immaturity of liver, which cannot process the yellow pigment bilirubin (a by-product of continuous breakdown of red blood cells) fast enough. Both skin and white of eyes turn yellow, and baby may become lethargic and half-hearted about feeding; in an otherwise healthy baby, jaundice fades after a few days. Standard treatment is to give baby plenty to drink to flush out excess bilirubin; if bilirubin level remains high, baby may be exposed to ultraviolet light to make bilirubin water-soluble so kidneys can eliminate it (there is a risk of very high bilirubin levels causing brain damage); in very severe cases, baby may need a blood transfusion.

In a few cases, jaundice may be due to haemolytic ANAEMIA caused by RHESUS INCOMPATIBILITY (baby's red blood cells come under attack from mother's antibodies) or bile duct atresia; former is referred to as haemolytic jaundice, and appears within 24 hours of birth; latter is known as obstructive jaundice, and usually onsets a week or so after birth, accompanied by DIARRHOEA and loss of weight. Haemolytic jaundice may require a blood transfusion, or no treatment at all, but the outlook for obstructive jaundice is poor unless the bile ducts can be surgically repaired.

Special remedies to be given every 2 hours for up to 10 doses when first signs of jaundice appear:

- First choice *Chamomilla 6c*
- If Chamomilla is not effective *Mercurius 6c*
- If jaundice is due to Rhesus incompatibility *Crotalus 6c*

Screaming
see CRYING AND SCREAMING

Seborrhoeic eczema
Common during first 3 months of life, affecting scalp, face, neck, armpits, or nappy area; scurfy patches on scalp are known as 'cradle cap'; these may become yellow and soggy-looking, and extend to eyebrows and ears; on face and elsewhere condition causes red blotches and pimples which become angry-looking when baby cries or gets hot; cause is not known, but condition is occasionally triggered off by NAPPY RASH (whereas nappy rash is confined to nappy area, eczema may involve abdomen and thighs as well). Severe seborrhoeic eczema can lead to infantile eczema, but most cases heal of their own accord. If homeopathic remedies and self-help measures given below produce no improvement within 3 weeks, see your homeopath. Antibiotics and steroids should be avoided unless general health is suffering, and then only used for as short a time as possible.

Specific remedies to be given every 4 hours for up to 14 days:

- Affected areas of skin weepy, encrusted, and easily become infected *Graphites 6c*
- Eczema mainly affects scalp and face, lesions thickly encrusted, swollen glands *Viola 6c*
- Skin dry and scaly, but not infected; Calendula ointment seems to have no effect *Lycopodium 6c*
- Scabby patches on scalp which ooze and mat hair together *Vinca 6c*

Self-help
Keep affected areas clean with regular washing and thorough drying. After washing, apply

Calendula ointment. Gently rub skin with olive oil to loosen scales before washing.

Sleep problems

Generally speaking, newborn babies spend most of their time sleeping or dozing, waking only for feeds, nappy changes, and cuddles. By end of first year, most babies are awake for 8 hours out of 24, although they may spend 2–3 hours sleeping during the day; by the time they are 7–10 months old most babies, and their parents, sleep through the night without waking. Ideally, a baby should be allowed to sleep whenever he or she is tired, wherever that happens to be; a certain amount of background noise is no bad thing.

Most night-time sleep problems in babies under 6 months old are caused by hunger, so first resort should be the breast or the bottle. If this does not have a sedative effect, problem may be wind or a dirty nappy; winding the baby or changing the nappy usually does the trick. Discomfort of COLIC or NAPPY RASH, or running a temperature, can also cause night-time grizzling. In the long run, taking baby back to bed with you, or giving too many cuddles in middle of night, may create more problems than it solves.

Occasionally babies wake in middle of night because they have kicked all their bedclothes off and feel cold; a sleeping bag or sleeping suit usually solves the problem.

Once the need for night-feeding stops, around age of 7–10 months, baby should sleep through the night; if she starts crying, don't immediately rush in to give reassurance; she will probably go back to sleep within a few minutes. If attention is always given on demand, baby may start to exploit the situation! That said, changes in routine can be very upsetting to babies, and at such times they genuinely need extra cuddling and reassurance.

Specific remedies to be given every 30 minutes starting 1 hour before baby's bedtime and every 30 minutes if baby wakes; 10 doses is maximum:

- If baby has had a shock or a fright *Aconite 30c*
- Baby irritable and impossible to please, only stops crying when picked up and carried around *Chamomilla 30c*
- Baby too excited or overwrought to sleep *Coffea 6c*
- Baby who wakes crying around 4 am and refuses to be pacified *Nux 6c*

Self-help
Make sure the baby's room is warm, but not too warm (around 20°C [68°F] is about right), and relatively quiet.

The baby should be woken up and given a late-night feed when parents go to bed. If the baby wakes up hungry in middle of night, give a feed immediately – if you are bottle-feeding, have everything ready you are likely to need. Give a proper feed, not water, as water will only temporarily allay hunger. If you find it difficult to get back to sleep, drink some chamomile tea – keep a thermos of it next to the bed. If you and your partner can take turns night-feeding, so much the better.

If sleepless nights are really getting you down, and the baby is over 12 weeks old and going about 5 hours between feeds during the day, it may be worth leaving the baby to cry for about 20 minutes before you take action; hunger crying is likely to continue, but habit crying will probably stop.

If the baby sleeps through the night but wakes very early, the best thing to do is change the nappy and give him or her some toys to play with, while you go back to sleep for an hour or two. You could also try adjusting your baby's internal 'clock' by making bedtime 15 minutes later each night until he or she wakes at a civilized hour.

Babies are very conservative and like to have a routine, so try to keep things in the same sequence and at roughly the same times each day. Avoid over-excitement in the hour or so before baby's bedtime. Have toys and mobiles nearby.

Slow weight gain

Most babies lose weight, often as much as 140 g (5 oz), in first few days, but by 10 days old they should have regained their birth weight; they should weigh twice as much by 5 months and 3 times as much at one year old (see chart on p. 156). Steady weight gain, without troughs or plateaux, is the desideratum; even a low birth weight baby should make steady progress, albeit on a lower level.

Breastfed babies who are losing weight should be fed on demand, if possible, and be allowed to suck for as long as they want; if bottle-feeding, check that you are giving correct amount and concentration of feed (see FEEDING PROBLEMS). If the baby is over 3 months old, he or she may need solids; this should be discussed with your health visitor or GP.

If slow weight gain is associated with periodic VOMITING, or with undue sleepiness, irritability, or reluctance to feed, see your GP; if it is associated with loose, pale, smelly stools, the baby may have a digestive problem such as lactose intolerance or COELIAC DISEASE; these problems also require attention of GP. Constitutional homeopathic treatment may also help.

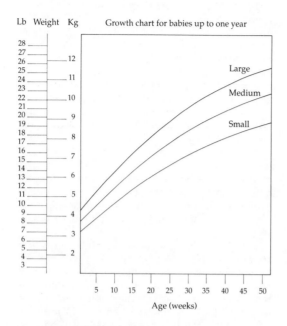

Lb Weight Kg   Growth chart for babies up to one year

Age (weeks)

Growth chart for babies up to one year

Teething

Sore gums, irritability, and stomach upsets can occur during eruption of milk teeth. Babies cut their first teeth around age of 6 months, and all 20 milk teeth (8 incisors, 4 canines, 8 molars) are usually through by the end of the third year. Homeopathic remedies are extremely effective against the pain and discomfort of teething. The small flaps of skin pushed aside as the molar teeth come through are quite natural; they separate from the gum in due course.

Specific remedies to be given every 30 minutes, or more frequently if pain is severe, for up to 10 doses:

- Child irritable, wants to be carried around, makes a fuss when put in cot, one cheek hot and red, the other pale *Chamomilla 30c*
- Child flushed and hot, pupils wide and staring *Belladonna 30c*
- Child thin, with a big head, tends to have sweaty feet and head, dislikes milk *Silicea 6c*
- Child nervous, restless *Actaea 6c*
- Child has mouth ulcers, is startled by sudden noises, dislikes downward motion *Borax 6c*
- Teeth have poor enamel and decay easily and quickly *Kreosotum 6c*
- Sore gums and diarrhoea, or copious salivation *Mercurius 6c*
- Acute pain and high temperature *Aconite 30c*

- Sore gums, child fretful and colicky *Colocynth 6c*
- Teething symptoms accompanied by constipation and ineffectual straining to pass stools *Nux 6c*

Self-help
Give Calc. phos. and Calc. fluor. (see Tissue Salts, p. 24) throughout teething period.

Umbilical hernia
Soft bulge of tissue around navel due to weakness in abdominal wall; bulge can be pushed back into tummy but tends to reappear when baby cries. There is little danger of underlying section of intestine becoming strangulated. Most such hernias are painless and heal of own accord during first year; if surgery is necessary, it is usually done between age of 3 and 5. If homeopathic remedies below do not produce some improvement within 2 months, see your GP.

Specific remedies to be given 3 times a day for up to 3 weeks:

- Infant or toddler who is overweight, very quiet, prone to head sweats at night, especially if he or she likes to eat earth or worms *Calcarea 6c*
- Infant or toddler who is thin and weedy, with a large head and sweaty feet *Silicea 6c*
- In all other cases *Nux 6c*

Vomiting
Main cause of vomiting is wind. Every time a baby swallows a mouthful of milk some wind enters as a protective mechanism to clear any milk from the pharynx into the oesophagus. After a little while a significant air bubble comes out as wind, often bringing a bit of milk with it. To counteract this, wind the baby by sitting her or him upright after feeding and rubbing their back, which will encourage the air to rise up the gullet and out.

Vomiting can also be caused by over-feeding, although regurgitating small amounts of feed is quite normal (see FEEDING PROBLEMS). If all the food is regurgitated, or vomiting has been going on for more than 24 hours, call your GP. If vomiting occurs immediately after a feed it may be due to passage of stomach contents up into the gullet. Your GP may suggest propping the baby up for an hour after each feed, and thickening feeds. If there is blood in the vomit it may be a hiatus hernia. Vomiting can also be caused by infections, but is seldom due to milk allergy. If, however, you feel that the cause is milk allergy, withdraw all cow's milk; do this under the supervision of your GP, health visitor or homeo-pathic doctor in order to prevent malnutrition.

If vomiting is accompanied by bouts of scream-ing, or if vomit is greenish-yellow, the cause may be obstruction to outflow of stomach (pyloric stenosis), especially if vomit shoots across the room, or INTUSSUSCEPTION; appropriate action is ②, and Aconite 30c every 5 minutes for up to 10 doses. Vomiting can also be a symptom of GASTROENTERITIS (with fever and frequent, watery stools), WHOOPING COUGH (slight fever, runny nose, paroxysms of coughing), and pyloric stenosis; in latter case, baby may vomit with such force that stomach contents are propelled some distance across room. If any of these conditions is suspected, 12.

Repeated vomiting is very dehydrating for a young baby; if signs of dehydration are present (dry mouth, sunken eyes, depressed fontanelle), ② and try to give sips of water with a little glucose and salt dissolved in it (1 teaspoon glucose and ½ teaspoon salt to 0.5 litre [1 pint] boiled cooled water).

Specific remedies to be given every hour, or every 15 minutes if vomiting is severe, for up to 10 doses:

- For vomiting generally *Ipecac. 6c*
- Waxy pallor, no crying, bluish rings around eyes *Phosphoric ac. 6c*
- Vomit full of green or yellow curds, perhaps because baby has developed intolerance of milk, baby exhausted and very distressed *Aethusa 6c*
- Vomiting in a fat, flabby baby who is prone to sour-smelling head sweats during sleep, fontanelle slow to close, teeth late in coming through *Calcarea 6c*
- Marked distension of abdomen *Lac can. 6c*
- Vomiting accompanied by constipation, stools pale, dry, and crumbly *Magnesia carb. 6c*
- Baby's stomach full of wind and rumbling which obviously cause pain *Natrum carb. 6c*
- Baby refuses breast, has sweaty head and cold smelly feet *Silicea 6c*
- Vomiting caused by fruit or food which has gone off slightly *Arsenicum 6c*
- Vomiting caused by fright *Aconite 30c*
- Vomiting brought on by rich or fatty foods, baby irritable and wants to be left alone *Bryonia 30c*
- Vomiting accompanied by craving for cold water, which is vomited up as soon as it becomes warm in stomach *Phosphorus 6c*

Whooping cough (pertussis)

A highly infectious illness caused by bacteria, serious in very young children and occasionally fatal in babies. Incubation is 1–2 weeks. Child is most infectious during first week of infection, and remains infectious for up to 3 weeks after onset of infection. First stage is runny nose and mild FEVER. Second stage is a cough which becomes more and more severe, beginning with a spasm and ending with a characteristic whoop as child fights to regain breath. Coughing may be violent enough to cause cyanosis (blue extremities), nose-bleeds, burst blood vessels in the eyes, and vomit-ing, and can last for anything from 2–10 weeks. Complications include pneumonia, leading to permanent lung damage, and also brain damage due to burst blood vessels in the brain. A second attack may be triggered off within a year of the first if the child is prone to COLDS and is in poor health.

If you suspect your child has been in contact with whooping cough or may be developing it, 48. GP may decide to give an antibiotic, which will kill bacteria before they take hold or at least reduce severity of attack. Give child live yoghurt daily for 5 days after the course of antibiotics finishes; this restores beneficial intestinal bacteria destroyed by antibiotics. If child's lips or fingers turn blue during coughing bouts, ②.

Specific remedies to be given after every attack of coughing for up to 2 days; if no improvement, or if unsure which remedy to give, consult your homeopath:

- Throat feels dry and tickly, impulse to cough is so violent that child vomits and can scarcely breathe between coughs, clasps stomach in pain when coughing, feels chilly and restless, symptoms worse after midnight *Drosera 6c*
- Hard, dry, hacking cough comes on around 3 am, child very chilly and exhausted, eyelids puffy *Kali carb. 6c*
- Coughing worse at night when child is warm in bed, alleviated by drinking cold water, vomited mucus is transparent and stringy *Coccus 6c*
- Paroxysms of coughing leave child breathless and exhausted, whooping intakes of breath cause lips to turn blue, cramps in toes and fingers (typically, thumbs are tucked into palms), drinks of cold water seem to help *Cuprum 6c*
- Stringy, yellow mucus coughed up *Kali bichrom. 6c*
- Child cries and complains of stomach pains before coughing attack comes on, has bursting feeling in head, cough worse at night and when lying down, better after coughing up mucus, then dry tickling in throat starts again and attack is repeated, with whooping and retch-

ing, child red in face, eyes puffy and bulging *Belladonna 6c*

- Child feels sick most of the time, becomes rigid, pale and breathless, then relaxes and vomits, which ends attack *Ipecac. 6c*

Immunization Orthodox immunization is offered as part of 'triple' vaccine (diphtheria, tetanus, whooping cough). Adverse reactions are exceedingly rare, despite reports in the popular press. The 'triple' gives 60-80 per cent protection but should not be given if your child has a fever or if the child had breathing difficulties after birth or a bad reaction to a previous immunization. There has been no research comparing the efficacy of orthodox and homeopathic immunization, but there is plenty of anecdotal evidence that Pertussin 30c nosode (see p. 19 for definition of nosode) prevents the graver complications of whooping cough.

Self-help
Do not give cough suppressants. Encourage child to eat little and often, and to sit up and lean forward during bouts of coughing. If child vomits frequently, keep a bowl within easy reach, and wash it out each time child is sick. Keep child away from other children until infectious stage is over.

Menopause

The menopause is not a disorder but, like puberty, a period of physical and emotional change which affects some women far more than others. The first definite sign is disruption of the menstrual cycle, an early warning that the delicate balance between ovaries, hypothalamus, and pituitary gland which ensures fertility is beginning to change. Most women have their last period (strictly speaking menopause means cessation of periods) around the age of 50, but for some women periods cease as early as 40 or as late as 58.

Symptoms
These fall into 3 main categories.

1 *Vasomotor symptoms* These occur when the nervous mechanism controlling the opening and closing of blood vessels is impaired, with resulting instability of blood supply to the skin. The most frequent and most severe symptom is hot flushes. According to surveys 55–90 per cent of women experience these, of which 25 per cent still have them 5 years after the onset. Flushes may start some time before the signs of menstrual irregularity. The sensation of heat covers the whole body, but is most intense on the face. On a reassuring note, although some women may feel like they are on fire it is most unlikely that others will notice. Most people are remarkably unobservant so do not allow embarrassment to create even worse problems for you. The hot flushes may be accompanied by shivering or heavy sweating, which can be offensive. Although harmless, if frequent they are likely to be associated with FATIGUE (see below, plus p. 50), DIZZINESS, HEADACHES and poor sleep (see below, and SLEEP PROBLEMS). Other vasomotor symptoms experienced may be palpitations, and formication, which is an unpleasant sensation of crawling in the skin.

2 *Genital symptoms* These symptoms relate to shrinkage, loss of tone and elasticity of tissues affecting the womb, vagina and urethra. The result of this is dryness, which may affect bladder functioning and sexual activity. The thinned vaginal walls are more predisposed to infection, and itching may develop around the vaginal opening (see PRURITIS VULVAE).

Reduced lubrication and elasticity may lead to discomfort on intercourse.

In our survey women also reported an increase in CERVICAL EROSION, unusual VAGINAL DISCHARGE and BREAST SWELLING during the menopause.

Since the urethra is also affected it may be irritable, as may the bladder, making the passage of urine frequent and uncomfortable. In addition the loss of tone supporting the bladder may cause STRESS INCONTINENCE.

3 *Psychological symptoms* Most frequently reported symptoms are FATIGUE, anxiety, SLEEP PROBLEMS, DEPRESSION, anger and irritability. Women also very often reported memory loss and poor concentration, PANIC ATTACKS and FRIGHT, confusion, and EXCITABILITY (see General Remedy Finder). For one or two women these symptoms were intense enough for them to fear insanity.

Of these symptoms fatigue, anxiety and irritability are more likely to appear some time before the menopause. Sleeping problems and possibly depression follow the end of periods, acting together to undermine general well-being.

Other symptoms

These generally include muscle and joint pains, with the onset of OSTEOPOROSIS. Lack of oestrogen can also result in thinning and drying of skin (see below), and may affect quality and quantity of hair (see below). Other symptoms reported by our women included FAINTING, CRAVING FOR SUGAR (see WEIGHT PROBLEMS Remedy Finder), ABDOMINAL PAIN, fluid retention (OEDEMA), NAUSEA, POOR APPETITE (see WEIGHT PROBLEMS, p. 35), CONSTIPATION, weight gain (see WEIGHT PROBLEMS, and COLDNESS (see General Remedy Finder), bruising of skin, tinnitus, itchy scalp and dandruff, URTICARIA and boils.

On reading the baffling list of symptoms it may appear that the end of life is at hand. Obviously, though, no woman is likely to get all these symptoms. Indeed some women go through the menopause with hardly any symptoms, or no symptoms at all. However, it is reassuring if you are troubled by a number of symptoms that it isn't just neurosis, but that your symptoms are very real, and are being experienced due to a change in hormone balance.

Artificial menopause

This is induced when the ovaries are removed surgically because of disease or are damaged by drugs or radiation. It can lead to fairly immediate symptoms of the menopause. These are likely to be more severe than a normal menopause; for instance flushing, depression and joint pains may be more pronounced. A menopausal state may follow removal of the womb (HYSTERECTOMY) without removal of the ovaries. In this case, since there are no periods to herald the onset of the menopause, such symptoms may be ill-understood and mis-managed.

Attitudes to menopause

Menopause comes at a time when a woman is already likely to be stressed by a variety of demands on her, such as children asserting their independence, ageing parents, or her own career. Regardless of increased life expectancy and social or environmental change, the ovarian timing mechanism still switches off at the same point. The average woman is therefore increasingly likely to live as many adult years post- as premenopausal, which makes it extremely important for her to prepare for, and optimize, the post-menopausal years. Research has shown that certain menopausal symptoms may be more pronounced in some personality types than in others. For instance, women with long-term emotional problems are more likely to fall victim: examples of this might be the married woman who decides that with the onset of the menopause her most valuable years are over; or the woman who fears that her femininity is reliant on her female biological functioning, i.e., menstruation, pregnancy and motherhood.

In contrast, those women who accept the menopause as a natural milestone are less likely to suffer complications, and it is often the case that those with fulfilling careers, intellectual or creative outlets and valued goals will fall into this category.

Such acceptance can be particularly difficult in the face of the superficial values imposed by our 'youth culture', in which older men are regarded as attractively rugged, but older women are written off. In cultures where women have a higher status menopausal depression is relatively nonexistent, although other factors such as nutrition and stress levels may play a part. Women, therefore, who cannot accept the ageing process, or who cannot regard the post-menopausal years in a positive fashion, are more likely to have exaggerated post-menopausal symptoms.

In general the menopause is a message from mother nature to a woman and her partner – if she has one – that she is now able to retire from the turbulent years of reproduction, with its emotional and physical stresses. Even for the reluctant childless, there is no further point in worrying about it. However, as much as it is an end, it is also a new beginning. Women who previously identified themselves mainly as wife and mother may at first find the menopause very challenging. Gradually, however, they discover a new independent identity, much to their own delight. Like all growth, ultimately the menopause is spiritually strengthening. It seems entirely appropriate that nature balances the helter-skelter phase of sexual pairing and probable child-care with an opportunity for entirely personal reflection of valuation in growth.

Onset of the menopause

The age at which a woman undergoes the menopause is thought to be linked to a number of factors, including:

1 *Smoking* – heavy smokers are more prone to an early menopause.
2 *Body size* – small, thinner women are more prone to an early menopause.
3 *Age of a woman at her last pregnancy* – a pregnancy after the age of 40, or no pregnancies

at all, would both be associated with a later menopause.

4 *Heredity* – some of the symptoms you experience during the menopause, or the degree to which you experience them, could be pre-ordained by your genetic inheritance. This means that natural therapies may not be entirely effective, and you may simply have to learn to live with certain changes.

Nutrition

It was first proposed in 1931 that HORMONE IMBALANCES could be linked to poor nutrition. Further research has confirmed and extended this proposal. In particular, micronutrients such as vitamins and minerals are increasingly used as a corrective factor in hormone imbalances. However, as these vitamin and mineral supplements have increased in popularity, signs of hormone imbalances such as PRE-MENSTRUAL SYNDROME continue to rise on account of dietary imbalance. It stands to reason that a woman experiencing nutritionally related pre-menstrual syndrome in her 20s–30s is likely to experience an earlier and more symptomatic menopause. This relates to the fact that the dynamic equilibrium between different hormones is coordinated by regulatory systems under the overall control of the pituitary gland. All the components required for the production of a particular substance must be available at the right time; for example, all the enzymes involved in production, metabolism and in transport systems. The amounts required all vary in individuals, due to various factors such as emotional and toxic stresses. As the menopause proceeds and the adrenal glands and fat tissues take over production of sex hormones, optimum nutritional supplies are necessary to minimize oestrogen withdrawal symptoms as the ovaries fail.

Self-help

1 *Hot flushes* Avoid tight clothing, especially around the neck. Try to control stress. Taking regular exercise (see WEIGHT PROBLEMS) can help to stabilize the temperature control mechanism; for instance, 20 minutes a day walking uphill, running, aerobics, dance, or cycling, as long as the exercise is vigorous enough to induce and maintain a sweat (this appears to reduce follicle stimulating hormone and luteinizing hormone levels). Exercise measures are more effective if started well before the menopause.

Hot flushes may be associated with HYPO-GLYCAEMIA, and it is important to minimize coffee, tea, alcohol and sugar intake, and have frequent protein snacks. A lack of vitamin E appears to have a de-stabilizing effect on oestrogen levels. It is more likely to occur in women on a predominantly processed food diet. It should be taken in combination with SELENIUM for maximum effect. Other beneficial nutrients include VITAMIN C and CALCIUM.

Meditation and relaxation techniques help to calm the mind, whilst benefit may be obtained from the visualization technique of channelling the heat of the hot flushes out of the body through the hands.

2 *Sleeping problems* (see also SLEEP PROBLEMS p. 237) Have a warm milk drink at bedtime; the warmth helps digestion, the calcium content contributes to optimum nerve function, and the small amounts of Tryptophan which are present are a natural tranquillizer. Women who are particularly anxious, agitated, restless and very sleepless may be deficient in magnesium, and benefit from supplements. Herbal teas such as lemon verbena, chamomile, woodruff, hawthorn, hops and passionflower could help.

Avoid eating large meals within 4 hours of bedtime; do some form of relaxation technique before going to bed, or have a bath. Sexual intercourse also helps to induce sleep in many people. Exercise regularly, as this appears to increase the amount of slow wave (good quality) sleep. Finally don't bottle up your feelings, going to sleep with a background of resentment, anger and anxiety. Try instead to discuss them with a confidante or your partner.

3 *Fatigue* (see also FATIGUE)

a Try to minimize the effects of possible related HYPOGLYCAEMIA. Low blood sugar can be relative, i.e., the symptoms may be experienced even if the blood sugar is within a normal range, as the symptoms relate to a sudden fall in level of blood sugar. Possible symptoms include sudden nervousness and irritability, energy spurts after meals, followed by exhaustion. Alternatively there may be excessive sleepiness after meals, depressive bouts and crying, forgetfulness, confusion and indecisiveness.

b Correct any possible anaemia. Most women's iron intake is only a third to a half of the total daily requirement, as a result of low intake of iron-rich foods and sub-optimum absorption. In fact only 10 per cent of the iron actually swallowed is absorbed (see also IRON).

c Consider the possibility of HYPOTHYROIDISM, if, for example, the fatigue is associated with an increased susceptibility to infection or disease, unexplained weight gain, sensitivity to cold, constipation, hair loss, puffy eyes and dry skin. The symptoms may be very similar to hypoglycaemia, because when the thyroid is underactive the liver appears to have impaired ability to mobilize sugar stores. Under-active thyroid may be detected by a low basal body temperature, i.e., the temperature of the body at rest. This is measured by taking your temperature, before getting up, on several mornings at least 10 minutes before having a cup of tea or going to the loo. Shake the thermometer down the night before. If the average is less than 97.8 this may indicate an under-functioning. The nutrients suggested for optimum thyroid function include: IODINE, VITAMIN B COMPLEX, CHOLINE, VITAMIN C, VITAMIN D, VITAMIN E, VITAMIN A, ZINC.

4 *Skin and hair* Although to some extent the ageing of skin is influenced by heredity it is also a function of lifestyle, including diet, exercise, smoking, ALCOHOL, sun exposure (see BEAUTY CARE) and sleep (see SLEEP PROBLEMS). At around 35 years visible signs of ageing appear. Regeneration of skin cells is at a slower rate, so the outer covering is exposed to the elements for a longer period of time. Loss of oil and moisture causes thinning and reduced elasticity, and fine lines and wrinkles appear as a result.

At the menopause many women have a generalized HAIR LOSS, and others may find hair appears in unfamiliar sites, e.g., FACIAL HAIR. This reflects a reversal in the ratio of male/female hormones caused by the falling oestrogen. See BEAUTY CARE for possible measures to take.

General rules for healthy skin and hair

1 Avoid smoking.
2 Drink plenty of water and minimize intake of coffee, tea, alcohol and fizzy drinks.
3 Minimize exposure to the sun.
4 Eat high quality and complex carbohydrate meals, and reduce refined sugars.
5 Minimize saturated fats and oil intake.
6 Humidify home and work atmospheres.
7 Exercise regularly.
8 The following nutritional supplements may be beneficial: VITAMIN A, VITAMIN B COMPLEX, PABA, VITAMIN C, VITAMIN E, ESSENTIAL FATTY ACIDS, IODINE, and IRON.

Libido and sexual activity

Sexual enjoyment after the menopause is probably determined more by psychological outlook than physical change. Some women can use the menopause as a reason to curtail sexual relationships in relationships in which there have been long-standing problems. Middle-aged men will also undergo sexual changes, with a resultant delay in arousal and orgasm. This means it is important to create time and atmosphere for sexual expression, and to communicate your needs.

Since the testosterone levels become proportionately greater after the menopause, sexual interest may in fact be heightened. Sex after the menopause can be enjoyed for its pure pleasure and the closeness it affords; if it has come to be associated only with reproduction then it is unlikely to be valued. On the other hand, the freedom from pregnancy the menopause presents can lead to an increase in interest, spontaneity and pleasure.

Other common problems associated with the menopause

Dry vagina Some women dread the decreased elasticity of the vagina; the reduced ability to lubricate may cause severe vaginal dryness and painful intercourse. A dry vulva may respond to Calendula ointment; KY jelly is very effective in treating dryness of the vagina if it affects intercourse. Small-dose oestrogen treatments are available locally if these do not work, and HRT is effective if it is still a major problem.

Vaginal and urinary tract infection There is an increased susceptibility to these (see CYSTITIS and VAGINITIS). Since vaginitis relates to some extent to the change in the internal environment from acidic to alkaline, douching with live yoghurt can be protective (one part live plain yoghurt to 3 parts boiled cooled water used as a douche, or soak tampon in yoghurt and then insert in vagina), twice daily for up to 1 week, then as required.

To help prevent urinary tract infection

1 Drink water regularly to flush the urinary tract clean of bacteria.
2 Empty the bladder immediately after intercourse.
3 Avoid tight fitting underclothes and jeans, and ensure the wearing of cotton crotch underwear.
4 Decrease sugar and refined carbohydrates. These tend to lead to a deficiency of valuable disease-fighting nutrients, and to encourage the growth of yeast and some bacteria.

Prolapse (see also p. 236) and stress incontinence (see also p. 238)

Exercising the vaginal, stomach and back muscles will help to extend the years of sexual pleasure, protecting against backache, prolapse and passing urine involuntarily. Most commonly recommended exercises are pelvic floor exercises, which strengthen the pubococcygeus muscle (PC), which extends from the pubic bone to the coccyx. You can feel your own PC muscle working by stopping and starting your flow of urine. To tighten the whole pelvic floor, pull up the vagina as well.

Pelvic floor exercises

1 Contract PC muscle tightly and hold for 3 seconds, relax for 3 seconds and repeat; build up gradually to 10 seconds.
2 Contract and release rapidly, working up from 30 to 200 gradually.
3 Lie on back, legs bent, feet on floor; raise pelvis until pull felt, then squeeze rhythmically.
4 It has been found that 5–10 sessions of 10 muscle contractions each day are most beneficial.

Osteoporosis

Because of the correlation between oestrogen decline and osteoporosis, HRT is routinely prescribed at the menopause with the aim of preventing loss of bone; this is its main proven advantage in addition to general symptom relief. 50 per cent of white female Caucasians are liable to get osteoporosis-related fractures (this is 10 times the male risk). Thus it has been predicted that if HRT were targeted on women with the least bone mass at the menopause, the incidence of fractures of the femoral neck (which carry a mortality rate of 20 per cent) could be decreased by up to 45 per cent. The cost to the NHS of osteoporosis-related fractures is approximately £500 million a year. It is estimated that at least 30 per cent of this figure could be saved by preventing and treating osteoporosis.

Prevention, however, begins 30–40 years before the first fracture. A number of factors are involved in osteoporosis, but the one which has received the most attention is the role of calcium; it is the loss of calcium from the bone that leads to its thinning, and eventual collapse or fracture. It is the collapse of the vertebral bodies, especially in the upper back, that leads to the characteristic bowed-over appearance of some old women that is popularly known as dowager's hump. Certainly an adequate amount of calcium in the blood appears to be essential to maintaining the long-term health of bone. The present Recommended Daily Allowance (RDA) for pre-menopausal women is 1,000 mg and for post-menopausal women 1,500 mg.

Calcium supply in the diet

Unless dairy products constitute a substantial part of the diet it may be difficult to achieve the RDA from other sources (particularly if you live in a soft-water area). In any case milk is not always an ideal source because of the relatively high incidence of cow's milk protein and lactose intolerance, and the fact that milk is low in magnesium which is essential for calcium absorption and assimilation.

Other high-calcium foods

Sardines 4 oz	496 mg
Salmon with bones 3 oz	275 mg
Almonds 4 oz	333 mg
Tofu 4 oz	154 mg
Broccoli 4 oz	130 mg

(this compares with the calcium content of dairy products)

Whole milk ⅓ pint	224 mg
Semi-skimmed milk ⅓ pint	235 mg
Yoghurt 5 oz	250 mg
Edam cheese 2 oz	414 mg
Cheddar cheese 2 oz	414 mg

Absorption of calcium

Whilst absorption of calcium varies with individuals, only 20–40 per cent of calcium in the diet is actually absorbed, and this decreases with age. The factors involved include:

1 Genetic make-up, which determines the efficiency of the absorption.
2 Exercise, which increases absorption.
3 Stress or illness, especially chronic illness such as liver and kidney disease, decreases the amount of stored calcium in the body.
4 Lack of specific nutrients, such as manganese, copper, zinc and boron and vitamins C, D, K may decrease absorption.
5 Certain medications, such as steroids, including the Pill, diuretics, aluminium antacids and anti-convulsants, smoking, coffee, alcohol, tea, bran and laxatives, may impair absorption and increase excretion.
6 High phosphate foods, i.e., processed cheeses, meat, fizzy drinks, instant soup and puddings, etc., can accelerate bone demineralization.
7 Lactose intolerance.
8 Increase in protein leads to a decrease in calcium, especially if the protein is of animal origin.
9 Calcium absorption is decreased in exercise-induced cessation of periods.

Supplementation of calcium

If indicated it is probably best to supplement calcium and magnesium in a ratio of 2 : 1. The dose is not universally agreed. It is probably around 1,500 mg of calcium for post-menopausal women and those with established osteoporosis, decreasing to 400 mg for elderly people. The latter could largely be provided by an extra ½ pint of semi-skimmed milk a day.

Other supplements to consider include:

1 *Vitamin D* This is only really necessary for the housebound who are rarely exposed to sunlight, which converts vitamin D to an active form.
2 *Boron* This has a calcium, magnesium and phosphorus-sparing effect.
3 *Digestive enzymes* A significant proportion of post-menopausal women have been shown to have a complete absence of hydrochloric acid in the stomach; some remain acid-free even after stimulation of the stomach. The addition of enzymes, particularly from sources such as papaya, may assist in the digestion and absorption of minerals like calcium. Hydrochloric acid supplements may also be required; see your homeopath or a nutritionally trained doctor.
4 *Potassium* Involved in maintaining bone density. Low magnesium may lead to a loss of potassium from the cells. Intake should be adequate if fruit and vegetables are eaten.
5 *Fluoride* Supplementation can lead to adverse side-effects, so should only be given under medical or dental supervision. Obtainable from fluoridated water and sea foods.
6 *Vitamin C* Necessary for the manufacture of collagen, found in collective tissue and cartilage and essential for bone formation. As stomach acid decreases with age, vitamin C can help calcium absorption by creating a weak acid medium.

Exercise
Bone density relates to how much bone is stressed; thus the bones of athletes and the physically active are considerably heavier than people who do not take any exercise. Although to gain maximum effect exercise should be a habit from early adulthood, it is never too late to start. The best exercises are weight-bearing, e.g., gentle jogging, dancing or skipping or vigorous walking. It is important to include the upper body by working with weights or doing aerobic exercises for the arms; these bones, especially the forearm and spine, are particularly affected in post-menopausal women.

Symptoms of collapse of the body and spine include:

1 Bad attacks of back pain.
2 Loss of height of up to 9 inches and a stoop.
3 Loss of rib cage and spinal movement leading to intolerance of exercise.
4 Weakness in the pelvic floor.

Screening for osteoporosis
Bone density should be at a peak in pre-menopausal women aged approximately 35, so screening women 45–50 should be an accurate predictor of risk. In men bone mass loss averages about 1 per cent per year. This is accelerated in women at the menopause, and for approximately 10–15 years after it, to 3–5 per cent, after which it falls back to 1 per cent. Several projects are presently being tested using a bone densitometer, which measures bone density at two sites in the spine and hip. Scores are aggregated and the lowest 30 per cent are advised to have HRT. So far more than a third appear to be at high risk. However, it must be demonstrated by a large, population-based study that screening and intervention is acceptable to women, and that it significantly reduces the long-term fracture rate. Attempts in the meantime are being made to predict which individuals are more likely to have low bone mass. These have used weight and lifestyle risk scores, including calcium intake, exercise time and alcohol intake; no practical formula has yet been agreed.

Risk factors for osteoporosis

1 Approaching menopause (under 45 years).
2 Amenorrhoea or lack of periods, e.g., from anorexia nervosa or too high levels of prolactin (a hormone secreted by the pituitary; it stimulates the breast to secrete milk – all women stop periods if breastfeeding on demand).
3 Underweight.
4 Strong family history of post-menopausal fractures.
5 Physical inactivity.
6 Poor diet which is lacking calcium.
7 Heavy smoking or drinking.
8 Someone who has had a Colles fracture (fracture of wrist) between ages 40–60.
9 Fair skin.
10 Never had a pregnancy.
11 Bowel problems which result in a significant mal-absorption of food.
12 Steroid therapy.
13 Long-term thyroxine treatment.

Hormone Replacement Therapy (HRT)

Advantages

1 *Prevention of osteoporosis* Oestrogen is the most effective method of retarding bone loss in post-menopausal women, but the dose has to be maintained for at least 5 years to effect a significant reduction in fractures. Remember accelerated bone loss in post-menopausal women is for up to 15 years.
2 *Relief of 'short-term' menopausal symptoms* (e.g., hot flushes, sweats and sleeping problems, tiredness, changes in personality and emotions). Skin may also look healthier due to collagen and fluid

conservation, and hair growth may improve. It also may be used to treat psychological factors such as depression, anxiety, irritability, agoraphobia, loss of confidence and treatment of local symptoms such as vaginal dryness and discomfort on intercourse.

3 *Reduced risk of heart disease* This is 5 times less common in pre-menopausal women than in men. After the menopause there is an increased incidence in ischaemic heart disease, where the blood supply to the heart gets gradually cut off; by the age of 70 years male and female incidence is the same. Several studies have shown a decrease in incidence of this following HRT, and there is evidence that patients who have had previous heart attacks benefit from oestrogen therapy. The protective effect, however, is lost when HRT is stopped. There may also be a considerable reduction in the risk of stroke. These views have recently been put in doubt by American research showing that it is men who are at excess risk at a younger age. The apparent protection from HRT may be no more than an erroneous interpretation of statistics.

Disadvantages

Long-term risks As recently as 1989 many doctors were worried about possible increased risk of heart attack, stroke, diabetes, BREAST CANCER and CANCER OF THE WOMB. However, it is now clear that only breast cancer remains as a source of anxiety and in fact the incidence of most of the other complaints has been reduced by long-term oestrogen therapy. The risk of cancer of the womb have been reduced to below that of an untreated population by using a combined progesterone and oestrogen pill in women unless they have had a hysterectomy. There is no convincing evidence from over 20 studies to implicate HRT in causing breast cancer in the short term, although one large study did show an increased relative risk of 1.5 times after 20 years of oestrogen use.

The consensus of medical opinion is currently that, in the long term, HRT increases the risk of developing breast cancer; a leading specialist has advised all women to have a mammogram before going on HRT.

Side-effects and acceptability

Cessation of the monthly period is the only benefit provided by the menopause, and the use of combined HRT loses this advantage. However, the periods tend to become lighter with age, and after 5 years on HRT consist of only a few days of spotting.

Other possible side-effects of 7–13 days of progesterone therapy per month include headache, depression, loss of energy and libido and bloating, symptoms similar to PRE-MENSTRUAL SYNDROME. Some side-effects may be modified by altering the dose and type of progesterone. HYPOGLYCAEMIA is another major side-effect of progesterone, and can be avoided by cutting down on refined carbohydrates, caffeine and alcohol, and by snacking on protein regularly.

Contraindications to HRT

Absolute Patients with these diseases should never use HRT:

1 BREAST CANCER.
2 CANCER OF WOMB.
3 SEVERE LIVER DISEASE.

Relative Where the patient and physician must use judgement, as there is some risk:

1 Heavy smoking.
2 FIBROIDS.
3 ENDOMETRIOSIS.
4 OTOSCLEROSIS.
5 Heart disease and history of blood clots
6 Hyperlipidaemia, especially if it runs in the family.

N.B. High blood pressure is not now considered a contraindication.

Types of HRT

Oestrogen can be administered by mouth, by skin patches, by cream or by implant. By itself oestrogen causes the lining of the womb to become thickened, and therefore shedding is necessary by use of progesterone to prevent disease such as cancer of the womb.

1 *Creams and pessaries* Suitable for treating superficial pain on intercourse and irritation around the opening of the urethra. The weakest possible preparation should be used to lessen the chance of absorption and metabolic side-effects.

2 *Skin patches* These are probably the best form, since they avoid the initial breakdown in the liver, so reducing undesirable side-effects; they can easily be stopped if they are causing side-effects. They are safer than tablets for diabetics, and for women prone to blood clotting, or with a history of liver disease.

3 *By mouth* If this is chosen, natural not synthetic oestrogen is best. Women who still have a womb must use combined oestrogen and progesterone, while women without a womb just use oestrogen. The progesterone dose should be as low as possible, as it counteracts to some extent the beneficial effects of oestrogen

in protecting against heart disease and stroke.

4 *Implants* Once oestrogen is found to be effective, then implants can be used. The advantage is that there is no daily medication to remember; the disadvantage is they have to be surgically implanted under local anaesthetic and are difficult to remove in the case of complications. They may also lead to the need for more and more frequent implants, which is not a feature of skin patches.

Future developments are as follows:

1 *A combined patch* At present the problem of absorption is such that the patch would have to be so large it would cover half the area of the trunk.

2 *Continuous progesterone and oestrogen* Overcomes the need for a cyclical bleed. It is not satisfactory at present as it results in irregular spotting in many patients who may then need a D & C to exclude other causes.

3 *Oestrogen skin creams* Used on the continent but absorption is very variable.

Conclusions about HRT

There can be no doubt that HRT has benefited the lives of many women, and produced spectacular results in well-being in some. It may not, however, be suitable for all women, and some women do experience unpleasant side-effects. The basic philosophy adopted by some proponents of HRT that the menopause is not a natural phenomenon, but rather a disease process, is highly suspect. The authors subscribe to the view that the menopause is a natural event; and it would be unnatural for women to go on child-bearing into their 80s and 90s because of other health problems which increase with age. This is not to mention the psychological effects on any child born to such an elderly parent.

We prefer to believe that HRT is essential in some women, for example, those who have had ARTIFICIAL MENOPAUSE or who seem to be completely incapable of producing oestrogen from any other source apart from the ovaries, possibly for genetic reasons. These women should be treated along the lines of an insulin-dependent diabetic. The majority of women suffering these days with the menopause are having problems because of cultural, life-style, nutritional and other reasons, many of which can be avoided by proper preparation before the onset of the menopause. Thus we feel that using HRT as a substitute for adopting a healthy lifestyle is a misguided viewpoint, and there may well be a change of heart in the medical profession towards its use in another 20 or 30 years' time. It is sobering to reflect that the oral contraceptive has been around for at least 2 decades longer than HRT, and a leading specialist recently announced that it would be another 20 years before we know the full extent of side-effects from oral contraception.

Homeopathic treatment

The homeopathic view of menopausal problems is that they represent imbalances which have been present for a long time; treatment is therefore constitutional; however, the remedies given below should be tried first. We would also encourage women to prepare for the menopause by looking to their nutrition, exercise and correcting any PMS symptoms, along with the development of a positive attitude and self value before its onset. There are remedies which can be used as a homeopathic Hormone Replacement Therapy, but the authors advise that this should only be done under the guidance of an experienced homeopath.

Finally, if periods are prolonged, or if spots of blood appear between periods or if the last period is followed 6 months or later by another period, see your GP. The source may be FIBROIDS, UTERUS PROBLEMS, CANCER OF THE UTERUS or CANCER OF THE CERVIX.

Specific remedies to be taken in the 30c potency every 12 hours for up to 7 days.

Please remember to check your choice against the Remedy Pictures (p. 305) where possible.

Sepia

Poor memory; difficulty in concentrating – worse for stress; agoraphobia; depression; weepiness; changeable moods; fearful; anxiety attacks during hot flushes; irritable; hair falling out; itchy scalp; left-sided headache; migraine; pain in temples; craving for sweets; lack of appetite generally; sinking feeling in pit of stomach; heavy periods with flooding; irregular periods; tendency to vaginal thrush; possible cervical erosion; vaginal dryness; pain in vagina during sexual intercourse; difficulty in breathing; backache – better for motion; hot sweats worse at night; offensive perspiration.

Generalities: Weariness; flushes of heat worse at night; in the evening – worse for slightest exertion; with perspiration; sudden fainting spells – worse before periods; sudden weakness – worse in a room full of people; arthritis; chilly.

Sulphur

Poor memory, worse for stress; depression; itchy scalp; left-sided headaches – worse before periods; left-sided migraines; noises in the ear; craving for sweets especially pre-menstrually;

lack of appetite; wind; stools like balls; heavy periods; pain in vagina during sexual intercourse; difficulty in breathing; legs tingling, prickling or asleep; rheumatic pains in extremities; sleeplessness; hot sweats day and night; bruises easily; urticaria; rashes and boils.

Generalities: Weariness; flushes of heat – worse in evening, at night, in warm room or room full of people; hot sweats generally worse before periods; tendency to put on weight.

Calcarea
Poor memory; irritability; panic attacks, agoraphobia; anxiety; depression; weepiness; changeable moods; claustrophobia; fearful; confusion; itchy scalp; left-sided headaches – headaches worse before periods; migraines; noises in ear; perspiration on face; feeling of anxiety in pit of stomach; craving for sugar and sweets; lack of appetite; heavy and/or irregular periods; tendency to thrush and cervical erosion; swelling of breasts before periods; backache – worse for damp weather; swelling of the finger joints; tingling; prickling; legs feel asleep; sleeplessness; hot sweats; urticaria.

Generalities: Hot flushes – worse before periods; feeling of weakness; tendency to put on weight; varicose veins; arthritis.

Lycopodium
Poor memory; irritability; difficulty in concentration – worse for stress; anxiety; depression; tearfulness; changeable mood; claustrophobia; fearful; itchy scalp; headaches before periods; pain in temples; right-sided migraines; noises in ear; chronic catarrh; perspiration; hot flushes on face; feeling of anxiety in pit of stomach; desire for sugar; desire for sweets; lack of appetite; wind; irregular periods; dryness in vagina; difficulty in breathing; backache – better for motion; swelling of finger joints; rheumatic pain in extremities, especially in hip and knee; offensive smelling sweat; boils.

Generalities: Weariness – worse before periods; tendency to overweight; hot flushes – worse in evening – with fainting – worse in warm room, room full of people; arthritis.

Lachesis
Poor memory; difficulty in concentrating; depression; over-excitement with talkativeness; confusion; dizziness; headache in general – worse on waking; worse on left side; worse before periods; pain in temples; left-sided migraine; hot flushes on face; constricted feeling round abdomen; heavy and/or irregular periods; flooding; difficulty in breathing; sleeplessness; hot

sweats in night; bruises easily; urticaria and boils.

Generalities: Weariness; hot flushes and sweats – worse before periods; tendency to faint.

Pulsatilla
Depression and weepiness; changeable moods; claustrophobia; over-excited; headache premenstrually; pain in temples; left-sided migraines; noises in ear; perspiration and hot sweats on face; feeling of anxiety in pit of stomach; desire for sweets; poor appetite; irregular periods; tendency to vaginal thrush and cervical erosion; difficulty in breathing; backache – better for motion; rheumatic pains in extremities, especially in hip; sleeplessness; hot offensive smelling sweats – worse at night; skin bruises easily.

Generalities: Weariness – worse before periods; tendency to put on weight; varicose veins; fluid retention; fainting with hot flushes – worse in warm room; worse in room full of people; arthritis; chilliness when not flushed.

Belladonna
Poor memory; irritable; anxiety; changeable moods; over-excitable; fearful; confused; headaches – worse before periods; pain in temples; left-sided migraine; noises in ear; sweating face; irregular periods; tendency to thrush; vaginal dryness; boils.

Generalities: General weakness before periods; tendency to put on weight, especially due to fluid retention; arthritis.

Carbo veg.
Irritability; difficulty in concentrating; confused; itchy scalp; headaches before periods; right-sided migraine; perspiration on face; feeling of anxiety in pit of stomach; desire for sweets; pain in back passage; wind; tendency to thrush and cervical erosion; difficulty in breathing; skin bruises easily.

Generalities: Hot sweats; weakness; varicose veins; alternating hot flushes and chilliness; fainting – worse in warm room; hot flushes at night.

Graphites
Irritability; difficulty in concentrating; depression; weepiness; over-excitable; fearful; itchy scalp; left-sided headache, and migraines; nose bleeds; noises in ear; wind with cutting pains; irregular scanty and/or heavy periods; tendency to vaginal thrush; dryness of vagina; skin rashes on back of neck; offensive smelling sweat.

Generalities: Weariness; tendency to put on weight; sudden weakness; fainting – worse in warm room.

Phosphorus
Poor memory; panic attacks; changeable mood; over-excitable; fearful; confused; itchy scalp; left-sided headaches, or migraines; desires salt; desires sweets; poor appetite; wind; difficulty in breathing; sleeplessness; bruising.

Generalities: Weariness; hot flushes; sudden fainting spells; tendency to put on weight, especially with fluid retention; general fainting – worse in warm room.

Bryonia
Irritability; anxiety; mental confusion; head-aches before periods; right-sided migraine; desire for sweets; constipation with hard, burnt-looking stools; dryness of vagina with thinning of walls; difficulty in breathing; worse after exposure to cold conditions; swelling of finger joints; rheumatic pains in extremities, especially in the knee; sleeplessness; bruises easily.

Generalities: Fluid retention; faintness – worse in a warm room; arthritis.

Natrum mur.
Worse for stress; depression; weepiness; claustrophobia; over-excited; confusion; itchy scalp; headaches before periods; right-sided migraines; poor appetite; stools like balls; tendency to vaginal thrush; dryness in vagina; pain during intercourse; greasy skin; urticaria.

Generalities: Weariness – worse before periods; weakness before periods; fainting; arthritis.

Other remedies to consider
- Hot flushes which come on very suddenly *Amyl nit. 30c*
- Hot flushes, loss of appetite, backache, feeling very taut and nervous, palpitations, symptoms worse around 3 am *Kali carb. 30c*
- Hot flushes worse in evening and after exercise, great weariness *Sulphuric ac. 30c*

Remedy Finder for Menopause

Pain in womb
Cimicifuga
Sepia

Vaginal discharge during menopause
Graphites
Sepia

Painful periods near menopause
Psorinum

Heavy periods during menopause
Calcarea
Crotalus
Graphites
Lachesis
Psorinum
Sanguinaria
Sepia
Sulphur

Weepiness during menopause
Sulphur

Depression during menopause
Sepia

Heat at top of head
Lachesis

Heat in head generally
Sulphur

Hair falling out
Sepia

Dizziness during menopause
Crotalus
Glonoinum
Sanguinaria
Ustilago

Fear of insanity
Cimicifuga

Fear generally
Cimicifuga

Anger with delusions about people or things
Colocynth
Nux
Zinc

Anxiety about disease
Kali brom.

Becomes very complaining
Kali brom.

Fear of public places and crowds
Glonoinum

Forgetfulness
Lachesis

Hysterical behaviour
Ignatia
Lachesis
Phosphoric ac.

Indifference
Cyclamen

Irritability
Cimicifuga
Lachesis
Psorinum

Cross and morose
Psorinum

Nose bleeds
Hamamelis
Lachesis
Pulsatilla
Sepia
Sulphur
Sulphuric ac.

Red face
Graphites
Kali bichrom.
Lachesis
Sulphuric ac.

Hot flushes in face
Graphites
Kali bichrom.
Lachesis
Lycopodium
Psorinum
Sulphuric ac.

Weak empty feeling in stomach
Crotalus
Lachesis
Tabacum

Nausea
Glonoinum

Sinking feeling
Ignatia
Sepia

Diarrhoea
Lachesis

Haemorrhoids
Lachesis

Frequent urge to pass water
Sarsaparilla

Burning pain in urethra
Berberis

Heavy feeling in chest
Lachesis

Breast swelling
Silicea
Sulphur

Pain underneath breasts
Cimicifuga

Swollen tender breasts
Sanguinaria

Palpitations of the heart
Calcarea ars.
Crotalus
Lachesis
Tabacum

Burning feet – especially soles
Sanguinaria
Sulphur

Sleeplessness
Aconite
Arnica
Belladonna
Cimicifuga
Coffea
Gelsemium
Kali brom.
Sulphur
Zinc

Clammy sticky sweats
Crotalus
Lachesis
Lycopodium
Sulphuric ac.
Terebinth

Profuse sweats
Sepia

Itchy skin
Caladium

Fainting
Aconite
Coffea
Glonoinum
Kali carb.
Lachesis
Moschus
Nitric ac.
Sulphur
Veratrum

Aggravation from coffee
Lachesis

Haemorrhage
Phosphorus

Hot flushes at night
Carbo veg.
Fluoric ac.
Hepar sulph.
Kali iod.
Lachesis
Rhododendron
Sepia
Sulphur
Sulphuric ac.
Tuberculinum

Hot flushes in general
Glonoinum
Lachesis
Manganum
Platina
Sepia
Sulphur
Sulphuric ac.

Permanent feeling of coldness
China

Feeling as if whole body is numb
Cimicifuga

Weight gain
Graphites
Sepia

Lack of sexual desire
Conium

Trembling all over body
Kali brom.

Trembling inside
Caulophyllum
Sulphuric ac.

Weakness
China
Cocculus
Conium
Crotalus
Kali phos.
Lachesis
Sepia

Weariness
Bellis
Calcarea

Involuntary urination
Apis
Argentum nit.
Arsenicum
Belladonna
Causticum
Dulcamara
Lycopodium
Natrum mur.
Nux mosch.
Phosphorus
Psorinum
Pulsatilla
Rhus tox.
Sepia
Staphisagria

Brittle fingernails
Graphites
Psorinum

Cramps during night
Calcarea
Lycopodium
Sulphur

Numbness of hands
Carbo an.
Cocculus
Graphites
Kali carb.
Kali nit.
Lycopodium
Phosphorus

Headaches
Carbo veg.
Lachesis
Sanguinaria
Sepia

Mental overexcitement
Aconite

Anacardium
Argentum nit.
Aurum
Belladonna
Causticum
Chamomilla
Coffea
Collinsonia
Graphites
Hepar sulph.
Hyoscyamus
Kali brom.
Kali iod.
Lac can.
Lachesis
Moschus
Natrum mur.
Nitric ac.
Nux
Opium
Phosphoric ac.
Phosphorus
Pulsatilla

Over-fantasizing
Belladonna
Cannabis ind.
Hyoscyamus
Lachesis
Stramonium

Asthma starting during menopause
Ambra
Argentum nit.
Arsenicum
Arsenicum iod.
Cuprum
Ipecac.
Kali ars.
Kali nit.
Lobelia
Pulsatilla
Sambucus
Silicea

Spongia
Stramonium
Sulphur

Dry skin
Arsenicum
Belladonna
Bryonia
Calcarea
Chamomilla
China
Colchicum
Dulcamara
Eupatorium
Kali ars.
Kali carb.
Ledum
Lycopodium
Nux mosch.
Oleander
Opium
Petroleum
Phosphorus
Plumbum
Silicea
Stramonium
Sulphur
Verbascum

Arthritic lumps
Apis
Benzoic ac.
Calcarea
Calcarea fluor.
Graphites
Ledum
Lycopodium

Varicose veins in legs
Carbo veg.
Causticum
Hamamelis
Lycopodium
Pulsatilla
Zinc

Fast pulse
Aconite
Apis
Arnica
Arsenicum
Arsenicum iod.
Belladonna
Berberis
Boron
Bryonia
Collinsonia
Conium
Cuprum
Ferrum phos.
Gelsemium
Glonoinum
Iodum
Mercurius
Natrum mur.
Nux
Opium
Phosphoric ac.
Phosphorus
Pyrogenium
Rhus tox.
Silicea
Spigelia
Stramonium
Sulphur
Zinc

Osteoporosis
Belladonna
Calcarea
Hepar sulph.
Lycopodium
Mercurius
Nitric ac.
Phosphorus
Pulsatilla
Sepia
Silicea
Sulphur

Mental and Emotional Problems

As you read through the ailments described in this book, remember that 'depression', and 'grief', and the symptoms which constitute them, are only labels of convenience. Psychology and psychiatry have divided and sub-divided human behaviour into hundreds of categories, and gained valuable knowledge by doing so. Homeopathy makes use of such labels because they are common currency, but never loses sight of the whole individual behind the label.

Very few diseases are wholly psychological or wholly physical. 'Mind' and 'body' affect one another interminably. The dichotomy is convenient, even useful in some circumstances, but it is false – who can say where the one begins and the other ends? Homeopathy treats only one entity, the Vital Force, the engine which drives every aspect of individual behaviour, and as clues to the state of that force, thoughts and feelings are just as important as lumps and bumps.

It is impossible to draw a line between balance and imbalance on the mental and emotional level. Mental health is a relative thing, depending entirely on what is acceptable or tolerable to the individual and to the community he or she lives in. If you find your thoughts and emotions uncomfortable, or are worried by certain aspects of your behaviour, that in itself is a recognition of imbalance; if your family, or society at large, finds your behaviour outrageous or damaging you may be labelled as mentally ill whether you agree with the label or not.

If you recognize in yourself, or in members of your family, tendencies which are life-denying – unsociability, apathy, insecurity – go and see a homeopathic physician. The earlier such tendencies are treated constitutionally the better; untreated, they may deepen or interfere permanently with your enjoyment of life. The remedies given during constitutional treatment will act on your Vital Force, giving you more energy and more confidence to sort out your problems. You may, in addition, be advised to make changes in diet, exercise, and lifestyle.

More than anything else, try to be kind to yourself and accept the way you are. Try to accept that there is a place inside you which has remained unchanged since babyhood. It is innocent, it trusts, it knows no fear, and needs only love. If that sounds saccharine and woolly-minded, perhaps you are not allowing yourself to get in touch with those feelings. At a very early age we learn that love is not always returned. Indeed it often has to be earned. This hurts, and so we close up and pretend that we do not want to love or be loved. In later life these dammed-up feelings prevent us opening up to other people, and lead to fear, anxiety, insecurity, loneliness, and depression.

Whenever you feel tempted to close down, shut off, hide away, give up . . . try to open up. *There are always alternatives*. A lot of problems are the result of getting it into our heads that there is no alternative, no escape, and we are left feeling helpless and hopeless. This has a profoundly weakening effect on the whole mind–body continuum. Try to give priority to your creative, life-seeking instincts; try to focus on other people's problems for a change. If you are unable to sit down and clear your mind and experience the contentment of just being alive, then you should consider learning some form of relaxation or meditation, which will give you that experience.

Although most mental and emotional problems are rooted in upbringing and childhood experiences, illness and various stressful life events also take their toll. Depression is quite common after viral illnesses such as influenza, glandular fever, shingles, and hepatitis. Bereavement, redundancy, family pressures, and pressures at work also place a severe strain on a person's ability to adapt.

Orthodox treatment of emotional and mental problems consists of drugs, often combined with some form of psychotherapy. If you wish to switch to constitutional homeopathic treatment, consult your GP first.

Severe mental problems requiring psychiatric treatment in hospital are rare, but if you find yourself in this situation and wish to have homeopathic treatment – homeopathically trained psychiatrists being very few and far between – ask your psychiatrist if he or she would have any objections to your taking homeopathic remedies or extra vitamins; these will not interfere with any drugs you are taking. When you are discharged, your psychiatrist may rarely agree to tail off your drugs so that you can switch fully to constitutional homeopathic treatment.

Agoraphobia see also PHOBIA

Extreme anxiety attached to being in public or crowded places. By avoiding such places anxiety is reduced to a tolerable level, but the anxiety is also reinforced. Being accompanied may make you feel less fearful, but anxiety increases the further away from home you go and the more crowded the situation. You may even develop claustrophobia as well. Agoraphobia is commonly accompanied by PANIC ATTACKS, especially at the beginning. The onset of these attacks is often associated with anxiety or depression following the death of a close relative (see GRIEF), a loss, or a major family argument. Most sufferers of agoraphobia are women in their late teens or early 20s. Since panic feelings can be made worse by HYPERVENTILATION or HYPOGLYCAEMIA, simply treating these may help to keep phobia under control. If not, behaviour therapy may be effective. Behaviour therapy involves the setting of tasks, which should be written down clearly, e.g., 'walk 50 yards, by myself, looking back at the house frequently', progressing to 'walk half a mile to the local shops, have a cup of tea in a café and walk home'.

Homeopathic treatment is constitutional, but in the meantime try the following.

Specific remedies to be given 4 times daily for up to 7 days, or ½ hourly for up to 10 doses if phobia is acute and disabling:

- Condition onsets after the death of a loved one *Natrum mur. 6c*
- Woman terrified of dying or collapsing if she goes into a shop, gets on to a bus, etc. *Aconite 6c*
- Fear brought on by an accident *Arnica 6c*
- Woman chilly, exhausted, restless *Arsenicum 6c*
- In an emergency, where no other remedy seems to be indicated *Sulphur 6c*

Blushing

Increased blood flow to face, ears, neck, etc. accompanying shame, embarrassment, and other thoughts/emotions which the blusher would prefer to hide; usually a passing phase, often linked with sexual inexperience or insecurity, and with emotional problems generally. Homeopathic constitutional treatment is recommended if blushing is part of a wider picture; if not, the remedies below may help.

Specific remedies to be taken as required for up to 10 doses:

- Face normally pale, personality outgoing and rather excitable, fear of thunder and the dark *Phosphorus 6c*
- Where woman is fair-haired, timid, cries easily, craves affection, and dislikes hot stuffy rooms *Pulsatilla 6c*
- Blushing causes faintness, especially if woman has tendency to become anaemic *Ferrum phos. 6c*

Depression see also POSTNATAL DEPRESSION

A small word that describes a huge range of negative thoughts and feelings from sadness to utter hopelessness, and an equally broad spectrum of physical symptoms. If the cause is a specific external event, such as bereavement, depression is usually temporary; it has a natural timespan, and after a while life regains its interest and colour. Depression can also follow childbirth (see POSTNATAL DEPRESSION). It can also occur after GLANDULAR FEVER and other viral infections (see CHRONIC FATIGUE SYNDROME), or be brought on by changes in body chemistry produced by ADDICTION to drugs or alcohol. Some people only experience depression in the winter months (Seasonal Affective Disorder, or SAD), possibly due to lack of light exposure. Occasionally it is a symptom of developing SCHIZOPHRENIA. But far more often it is the mind which manufactures causes for depression, in the form of rather fixed, life-denying attitudes and beliefs which lead to fear, anger, guilt, frustration, a sense of persecution, loneliness, hopelessness . . . These then affect the body, which in turn affects the mind, and so the vicious circle is established. One person in 25 feels depressed enough to seek professional help at some point in his or her life, and on average twice as many women seek help as men.

Depression in elderly women is often associated with loneliness, low income, losing friends and relatives, feeling left behind and out of touch, becoming dependent on others, worries about health, fear of death and dying . . . Occasionally symptoms of depression – lethargy, social withdrawal, lack of concentration, forgetfulness, poor sleep, loss of appetite etc. – are mistaken for senile dementia; unlike senile dementia, however, depression is treatable.

Depression is not something to be ashamed of; it is a recognized illness. Depression is diagnosed when a person has been feeling down for a significant length of time, for months rather than weeks, and when some of the following symptoms are also present: a significant increase or decrease in appetite or weight, excessive sleep or an inability to sleep, a marked slowing down of movement and thinking, a marked lack of energy, inability to concentrate or make decisions, general loss of interest in activities once considered enjoyable, recurrent thoughts of DEATH or SUICIDAL TENDENCIES. If several of these symptoms are present, don't delay in seeking professional help. Severe or prolonged depression yields more surely to professional help than to self-help or help from friends or relatives; the sufferer (and to some extent those around him or her) is too locked inside the depression to be objective about it.

It is not true that people who talk of suicide do not attempt suicide; they can and do. If you feel that life is no longer worth living, and start thinking about suicide and the methods you are going to use, call the Samaritans or your doctor immediately. You need help, fast.

The symptoms described above are one aspect of a form of depression called manic depression, in which mood alternates between depression and mania. In manic phases the person is reckless and impulsive, highly energetic, even euphoric.

If your GP diagnoses mild depression, he or she will probably prescribe antidepressants or refer you to a psychotherapist. Antidepressants do not cure depression; they merely relieve distressing symptoms until the underlying causes resolve themselves. If depression is severe you will be referred to a psychiatrist; again the options are anti-depressants and psychotherapy, and in extreme cases ECT (electroconvulsive therapy) which requires a stay in hospital, and perhaps occupational therapy to re-establish a normal pattern of life. You should think long and hard before agreeing to ECT as it can impair long-term memory and its effects may not be permanent. Where there is a marked chemical component to depression a change in diet may be recommended (excess vitamin D, zinc, copper, and lead are known to contribute to depression).

Both chronic and acute depression will respond to constitutional treatment from an experienced homeopath, but if you, or a friend or a relative, feel suicidal, call the Samaritans or your doctor immediately.

Specific remedies to be taken 3 times daily for up to 14 days during episodes of mild or moderate depression or while waiting for constitutional treatment:

- Woman restless, chilly, exhausted, obsessively neat and tidy *Arsenicum 6c*
- Feeling chilly, suffering from wind, on edge, oversensitive to noise, light and other stimuli, racing thoughts get in the way of sleep, vivid dreams leave you exhausted on waking *China 6c*
- Lack of energy and stamina after viral illness such as flu or glandular fever *Cadmium phos. 6c*

- Feeling totally worthless, suicidal, disgusted with oneself *Aurum 6c* (if suicidal, also phone the Samaritans or your doctor)
- Depression follows deep grief or heartbreak after a love affair *Ignatia 6c*
- Bottling up emotions, rejecting sympathy because it embarrasses you and makes you want to break down and cry, wanting to hide away *Natrum mur. 6c*
- Bursting into tears at the slightest provocation, wanting a lot of reassurance and attention *Pulsatilla 6c*
- Extremely irritable, finding fault with everyone around you *Nux 6c*
- Feeling irritable, tearful, chilly, very turned off even by the idea of sex *Sepia 6c*

Self-help

Mild depression can often be relieved by making minor changes in lifestyle. If you feel under too much pressure, give up one or two activities that are not essential. If you feel isolated or out of touch, try to get out more or take up a new interest so that you meet other people. If you have children, organize a babysitter so that you can have at least one night a week to yourself. Make sure your diet does not include excessive amounts of vitamin D, zinc, copper, or lead, and avoid tea and coffee. In some women, oral contraceptives seem to contribute to depression; the obvious course is to discuss alternatives with your GP. Increase your intake of vitamins B_1, B_2, B_3, B_5, B_6, and C, folate, biotin, bioflavinoids, calcium, potassium, and magnesium.

Grief

A natural reaction to the loss of a person, animal, or object in whom or in which one has invested much love and affection; not a reaction to be underestimated or bottled up. Grieving is a process which has several fairly distinct stages. First, there may be a sense of unreality, numbness, a refusal to believe that the loved one is dead; then there may be a mixture of complex emotions such as guilt (at not having been close enough to the person or done enough for them, for example) and anger (that the hospital or doctor did not do enough, that the person had no right to die, etc.). Then DEPRESSION may set in. Finally, life becomes bearable again, even enjoyable. The whole process may take from one to two years, and even then there may be a painful anniversary reaction when the anniversary of the person's death comes round.

How well we cope with grief depends partly on our relationship with the dead person; if there were elements in the relationship that gave rise to strong feelings of guilt or anger, grief may be blocked. A lonely, isolated woman may also find grief difficult to cope with; she has no one to express grief to. There is also a theory that in grieving we relive the experience of being separated from the nipple; if our infantile reaction was rage and desolation, our adult reaction to the loss of love may be the same, making it very difficult to progress through the various stages of grief to full recovery. If grief lasts for longer than about 18 months, professional help may be necessary to prevent depression becoming chronic.

Most women receive a lot of attention and kindness in the weeks immediately after bereavement, but it is often 4 or 5 months later that they need most support; that is often the worst time, when they finally accept that the person is dead. Give as much practical help as you can, and allow the woman to talk about her loss even if it is painful; if she so much as hints at suicide (see SUICIDAL TENDENCIES), seek professional help. And continue your support for as long as you can.

Orthodox treatment of grief is based on antidepressants and psychotherapy, or both. Homeopathy offers specific remedies during the various stages of grief, and also constitutional help if there is a failure to progress from one stage to the next.

Early stages

Specific remedies to be taken 4 times daily for up to 14 days, or every 2 hours for up to 10 doses if feelings of grief are overpowering:

- Woman wants to be left alone, insists that she feels all right, doesn't want to be touched, reactions are those of someone in shock *Arnica 30c*
- Woman fearful, on verge of collapse *Aconite 30c*
- Woman very frightened by death of loved one, numb with grief *Opium 6c*

Later stages

Specific remedies to be taken 3 times daily for up to 14 days, or every 2 hours for up to 10 doses if feelings are disrupting normal life:

- Woman extremely angry and critical of others *Nux 6c*
- Woman very depressed and apathetic *Phosphoric ac. 6c*
- Sleeplessness, helpless weeping, catarrh *Pulsatilla 6c*
- Woman rejects consolation and sympathy because it makes her cry, prefers to hide feelings *Natrum mur. 6c*
- Woman finds emotions difficult to control, and laughs, sighs, or cries at inappropriate moments *Ignatia 6c*

Final stages

See remedies listed under DEPRESSION.

Self-help

Talk, say how you feel, ask for help. A stiff upper lip may look dignified, but the cost may be chronic depression and lowered resistance to illness. Organizations such as Cruse (address p. 335) offer counselling and support to the bereaved. Your homeopath or GP may be able to recommend a psychotherapist who can help you to get over the worst. Some people seek comfort in spiritualism, but it takes an experienced spiritualist, and one who has some knowledge of basic psychotherapy, to assist a woman through the mourning process; satisfying a desire to communicate with the dead may prolong grief rather than assuage it and make it difficult to move on. Above all, be patient with yourself.

Obsessions and compulsions

An obsession is a thought or idea that seizes the mind and won't let go; a compulsion is an irresistible urge to act out a thought or idea, however absurd. Hypochondria, for example, is an obsession with health which is translated into buying cupboardfuls of medicines; ANOREXIA is an obsession with physical appearance which translates itself into self-starvation. Most women develop relatively harmless obsessions and compulsions at some time or other, commonly to do with diet, health, hygiene, and personal safety. But if certain thoughts or actions begin to dominate behaviour and disrupt work, family, and social life, treatment should be sought, initially through your GP. A combination of psychotherapy and drugs is the conventional solution, although in extreme cases surgery may be used to cut certain nerve pathways in the brain. Homeopathic treatment is constitutional and longterm, and compatible with psychotherapy but not always with psychoactive drugs.

Specific remedies to be taken every 2 hours for up to 10 doses only if an obsession or compulsion becomes overwhelming:

- Thoughts of death and dying, feeling utterly worthless (999), then *Aurum 30c*
- Woman feels as if body and mind are separate, or that her mind is being controlled by some superhuman agency *Anacardium or. 30c*
- Unshakeable feelings of inadequacy, overwhelming urge to sit on floor and count small objects *Silicea 30c*
- Woman convinced there are live animals wriggling round in stomach, or that limbs are made of glass and so brittle they will break, especially if she has warts *Thuja 30c*

Panic attacks

Usually associated with anxiety or phobia, experienced as a sudden surge of extreme anxiety with palpitations, sweating, tremor, unsteadiness, empty feeling in the chest and pins and needles. You may think you are going to die, become insane, collapse, have a heart attack or do something very embarrassing. The symptoms are often due to a combination of HYPOGLYCAEMIA and HYPERVENTILATION, whatever the mental trigger. Realizing this and controlling it by good diet and proper breathing techniques will do much to help bring the attacks under control: think chemicals!

Specific remedy to be taken as often as required up to 10 doses in an acute attack:

• *Aconite 30c*

Phobia see also AGORAPHOBIA

A phobia is a more or less disabling fear attached to a specific object or situation which is, on the face of it, not at all threatening. A fear of snakes is reasonable in the middle of Africa, less so in Britain, but when a picture or even a shape suggestive of a snake causes intense physical loathing, the fear is irrational, phobic. Most of us have a phobic reaction to something, but in the normal course of events either manage to avoid it or to keep our fear in check.

A phobia may be the result of an unpleasant personal experience, but it can also be a fear copied from parents, a fear transferred from quite another object or set of circumstances, or a fear dredged up from the deepest levels of consciousness where Jung imagined the collective memory of the human species to exist. More prosaically, though rarely, phobias can be due to organic disease, to epilepsy, brain tumours, or brain injury. Acute panic states can also be brought on by HYPOGLYCAEMIA (low blood sugar levels) or HYPERVENTILATION (fast, shallow breathing which starves the brain of oxygen).

Where no organic cause can be found, conventional treatment is by drugs (to control the anxiety), and various forms of behaviour therapy, notably desensitization (step by step exposure to the feared object or situation, coupled with relaxation techniques) and flooding (very unpleasant, full-scale exposure to it). Homeopathy offers constitutional treatment, and a number of remedies for specific situations. See also remedies listed under FRIGHT.

Fear of heights

Specific remedies to be taken 4 times daily for up to 14 days, or ½-hourly for up to 14 doses if fear is intense:

• Fear associated with impulse to jump *Argentum nit. 6c*
• Fear associated with sensation of falling *Borax 6c*
• Fear associated with extreme giddiness *Sulphur 6c*

Fear of the dark

Specific remedies to be taken 4 times daily for up to 14 days, or ½-hourly for up to 10 doses if fear is acute:

• Woman talks and prays continuously *Stramonium 6c*
• Woman nervous and highly strung, responds immediately to affection and reassurance *Phosphorus 6c*

Stage fright, fear of performing in public

Specific remedies to be taken 4 times daily for up to 14 days, or ½-hourly for up to 10 doses if fear is acute:

• Great apprehension, although person performs well once she has started, or person who, when eating in company, feels full after a small amount of food and socially inadequate *Lycopodium 6c*
• Woman feels weak at the knees *Gelsemium 6c*
• Where woman is a musician and prone to stomach upsets *Anacardium 6c*
• Fear acute enough to cause flatulence and diarrhoea *Argentum nit. 6c*

Self-help

With certain phobias, if motivation is strong enough, it is possible to desensitize yourself to some extent; this is true of some animal phobias, and of claustrophobia and AGORAPHOBIA. Take things very slowly, exposing yourself to the thing you fear step by step; learn a few simple breathing and relaxation techniques so that you can defuse anxiety each time it threatens to get the better of you.

Psychotic illness

Severe disturbance of thoughts and emotions in which person is completely out of touch with reality as other people perceive it. Symptoms include complete social withdrawal, profound apathy, delusions, hallucinations and other sensory distortions, and wildly inappropriate speech, behaviour, thoughts, and feelings. Manic depression, schizophrenia, and paranoia are classed, by the psychiatric profession, as psychoses or psychotic illnesses. There is much debate about causes, ranging from the genetic and biochemical to the environmental and frankly existential. Some psychotic states, however, can be fairly clearly related to damage or injury to the brain. These are known as *organic psychoses*, to distinguish them from other forms of psychosis which appear to have no physical cause. Psychotic behaviour can be triggered off, for example, by an impact injury to the brain, by a brain tumour, by toxic metals (lead, mercury, copper), by certain prescription drugs, or by lung infections such as pneumonia. In such cases, treatment or removal of the apparent cause may relieve psychotic symptoms. Conventional treatment of non-organic psychoses is by anti-psychotic drugs, with or without admission to hospital.

Once the cause has been found and treated, or once orthodox drugs have stabilized behaviour, constitutional homeopathic treatment and nutritional manipulation are recommended.

Shyness

A defence against being thought uninteresting, silly, inexperienced, etc. In reality, most 'shy' people are thoughtful and sensitive – traits which are much more attractive than brashness and loudness – but they reject themselves rather than risk the pain of being rejected by others; the signals that go with shyness – avoidance of eye contact, folded arms, crossed legs, muttered or monosyllabic replies to questions – are also those which tell other people 'I am not interested in you'.

Constitutional homeopathic treatment is recommended if shyness is part of general in-security and lack of self-confidence. If shyness is only a problem in certain situations, select an appropriate remedy from the list below.

Specific remedies to be taken hourly for up to 10 doses before or during situation which causes apprehension:

- Woman quiet and sensitive, cries and blushes easily, panics in hot stuffy rooms *Pulsatilla 6c*
- Woman timid, inclined to break down in tears, sometimes obstinate, feels the cold, especially cold winds *Silicea 6c*
- Woman very pale, highly strung, fearful, desperately in need of affection and re-assurance *Phosphorus 6c*
- Great nervousness about new situations, tendency to conceal nervousness by bragging and behaving outrageously or violently *Lycopodium 6c*

Self-help

It often helps to admit being shy; that way, other people make a little more effort to break the ice and draw you out. Try to concentrate on the other person, not on yourself. Relax. Watch and listen. Is everyone else consistently brilliant and witty? Of course not. Ask open questions like 'What do you think of . . .?' or 'How do you feel about . . .?' rather than questions like 'What do you do?' or 'Have you been to see . . .?' which invite factual, potentially conversation-stopping answers.

Stress

Notoriously difficult to define since similar events affect people differently; one person's 'enjoyable challenge' may be another's 'last straw'. Psychologist Hans Seyle has theorized that we all make some attempt to improve per-formance under pressure, but that at some point we all begin to suffer from overload; if the pressure continues, we lose our resilience, tire, and fall into ill health.

It has been thought for some time that people who have psychiatric illness such as depression, or who have experienced some form of stress, tend to get ill because their immune system has been weakened. Research into psychoneuro-immunology has shown this to be true, and has started to unravel some of the connections be-tween all of them.

In homeopathic medicine, ailments such as food ALLERGY, asthma, HYPOGLYCAEMIA, digestive disorders, high blood pressure, etc., are looked on as manifestations of stress. Accordingly, treat-ment is long term and constitutional. However, in acute circumstances, one of the remedies below may be appropriate.

Specific remedies to be given every 4 hours for up to 10 days:

- Stress due to grief or bad news *Phosphoric ac. 30c*
- Stress due to overwork *Picric ac. 30c*
- Stress following emotional upset, a broken love affair, etc. *Ignatia 30c*
- Stress brought on by 'burning candle at both ends', especially by smoking, eating, or drink-ing too much, person irritable *Nux 30c*

Self-help

Learn some form of relaxation or meditation, even if it is only 10 minutes a day. Shed one or two burdens/obligations and don't take on any new ones until you feel better – learn how to say no. Eat at regular times, and get a proper night's rest. Take vitamin B complex. Take more exercise, but don't exercise to the point of tired-ness. If you need emotional support, try coun-selling; the counsellor's job is to work *with* you, pinpointing areas of stress and helping you deal with them.

Suicidal tendencies
see also DEPRESSION

Thoughts of suicide, and talk of suicide, are danger signals which should never be ignored. If someone is feeling suicidal, give Aurum 6c once every 5 minutes for up to 10 doses. Phone Samaritans or your doctor immediately.

Suicide is less frequent among married people than among single, widowed or divorced people, which clearly suggests that the factors leading to it – DEPRESSION, anxiety, INSECURITY, GRIEF – are aggravated by loneliness, or at least by the lack of close, continuing relationships.

Beauty Care Problems

We have stressed in the introduction to this book that true beauty shines through the eyes of the woman who is at peace within herself, and who has come to terms with both her talents and her shortcomings.

In many ways, however, this is a superficial age, and flawless skin, lustrous hair, and an immaculate figure are the hallmarks of supposed beauty. If you are afflicted with some disease which is instantly visible you have an added obstacle to overcome in the struggle to find your place in this world. For this reason, we decided to include a section on the hair, eyes, face, skin and feet.

As you will see, although homeopathic remedies and beauty therapies can help, very often you also have to work hard at lifestyle, diet and so on in order to both look and feel your best. If you are as fit and healthy as possible physically this will translate into a state of general well-being which will be apparent to the outside world. Bear in mind that many of the beautiful models you see in glossy magazines are not really so perfect in real life. You don't have the benefit of professional photographers with soft lenses and computer enhancement like they do. Just be yourself and be content: that will make you really attractive.

Hair

Just as the coat of an animal may give the first indication of poor health, so our hair reflects our general well-being, level of stress and state of nutrition. However, most of the damage that we do to our hair is from external things that we put on it and do to it. Chemicals, sunlight, chlorine and too frequent use of heated appliances can all cause the hair to become dry and dull, making the scalp itchy and flaky. Your hairdresser – or beauty therapist if you feel you need one – can suggest the best products to use on your hair, and it is recommended that you change brands fairly often. More detailed information can be obtained by reading *A Way of Looking* (Bibliography, p. 342).

Baldness
see HAIR LOSS

Dandruff

Excessive amounts of flaking skin on scalp, sometimes with itchiness and redness; may be a symptom of SEBORRHOEIC ECZEMA, a mild form of eczema which can also affect face and chest; more rarely, condition is a feature of PSORIASIS, involving knees and elbows as well, or a sign of a fungal infection. Hair growth is not usually affected.

More simply, dandruff may just be due to a build-up of hair care products that haven't been properly rinsed away. Occasional use of a special shampoo such as Neutrogena will help to remove this. You can prevent the problem by combing your hair before washing it, and making sure you rinse it thoroughly. Dandruff may be aggravated by stress.

If possible, try the homeopathic remedies and self-help measures given below, or try a beauty salon, before resorting to scalp preparations containing steroids. If appropriate, use remedies given for SEBORRHOEIC ECZEMA and PSORIASIS.

Specific remedies to be taken 3 times daily for up to 2 weeks:

- Scalp dry, sensitive, and very hot, unbearably itchy at night, round bare patches of scalp show through hair *Arsenicum 6c*
- Scalp moist, greasy, and sensitive around hair roots *Sepia 6c*

- Dandruff thick, a lot of scratching at night, which causes skin to burn, scalp made even drier by washing hair *Sulphur 6c*
- Intense itching, thick leathery crusts with pus underneath and white scabs on top *Mezereum 6c*
- Flaky scalp, hair loss *Fluoric ac. 6c*
- Scalp moist, encrusted, and smelly, crusting worse behind ears *Graphites 6c*
- Itching like insect bites all around hairline of forehead, moist, smelly spots behind ears, itchiness made worse by heat *Oleander 6c*
- White crusting around hairline, hair lank and greasy *Natrum mur. 6c*

Self-help
In addition to the remedies above, take Kali sulph. (see Tissue Salts p. 24) 3 times daily for up to 1 month, then 3 times daily for only 5 days out of 7 until scalp improves. Reduce intake of refined carbohydrates and animal fats, and take extra vitamins B, C, and E, zinc and selenium.

Dandruff which sticks to the hair and scalp can be loosened by rinsing scalp with sour milk or a mild solution of lemon juice (2 tablespoons lemon juice to 0.5 litre [1 pint] boiled cooled water). As for shampoo, use pure soap. Apply Calendula ointment to itchy areas around hairline. If whole scalp itches, apply cold-pressed linseed oil, cod liver or olive oil (cold-pressed) overnight (sleep on an old towel) and wash it off with pure soap shampoo in the morning. If all else fails, wash hair in shampoo which contains Selenium, but follow the instructions carefully.

Scalp exercises are recommended, and it is important they are practised at home as part of your routine – they will improve circulation and stimulate hair growth at the same time. Treatment in a salon would consist of scalp massage with exfoliating creams and oils, possibly an aromatherapy oil, first removing the dry flaky skin then relaxing and moisturizing the scalp.

Greasy hair
Caused by overactivity of the sebaceous glands, which produce a waxy substance called sebum to keep hair supple and waterproof (see diagram 17); often associated with other skin problems, and in youngsters with either ACNE or the general hormonal upheaval of adolescence. Can be aggravated by over-frequent washing with strong shampoos which destroy acid balance of scalp. Constitutional treatment is recommended if the specific remedies and self-help measures below do not improve matters.

Specific remedies to be given every 12 hours for up to 1 month:

- As first resort *Bryonia 6c*
- Greasiness associated with tight sensation in scalp, which feels sweaty, over-production of saliva, intolerance of heat and cold *Mercurius 6c*
- Greasiness associated with thinning hair, especially after prolonged emotional stress or grief *Phosphoric ac. 6c*

Self-help
Cutting down on refined carbohydrates (sweets, chocolates, soft drinks) often helps, and so does frequent washing with mild or very dilute shampoo (try a herbal shampoo such as seaweed or rosemary).

Greying hair
Essentially, we all go grey when our genes say so, when they turn off the pigment-producing cells in our hair follicles. However, premature greying may be due to a lack of vitamin B_5 or PABA (para-aminobenzoic acid), or to severe STRESS; it can also be an indicator of increased risk of auto-immune disease. If associated with ECZEMA or HAIR LOSS, constitutional treatment would be appropriate, but the remedies given below should be tried first.

Specific remedies to be given every 12 hours for up to 1 month:

- Greying associated with hair loss, especially after grief or prolonged mental stress *Phosphoric ac. 6c*
- Greying associated with baldness and eczema behind ears *Lycopodium 6c*
- Greying associated with hot flushes and painful scalp *Sulphuric ac. 6c*

Self-help
Vitamin B_{12} and B complex and also zinc are recommended.

Hair loss
Hair grows from follicles in the scalp. Normally about 90 per cent of the hairs are in a growing phase and 10 per cent in a resting phase, which lasts about 100 days. Every day about 100 hairs are pushed out by the new hairs. If these are fine, short and colourless they are not obvious, but if they are long and black they can look like a very alarming volume indeed.

Hair growth temporarily slows down and it is quite common, after a feverish illness, for hair to be lost faster than it can be replaced, causing some thinning. Other causes include operations, accidents and crash diets. In pregnancy, more hairs are produced than usual as more follicles are in the active phase and hair gets thicker. After delivery, however, more hairs enter the resting phase and remain there, for the usual period. They are then replaced, causing an alarming loss of hair, with actual thinning, but this is only temporary. Slight thinning is also common in women as they get older.

Baldness is predominantly a male phenomenon, tending to run in families; in men a receding hairline generally meets a thinning crown, producing a tonsure effect; in women only the crown thins. In babies, rubbing can cause hair loss, but the hair regrows.

Rarely hair loss is caused by deficiency ailments such as hypothyroidism (see THYROID PROBLEMS) or iron-deficient ANAEMIA, by a lack of zinc or B vitamins, especially biotin, and inositol, or by cytotoxic drugs used to treat CANCER; too much vitamin A or selenium, and also oral contraceptives and anticoagulant drugs, can have the same effect. Generally speaking, once the cause is removed, hair starts growing again. Conditions which destroy hair follicles, however, such as ringworm and LICHEN PLANUS, cause permanent patches of baldness. In *alopecia areata* patches of baldness appear quite suddenly, with all but a few hair follicles becoming inactive; the cause is not known.

Hairdressing techniques – notably perms or if excessive force is used – can cause problems with hair. For example, if a home perm is done, followed by a hairdresser's perm, the hair is very likely to be damaged. However, it is very unusual for the actual follicle to be damaged, so the hair will eventually grow back. It is recommended that before dyeing hair a patch test is done against the hair dye. Most hair dyes are chemically similar, whether they are called tints, rinses or colours, except for henna. So if you become allergic to hair dye the only dye you will be able to use is henna. Orthodox medicine has little to offer that is harmless in the treatment of hair loss, except for treating infection where it is present. There is a drug called Minoxidil, which was originally developed to treat high blood pressure but was found to cause hair growth. It needs to be applied continuously, and when it is stopped the hair falls out; the drug's long-term safety is also in some doubt.

Constitutional treatment can be helpful for thinning hair, giving a boost to the metabolism generally, but the remedies below should also be tried.

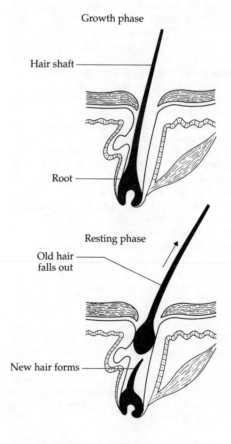

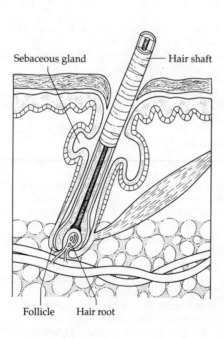

The structure of a hair

Hair growth

Specific remedies to be taken in the 6c potency every 12 hours for up to 1 month.

Please remember to check your choice against the Remedy Pictures (p. 305) where possible.

Lachesis
Hair falling out – worse before periods.

General symptoms: Difficulty in concentrating; difficulty in coping with bereavement; chronic headaches; sensation of plug or lump in throat; bloating of stomach; hot flushes; tendency to PMS; lack of energy.

Lycopodium
Hair falling out – worse before periods – worse after bereavement or childbirth; premature baldness or grey hair.

General symptoms: Difficulty in concentrating; chronic headache; acne; bloated abdomen; lack of periods; fatigue; tendency to PMS.

Sepia
Hair falling out – worse after childbirth and at menopause.

General symptoms: Difficulty in concentrating; indifferent to loved ones; chronic headache; acne; lack of periods; hot flushes and hot sweats; PMS; fatigue.

Sulphur
Hair falling out – worse after bereavement.

General symptoms: Chronic headache; bloated abdomen; lack of periods; hot flushes; lack of energy; tendency to PMS.

Calcarea
Hair falling out – worse before periods.

General symptoms: Difficulty in coping with grieving process; chronic headache; bloated abdomen; sleeplessness; hot flushes; tendency to weight gain; fatigue.

Phosphorus
Hair falling out in handfuls.

General symptoms: Difficulty in concentrating; difficulty in coping with grieving process; chronic headache; acne; bloated abdomen; hot flushes; fatigue; tendency to PMS.

Causticum
Hair loss before periods and following bereavement.

General symptoms: Difficulty in concentrating; difficulty in coping with grieving process; chronic headache; acne; sensation of lump in throat; hot flushes; fatigue; tendency to PMS.

Graphites
Hair falling out – worse after bereavement.

General symptoms: Difficulty in concentrating; difficulty in coping with grieving process; chronic headache; fatigue.

Pulsatilla
Hair falling out – worse before periods, after bereavement.

General symptoms: Difficulty in coping with grieving process; chronic headache; lack of periods; hot flushes; fatigue; tendency to PMS.

Natrum mur.
Hair falling out – worse before periods, and after bereavement; hair loss associated with dandruff and white crusts on scalp, especially round hairline.

General symptoms: Difficulty in coming to terms with coping with grieving process; chronic headache; sensation of lump in throat; bloated abdomen; tiredness; tendency to PMS.

Silicea
Hair falling out.

General symptoms: Difficulty in concentrating; chronic headache; acne; lack of periods; fatigue.

Kali carb.
Hair falling out – falling worse before periods, associated with dryness of hair and scalp.

General symptoms: Chronic headache; abdominal distension; lack of periods; sleeplessness; fatigue; tendency to PMS.

Arsenicum
Hair falling out – worse after bereavement.

General symptoms: Chronic headache; abdominal distension; sleeplessness; fatigue; tendency to overweight.

Other remedies to consider
- Hair loss associated with boils on scalp and headaches which become more insistent at night, person very depressed *Aurum 6c*
- Scalp feels painful when touched, loss of body hair as well *Selenium 6c*
- Hair loss after grief or extreme emotion, predominant feelings are indifference and exhaustion *Phosphoric ac. 6c*
- Hair loss follows severe injury *Arnica 6c*

• Hair loss in an elderly person who has poor circulation and is mentally slow *Baryta carb. 6c*

Self-help
Over-frequent washing and conditioning encourage dryness and make the hair look greasy quickly. One application of shampoo is quite enough to remove dirt and grime; if possible let hair dry naturally. Scalp massage may be beneficial in some cases since it encourages circulation. Vitamin B complex, vitamin C, zinc, and iron are recommended. Also, make sure diet contains sufficient protein (from vegetable as well as animal sources).

Specific Remedy Finder for Hair

Ailments after cutting hair
Belladonna
Glonoinum
Kali iod.
Phosphorus

Baldness
Anacardium
Apis
Baryta
Fluoric ac.
Graphites
Phosphorus
Sepia
Silicea
Zinc

Baldness in patches
Apis
Arsenicum
Calcarea
Graphites
Hepar sulph.
Phosphorus

Baldness in young women
Baryta
Silicea

Brittle hair
Kali carb.
Psorinum

Hair changes colour
Kali iod.

Hair becomes curly
Mezereum

Hair feels as if it has been drawn upwards
Muriatic ac.

Dry hair
Ambra
Calcarea
Fluoric ac.
Kali carb.
Medorrhinum
Phosphorus
Plumbum
Psorinum

Sulphur
Thuja

Static electricity in hair
Medorrhinum
Veratrum

Hair falling out
Aurum
Carbo veg.
Carbon sulph.
Fluoric ac.
Graphites
Kali carb.
Kali sulph.
Lachesis
Lycopodium
Natrum mur.
Nitric ac.
Phosphorus
Sepia
Silicea
Sulphur
Thuja

Hair falling out all over head
Selenium

  after disease
  Lycopodium
  Manchinella

  due to dandruff
  Ammonium mur.
  Thuja

  from grief
  Phosphoric ac.

  in handfuls
  Mezereum
  Phosphorus

  in menopause
  Sepia

  after childbirth
  Calcarea
  Cantharis
  Carbo veg.
  Lycopodium
  Natrum mur.

Nitric ac.
Sepia
Sulphur

  during pregnancy
  Lachesis

  after pregnancy
  Sepia

  better at seaside
  Medorrhinum

Hair falling out in spots
Apis
Arsenicum
Calcarea
Fluoric ac.
Hepar sulph.
Phosphorus
Psorinum

Hair falling out

  more marked on forehead
  Hepar sulph.
  Mercurius
  Natrum mur.
  Phosphorus

  on back of head
  Carbo veg.
  Chelidonium
  Petroleum

  on sides
  Graphites
  Staphisagria

  on temples
  Kali carb.
  Natrum mur.

  when it becomes grey
  Arsenicum
  Kali iod.
  Lycopodium
  Phosphoric ac.
  Silicea
  Staphisagria
  Sulphur

  all over body
  Alumina

Greasy hair
Bryonia
Causticum
Medorrhinum
Natrum mur.
Phosphoric ac.

Lustreless
Medorrhinum
Psorinum
Thuja

Moving sensation
Stannum

Painful when touched
Apis
Arsenicum
Selenium

Pulled out sensation
Lycopodium
Magnesia carb.

   especially on top of head
   Aconite
   Argentum nit.
   Phosphorus

Hair sticks together
Mezerium
Natrum mur.
Psorinum

Hair sticks together at ends
Borax

Stiff hair
Nux mosch.

Hair tangles easily
Borax
Fluoric ac.

Cannot bear weight of hair
Glonoinum

Eyebrows falling out
Kali carb.
Nitric ac.

Eyelashes falling out
Apis
Arsenicum
Calcarea sulph.
Chelidonium
Euphrasia
Mercurius
Rhus tox.
Selenium
Staphisagria
Sulphur

Sensation of hairs on face
Graphites

Tears hair from jealousy
Lachesis

Hair loss from skin eruptions
Lycopodium
Medorrhinum
Mercurius
Mezereum
Rhus tox.

Eczema on hair margin from ear to ear at back of head
Natrum mur.
Sulphur

Impetigo in margins of hair
Natrum mur.

Moist eruptions eating away hair
Kali bichrom.
Mercurius
Natrum mur.
Rhus tox.

Pimples in margin of hair in front
Nitric ac.

Sensitivity of brain from brushing hair
Arnica
Silicea

Headache from binding up the hair
Argentum
Belladonna
Carbo veg.
China
Cina
Glonoinum
Hepar sulph.
Kali nit.
Mezereum
Nitric ac.
Nux
Phosphorus
Pulsatilla
Silicea
Sulphur

Headache from combing hair
Bryonia
Mezereum

   after cutting hair
   Belladonna
   Sepia

Pressing pain in temples from touching hair
Agaricus

Pressing pain in top of head from touching hair
Carbo veg.

Sensation as if hair being pulled
Aconite
Alumina
Argentum nit.
China
Kali carb.
Laurocerasus
Phosphorus
Rhus tox.
Sulphur

Tenderness of scalp from combing hair
Arsenicum
China
Hepar sulph.
Rhus tox.
Silicea
Sulphur

Pain in eye from combing hair
Nux

Colds after cutting hair
Belladonna
Nux
Sepia

Hair falling out of nostrils
Causticum
Graphites

Sensation on left side as if hair being pulled
Platina

Sneezing from combing or brushing hair
Silicea

Eczema on margins of hair
Sulphur

Moustache in women
Natrum mur.
Sepia
Thuja
Thyroidinum

Diarrhoea after cutting hair
Belladonna

Pubic hair falling out
Natrum mur.
Nitric ac.
Selenium
Zinc

Hair falling out on labia and vulva
Mercurius
Nitric ac.

Pubic hair falling out associated with vaginal discharge
Lycopodium
Natrum mur.

Hairy back
Tuberculinum

Pus spots on arms with hair in middle
Kali brom.

Sensation of hair on arms
Medorrhinum

Sensation of hair on the backs of fingers
Fluoric ac.

Sensation of hairs on forearm being pulled
Thuja

Shooting pain like a splinter on touching hair on hand
Ignatia

Dreams of hair
Magnesia carb.

Chilliness and sensation of hair standing on end
Baryta
Silicea

Sensation like ants crawling around root of hairs
Phosphoric ac.

Itching and burning skin on hairy parts
Rhus tox.

Sensitivity in hair when touched
Apis

Eyes

The eye is designed to bend (refract) light rays and bring them to a focus on the retina. When we want to focus on near objects, tiny circular muscles around the lens contract, making the lens fatter; when we focus on distant objects, another set of muscles, radial muscles, contracts and pulls the lens flatter. All the transparent elements of the eye – the conjunctiva, the cornea, the fluid-filled chamber in front of the lens and the gel-filled chamber behind it – contribute something to refraction but only the lens is capable of 'accommodation', changing its focusing power.

In a woman who is short-sighted images of distant objects are brought to a focus just in front of the retina. This happens if the eyeball is too long from back to front, or if the ligaments which attach the radial muscles to the lens become slack. In a long-sighted woman, the opposite occurs; near objects are focused just behind the retina, either because the eyeball is too short from back to front or because the radial muscles become lazy. In either case, the result is a fuzzy image. These and other refractive errors are relatively easy to correct.

The eyeball consists of three distinct layers of tissue: a tough, opaque outer layer called the sclera, in which the cornea is a transparent window; the choroid layer, liberally supplied with tiny blood vessels and heavily pigmented to stop light escaping through the back of the eye or setting up reflections within the eyeball; and the light-sensitive retina, literally a carpet of nerve fibres with specialized endings. Pigments in these nerve endings (photoreceptors) change their chemical composition in response to various wavelengths and intensities of light, and as these changes take place electrical impulses are generated and transmitted to the optic nerve and then to that part of the brain which makes sense of visual stimuli. Objects are upside down when projected on to the retina, but 'seen' the right way up because certain fibres in the optic nerve cross over before they reach the brain. The retina is easily damaged – by leaking blood vessels in the choroid, for example, or by a build-up of pressure within the eye.

In dim light, which stimulates the 125 million or so rod receptors around the edge of the retina, we see things in monochrome, in shades of black, white, and grey. In bright light, which stimulates the 7 million or so cone receptors packed in the central area of the retina, we see things in colour and with great sharpness. There are three kinds of cones, sensitive to the red, blue, and green wavebands of the visible spectrum; the marvellous variety of colours we see is the result of differential stimulation of these three kinds of receptors. The light sensitive pigment inside them, called rhodopsin, is replaced during sleep, a process which requires vitamin A. Whereas rod receptors, which contain a different pigment, wear out every 2 weeks or so, cones remain functional for 9–12 months. At the end of their useful life, rods and cones are replaced, but after the age of 40 cone replacement becomes less efficient, leading in severe cases to macular degeneration.

The pigmented, muscular iris controls the amount of light reaching the retina. In dim light the iris aperture, the pupil, is large; in bright light it shrinks to pinhead size. Iridologists diagnose many different ailments from the state of the iris. Eye movement is controlled by three pairs of muscles originating from the bony orbit of the eye and attached to the sclera. Under normal circumstances both eyes swivel in unison, receiving two almost identical pictures of the world which we 'see' as one.

The conjunctiva, a continuation of the epidermis, is continuously cleansed and lubricated by salty, bactericidal fluid produced in the tear glands just above the eye. If dust, bacteria, and irritants are not constantly removed, the conjunctiva becomes scratched and sore, and sometimes infected. The duct which drains away this cleansing fluid opens into the back of the nose. Small wonder that our noses run when we start slicing onions! The fluid in the front chamber of the eye nourishes both lens and cornea; it too is constantly replenished. Blockage of the duct through which it drains can lead to glaucoma, a rise in pressure inside the eyeball.

Since the Government introduced charges for testing eyesight in 1989, there has been a significant falling off in the number of tests carried out. The authors recommend that you have your eyes tested at least every 2 years, more frequently if you have any trouble whatsoever. This is particularly important if you are driving; in Europe an eyesight examination has to be carried out before getting a full driving licence.

Sunglasses protect both the eyes themselves from ultraviolet light, and the delicate skin around the eyes; they also help to prevent lines around the eyes caused by squinting. It is important to get a good quality lens that will absorb light across the spectrum.

General self-help
Massage around the eyes to tone up that area. Moisturizing is very important, as there is no natural moisture here – it is borrowed from the rest of the face, so from the age of about 25 onwards we should supplement moisture on the face. A very light moisturizer is best, as anything too heavy will just sit on the surface of the skin, soaking up bacteria. When moisturizing this area remember to work from the temples towards the nose and over the browbone. Creams are preferable to gel, as gels contain spirit, causing them to evaporate; this leads to a tightening effect.

Conjunctivitis
Inflammation of the conjunctiva, the transparent covering of the eye, due to infection or ALLERGY; uncomfortable but not serious except in newborn babies. Gummy, yellow discharge on waking in the morning is usually a sign of infection. When caused by hay fever and allergic rhinitis, or by a food allergy, the whites of the eyes become red and gritty (the 'ground glass in the eyes' feeling) but there is no discharge. Occasionally condition is caused by cleaning solution used with soft contact lenses (see CONTACT LENS PROBLEMS).

Specific remedies to be taken every hour for up to 10 doses; if condition does not improve within 24 hours, see your homeopath or GP:

- Symptoms come on after injury or exposure to cold *Aconite 30c*
- Copious discharge *Argentum nit. 6c*
- Little or no discharge *Euphrasia 6c*

Self-help
Bathing the eyes with Euphrasia (10 drops of Euphrasia mother tincture and 1 level teaspoon salt to 0.25 litre [½ pint] warm water) is very soothing, whether condition is caused by infection, allergy, or lens cleaner; bathe them every 4 hours, but not more than 4 times a day, and use a disposable eye bath. Never use anyone else's face cloth or towel on your face, and be scrupulous about washing your hands before and after touching your eyes.

Contact lens problems
Contact lenses do not suit all eyes; if you suffer from hay fever or bouts of CONJUNCTIVITIS, for example, spectacles may be more suitable.

Many people find soft contact lenses more comfortable than hard ones, and leave the lenses in for several days at a time. The lenses usually need replacing within a couple of years. More recently, soft, disposable contact lenses have been available; these can be left in for up to 2 weeks at a time and then thrown away. Hard lenses are less comfortable, and take some getting used to, but they are cheaper and last 6–8 years. Vision tends to be better with them, and they can be prescribed for a wider range of sight problems; they are also easier to keep sterile. Recent evidence from Moorfields Hospital, however, suggests that soft lenses – either extended-wear or disposable lenses – are 15 times more likely to cause dangerous bacterial infection to the eyes than hard, gas permeable lenses. These eye infections can be sight-threatening, and Moorfields are now suggesting that lenses should not be left in overnight, as doing so affects the ability of oxygen to get to the cornea and nourish it; if the cornea is starved of oxygen it is more liable to infection.

Soft lenses are attractive to sportswomen, however, as they can be put in for a couple of hours without your eyes needing time to get used to them. Drivers also like them as they don't cut out side vision as spectacles do.

Once you have become used to wearing contact lenses, the main problems are irritation and infection. Foreign particles trapped between the lens and the conjunctiva can cause irritation; so can hot, dry, or smoky atmospheres. Infection of the conjunctiva is usually caused by poor hygiene or by wearing lenses for too long. Always wash your hands before putting lenses in or taking them out, and always follow your optician's instructions about cleaning and soaking your lenses. A few people, especially if they have some form of ALLERGY already, become allergic to contact lenses or to soft lens cleaning solutions, in particular those containing the preservative Thiomersal; in such cases, alternative cleaning methods are available.

See CONJUNCTIVITIS for specific remedies and self-help measures.

Dry eye

Lack of lubrication from the tear glands above the eyes, causing eyes to feel gritty and the whites to turn red; mainly affects women, usually in middle age; sometimes linked to rheumatoid arthritis or to an ALLERGY (especially to gluten, house dust, and pets), but can also be a drug side-effect. Your GP will prescribe artificial tear drops. Hot rooms filled with cigarette smoke should be avoided.

Self-help

Euphrasia eye baths (see CONJUNCTIVITIS) can relieve soreness temporarily, but extra vitamin C, B_2, B_6, and A, and evening primrose oil, may have longer-lasting effects.

Eyelid problems

see also STYE

Blepharitis

Crusting and redness around the edge of the eyelids, often associated with DANDRUFF. Untreated, flakes of skin may enter the eye and cause CONJUNCTIVITIS, or the eyelashes may fall out. Like dandruff, the condition is deep-rooted and best treated constitutionally. Orthodox treatment is by antibiotic or steroid ointments which suppress rather than cure the condition.

Specific remedies to be taken every 4 hours for up to 2 weeks:

- Eyelids red and gummy *Hepar sulph. 6c*
- Eyelids red and swollen, gummy in morning *Graphites 6c*
- Where itchiness is main complaint *Calcarea 6c*
- Lids sore and burning, with tiny ulcers, made worse by bathing eyes in water *Sulphur 6c*

Self-help Last thing at night, bathe eyelids with saline solution (1 teaspoon salt to a glass of warm water) and lightly apply Calendula ointment. Reduce intake of animal fats, and take 1 tablespoon cold-pressed linseed oil daily. Vitamins B and C and zinc may also be beneficial.

Drooping eyelids (ptosis)

Caused by damage to the lid muscle or to the nerve controlling it; damage may be a consequence of injury, myasthaenia gravis, diabetes, or an aneurysm within the skull, or simply the result of ageing. Can block vision, and is often accompanied by double vision; sometimes correctable by surgery. Constitutional homeopathic treatment should certainly be tried.

Specific remedy to be taken every 12 hours for up to 10 doses while constitutional treatment is being sought:

- *Gelsemium 30c*

Ectropion

A turning outwards of the lower lid as the lid muscles become lax, exposing the lower part of the eyeball and preventing tears from draining into tear duct; tears run down cheek instead, lower lids become dry and sore, and lower part of conjunctiva thickens, pushing lid further away from eyeball; usually a complaint of old age. Untreated, a corneal ulcer may form; in severe cases, minor surgery may be necessary.

Specific remedy to be taken 4 times daily for up to 2 weeks:

- *Borax 6c*

Self-help Bathe eyes with Euphrasia solution (see CONJUNCTIVITIS).

Entropion

A turning inwards of the lower lid due to contraction of the muscles around the lid margin, causing CONJUNCTIVITIS or a corneal ulcer as inturned lashes irritate and scratch the eyeball; condition mainly affects old people, and can be caused, and made worse, by screwing up and rubbing eyes. Can be corrected by minor surgery.

Specific remedy to be taken every 4 hours for up to 2 weeks:

- *Borax 6c*

Self-help Bathe eyes with Euphrasia solution (see CONJUNCTIVITIS).

Eyestrain

If you are aware of tightness around the eyes, or if you habitually screw up your eyes or have difficulty focusing on distant objects after focusing on near ones for any length of time, or vice versa, have your eyes tested by a qualified optician. If you wear spectacles or contact lenses, your eyesight should be tested once a year.

Specific remedies to be taken 4 times daily for up to 7 days:

- Ciliary muscles tired from looking into distance for a long time *Arnica 6c*
- Eyes ache when you look up, down, or sideways *Natrum mur. 6c*
- Eyes burn and feel strained after close work or reading *Ruta 6c*
- Tired eyes associated with great nervousness and apprehension, or with sexual overindulgence *Phosphorus 6c*

Self-help

Palming If you are studying a great deal, or using a VDU, do this exercise every half an hour.

Place the palms of your hands gently over your eyeballs. This should exert enough pressure to stop the eyeball from flicking around, but not cause any tenderness. Support your arms on the desk and allow the eyes to relax for a couple of minutes. Then do the following exercise: hold one finger about 6 in from the eyes and a pencil at full stretch, look at the finger then the pencil, then back to the finger again. Repeat for 2 minutes.

Floaters

Small objects which seem to drift across field of vision when eyes or head are turned; in the elderly, cause may be degeneration of vitreous humour inside the eyeball; other causes may be detached retina or bleeding into the eye. In naturopathy, if the above causes have been ruled out, floaters are taken to be a symptom of a sluggish liver and a build up of toxins in the body. If condition worsens, or if vision starts to blur, ②.

Specific remedies to be taken 3 times daily for up to 7 days:

- If symptoms come on after an accident *Arnica 6c*
- Where specialist has diagnosed bleeding from back of eye *Hamamelis 6c*
- Floaters associated with misty vision *Phosphorus 6c*

Self-help

If the above remedies do not help, and if retinal detachment has been ruled out, follow the LIVER DIET (pp. 264–5) for 1 month.

Puffy eyes

Chronic puffiness under the eyes may be a sign of kidney problems, therefore if you are also feeling unwell, see your GP or homeopath. Simple puffiness can be reduced by the use of cold compresses, or you can use an eye mask (made in this country by Optrex), which can be left in the fridge. It should be left on for 10–15 minutes.

Stye

An infection which develops at the root of an eyelash; looks rather like a boil to begin with, then develops a head of pus; red and painful, but usually clears up of its own accord within 7 days. For recurrent styes, conventional treatment is antibiotics; the homeopathic approach is constitutional, intended to boost general resistance to infection.

Specific remedies to be given every hour for up to 10 doses:

- *Pulsatilla 6c*
- If Pulsatilla produces no improvement *Staphisagria 6c*

Self-help

To disperse a stye, try hot spoon bathing: wrap cotton wool round handle of a teaspoon, then repeatedly dip spoon in very hot water and put it against stye. You should not try to burst the stye by squeezing it. Tighten up on personal hygiene; for example, never touch or rub your eyes with dirty hands.

Twitching eyelids

Brief flickering of one eyelid, with no other signs of twitching or trembling, is usually an indication of tension or tiredness, and nothing to worry about. Constitutional treatment would be appropriate.

Specific remedies to be taken every 4 hours for up to 6 doses if twitch persists:

- Twitching of eyelid only *Codeinum 6c*
- Twitching of eyelid and eyeball *Agaricus 6c*
- Twitching and inflammation of eyelid *Pulsatilla 6c*

Watering eyes

Continuous watering of the eyes is fairly rare and usually the cause is blockage of the tear ducts due to infection or injury, especially injury to the bridge or side of the nose. If condition is not relieved by the remedy given below, see your GP;

conventional treatment is to syringe blocked duct, give antibiotics if infection is present, or re-establish drainage from the eye into the nose by surgery. In newborn babies the tear ducts sometimes fail to open; gentle massage up the side of the nose to the inner corner of the eye may encourage them to do so, but sometimes a probe is necessary.

Specific remedy to be given 4 times daily for up to 7 days:

• Tear duct infected *Silicea 6c*

Remedy Finder for Eyes

Bright light upsets
Aconite
Argentum nit.
Arsenicum
Baryta
Belladonna
Calcarea
Carbon sulph.
China
Conium
Euphrasia
Graphites
Lac can.
Lycopodium
Mercurius
Natrum mur.
Natrum sulph.
Nux
Opium
Rhus tox.
Sulphur

Pain in eye from reading or sewing
Bryonia
Natrum mur.
Ruta

Sight of blood makes symptoms worse
Alumina
Nux
Veratrum

Sight of needles makes symptoms worse
Silicea

Heavily infected discharge from eyes
Argentum nit.
Calcarea
Hepar sulph.
Lycopodium
Mercurius
Pulsatilla

Burning discharge
Carbon sulph.
Chamomilla
Euphrasia
Graphites
Hepar sulph.
Sulphur

Mucus or pus
Calcarea
Calcarea sulph.
Causticum
Mercurius
Pulsatilla
Tellurium

Tears
Allium
Belladonna
Calcarea
Euphrasia
Fluoric ac.
Lycopodium
Mercurius
Natrum mur.
Nitric ac.
Opium
Phosphorus
Pulsatilla
Rhus tox.
Ruta
Staphisagria
Sulphur

Face

We are born with an acid mantle on our skin, keeping it soft and supple, to protect it from bacteria and the elements. As we age, this mantle becomes vulnerable and damaged by sun, wind, pollution and general abuse. All this contributes to the ageing process – the drying out of the skin, and the slowing down of the rejuvenation of elastin and collagen fibres. There are normal changes, through puberty, the menstrual cycle, pregnancy and the menopause, which all contribute to degeneration of the skin.

From the age of 20 our skin starts to dry out, so ideally cleansing, toning, moisturizing and nourishing of the skin should be done morning and night. Finding the correct Ph-balanced preparations for your skin type is daunting when faced with the huge range of products available.

Finding the right preparation can be a life-long and expensive quest!

Remember that skin can get bored with the same preparation, i.e., something you have used for years suddenly brings you out in spots – change is then obviously sensible. A beauty therapist can advise you on your skin type, how to improve it, and maintain it in good condition.

If a spot appears when least wanted, i.e. a very special occasion, a beauty therapist can cleanse and condition the area, drying up the spot. Using a peeling mask to iron out the surface of the skin, dead cells are removed, leaving the area clean and as mark-clear as possible for applying make-up to cover the mark if you wish to. If make-up is used it should be cleansed off with care at night prior to moisturizing.

To keep your face in trim we recommend facial exercises.

Acne

Spotty skin on face, neck, or back caused by the boost which higher hormone levels give to the production of oily sebum and the growth rate of cells in the epidermis; clogged by a mixture of dead cells and sebum, some sebaceous glands become inflamed, forming raised, red spots or pus-filled pimples; squeezing and picking do not improve matters. Condition is often more severe in boys than girls, but skin usually clears in late teens or early twenties. Lasting scars are rare. In some cases foods such as chocolate, cheese, and nuts, and fizzy citrus drinks and junk foods in general seem to aggravate condition; STRESS, steroids, and anti-epilepsy drugs may also play a part. In severe cases GP may prescribe an anti-septic lotion which peels the top layer of skin, or antibiotics, hormones, or drugs based on vitamin A. Homeopathic medicine regards acne as a symptom of fundamental imbalance, so treatment is long-term and constitutional; however, the remedies and self-help measures below may produce some improvement.

Specific remedies to be taken in the 6c potency 3 times daily for up to 14 days.

Please remember to check your choice against the Remedy Pictures (p. 305) where possible.

Calcarea

Pustules; acne on cheeks – worse before periods, worse in warm conditions, after drinking alcohol; blackheads on face and nose; pustules on chest; pimples on face; acne worse on cheeks, in winter; blind boils on face, with spots that are itchy; chapping and cracking of lips; pale, sickly yellow face colour; eruptions and ulcers in corner of mouth; crusty lesions; eczema and inflammation of face; itching and sweating of face with swelling.

General symptoms: Weakness; hot flushes; swelling of ankles.

Lycopodium

Acne on cheeks – worse before periods, in warm conditions, in cold conditions and after drinking alcohol; pimples on face – worse from stress, in winter; blind boils after eating chocolate; bluish discoloration of eyes and lips; greyish pale, red or yellow discoloration of face; moist eczema on face; sores around mouth; freckles; inflammation of face; swelling of face with twitching and perspiration.

General symptoms: Swelling of the ankles.

Sulphur

Longstanding acne – worse before periods, from warmth, after drinking alcohol; acne on nose; blackheads on face and nose; pimples – worse for stress; spots very painful and itchy; acne – worse when recovering from illness; chapped, cracked lips; pale or red discoloration of face; red spots; unusual redness of lips with dryness; ulceration round mouth; freckles; itchy chin; painful eruptions on chin; swelling of the upper lips; flushing of face with shivering; symptoms worse for washing.

General symptom: Hot flushes.

Sepia

Acne on cheeks – worse before periods, in cold weather; blackheads on face; pustules on back; acne worse for stress, worse on cheeks, with infertility; itchy spots, worse after periods; cracking of lower lips; earthy, pale, yellowy complexion; eruptions around lips, mouth and nose; acne on forehead; herpes on face; blisters on face; saddle across nose, usually yellow; swelling of the lips.

General symptom: Hot flushes.

Lachesis

Acne on cheeks – worse before periods, worse in warm weather, after drinking alcohol; pustules on back; pimples on chest; tendency to scar – worse during and after periods.

General symptoms: Hot flushes; swollen ankles.

Silicea

Acne on cheeks – worse in cold weather, after drinking alcohol; blackheads on face; painful pustules on back; pustules on chest; tendency to scar; acne more pronounced when recovering from illness.

Natrum mur.

Acne on cheeks – worse before periods, in warm weather; after drinking alcohol; blackheads on face – worse for stress; pimples on back, with infertility; spots itchy; greasy face.

Phosphorus

Acne worse in warm and in cold conditions, after drinking alcohol; pustules on nose.

General symptoms: Hot flushes; swollen ankles.

Causticum

Pustules on face; pimples on face; acne on cheeks and nose – worse in cold weather, and after drinking alcohol.

General symptoms: Hot flushes; sore pain in jaw.

Graphites
Acne worse for warm and cold weather; black-heads on face and nose; pimples on chest; pustules on face; pimples on face; tendency to scar – worse after periods.

General symptoms: Irregular periods; swollen ankles.

Kali carb.
Acne – worse before periods, and in cold weather; pimples on chest, back and face – worse for stress and in winter; blind boils on face.

Mercurius
Pustules on face – worse in warm conditions, and after drinking alcohol; pimples on face – worse for stress; greasy skin.

General symptom: Swollen ankles.

Nitric ac.
Pustules on face – worse in cold; blackheads on face and nose; pimples on face – worse for stress; tendency to scar.

Belladonna
Pustules on face; acne on cheeks – worse in warmth, and after drinking alcohol; blackheads on face; painful spots.

Hepar sulph.
Large pustules like boils on nose, face, and chest – worse in cold; blackheads on face; pimples on chest, aggravated by lack of sleep; pimples on face; spots very painful even when touched very lightly – worse in winter.

General symptoms: Hair falling out; piles; fatigue; swollen ankles; great anger; violent hunger.

Pulsatilla
Acne – worse before periods, in the warm, cold and after drinking alcohol; pimples on back – worse in winter, and after eating chocolate and rich fatty foods.

General symptoms: Infertility; irregular periods; piles; fatigue; trembling in hands; hot flushes; swollen ankles.

Rhus tox.
Acne on cheeks – worse in cold weather and after drinking alcohol; pimples and pustules on chest; pimples on face – worse for stress and in winter; itchy spots; greasy skin.

General symptoms: Piles; fatigue; hot flushes; swollen ankles.

Psorinum
Acne worse in cold and aggravated by hand against the skin; pustules on chest and chin; pimples on face – worse for stress and in winter; greasy skin on face.

General symptoms: Piles; fatigue; trembling hands; hot flushes; swollen ankles.

Carbo veg.
Pustules on face – worse before periods, in the cold and after drinking alcohol; blackheads on face; pimples on face – worse for stress and in winter – better in warm, wet weather; hair falling out.

General symptoms: Piles; fatigue; hot flushes.

Conium
Pustules on face – worse before periods, in the cold, after drinking alcohol, and if not sleeping properly; pimples on face – worse for stress and in winter.

General symptoms: Infertility; dull aching pain in abdomen – worse after periods; hair falling out; weakness; fatigue; trembling hands.

Antimonium
Pustules on face; acne on cheeks – worse for warm and cold weather, and after drinking alcohol; pimples on chest; pimples on face – worse for stress; itchy eruptions.

General symptoms: Hair falling out; piles; weakness; fatigue; trembling hands.

Aurum
Pustules on face – worse in cold weather and if overtired; pimples on face – worse from stress, in winter and with infertility.

General symptoms: Hair falling out; weakness.

Arsenicum
Pustules on face – worse for cold and after drinking alcohol; blackheads on face; pimples and pustules on chest – worse in winter; swelling of ankles.

Other remedies to consider
- Itchy spots, fidgety feet, restless sleep, unpleasant dreams *Kali brom. 6c*
- Blind pimples and weeping pustules which form yellow crusts, spots slow to heal *Calcarea sulph. 6c*
- Where pus-filled pimples are main feature *Antimonium tart. 6c*

Remedy Finder for Acne

Acne in general
Aurum
Calcarea sil.
Carbo veg.
Carbon sulph.
Causticum
Hepar sulph.
Kali brom.
Nux
Sepia
Silicea

With boils
Belladonna
Calcarea
Hepar sulph.
Kali iod.
Silicea
Sulphur

Blackheads
Arbrotanum
Arsenicum
Belladonna
Bryonia
Calcarea
Carbo veg.
Carbon sulph.
Graphites
Hepar sulph.
Natrum ars.
Natrum carb.
Natrum mur.
Nitric ac.
Sabadilla
Selenium

Sepia
Silicea
Sulphur
Tuberculinum

Blackheads that ulcerate
Selenium
Tuberculinum

Blackheads on chin
Tuberculinum

Blind boils
Calcarea
Crotalus
Gelsemium
Kali carb.
Kali iod.
Lycopodium
Petroleum
Picric ac.

Pimples
Calcarea
Carbon sulph.
Causticum
Graphites
Kali carb.
Kreosotum
Lycopodium
Mercurius
Natrum mur.
Nitric ac.
Nux
Sulphur

Pustules
Antimonium tart.
Aurum met.
Belladonna
Cicuta
Tuberculinum

Pus coming out
Antimonium
Cicuta
Psorinum
Rhus tox.

Greasy face
Baryta
Bryonia
China
Magnesia carb.
Mercurius
Natrum mur.
Plumbum
Psorinum
Rhus tox.
Selenium
Tuberculinum

Hard scarring
Graphites

Oily sweats
Bryonia
China
Magnesia carb.
Mercurius
Stramonium
Thuja

Self-help
Sunlight, vitamins A and B_6, and zinc all have a beneficial effect, although zinc may interfere with the absorption of some orthodox drugs given for acne. Avoid refined carbohydrates and iodine (in some cough mixtures, seaweed, etc.). The LIVER DIET on p. 264, followed for 1 month, should also have a positive effect. (Check also for HYPOGLYCAEMIA.) Thoroughly wash affected areas twice a day – that will remove excess sebum and dead cells. Mildly antiseptic over-the-counter preparations should be used very sparingly as they can cause sensitization reactions.

Whiteheads can sometimes be removed by washing the face or by massage. If deep-seated, the sebaceous plug can be removed by a beauty therapist, using a lance or electrical diathermy needle.

The appearance of skin with acne can be very distressing, and it is not always successful to use a cover stick or foundation to cover the eruptions. This often aggravates the problem, especially if the acne is in a pustular condition, which causes the foundation to clog and possibly introduce bacteria into the skin. Resist the inclination to touch the lumps as this can cause a secondary pustule to erupt on the surface of the skin.

Scar tissue of varying dimension and depth may form, and you may wish to visit a beauty salon. The treatment in a salon consists of softening the skin, massage to help the skin's metabolism and increase the circulation, peeling masks to stimulate new cell growth, and camouflage. In some cases dermal abrasion (surgical removal of the layer of deep scar tissue) may be recommended by a dermatologist.

If the skin is painful apply a hot compress; this will ease the pain, increasing circulation. The skin may visibly suffer and crack, but avoid using products that are too strong to alleviate the problem. Drying out the skin too viciously causes more keratinization, and clogging of the follicles. Glands that are still over-producing sebaceous oil begin the problem again, thus never actually clearing the follicle so that skin can function more efficiently.

Chloasma

Patches of darker skin on face, especially on cheeks, which appear during pregnancy or while on the pill; once hormones settle down after childbirth or discontinuation of the Pill, patches usually fade. If the remedy below produces no improvement within 1 month, consult your homeopath.

Specific remedy to be taken every 12 hours for up to 2 weeks:

- *Sepia 6c*

Self-help
Take extra Vitamin C and E.
    Elimination can be speeded up by a treatment requiring desquamation – a peeling and drying of the surface cells. This can be done at a beauty salon; a facial massage is incorporated, and advice on what creams to use at home. Treatment may involve more than one visit but is generally quite successful.

Cold sores

Culprit is the extremely infectious *Herpes simplex* virus, which can also cause corneal ulcers and genital herpes (see SEXUALLY TRANSMITTED DISEASES), so do not touch eyes or genitals after touching cold sores. In first stage of infection, blisters and then ulcers form *inside* the mouth or on the face, accompanied by red, swollen gums, a furry tongue, mild fever, and feeling generally under par. Though these symptoms clear up within a few days, the virus may not be destroyed, so whenever immunity is at a low ebb infection tends to reappear around mouth and lips, causing blisters which weep and then become encrusted; these usually clear up within 5–7 days. Though antiviral ointments are often effective, the authors advise against all external applications whilst undergoing homeopathic treatment if possible. Outbreaks can be treated using the remedies given below, but constitutional treatment is the proper solution.

Specific remedies to be given 4 times daily for up to 5 days:

- Many ulcers inside mouth, gums bleed easily, whole mouth very sore, worse at night *Sempervivum 6c*

- Deep crack in middle of lower lip, mouth very dry, sores puffy and burning, pearl-like blisters on lips *Natrum mur. 6c*
- Mouth and chin infected, ulcers at corner of mouth *Rhus tox. 6c*
- Cracks at corners of mouth, lips pale, red itchy rash on chin, burning blisters on tongue, breath smells nasty *Capsicum 6c*
- Eruption around the nose *Aethusa 6c*

Self-help
Take extra lysine (an amino acid), vitamin C, zinc and bioflavonoids, and avoid foods containing arginine (another amino acid, found in peanuts, chocolate, seeds, and cereals).
    Avoid sunbathing.

Facial hair problems

In men, facial hair is a secondary sex characteristic marking the transition from juvenile to adult; in women, facial hair commonly increases after the menopause or it may run in the family. Excessive hairiness generally may be a sign of hypopituitarism, which is usually accompanied, in women, by weight gain (see WEIGHT PROBLEMS), deepening of the voice, and cessation of periods. Certain drugs can also cause facial and body hair to increase; if this is the case, see your GP.
    If facial hair causes embarrassment, plucking, waxing, shaving, or special depilatories will temporarily remove it; electrolysis may or may not remove hair permanently, and needs to be done by an expert. Constitutional homeopathic treatment may help, but there are no specific remedies apart from the one given below.

Specific remedy to be given every 12 hours for 3 doses and observe for 1 month:

- Hair confined to upper lip, especially if growth increases after vaccination against smallpox or after a bad reaction to some other vaccine *Thuja 30c*

Self-help
Plucking may distort the follicle, causing the hair to grow at a different angle, or it may cause in-growing hair. The hair may break off half-way up the follicle, causing it to be stubbly when it comes through. Only a hormone imbalance, however, can change the growth of hair or determine whether you have hair or not.
    Bleaching hair obviously takes out the colour, making it less obvious, but some bleaches dry and swell the hair, making it coarse to the touch. Shaving the hair only keeps it in good condition, like a regular visit to the hairdressers. The same applies to depilatory creams which will sink into

the top of the follicle and take a little more of the hair than shaving. This is a chemical reaction, and if it is melting the hair, what is it doing to the skin?

So what can be done? Tampering with hormones is something doctors do not recommend unless your health is at risk. A beauty therapist can help with the following treatments: waxing, electrolysis and tweezer epilation.

Waxing is removal of the hair with a sticky substance placed on the hair, removing it against the growth. There are several forms of waxing: hot wax, cool wax and sugaring. If applied and removed correctly any of these will be successful. Once the hair has been removed a soothing cream is applied to the skin and you will be told not to go in the sun, have a hot shower or bath, or swim in chlorinated water until the following day. This is simply because the natural oils on the surface of the skin have been removed with the dead cells and the hair, and the surface of the skin has to repair itself. If you should suffer from in-growing hair due to the dryness of the skin after waxing, use a loofah or a body brush to get rid of the dead cells on the surface of the skin the night before waxing. This allows hairs that may be trapped under the surface to break free. Follow this with a hot bath, and massage a rich moisturizing cream into the skin. Overnight the skin will be moist and the hair ready for waxing in the morning. Don't, however, moisturize the skin on the day of waxing. There are home kits available from most chemists, but you have to be very positive when doing your own waxing as it is rather like removing a plaster. If it is not removed at the correct angle you will more than likely break the hair off, leaving stubble.

Acne rosaceae

Produces ACNE-like symptoms, but occurs in middle age; cheeks and nose flush easily, becoming permanently red, with small pus-filled spots; usually aggravated by hot spicy foods, tea, coffee, and alcohol (see also ALCOHOLISM), and by STRESS, but causes are thought to be oral contraceptives, steroid ointments, and possibly a deficiency of vitamin B_2 (riboflavin). Antibiotics are usually prescribed.

If stress is the major factor, homeopathic treatment is constitutional. However, the remedies listed below may be beneficial.

Self-help

Take extra vitamin B_2, and try the LIVER DIET (pp. 264–6) for 1 month. If you are on steroids, stop taking them if possible after discussion with your GP. Cut out spicy foods, coffee, smoking and alcohol.

Specific remedies to be taken in the 6c potency 3 times daily for up to 3 weeks:

Please remember to check your choice against the Remedy Finder (p. 305) where possible.

Arsenicum

Pimples on the head; swelling of the face; facial rash; pustules on the face; itchy eruptions; skin flaking and scaly; moist eruptions; eruptions burn.

General symptoms: Headaches from alcohol; anxiety and restlessness; vaginal discharge – worse for drinking alcohol, from exposure to wind and cold applications, for changes in temperature, from eating meat.

Sulphur

Pimples on the head; facial rash; itching, painful, moist eruptions.

General symptoms: Headaches – worse after drinking alcohol, for stress; vaginal discharge; skin worse after drinking, for drinking warm or hot drinks, before periods, in warm weather.

Calcarea

Facial swelling; pustules on face; eruptions itchy, flaky, and can be moist – worse on cheeks; spots.

General symptoms: Worse for stress; anxiety; headaches – worse after drinking alcohol; Eustachian tube catarrh; vaginal discharge; face worse after drinking alcohol, before periods, in warm weather, after eating meat.

Sepia

Swelling of face; eruptions burning, itchy, flaky or moist – worse on cheeks; spots on face.

General symptoms: Worse for stress; headache; vaginal discharge with eating fish – worse before periods.

Rhus tox.

Swelling of face; rash on face; itchy burning, or moist eruptions – worse on cheeks.

General symptoms: Worse for stress; headache made worse by drinking alcohol; rash aggravated by drinking alcohol; skin worse for warm drinks, windy cold or wet weather; aching pains in limbs.

Lachesis

Facial swelling; eruptions on cheeks; flaky rashes; worse in morning; face reddish purple and mottled.

General symptoms: Worse for stress; anxiety; headaches – worse for drinking alcohol; vaginal discharge; rash worse for drinking alcohol, for warm drinks, before periods, in windy weather, from exposure to the sun, for warm conditions after changes in temperature.

Lycopodium
Facial swelling; itchy, flaky or moist eruptions – worse on cheeks.

General symptoms: Worse for stress; anxiety; headaches – worse for drinking alcohol; rash worse for drinking alcohol; vaginal discharge – worse before periods, for windy weather, for warm conditions.

Mercurius
Facial swelling; rash on face; pustules on face; itchy, flaky, moist eruptions; spots on face.

General symptoms: Worse for stress; anxiety; headache; Eustachian tube catarrh; vaginal discharge; rash worse for drinking alcohol, before periods, in warm conditions.

Phosphorus
Pimples on head; facial swelling; itchy, flaky eruptions.

General symptoms: Worse for stress; headache, especially after drinking alcohol; Eustachian tube catarrh; vaginal discharge; rash worse after drinking alcohol, after warm drinks, before periods, in windy weather, for warm conditions, for change in temperature.

Causticum
Pustules on face; itchy, burning eruptions – worse on cheeks.

General symptoms: Worse for stress; anxiety; Eustachian tube catarrh; vaginal discharge; headache; rash worse after drinking alcohol, before periods.

Natrum mur.
Pimples on head; facial swelling; rash on face; itchy eruptions – worse on cheeks.

General symptoms: Worse for stress; anxiety; headache, especially after drinking alcohol; Eustachian tube catarrh; vaginal discharge; rash

worse after drinking alcohol, before periods, from exposure to the sun, in warm conditions.

Pulsatilla
Facial rash.

General symptoms: Headache, especially after drinking alcohol; Eustachian tube catarrh; vaginal discharge; rash worse for drinking alcohol, for eating fish, warm drinks, before periods, in windy weather, from exposure to the sun, for changes in temperature or warm conditions generally, for eating meat.

Belladonna
Swelling of face; rash on face; pustules on face; eruptions on cheeks; painful spots; early stages face red, dry and burning hot.

General symptoms: Stress; anxiety; headache, especially after drinking alcohol; rash worse after drinking alcohol, in windy weather, from exposure to the sun, in warm conditions.

Antimonium
Facial rashes; pustules on face; itchy flaky eruptions, especially on cheeks.

General symptoms: Worse for stress; anxiety; headache, especially after drinking alcohol; rash worse after drinking alcohol, from exposure to the sun, in warm conditions.

Graphites
Facial swelling; rash on face; itchy, flaky or moist eruptions.

General symptoms: Stress; anxiety; headache; vaginal discharge, symptoms worse for warm conditions.

Other remedies to consider
- Face always red and dry, with pimples and pus-filled spots *Sulphur iod. 6c*
- Burning and itching aggravated by heat, especially in women with scanty periods *Sanguinaria 6c*
- Condition made worse by alcohol, tea, and coffee; person constipated, irritable, and chilly *Nux 6c*

Remedy Finder for Acne Rosaceae (Facial Rash)

		on nose
Calcarea sulph.	**Bluish lesions**	Causticum
Carbo an.	Lachesis	Psorinum
Carbo veg.	Sulphur	
Causticum		
Lachesis		**Facial rash**
Psorinum	**in groups**	Belladonna
Rhus tox.	Causticum	Pulsatilla

Rhus tox.
Sulphur

Bluish rash
Lachesis
Phosphorus

Burning rash
Causticum
Teucrium

Purple rash
Hyoscyamus
Sepia

Worse for scratching
Alumina

Worse for warmth
Euphrasia
Kali iod.

Worse after washing
Glonoinum

Rash on chin
Ammonium carb.

Itching on forehead
Rheum

Blotchy rash
Carbo an.
Fluoric ac.
Graphites
Guaiacum
Hepar sulph.
Kali bichrom.
Kali iod.
Ledum
Lycopodium
Phosphorus
Rhus tox.

Burning or smarting
Anacardium
Arsenicum
Causticum
Cicuta
Rhus tox.
Sarsaparilla
Sepia

Coppery coloured
Arsenicum
Arsenicum iod.
Aurum
Carbo an.
Graphites
Kali iod.
Lycopodium
Psorinum

Crusty and scabby rash
Arsenicum
Calcarea
Dulcamara
Petroleum
Rhus tox.

Skin flaking off
Arsenicum
Belladonna
Kali ars.
Mercurius
Psorinum
Rhus tox.
Sulphur

*Facial Rash (apart from
    Acne Rosacea)*

Dry rash
Arsenicum
Lycopodium

Eczema
Arsenicum
Calcarea
Cicuta
Croton
Dulcamara
Graphites
Hepar sulph.
Psorinum
Rhus tox.
Sarsaparilla
Sulphur

Eczema worse for heat of stove
Antimonium carb.

   like dried honey
   Cicuta

   in margins of hair
   Sulphur

Moist eczema
Cicuta
Graphites
Lycopodium
Petroleum
Psorinum
Rhus tox.

   in nursing mothers
   Sepia

   around the mouth
   Mezereum
   Natrum mur.

   in corners of mouth
   Arundo
   Graphites

Hepar sulph.
Rhus tox.

Excoriating rash
Mercurius
Petroleum

Fissures
Graphites

Herpes
Lachesis
Ledum
Natrum mur.
Rhus tox.
Sepia

Itching
Mezereum
Rhus tox.
Sepia
Sulphur

Moist rash
Dulcamara
Graphites
Lycopodium
Mezereum
Rhus tox.

Moist rash on nose
Graphites

Painful especially on chin
Sulphur

Pimples and pustules
   see ACNE, p. 187

Ringworm
Sepia

Crusty and scaly
Antimonium
Arsenicum
Baryta
Causticum
Lachesis
Psorinum
Sepia

Urticaria and hives
Apis
Arsenicum
Copaiva
Sulphur

Blisters
Croton
Manchinella
Natrum mur.
Psorinum
Rhus tox.
Sepia

Complexion bluish
Arsenicum
Asafoetida
Baptisia
Belladonna
Bryonia
Camphor
Cannabis ind.
Carbo veg.
Conium
Cuprum
Digitalis
Hyoscyamus
Ipecac.
Lachesis
Morphine
Opium
Veratrum
Veratrum vir.

dirty-looking
Argentum nit.
Lycopodium
Psorinum
Sulphur

earthy
China
Ferrum
Ferrum iod.
Ferrum phos.
Graphites
Mercurius
Opium
Sepia

pale
Anacardium
Antimonium tart.
Argentum
Arsenicum
Berberis
Calcarea

Calcarea phos.
Camphora
Carbo veg.
Carbon sulph.
China sulph.
Cina
Clematis
Cuprum
Digitalis
Ferrum
Ferrum phos.
Graphites
Lobelia
Lycopodium
Manganum
Medorrhinum
Natrum ars.
Natrum carb.
Natrum mur.
Natrum phos.
Opium
Phosphoric ac.
Plumbum
Secale
Sepia
Sulphur
Tabacum
Tuberculinum
Veratrum
Zinc

red
Apis
Baptisia
Belladonna
Bryonia
Capsicum
Chamomilla
Chelidonium
China
Cicuta
Cina

Ferrum
Hyoscyamus
Lachesis
Melilotus
Mezereum
Nux
Opium
Phosphorus
Rhus tox.
Sanguinaria
Stramonium
Veratrum vir.

sallow
Argentum nit.
Carbo veg.
Chelidonium
Medorrhinum
Natrum mur.
Plumbum
Sulphur

yellow
Argentum
Argentum nit.
Arsenicum
Cadmium
Calcarea
Calcarea phos.
Causticum
Chelidonium
Conium
Ferrum
Ferrum iod.
Gelsemium
Lachesis
Lycopodium
Mercurius
Natrum sulph.
Nux
Plumbum
Sepia
Sulphur

Skin

The skin accounts for 16 per cent of total body weight and is therefore the largest organ in the body. Stretched out, it would cover 2.0–2.6 m^2 (21–27 ft^2). Skin is lost and renewed at the rate of 30 g (1 oz) a month, which adds up to about 18 kg (40 lb) in an average lifetime. The outer layer, the epidermis, is effectively lifeless; it consists of flattish cells which are dying or already dead. These cells waterproof the skin and protect it from infection, and are continuously manufactured in the underlying layer of skin, the dermis. In this deeper, living layer lie blood vessels, lymph vessels, nerve endings sensitive to heat, cold, pain, and pressure, glands which manufacture sebum to keep the skin supple and waterproof, follicles which manufacture hair and nails, glands which eliminate toxins and wastes as perspiration, cells which synthesize vitamin D if the skin is exposed to sunlight, and cells which contain the dark pigment melanin which protects the skin from harmful wavelengths in sunlight. Binding them all together, and giving the skin its softness and resilience, are two more kinds of tissues, fatty (adipose) tissue and elastic con-

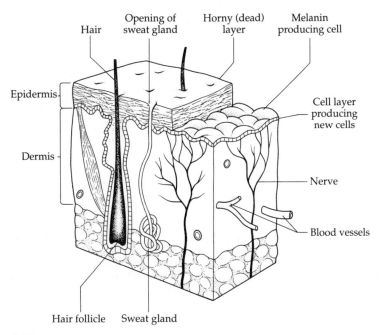

The structure of skin

nective tissue. Wrinkles represent a loss of fat and elasticity. Beneath the dermis and attached to it by flexible fibres lie muscles, tendons, ligaments, and bones.

In homeopathic medicine skin conditions, which include conditions affecting hair and nails, are viewed as manifestations of general imbalance, of poor metabolic function. Rather than treating the obvious and visible symptoms – itchiness, blisters, scaliness, etc. – the whole constitution is treated. Suppressing symptoms at skin level may cause the underlying imbalance to express itself in an internal, and often more important, organ. This is why externally applied potions like retin-A are viewed with suspicion, although it only appears to be active against conditions caused by excessive sun exposure. It is ineffective against conditions determined by the health and age of the body as a whole.

Skin tone and colour tell a trained homeopath a great deal about a person.

In general, skin problems are not helped by sugar, refined carbohydrates, chocolate, tea, coffee, alcohol, spices, or perfumed cosmetics, or by constipation and lack of exercise, both of which slow down the elimination of toxins.

To moisturize dry skin, use pure olive oil or Calendula cream; if using these on the face, apply them very sparingly. Excessive washing tends to dry the skin, but skin brushing – with a dry loofah or soft bristle brush – is very beneficial;

it removes dead cells from the epidermis and because it gently massages the blood and lymph vessels in the dermis it speeds up the elimination of toxins. (See FACE, p. 186.)

Oils in the bath are all right, although most just tend to oil up the bath itself, without doing a great deal for the skin. A preparation which dissolves in the water is better. Try putting oatmeal in a muslin bag and tying it over the hot-water tap when filling the bath. After a bath use a rich moisturizer, massaged into the skin.

Aromatherapy

Certain aromatherapy oils should not be used when taking homeopathic remedies, as they may antidote the remedies. Those to beware of are Peppermint, Camphor, Eucalyptus, Rosemary and the Thymes. Lavender is acceptable only in a less than 2 per cent solution.

Birthmarks

see under SPECIAL PROBLEMS IN INFANTS

Blushing
see p. 171

Boils and carbuncles

Infections of the hair follicles, usually the work of *Staphylococcus* bacteria, also responsible for food poisoning; a carbuncle is a particularly large boil or a close-knit group of boils sited somewhat deeper in the dermis than the average boil. As white cells attack bacteria, thick white or yellow pus accumulates, causing pain and swelling, and the boil develops a head; after a day or two the boil either bursts or slowly reduces and heals. Recurrent boils can be a symptom of diabetes. Orthodox treatment is antibiotics and, if necessary, lancing. Homeopathic treatment is constitutional, but the remedies below can be used to relieve pain and swelling.

Specific remedies to be given every hour for up to 10 doses:

- Boil in early stage, skin very red and tender *Belladonna 30c*
- If boil weeps easily and is sensitive to the slightest touch, or to bring boil to a head *Hepar sulph. 6c*
- To cleanse a boil which has burst, or to help heal a boil which has been slow to develop and slow to disperse *Silicea 6c*
- Skin over boil bluish, blistered, and very angry-looking, with a black centre *Anthracinum 6c*
- Skin over boil burning hot, aggravated by application of heat *Arsenicum 6c*
- Boil weeps but causes little pain *Gunpowder 6c*

Self-help
At first sign of inflammation, bathe affected area with Hypericum and Calendula solution (5 drops of mother tincture of each to 0.25 litre [½ pint] boiled cooled water). A pad of cotton wool soaked in hot salt water (1 teaspoon to 0.25 litre [½ pint]) and applied to the boil every few hours reduces pain. Never squeeze a boil. If it bursts, let it drain by itself. If possible, avoid handling food.

Cancer of the skin
see also CANCER

Skin cancer can take the form of a rodent ulcer, a squamous cell carcinoma, or a malignant melanoma. Of these, rodent ulcers are the most common, and malignant melanomas potentially the most serious. Women most at risk are over 50, with fair skins, who have had long exposure to strong sunlight. Any lump or 'bite' which does not heal within a week or two, or any change in a mole or wart, should be investigated by your GP.

Malignant melanomas
These are usually confined to the legs although they can also occur on soles of feet; unfortunately, chances of this form of cancer spreading to other parts of the body are high, unless it is caught in very early stages. Judging by doubling of the number of deaths from this form of cancer since 1950, short intense exposure to strong sun, the kind of exposure many people get on holidays abroad, may be a significant factor. Malignant melanomas develop from pigment cells, usually from pre-existing moles – see MOLES for danger signs. If you notice changes in a mole, or a new mole or new patch of pigment, 48 . If mole is malignant, immediate surgery and perhaps radio-therapy will be necessary. If cancer has already spread, alternative therapies, especially Gerson therapy, may be more beneficial than chemo-therapy – see CANCER for details.

Rodent ulcers
These often appear on the face, especially on the nose or around the eyes; other common sites are tops of ears, bald scalps and hands. They grow very slowly, and seldom if ever spread to other parts of the body, although they can be locally invasive and destroy an eye or ear, or erode a major artery, if not treated early. Some rodent ulcers are merely raised lumps with a scabby crust, others are like bright pink warts with a fissured centre, and others look like small fleshy cushions; they may bleed from time to time, but they never heal. Routine treatment is to freeze the ulcer and remove it, or destroy it by radiation. A rodent ulcer is not a sign that cancer is likely to develop elsewhere.

Squamous cell carcinomas
These most commonly appear on the lips, near the ears, or on the hands, and may take the form of enlarging open sores or wart-like lumps; sunlight, tars, and in some cases SOLAR KERATOSES are thought to be triggers. This form of cancer can metastasize, so early treatment is essential; options, depending on size and site of carcinoma, are freezing, radiotherapy, or surgical removal.

For all three forms of skin cancer, constitutional homeopathic treatment is recommended in addition to orthodox treatment.

Carbuncles see BOILS AND CARBUNCLES

Cellulite
Unsightly 'orange peel' skin and dimpling, especially on thighs and upper arms; due to fluid retention and hard accretions of fat cells; culprits are insufficient exercise, poor elimination of fluids and wastes through lymphatic vessels, being overweight, and not eating enough raw vegetables and fruit. Persistent, unsightly fat is often a depot for toxins, either environmental or dietary.

Self-help
Exercise, skin brushing, massage, and eating as many organic and as few processed foods as possible can help a lot. If you wish to speed up the whole process, treatment in a salon by a beauty

therapist may be helpful. Cellulite treatments are available in the form of a deep and powerful massage. Warming the body prior to treatment is beneficial.

It is claimed that creams using essential oils may actually penetrate the skin, breaking down the fat and fluid. Lymphatic drainage can be carried out by hand or machine at a beauty salon, with the additional use of aromatherapy oils (p. 185).

Chilblains

An extreme reaction to cold, in which superficial blood vessels contract excessively causing skin to go pale and numb, then red, swollen, and itchy; eventually skin may break; most common on hands and feet. Problems get worse with repeated exposure to cold and damp. If the remedies given below do not seem to be effective, see your homeopath.

Specific remedies to be taken every ½-hour for up to 6 doses:

- Chilblains which burn and itch, skin red and swollen, and not relieved by cold applications *Agaricus 6c*
- Chilblains get worse in cold weather, woman feels chilly, is prone to head sweats, and puts on weight easily *Calcarea 6c*
- Chilblains most painful when limbs hang downwards, veins swollen, warmth makes discomfort worse *Pulsatilla 6c*
- Chilblains itch and burn, skin weepy and watery, damp makes problem worse, woman prone to rough skin *Petroleum 6c*

Self-help

Keep affected parts as warm and as dry as possible during cold or damp weather. If skin is broken, apply Calendula ointment; if not, apply Tamus ointment, available from health-food shops or homeopathic pharmacies (see Useful Addresses, p. 338). Try not to scratch.

Cracks and fissures

For reasons which are not fully understood but which are generally labelled 'constitutional', some women are prone to cracked lips, finger tips, etc. If the remedies below do not improve matters, constitutional homeopathic treatment should be sought.

Specific remedies to be taken 3 times daily for up to 2 weeks:

- Cracks at corner of mouth, skin rough and red *Petroleum 6c*
- Cracking in folds of skin, especially if complicated by fungal infection in areas which are kept warm and moist, skin dirty-looking and very itchy, symptoms aggravated by washing *Sulphur 6c*
- Cracking in nostrils, on lips, behind ears, on nipples, or on fingertips *Graphites 6c*
- Cracking worse in winter, woman overweight, chilly and sweaty *Calcarea 6c*
- Cracks on finger tips become deeper in cold weather and are slow to heal, sweaty hands and feet *Silicea 6c*

Self-help

Apply Calendula ointment. Vitamin B complex, vitamins A and C, zinc, and essential fatty acids should be beneficial.

Eczema (dermatitis)

Local inflammation of the skin, accompanied by ITCHING, redness, weeping, blistering, and bleeding if scratched.

Contact eczema

This is caused by allergies to plants, fabrics, and metals and is often associated with asthma, hay fever and allergic rhinitis. Substances that can cause it are in the tens if not hundreds of thousands. The most common ones are: nickel (found in costume jewellery), chromate (found in wet cement), epoxy resins (used as surface coatings, adhesives and paints).

Cosmetics: Fragrances, biocides and preservatives are the usual culprits (colourings and anti-oxidants may cause a problem in lipsticks). Two strange effects are that the hardeners used in nail varnish very often cause eczema on the eyelids, face and neck rather than on the hands; and the arc-dye used to colour hair often causes marked eczema on the face, eyelids and ears but not the scalp to which it is actually applied.

Rubber can cause dermatitis – on the hands from gloves, and the feet from shoes (for substitutes see Self-help). Formaldehyde may cause problems for hairdressers from the shampoos they use. The type of phosphorus present in 'strike anywhere' matches can give an acute eczema on the face and eyelids. An extract of pine is the usual cause of sensitivity in sticking plasters. It is also found in solder.

Some drugs, such as local anaesthetics, some antibiotics and antiseptics and even antihistamines, can produce contact eczema. Lanolin, which used to be the main base of most ointments, has now been replaced.

If the eczema is inflamed and has blisters then a bath containing sodium bicarbonate is a good idea. Aromatherapy oils to use in massage are Fennel, Chamomile, Geranium, Sandalwood,

Hyssop, Juniper and Lavender (less than 2 per cent strength). If eczema is dry, Calendula oil, as a carrier, should be used with the aromatherapy in the morning and the evening.

Detergent eczema
An occupational hazard of housewives, catering workers, hairdressers, nurses, mechanics . . . anyone in fact who comes into daily contact with household cleaners, washing-up liquid, shampoos, grease removers, all of which contain detergents; hands become rough, red, scurfy, sore, and itchy, especially on knuckles.

Discoid eczema
Appears on arms or legs as itchy, round, red patches which proceed to flake, blister, weep, and form crusts; condition may last for several months, but it is rare and its cause is not known.

Pompholyx eczema
Causes itchy, weeping blisters on palms of hands and soles of feet, and is thought to be due to STRESS or poor diet; it is uncommon, and usually clears up of its own accord after 2 or 3 weeks.

Seborrhoeic eczema
This seems to be inherited, not linked to any allergy; it causes flakiness and itching in smile lines between nose and mouth, in the beard area, around hairline, on scalp (see DANDRUFF), on chest, and also in the groin or armpits, or between or under the breasts.

The orthodox approach to eczema is to prescribe steroid ointments to relieve inflammation, and if necessary antihistamines and antibiotics to control itching and infection; to discover the allergen(s) involved in contact eczema, a patch test may be necessary. However, steroid preparations should be avoided unless eczema is so bad that it is causing miserable, sleepless nights, which in turn are causing stress and aggravating the eczema.

Homeopathic treatment for eczema is constitutional, but the following remedies may be used while help is being sought or when itching is very bad.

Specific remedies to be taken 4 times daily for up to 2 weeks:

- Eczema mainly affects palms and area behind ears, honey-like discharge from skin *Graphites 6c*
- Skin red, dry, rough, and itchy, aggravated by heat and washing, especially if woman has diarrhoea which gets worse early in morning *Sulphur 6c*

- Affected skin cracks easily *Petroleum 6c*
- Blisters itch more at night or in damp weather, but improve with warmth *Rhus tox. 6c*
- Skin dry and itchy, woman constipated *Alumina 6c*
- Skin very sensitive and easily infected, feeling generally chilly and worse in cold *Hepar sulph. 6c*
- Skin dry and burning, but aggravated by cold applications *Arsenicum 6c*
- Skin irritated, dirty-looking, and prone to infection, general chilliness *Psorinum 6c*

Self-help Obviously, known irritants should be avoided. Wear rubber gloves for gardening, housework, washing-up, etc. If rubber gloves are the culprits, wear cotton gloves inside them or use plastic gloves. Always dry hands thoroughly after washing, and use Calendula cream as a moisturizer. If the culprit is stress, exercise, relaxation, or a simple form of meditation may help, as may a holiday in the sun, thanks to ultraviolet radiation. Try oatmeal baths (see introduction, p. 194).

You could also try rubbing evening primrose oil on to unaffected areas of skin. Take extra vitamins B and C, and also zinc. Add safflower oil capsules to diet. Going on the LIVER DIET (pp. 264–6) for 1 month would do no harm either.

Try to prevent eczema by breastfeeding your children, and taking care over weaning (see BREASTFEEDING).

Itching
If accompanied by a *rash*, may be due to ECZEMA (extensive patches of red, sore skin), URTICARIA (light red, raised weals), scratching (raised red weals following line of scratch), PSORIASIS (red patches covered in silvery scales), ringworm (red, ring-shaped patches fading in centre), scabies (red rash on trunk, also on hands and wrists, or genitals, with scabies mite burrows visible under magnifying glass), or LICHEN PLANUS (small, shiny, violet spots).

Among the conditions which cause itching, but no obvious rash, are threadworms, PRURITIS ANI, anal fissure, PILES, and sometimes DIARRHOEA (itching confined to anal area), jaundice (general itchiness, eye whites yellowish), icthyosis (skin dry and scaly, especially in cold weather), head lice, and DANDRUFF.

See conditions mentioned above for suitable homeopathic remedies.

Keloid
Excessive and sometimes unsightly growth of scar tissue after an injury, burn, vaccination, or operation, or after ear-piercing, most com-

mon in dark-skinned people; wound appears to heal normally at first, then scar begins to grow; occasionally, keloids develop from old scar tissue or from unscarred skin. Orthodox treatment is by steroid injections, freezing, radiotherapy, or cosmetic surgery. If specific remedies given below do not halt or reduce growth within a month or so, see your homeopath.

Specific remedies to be taken 3 times daily for up to 3 weeks:

- Keloid in early stages *Graphites 6c*
- Long-standing keloid *Silicea 6c* followed by *Fluoric ac. 6c*

Lichen planus

An itchy outbreak of small, shiny, purplish-red lumps, often on arms and legs, but occasionally on scalp, causing HAIR LOSS; can also lead to nail deformities (see NAIL PROBLEMS), or cause a white lacy pattern inside mouth. Cause is not known, but majority of people affected are over 50; condition is harmless, if annoying, and onsets suddenly, with spots fading to brown before disappearing. Conventionally treated with steroid tablets or ointment. Constitutional homeopathic treatment is recommended if the condition recurs, as it sometimes does once steroid treatment stops; however, the remedies below should be tried first.

Specific remedies to be given 4 times daily for up to 3 weeks:

- Remedy of first resort, whether condition is acute or chronic *Sulphur iod. 6c*
- Rash burns and itches *Arsenicum 6c*
- Outbreak worse on face and neck, spots feel prickly and itchy *Juglans 6c*
- Undressing makes itching worse *Rumex 6c*

Lumps or swellings

Innocuous bumps on hands or feet may be WARTS, corns or calluses, or ganglia; painful swelling may be an abscess or the after-effect of a vaccine; BOILS AND CARBUNCLES and bites and stings also cause painful swellings; potentially more serious are lumps in the lymph glands of the armpit, breast, or groin, suggesting the possibility of infection or irritation from anti-perspirants, CANCER OF THE BREAST, Hodgkin's disease, or lymphoma, and moles or warts which suddenly enlarge or become more prominent, suggesting some form of CANCER OF THE SKIN; swelling of the lymph glands at the back of the skull may be a symptom of German measles (with a pink rash and fever); if lymph glands in the neck are swollen, pharyngitis, tonsillitis, or

GLANDULAR FEVER (with sore throat) may be the cause; swelling between ear and jaw on one side of face may be mumps (sometimes glands under jaw swollen too, pain on swallowing, fever), a tooth abscess (jaw aches or throbs), or a salivary duct tumour; an unfamiliar small bulge on the abdomen or groin may be a hernia; swellings around joints, accompanied by stiffness, pain, and tenderness, may be bursitis, RHEUMATOID ARTHRITIS, or OSTEOARTHRITIS; fluid retention or OEDEMA may be due to kidney problems such as glomerulonephritis or kidney failure (swollen ankles, passage of small amounts of urine, nausea and vomiting, drowsiness).

If you suspect a lump or swelling may be malignant, 48; if either of the kidney problems mentioned above is suspected, 12. Otherwise see entries above for homeopathic remedies.

Moles

Dense collections of cells containing the skin pigment melanin – the rest of the pigment cells are evenly distributed and are only stimulated to produce melanin when the skin is exposed to the sun's ultraviolet rays. Moles can be flat, raised, or hairy, and usually develop in childhood; moles which develop later should be regarded with suspicion as they may be an early sign of malignant melanoma (see CANCER OF THE SKIN), a form of cancer which develops in pigment cells. Other danger signs in moles are a diameter of more than 1 cm, an increase in size, an irregular notched outline, inflammation in or around a mole, an irregular dark area within a mole, crusting or oozing, bleeding, or itching, or other change in sensation. Occasionally a seborrhoeic wart (see WARTS) may be mistaken for a mole. If a mole is considered unsightly, camouflage make-up can be used. If necessary a mole can be removed by a plastic surgeon, although often it can be an attractive feature.

Self-help

If a mole has hair growing out of it cutting the hair close to the surface is best as plucking it out may upset the natural cell structure. If the hair growth is a real problem, then ask a dermatologist if it is safe to have electrolysis to remove the hair.

Naevus

This appears as a central dilated blood vessel with smaller capillaries radiating from it, giving the appearance of a red spider – it is really a broken vein. It is often in the cheek area where the skin is fine and mature. Care can be taken to stop this condition worsening by using protective creams and blocks against extremes of temperatures, sun and wind. It is generally a hereditary condition, but can be caused by over-zealous cleansing and peeling on very fine skin.

Treatment in a beauty salon is called electrical diathermy coagulation – the use of an electrolysis needle. Obviously aftercare is important and advice should be given at the time of treatment. If the skin is prone to this condition the chances of it recurring are high if care is not taken.

Nail problems

Disorders specifically affecting the nails are few; more often, discoloration or deformity is the result of injury, or of nutritional, respiratory, or heart disorders.

Deformed nails

There are a variety of causes, including iron deficiency (nails become spoon-shaped), respiratory or heart problems (nails become clubbed, growing round swollen ends of fingers and sometimes toes), PSORIASIS (nails become pitted), injury (nails develop horizontal ridges), and infection, or simply old age (nails develop vertical ridges, possibly due to malabsorption of vitamins A, B complex, and C, calcium, magnesium, zinc, and essential fatty acids).

Self-help Preventive measures include keeping nails short, wearing gloves for gardening and rubber gloves if hands are repeatedly immersed in water, trimming toenails straight across to prevent them ingrowing (see below), and wearing shoes which do not press on toenails.

Stains on the nail may be the result of smoking, chemical cleansers such as bleach or even heavily chlorinated water from a swimming pool. Using lemon juice can help to eliminate these stains. Wearing nail polish in very strong sunlight can also cause staining, as the sun actually draws the colour into the nail. Psoriasis and eczema can cause pitting in the nails; this can be treated with fillers and strengtheners, provided a test patch is done to check for any allergic reaction.

Discoloured nails

Telltales of a variety of conditions, including ANAEMIA (nails very pale), liver problems (nails whitish) bacterial endocarditis (nails have dark flecks in them which look like splinters), and fungal infections (nails turn whitish and soft or crumbly); nails also turn purplish or black when hit (see sub-ungual haematoma below) or put under gentle but constant pressure for any length of time. White spots on nails are often a sign of zinc or vitamin A deficiency.

Fungal infections

These turn the nails white and crumbly, causing ridging and thickening afterwards. Orthodox medicine prescibes antifungal drugs or ointments. However, the homeopathic remedies below should be tried first.

Specific remedies to be taken 2 times daily for up to 6 weeks:

- Nails brittle, with horny thickening *Antimonium 6c*
- Nails deformed, with white spotting *Silicea 6c*
- Nails thickened, deformed, brittle or crumbly, inflamed and painful, with blackening *Graphites 6c*
- Nails brittle, with skin at base red and swollen *Thuja 6c*

Self-help Soak nails twice a day in Calendula solution (10 drops mother tincture to 0.25 litre [½ pint] boiled cooled water) or apply Calendula ointment. Rub small amount of Whitfield's ointment (available from chemists) round nail and nailbed twice daily.

Ingrowing toenails

Usually caused by ill-fitting shoes or by tapering nails at sides instead of cutting them straight across; occasionally they can be due to problems in the nailbed. As the sides of the nail curve under, surrounding skin becomes inflamed and tender. Orthodox treatment is minor surgery. In early stages, process can be arrested by working a small piece of lint between side of nail and skin over top of nail and nailbed underneath after thoroughly bathing toe with Hypericum and Calendula solution (5 drops of mother tincture of each in 0.25 litre [½ pint] boiled cooled water). If nail becomes infected, use remedies given for paronychia (see below).

Specific remedies to be taken every 12 hours for up to 1 month, then see your GP if no improvement:

- To strengthen nails which repeatedly ingrow *Magnetis austr. 6c*
- If nails are very brittle *Thuja 6c*

Paronychia

An acute bacterial or yeast infection which attacks growing tissue at base of nails, causing red, swollen cuticles, and sometimes blisters of pus (whitlows) alongside nails; can result in deformed or discoloured nails.

Specific remedies to be given hourly for up to 10 doses:

- Early stage, skin at base of nails hot, red, tender, and throbbing *Belladonna 30c*
- Base of nails yield pus when pressed, skin around nails very tender *Hepar sulph. 6c*
- Infection slow to heal *Silicea 6c*

Self-help See fungal infections (above). Also, take zinc, vitamin C, and vitamin B complex.

Sub-ungual haematoma

A very painful condition caused by crushing or trapping injuries; nail rapidly blackens as blood accumulates beneath it; only way to relieve pain is to relieve pressure of blood under nail. Your GP will do this by lancing the nail, but if medical help is not available, you can lance the nail yourself by heating a straightened paper clip with a match or lighter until red-hot and plunging it through the nail in the centre of the blackened area until blood appears. Also, immediately after the injury, take Arnica 30c every hour for up to 10 doses.

Whitlows

see Paronychia

Oedema

Abnormal accumulation of fluids in body tissues, showing as puffiness under the skin, especially around ankles; occurs in heart, liver, and kidney disease, and in protein malnutrition; many women, especially before periods (see PRE-MENSTRUAL SYNDROME), in hot weather, and as result of prolonged standing, develop a minor form of oedema. Exact cause of condition is not known; probably a combination of factors – hormonal, metabolic, nervous – is responsible, and in some cases ALLERGY may play a role.

Angioneurotic oedema

A complication of URTICARIA, an allergic reaction to nettles and other plants, thought to be aggravated by STRESS; swelling rapidly affects eyes and lips, and may extend to throat, obstructing breathing; appropriate action is ⑨⑨⑨ and Apis 30c every 5 minutes for up to 10 doses. Pulmonary oedema (breathlessness and coughing, with blood-flecked sputum, dramatically worsening in space of a few hours) is also life-threatening; again, appropriate action is ⑨⑨⑨.

Severe chronic oedema causes swelling of ankles, legs, abdomen, face, and hands; weight fluctuations during course of day; intense thirst and frequent urge to urinate, especially when lying down; bowel and bladder upsets; HEAD-ACHE, visual disturbances, fainting; mental

function may also be impaired. Orthodox treatment is restriction of carbohydrates, especially refined carbohydrates; diuretics are also used, but can cause dependency and further fluid retention. Homeopathic treatment is constitutional; in meantime, choose a remedy from the list below.

Specific remedies to be taken 3 times daily for up to 2 weeks:

- Swelling of feet and ankles, chilliness, restlessness, thirst for hot beverages taken in small quantities at frequent intervals *Arsenicum 6c*
- Swelling accompanied by inflammation and stinging pains, discomfort made worse by heat and even light pressure *Apis 6c*
- Mild swelling in hot weather or hot rooms *Natrum mur. 6c*

Self-help Cut down on salt and try to lose weight. Take extra vitamin B_6 and B complex, and magnesium. If swelling occurs mainly in hot weather, take Natrum mur. tissue salt (see p. 24) 3 times a day while weather remains hot.

Lymphoedema

This is swelling from fluid retention caused by blockage of the lymphatic system. It may be inborn or develop as a result of damage to the lymphatic system, principally as a side effect of cancer therapy. Caught early, it can be treated with support stockings, skin care and advice to prevent the swelling from worsening and to protect the limb from infection. If the limbs have become rock hard, more intensive treatment may be needed. For further information there is a booklet called 'Lymphoedema Advice and Treatment' available from the Sir Michael Sobell House (see Useful Addresses, p. 334).

Perspiration problems

Sweat glands (eccrine glands) are most plentiful on forehead and scalp, palms of hands, soles of feet, in groin and armpits, and around nipples; sweating reduces body heat and gets rid of various wastes. Naturopathically, it is not healthy to suppress perspiration with antiperspirants.

Excessive perspiration (hyperhidrosis), if not obviously due to hot surroundings or exertion, may be a sign of fever, OBESITY, thyrotoxicosis (loss of weight despite increased appetite, bulging eyes, trembling – see THYROID PROBLEMS), Hodgkin's disease (swollen glands, especially in neck, itchy skin), or tuberculosis (night sweats despite few bedclothes, weight loss, coughing);

tuberculosis and Hodgkin's disease require prompt medical attention.

Body temperature, and therefore sweating, can also be increased by alcohol or withdrawal from alcohol (see ALCOHOLISM), aspirin, vitamin B$_1$ deficiency, or wearing man-made fibres; anxiety produces sweating on forehead, upper lip, soles, and palms; hot flushes – suddenly feeling very hot and sweaty – are a common symptom of the MENOPAUSE; cold sweats can be a symptom of HYPOGLYCAEMIA. Adolescent concerns about increased sweating and BODY ODOUR are related to the fact that sweat glands under arms and in groin do not become active until adolescence. Appreciable amounts of sodium and zinc are lost in perspiration.

Scientists in Japan have recently discovered that the unpleasant smell from some people's feet is due to a particular fatty acid called isovaleric acid. It appears we all have this chemical, but most of us have it in a very mild form.

If excessive sweating is causing embarrassment, and does not seem to have any clear cause, constitutional homeopathic treatment may help. In the meantime, the remedies below should be tried; they should produce some improvement within about 2 weeks.

Specific remedies to be taken 4 times daily for up to 2 weeks:

- Woman overweight, cold and clammy, sweat smells sour, head sweats worse at night *Calcarea 6c*
- Woman thin, chilly, prone to sweaty feet which smell unpleasant *Silicea 6c*
- Hot sweating on head, with diarrhoea first thing in morning *Sulphur 6c*
- Sweating worse on head, sweat profuse and sour-smelling, cold weather and walking reduce sweating *Fluoric ac. 6c*
- Perspiration very pungent and sticky, made worse by heat or cold *Mercurius 6c*
- Perspiration smells unpleasant and is worst on feet and under arms, right foot may be hot and left foot cold *Lycopodium 6c*

Lack of perspiration (anhidrosis) is probably due to some fault in the autonomic nervous system (part of nervous system which is not under voluntary control); overheating and possibly heat stroke are risks in hot weather. Constitutional treatment is recommended, but one or both remedies below should be tried first.

Specific remedies to be taken 3 times daily for up to 3 weeks:

- *Aethusa 6c* or, if no improvement, *Alumina 6c*

Self-help
If you suffer from excessive perspiration, shower night and morning to remove stale sweat (body odour is mostly caused by bacteria, which thrive on sweat), and wear cotton underwear and shirts, and change them daily. The answer to smelly feet is to wash and dry them thoroughly at least once a day, avoid nylon socks and tights, and wear sandals rather than shoes. If you must use a deodorant/anti-perspirant, use one which does not contain aluminium (look in your local health-food shop).

Prickly heat
Acute itchiness most common among fair-skinned people in tropical or sub-tropical climates (dark-skinned people are not affected); due to a combination of damp heat, wearing clothes, being overweight, using soap too often, and a tendency to produce too much sebum. Itchy, prickling sensation is due to inflammation caused by bursting of sweat gland ducts blocked by sebum; if many sweat gland ducts are blocked, result may be heat stroke. If condition is particularly troublesome, constitutional treatment will be appropriate.

Specific remedy to be taken every 2 hours for up to 10 doses as soon as prickling sensation starts; if necessary, repeat dose daily, but not more frequently:

- *Apis 30c*
- As preventive, take *Sol 30c* 3 times daily during exposure for up to 3 weeks in every 4

Self-help
Avoid hot baths and showers, use soap once a day only, and try to acquire a protective tan (see SUNBURN). Avoid hot drinks, spicy foods, and meat extract. Increase vitamin C intake. Try bathing affected parts in dilute bicarbonate of soda. Drink plenty of coconut water, especially in the tropics.

Psoriasis
An inherited skin condition in which the epidermis produces new cells too fast for keratin formation to take place – keratin is a fibrous protein that forms a tough, protective covering over skin, nails, and hair. As a result, unsightly patches of flaking skin develop, on knees, elbows, sacrum, or scalp behind ears; patches are well-defined, slightly raised, deep pink beneath their silvery scaling, and not necessarily sore or itchy. Nails may also be affected, becoming thick, rough, or pitted, or separating completely from the nailbed (see NAIL PROBLEMS). In a few sufferers, joints of hands, fingers, knees, and ankles may become inflamed and swollen.

The condition is chronic, has a large genetic component and flares up at intervals. It is rare before the age of 5, and most common between the ages of 15 and 30; can be precipitated by infection (especially streptococcal sore throats), drugs such as chloroquine (used in treatment of malaria and some forms of arthritis), lithium, beta blockers and hormonal factors. The peak incidences for women are puberty and menopause, and it often improves during pregnancy and relapses after delivery. Although most patients improve with sunlight, a small number develop psoriasis when exposed to sun. The condition can also be brought on by stress or injury. Recent research has shown that selenium deficiency may play some part in psoriasis.

Orthodox treatments include steroid and coal tar ointments, cytotoxic drugs which slow down cell division, vitamin A and D derivatives (which can be highly toxic), and special ultraviolet therapy. The condition can be managed each time it recurs, but not cured. Constitutional homeopathic treatment, and the self-help measures below, usually prove beneficial. If the remedies given below do not produce some improvement within 2 weeks, see your homeopath.

Specific remedies to be taken 4 times daily for up to 2 weeks:

- Affected areas of skin burning hot, mentally restless but physically exhausted, feeling chilly *Arsenicum 6c*
- Dry, red, scaly, itchy patches worse after baths, especially if woman often feels too hot *Sulphur 30c*
- Skin behind ears affected, exuding honey-coloured pus *Graphites 6c*
- Affected areas extremely scaly, aggravated by warmth *Kali ars. 6c*
- Condition aggravated by cold and worse in winter *Petroleum 6c*

Self-help
Provided you do not have a sensitive skin, careful sunbathing (6 sessions starting at 10 minutes and increasing to 60 minutes) or several 10-minute sessions under an ultraviolet lamp may help to clear up an outbreak. To reduce stress, learn to relax or meditate. Try the LIVER DIET (pp. 264–6) for 1 month, and take extra zinc. Massage is recommended – as long as the skin is not broken – to soothe the nervous system, using Bergamot, Lavender oil (less than 2 per cent strength) in a lotion base or a Sandalwood oil. Aromatherapy is very calming and healing, and at the same time moisturizes the skin. To relieve tension, reflexology may also be a good idea.

Sebaceous cysts (wens)
Smooth, yellowish lumps under the skin, especially on the scalp, with small sacs of whitish fluid inside; painless and harmless unless infected by bacteria, in which case they may burst, releasing pus; if infection recurs, as it tends to, surgical removal may be recommended, otherwise conventional treatment is antibiotics. If remedies below do not clear up infection within 5 days, see your homeopath.

Specific remedies to be given every 8 hours for up to 5 days:

- Cyst on scalp which is sensitive and flaking *Baryta 30c*
- Cyst producing pus *Hepar sulph. 30c*

Solar keratoses
Rough red patches on skin which develop as result of prolonged exposure to strong sunlight; most common in people with fair or sensitive skin, and sometimes a precursor of squamous cell carcinoma (see CANCER OF THE SKIN).

If the homeopathic remedies given below do not reduce redness and roughness within 1 month, see your GP.

Specific remedies to be taken every 12 hours for up to 1 month:

- A general tendency to feel hot, fair skin which burns easily in sun, a tendency to bleed easily *Phosphorus 6c*
- Red patches which are dry, flaky, and burning hot, but rest of body feels cold *Arsenicum 6c*

If you are fair-skinned and about to take a holiday in the sun, take Sol 30c as a preventive; correct dosage is three times daily for 3 weeks out of 4 while exposed to the sun.

Sunburn
The sun's ultraviolet rays can cause a lot of damage to skin. Even dark skins wrinkle badly after prolonged exposure to the sun (ultraviolet light actually breaks down the elastic tissues). In skins unused to the sun, reckless exposure produces heat and redness – the boiled lobster look – and even blistering. Gradual exposure, however, encourages the skin to step up melanin production, giving natural protection against sunburn. In fair skins which have little melanin-producing capacity, exposure can produce SOLAR KERATOSES and malignant changes (CANCER OF THE SKIN).

Sensible sunbathing means exposing yourself to the sun gradually so that your skin has time to produce more melanin; sunbathe for 15 minutes on the first day, then increase sun time by 15 minutes each day. Suntan lotions without a screening factor – the factor which minimizes burning – are useless; buy one with a screening factor that suits your skin type.

Urticaria (nettle rash, hives)

Raised red patches or weals, sometimes with paler areas in centre, which cause intense itching; can be caused by food ALLERGY (to shellfish, strawberries, nuts, etc.), food additives, certain drugs (notably aspirin), scratching, insect bites, and extreme STRESS (grief at the death of a loved one, for example); in people with sensitive skin, heat, cold, or sunlight may raise weals. Regardless of the cause, stress and tension usually make condition worse. Conventional treatment is by antihistamines. In a few cases, eyes, lips, and throat may swell dramatically (see angioneurotic OEDEMA), leading to suffocation; this is an emergency situation, so ⑨⑨⑨ and give Apis 30c every minute until help arrives.

If, after avoiding known causes, condition recurs, constitutional homeopathic treatment would be worthwhile.

Specific remedies to be taken every hour for up to 10 doses during attack or while constitutional help is being sought:

- Burning and swelling of lips and eyelids, made worse by warmth *Apis 30c*
- Rash caused by stinging nettles or some other plant, made worse by touching, scratching, or bathing with water *Urtica 6c*

Varicose ulcers (venous ulcers)

In older people with poor circulation or VARICOSE VEINS, even a tiny crack or injury to the skin can be slow to heal; without a good supply of fresh blood to bring in infection-fighting white blood cells or take away toxins, the injury site may become ulcerated and take months to heal; a typical varicose ulcer has a pale, weeping centre, a red, itchy surround, and brown mottling around that; commonest site is on legs, just above ankles. Routinely treated by applying antiseptic dressings to prevent infection, and support bandaging to speed up blood flow; in severe cases, GP may recommend hospitalization, and vein surgery or a skin graft may be necessary.

The remedies given below promote healing, but if there is no improvement within 14 days, see your homeopath.

Specific remedies to be taken 4 times daily for up to 14 days:

- General remedy for varicose ulcers *Hamamelis 6c*
- Ulcers bleed easily and cause splinter-like pains *Nitric ac. 6c*
- Ulcers burn, especially between midnight and 2 am, but are less painful when heat is applied *Arsenicum 6c*
- Skin around ulcers bluish-purple *Lachesis 6c*
- Ulcers which are slow to form and equally slow to heal, with chronic mild infection *Silicea 6c*
- Early stages, before ulcer forms, when skin is hot, red, and throbbing *Belladonna 30c*
- Edges of ulcers clear-cut, as if made with a hole punch, white discharge *Kali bichrom. 6c*
- Ulcers oozing unpleasant-smelling pus and serum *Mercurius 6c*
- Ulcers form reddish scabs with pus beneath *Mezereum 6c*
- Ulcers bleed easily *Phosphorus 6c*
- Varicose ulcers in an elderly woman *Carbo veg. 6c*
- Ulcers at site of injury *Arnica 6c*

Self-help
If ulcers are due to varicose veins, raise legs above hip level when resting, avoid standing for any length of time, and go for a daily walk. Take extra vitamin C and zinc. Apply Hypericum and Calendula ointment to dressings, and change them daily.

Vitiligo

A rare condition in which white patches appear on skin due to a shutting down of pigment (melanin) production; since it occurs frequently in conjunction with pernicious anaemia (see ANAEMIA) and hypothyroidism (see THYROID PROBLEMS), it may be a disorder of the auto-immune system, but nutritional deficiencies or tropical fungal disease may also be responsible.

There are no specific homeopathic remedies for vitiligo, but constitutional treatment may help. If pigment loss is extensive and embarrassing, your GP may refer you to a dermatologist.

Warts

Caused by viruses which invade the skin and cause the cells to multiply rapidly, forming raised lumps; unable to kill the viruses, the body walls them off. In susceptible individuals, warts are contagious: touching warts can quite easily transfer viruses to new sites, and new warts develop (see vulval and penile warts – VAGINAL AND VULVAL PROBLEMS, PENIS PROBLEMS).

Common warts are small, horny, and flesh-coloured or whitish, and most commonly occur on hands; on soles of feet, where they are called verrucas, constant pressure causes them to harden and burrow inwards, making walking quite painful. Two other types of wart, most common in children, are planar warts (which usually occur in groups, and look like tiny, brownish, fleshy blisters) and molluscum contagiosum (small, pearl-like warts with depressed centres, which seldom occur singly). Persistent warts are conventionally treated with wart paint, or they can be burnt or frozen off, or dug out. Warts which form after the age of 45, particularly seborrhoeic warts, which look like large, rough-surfaced moles, should be shown to your GP as soon as possible; they may be completely innocuous, or they may be malignant (see CANCER OF THE SKIN).

Homeopathic medicine offers a number of specific remedies for warts, but if home treatment does not produce improvement within a month or so, consult your homeopath. Long-term constitutional treatment may be necessary to tackle the underlying problem.

Specific remedies to be given every 12 hours for up to 3 weeks.

Please remember to check your choice against the Remedy Pictures (p. 305) where possible.

- Soft, fleshy, cauliflower-like warts – chiefly on back of head – which ooze and bleed easily *Thuja 6c*
- Many warts, chiefly on face, eyelids, and fingertips, also painful verrucas *Causticum 6c*

- Cauliflower-like warts which itch and sting, and sometimes ooze and bleed, or become large and jagged-edged, upper lip most affected *Nitric ac. 6c*
- Many small, horny warts which itch, sting, weep, and bleed *Calcarea 6c*
- Horny warts associated with a callus *Antimonium 6c*
- Hard, smooth, fleshy warts, chiefly on back of hands *Dulcamara 6c*
- Warts on hands *Kali mur. 6c*
- Weeping, ulcerated warts on tips of toes *Natrum carb. 6c*
- Warts on palms of hands, tendency to sweaty palms *Natrum mur. 6c*
- Large black warts with hairs in them *Sepia 6c*
- Hard warts which burn and throb *Sulphur 6c*

Self-help
Apply Thuja mother tincture twice daily and cover with a plaster. Over-the-counter wart preparations can also be used, but never on facial or genital warts; apply them to the wart only, not to the surrounding skin, and be careful not to get them in your eyes.

Warts can sometimes be removed by using electrical diathermy by a beauty therapist. Skin tags are most commonly removed in this way; these are rounded fleshy stems protruding from the surface of the skin, usually found on the neck, armpit or cleavage areas. The electrolysis needle is used to cauterize and dry up the stem of the wart, causing it to shrivel and fall off.

Remedy Finder for Skin

Clammy skin
Arsenicum
Camphor
Chamomilla
Ferrum
Ferrum phos.
Lycopodium
Mercurius
Phosphoric ac.
Phosphorus
Veratrum

Cold skin
Arsenicum
Calcarea
Calcarea phos.
Camphor
Carbon sulph.
Digitalis
Helonius
Ipecac.
Laurocerasus

Nux mosch.
Oxalic ac.
Rhus tox.
Secale
Sepia
Sulphur

Cracks in skin
Calcarea
Carbon sulph.
Petroleum
Pulsatilla
Sarsaparilla
Sepia
Sulphur

Cracks after washing
Calcarea
Sepia
Sulphur

Cracks in winter
Calcarea

Carbon sulph.
Petroleum
Sepia
Sulphur

Dry skin
Arsenicum
Belladonna
Bryonia
Calcarea
Chamomilla
China
Colchicum
Dulcamara
Petroleum
Graphites
Kali ars.
Kali carb.
Ledum
Lycopodium
Nux mosch.
Oleander

Opium
Petroleum
Phosphorus
Plumbum
Secale
Senega
Silicea
Stramonium
Sulphur
Teucrium
Verbena

Feeling like ants on the skin (formication)
Lycopodium
Phosphoric ac.
Rhododendron
Rhus tox.
Secale
Sulphur
Tarentula

Freckles
Lycopodium
Phosphorus

Goose flesh
Helleborus
Nux
Veratrum

Skin that does not perspire properly
Anacardium
Conium
Kali carb.
Kali phos.
Lycopodium
Phosphoric ac.

Intertrigo (inflamed skin in folds, particularly under breasts)
Causticum

Graphites
Kreosotum
Sulphur

Itchy skin
Agaricus
Arsenicum
Bovista
Carbo veg.
Carbon sulph.
Causticum
Chelidonium
Graphites
Lycopodium
Magnesia carb.
Mercurius
Mezereum
Natrum mur.
Psorinum
Pulsatilla
Sepia
Silicea
Spongia
Staphisagria
Sulphur
Tarentula
Urtica

Itchiness relieved by scratching
Asafoetida
Calcarea
Cyclamen
Muriatic ac.
Natrum mur.
Phosphorus

Itchiness made worse by scratching
Anacardium
Arsenicum

Capsicum
Pulsatilla
Rhus tox.
Sulphur

Pale skin
Belladonna
Calcarea
Cocculus
Ferrum
Lycopodium
Nitric ac.
Platina
Pulsatilla
Secale
Sulphur
Veratrum

Red skin
Agaricus
Apis
Belladonna
Graphites
Mercurius
Rhus tox.
Stramonium

Sensitive skin
Apis
Belladonna
China
Hepar sulph.
Lachesis
Lyssin
Mercurius
Petroleum
Phosphoric ac.
Plumbum
Silicea
Sulphur

Feet

Because they are so far away from our eyes feet tend to be neglected. Diabetics especially, however, need to be careful of their feet, and have regular check-ups with a chiropodist, which can be done on the NHS. In addition to diabetics, pregnant women, the elderly, under 18s and the handicapped can automatically get NHS treatment.

Foot massage is a wonderful way to relax.

Athlete's foot
Fungal infection in which skin round toes be-

comes red and itchy, then white and soggy, and flakes or peels off; in severe cases toenails become yellow and distorted. Ringworm (red, itchy rash on scalp) is caused by the same fungus, which likes warmth and moisture found in swimming pools and changing rooms. Most GPs prescribe anti-fungal ointments, powders, or tablets. As with many skin conditions, homeopathic approach is to boost immune system generally, so treatment is constitutional.

Self-help
Wash feet regularly and dry them thoroughly (a hair dryer is good for drying between toes). Let as much air get to your feet as possible; if you must wear socks, wear cotton rather than nylon, and if you must wear shoes, wear sandals. Over-the-counter anti-fungal powder and Whitfield's ointment, available from chemists, may be used if condition is very persistent.

Corns and calluses
Under constant or repeated pressure, skin thickens and hardens; calluses are patches of hard skin on hands or feet, and are quite common with bunions; corns occur on the toes and are small areas of hard skin which have been pressed inwards. When pressed, both corns and calluses feel tender; ulcers can develop beneath calluses in diabetes. Culprits are ill-fitting shoes and high heels, or heavy manual work. If corns are very painful, your GP will refer you to a chiropodist.

Specific remedy to be taken 4 times daily for up to 2 weeks:

• *Antimonium 6c*

Self-help
Corns and calluses will not go away if you continue to wear the shoes which caused them. Wear flat, comfortable shoes – sandals would be better – and as a temporary measure place felt or rubber rings over the corns to relieve pressure. Regularly soften hard skin with Calendula ointment or cut it away with a corn file. To strengthen your arches and prevent your untramelled feet from splaying, try picking up rubber squash balls with your toes!

Verrucas see WARTS

PART 3

A–Z OF OTHER CONDITIONS

Please remember to check your choice of remedy in the Remedy Pictures (p. 305) and to look for further information, if required, in the Specific Remedy Finders after each 'Ailment or Condition' in PART 2, or in the General Remedy Finder (p. 269).

Abdominal distension (bloated abdomen)

see also ABDOMINAL PAIN

Usually due to retention of wind, faeces, or body fluids, as in IRRITABLE BOWEL SYNDROME (wind and pain, relieved by passing wind or stool), CONSTIPATION, or PRE-MENSTRUAL TENSION, or after eating too many pulses; can also be due to malabsorption (pale, greasy stools, weight loss), swallowing air, under-production of stomach acid, food intolerance, intestinal CANDIDIASIS, etc.

Perhaps the most serious conditions signalled by abdominal distension are obstruction (severe pain with or without vomiting, inability to pass wind, fever) and appendicitis (if appendix has burst); if obstruction or a burst appendix is suspected, (999).

Other distension-related conditions requiring prompt medical attention are retention of urine (relieved by passing urine), cirrhosis of the liver (with jaundice), congestive heart failure (with puffy ankles which pit when pressed, breathlessness which gets worse at night and during exercise) and glomerulonephritis (swollen ankles which pit when pressed, small amounts of urine); if any of these conditions is suspected, 12 .

Give specific homeopathic remedies appropriate to the cause; if none of the remedies listed elsewhere seems to answer the case, the remedies given below may be used.

Specific remedies to be given every ½ hour for up to 10 doses:

- Marked constipation, passing of wind *Lycopodium 6c*
- Passing wind, abdominal pain relieved by bending backwards, bowels loose *Dioscorea 6c*
- Hysterical distension of abdomen, particularly after grief *Ignatia 6c*
- Bowels feel as if there is a live animal in them, lots of wind and rumbling, abdomen distended, chronic diarrhoea *Thuja 6c*

Self-help

If wind is the problem avoid gas-producing foods such as pulses, nuts, onions, and cabbage.

Abdominal pain

Strictly speaking, the term abdominal pain covers all forms of pain (aches, cramps, colic, etc.) felt between diaphragm and groin; it therefore includes 'stomach ache', although pain due to ailments of the upper parts of the digestive tract – stomach, duodenum, pancreas, gall bladder, and liver – is likely to be felt in the upper abdomen, behind the lower ribs or between the ribs and the navel.

Acute abdominal pain, pain so severe that the slightest movement is agony, may be due to appendicitis (if appendix ruptures, there is severe pain in lower right abdomen, with vomiting and fever), obstruction of part of the intestine or bowel (abdomen distended, vomiting, constipation or diarrhoea, inability to pass wind), acute pancreatitis (severe pain in upper abdomen, radiating to back, with vomiting), a perforated peptic ulcer (sudden intense pain, followed by shock), diverticulitis (pain in lower left abdomen, fever, nausea), or internal injury, all of which can very swiftly lead to peritonitis. All are emergency situations, so (999); once in hospital, it may be necessary to open up the abdomen to find out what is wrong.

Self-help

If pain is severe, do not drink or eat until you have seen your GP, and do not take painkillers or drink alcohol. A hot water bottle or an ice pack applied to the site of the pain may help.

Specific remedies to be given, for up to 10 doses only, until medical help arrives:

- Suspected burst appendix *Lachesis 6c* every 5 minutes
- Suspected obstruction *China 6c* every 5 minutes
- Woman in state of fear and shock *Aconite 30c* every 10 minutes
- If pain follows injury *Arnica 30c* every 10 minutes

Acute abdominal pain can also be due to gastroenteritis or food poisoning (diarrhoea, vomiting, fever), renal colic (pain is intermittent and extends from small of back to groin), acute pyelonephritis (fever as well as pain), GALLSTONES or cholecystitis (pain under right ribs), CYSTITIS (painful or frequent urination), shingles (burning pain localized to strip down one side of abdomen, tenderness), indigestion (especially after alcohol or heavy meals), diverticulosis or diverticulitis (cramps and tenderness in lower left abdomen), CONSTIPA-TION, disruption to blood flow in the area of bowel and intestines (possibly caused by thrombosis, a haemorrhage, or an aortic aneurysm), or even a sudden change of diet (constipation, lots of wind). In pregnancy, acute lower abdominal pain, especially if associated with vaginal bleeding, may signal an ECTOPIC PREGNANCY or a MISCARRIAGE.

If pain is severe and continues unabated for more than 1 hour, or occurs during first 3 months of pregnancy, ②.

Among the many causes of chronic or recurrent abdominal pain are PELVIC INFECTION (smelly vaginal discharge), hiatus hernia (heartburn made worse by bending or lying down), indigestion and PEPTIC ULCER (pain relieved by antacids), pancreatitis (pain in upper abdomen), GALLSTONES (pain in upper right abdomen), Crohn's disease (cramps after eating, diarrhoea), HERNIAS in the abdominal wall in the area of the navel or groin, IRRITABLE BOWEL SYNDROME (often one-sided abdominal cramps), and ulcerative colitis (left-side abdominal pain relieved by passing stools).

If pain is localized between navel and breastbone and person is losing weight at rate of 0.5 kg (1 lb) or more per week, cause may be cancer of the stomach; if there is persistent pain in the lower abdomen, with fever, and alternate bouts of constipation and diarrhoea, cause may be cancer of the colon. In either case, appropriate action is 48.

If abdominal pain can be traced to any of the causes mentioned above, see relevant listed entry for homeopathic treatment. Where pain is recurrent but the cause cannot be found, constitutional treatment would be a sensible course.

Specific remedies to be given ½-hourly for up to 10 doses when pain comes on:

- Pain onsets and stops with equal suddenness, as if abdomen has been gripped by a hand and then released, face red and hot, abdomen tender and sensitive to slightest jarring *Belladonna 30c*
- Pain like a stitch, abdomen feels as if it is about to burst, pressure makes pain worse, pain so severe that woman cannot move, think, or talk, breathing shallow *Bryonia 30c*
- Cutting pain causes woman to double up and cry out, abdomen distended with wind, attack may follow anger outburst *Chamomilla 6c*
- Violent, cutting, twisting pain just below

navel, relieved by passing wind, bending forwards, or pressing on abdomen *Colocynth 6c*
- Pain so violent that woman cries out, relieved by warmth, friction, and pressure on abdomen *Magnesia phos. 6c*

Addiction
see also DRUG ADDICTION, ALCOHOLISM

An inability to do without something on the physical or psychological level, to the point where craving for it begins to destroy or dominate family, social, or working life.

We begin wanting things as soon as we are born – food, warmth, love – and we want them instantly. As children we exist in a broil of anticipation, of the next birthday, of the next trip to the seaside. As adults our needs are more varied and complex, but the world no longer revolves around us as it did when we were children; unsatisfied, those needs make us vulnerable to palliatives such as alcohol, drugs, tobacco, and so on. Not everyone succumbs, not because they are models of morality, or will-power, or emotional stability, or cushioned by circumstances, but because their brain chemistry is not affected by them in a sufficiently rewarding way.

The brain is receptive to pain-relieving and pleasure-giving substances because it manufactures similar substances itself; if the manufacture of these substances, collectively known as endorphins, is low, for congenital reasons or because their production has been depressed or disordered by drug-taking, the conditions exist in which drugs and other addictive substances will be gratifying. Unfortunately, the highs produced by most substances of abuse are shortlived, quickly followed by lows. The higher the highs, the lower the lows. The only cure for a low is another high . . . and so the destructive spiral of addiction sets in. So-called addictions to television, sweets, coffee, and so on are not in the same league as dependence on drugs or alcohol, but like life-threatening addictions they are often substitutes for needs which are not being met.

Patterns of addiction, and attitudes towards it, are changing. In the last 25 years, for example, the proportion of female to male alcoholics has increased from 1 in 8 to 2 in 5. The prevailing view today is that dependence on alcohol or drugs is a disease, precipitated by social and emotional factors certainly, but due primarily to constitutional factors.

The first step towards fighting addiction is to recognize that you are becoming addicted. Since addicts in bud have a great capacity for denying the truth, the first alarm bells are usually sounded by friends, relatives, or colleagues at work.

There is no definite point at which a casual

drug user becomes an intensive user or a heavy social drinker becomes an alcoholic, so it is no use saying to yourself: 'I'll stop when such and such happens.' When it becomes difficult to do without, physically or psychologically, you are already becoming dependent; the substance is controlling you, not you it. The only way to prevent dependence increasing, as it almost certainly will, is to stop now, with the help of family, friends, and support organizations.

Adolescence

The changes that initiate transition from child-hood to adulthood usually begin around the age of 10–11 years in girls. Girls reach sexual maturity earlier than boys, and have an earlier spurt in weight and height gain. Although the order in which the events of puberty occur is more or less the same in most girls, the age at which these events happen varies considerably.

The first sign of puberty is slight swelling of the breasts; this usually happens between the age of 10 and 11. Pubic hair begins to appear at around the same time, before underarm hair. Most girls have their first period (menarche) between the age of 12½ and 13½, just after their rate of height gain reaches its peak, but menarche at 11 or 14 is not at all uncommon. Menstruation is irregular at first, but usually settles down to a 26–28 day cycle by the age of 16. At the same age height gain levels off.

Adolescence is a time of great emotional and intellectual change too, a time when families need to give the most, and also take the most. A teenager has to negotiate some very tricky con-flicts, between dependence and independence, between values held by parents and those held by peers, between wanting to be as free as a bird and having to make commitments. If parents are not prepared to be very open about their own feel-ings, about their own attitudes to sex, drugs, politics, and the world in general, and about their own experiences of growing up, the conflicts of adolescence can be very painful and very lonely, and are likely to repeat themselves in later life. A balance has to be struck between over-strictness and laissez faire. Laying down the law too heavily is likely to cause humiliation and resentment, but not making any rules is likely to be misconstrued as not caring.

No matter how untidy, loud, rude, hostile, and rebellious adolescents may be in their efforts to achieve a sense of self, what they need most is love and understanding, and their own 'space', physically as well as emotionally. Once they realize and accept that parents also need their own space, the stage is set for healthy transition to adulthood.

Delayed periods (see also MENSTRUAL PROBLEMS)
Periods usually begin between age of 11 and 14, becoming regular at 15 or 16. If first period (menarche) has not occurred by age of 16, GP should be consulted; cause may be ANAEMIA, STRESS, or an imperforate hymen (sheet of tissue completely blocking outflow of blood from vagina). Constitutional homeopathic treatment may be necessary, but the remedies below should be tried first; if there is no improvement after 2 months, see your GP or homeopath.

Specific remedies to be given every 12 hours for up to 3 weeks:

- Girl prone to nosebleeds *Bryonia 6c*
- Girl who is timid, often feels chilly, cries easily, suffers from headaches, prefers being in open air, feels sick when she eats rich food *Pulsatilla 6c*
- Lack of periods associated with constipation and anaemia, especially if girl has pear-shaped figure, worries a lot, and hates sympathy *Natrum mur. 6c*
- Sinking feeling in pit of stomach around 11 am, hot flushes, tension headaches, craving for fatty foods *Sulphur 6c*
- Depression, chilliness, weakness, eczema be-hind ears, mucous discharge from vagina *Graphites 6c*
- Girl overweight, nervous, and worried, com-plains of unusual fluttering and throbbing of heart, suffers from abdominal pain around 3 pm, sour belching from indigestion, redness and smarting of vulva, face flushed and pale by turns *Kali carb. 6c*

Delayed puberty
Girls tend to follow their mothers in the time of puberty. Chronic illness and malnutrition can delay onset; puberty also comes later in girls who are very thin or small for their age. If growth spurt has not taken place by age of 15, there may be cause for concern. Constitutional homeo-pathic treatment may be necessary, but if girl is generally healthy one of the remedies below should be tried first; if there is no improvement after 2 months, see your GP or homeopath.

Specific remedies to be given every 12 hours for up to 3 weeks:

- Girl thin, with a large head, chilly, prone to head sweats, generally timid but can be obstinate at times *Silicea 6c*
- Girl flabby and overweight, chilly, prone to sour sweats, mentally and physically sluggish *Calcarea 6c*
- Girl mentally and physically immature for age,

plagued by sore throats, tonsillitis, and swollen glands, delayed periods *Baryta 6c*

Alcoholism

see also ADDICTION

The modern concept of alcoholism is that it is a disease which is curable. Individual tolerance to alcohol varies widely, even among alcoholics, but tolerance increases as drinking gets heavier. Patterns of drinking also vary; some alcoholics drink constantly, others have binges lasting for several days and then don't touch a drink for a week.

In the early stages, it may be difficult to tell whether someone is an alcoholic. There is no convenient borderline between 'social drinking' and alcoholism. Social drinkers, even heavy social drinkers, may be correct in assuming that they drink simply to be sociable; they may *not* be constitutionally predisposed to addiction. But alcohol is no respecter of motives. It is a powerful poison, affecting every cell in the body, especially those in the liver, heart, and brain, and it produces increasing tolerance. It also causes nutritional deficiencies because it disrupts appetite and destroys nutrients in the gut.

The upper limit of sensible drinking is now regarded as 21 units per week for men and 14 units for women. Alcohol can also cause foetal abnormalities.

Among the signs of growing dependence are a tendency to start drinking earlier and earlier in the day, and not just in public but also secretly; increasing irritability and aggression, blurred recall of events in the immediate past, even blackouts, unreliability, and a general drop in performance at all levels. At this stage the woman usually denies that she has a problem. The later signs of dependence are more difficult to deny. Socially there is an increase in road traffic and industrial accidents, vandalism and cruel activity, including violent behaviour.

Psychological problems may be: DEPRESSION, paranoia, marked difficulties with memory and concentration, sexual difficulties and family problems including child abuse. Physical problems may be: husky voice, flushed red face with prominent veins, contusions from falls, trembling hands, chronic stomach ache due to gastric erosion and cirrhosis of the liver. Alcoholism may also contribute to high blood pressure. If the craving for alcohol is not satisfied, withdrawal symptoms set in.

Various studies of twins have shown that heredity plays a more powerful part in alcoholism than environment. Most at risk are people who have a parent, or parents, with a drink problem. However, a diet poor in certain vitamins and minerals, or a tendency to HYPOGLYCAEMIA, also poses a risk, and recently it has been suggested that excess lead in the diet or environment may be a predisposing factor. Alcoholism is most common among people aged 35–50, but is not unknown among adolescents. The extent of the problem is not precisely known, since far more people are affected than are diagnosed or treated, but estimates range from 1 to 4 per cent of the population.

Alcoholism requires professional medical help. It is possible to wean a person off alcohol in the short term by using vitamins, tranquillizers, various forms of aversion therapy, counselling, and so on, but that is only the first step. As most ex-alcoholics will confirm, the hard work starts when a person leaves the hospital or clinic after detoxification, and realizes that he or she must never touch alcohol again. The right amount of alcohol for an ex-alcoholic is no alcohol. This is where Alcoholics Anonymous provides invaluable support.

Homeopathy does not offer treatment for alcoholism as such, although in emergencies

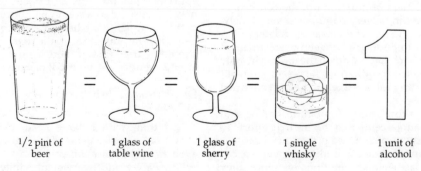

| 1/2 pint of beer | 1 glass of table wine | 1 glass of sherry | 1 single whisky | 1 unit of alcohol |

The units of alcohol

Each of the above drinks contains one unit of alcohol (one unit equals approximately 8 g alcohol)

various homeopathic remedies can be used to relieve the symptoms of withdrawal. However, it does offer constitutional treatment to boost general health, vitality, and self-confidence once the habit has been broken. The authors unhesitatingly recommend such treatment as part of staying alcohol-free. That said, homeopathy can offer a number of remedies for the effects of occasional over-indulgence in alcohol.

Specific remedies to be taken ½-hourly, or more frequently if necessary, for up to 12 doses:

- Hangover in morning, especially after drinking spirits, woman 'burning the candle at both ends' *Nux 6c*
- Stomach pain after heavy drinking *Capsicum 6c*
- Social bingeing, woman talks too much and hates tight clothing *Lachesis 6c*
- Woman more depressed and irritable than usual, near end of tether *Avena 6c*
- Woman apprehensive, trembling, lethargic, sensitive to noise *Zinc 6c*
- Solitary drinking, abnormal flatulence, nervous exhaustion *Sulphur 6c*
- Nausea and vomiting after drinking beer, tendency to profuse, stringy catarrh *Kali bichrom. 6c*

Self-help
The role of Alcoholics Anonymous (address p. 335) has already been referred to; meetings take place most nights of the week in most towns of any size, and anyone who thinks she has a drink problem can attend. There is a sister organization, Al-Anon Family Groups UK & Eire (address p. 335), which offers support and counselling to the families and friends of alcoholics.

After stopping drinking it is important to eat a healthy, varied diet and to make up deficiencies of vitamins A, B, C, D, K, folic acid, bioflavinoids, iron, manganese, potassium, and cysteine (an amino acid found in dairy products, whole grains, nuts and seeds). A high-dose multi-vitamin and mineral supplement would be the most convenient way of doing this in the first month after stopping drinking. Regular intake of all the nutrients mentioned above is advised even for moderate social drinkers. Evening primrose oil would also be beneficial.

Allergy
An allergy is conventionally thought of as an excessive reaction between an antigen (allergen) and an antibody. Some people, through their genetic inheritance, produce large numbers of the kind of antibodies which cause the release of large quantities of histamine when they bind to certain antigens (allergens); histamine causes large quantities of fluid to leak out of blood vessels and tissues, resulting in the distressing symptoms of allergy – local swelling, redness, and itching. Into this category of allergic reaction come hay fever and allergic rhinitis, COELIAC DISEASE, certain forms of asthma and CONJUNCTIVITIS, ECZEMA, and URTICARIA. In a few people the histamine reaction occurs throughout the body (anaphylaxis) and can cause death from shock or suffocation.

At the other extreme allergies are known to cause headaches and feelings of fullness in the head (see HEADACHE), excessive drowsiness after eating, insomnia (see SLEEP PROBLEMS), ringing in the ears, recurrent sinusitis and ear infections, sore throat, nausea and vomiting, DIARRHOEA, CONSTIPATION, flatulence, ABDOMINAL PAIN, chronic fatigue, aching joints and muscles, binge eating (see BULIMIA), anxiety attacks, DEPRESSION, tearfulness, unusually aggressive behaviour, apathy, confusion, hyperactivity, inability to concentrate. . . In such cases mechanisms other than the classic antigen-antibody response are almost certainly involved.

Among the many substances known to cause allergic reactions are dust, house dust mites, fur and feathers, tree and grass pollens, various plants, wool and other fabrics, nickel and other metals, gases and vapours given off by gas appliances, household cleaners, paints, solvents, plastics, pesticide residues, non-stick coatings, various drugs, including penicillin, and of course many foods and food additives.

Desensitization treatment – carefully controlled exposure to progressively stronger doses of the allergen concerned. Orthodox desensitization is permitted only in situations where full resuscitation facilities are available. Other forms discussed below involve very small quantities. It only works when one or two substances are involved and should only be tried if other measures fail. Most forms of desensitization work for some people for a while; the allergy then returns more violently than before, and is more difficult to treat. In the authors' experience all forms of desensitization carry a risk, although it is said that enzyme potentiated desensitization (EPD) is safer than other methods. It is thought to be about 80 per cent effective, but benefit may be delayed for up to 2 years.

EPD is a treatment using a complex mixture of extremely dilute extracts of a great variety of foods combined with an enzyme (beta glucuronidase) which activates the immune system so that it can respond to the dilutions of the food. It is either applied by injecting a very small quantity of the fluid under the skin, or the skin is scratched, a small quantity of liquid put on it, and a small plastic cup applied. To begin with doses are needed every 2 months, and then every 3 months. Often things get worse before they get better. There are few risks with this form of desensitization apparently, but several drawbacks.

Firstly, although it can be obtained on the National Health Service occasionally (particularly at the Royal London Homeopathic Hospital), it is usually given privately, costing between £200 and £400 per year. Secondly, there may be no improvement for 6 months. Thirdly, it will not deal with chemical allergies directly. Fourthly, according to various sources, there are some foods it will not desensitize the patient against – particularly chicken, raw apples, raw carrots and celery.

Suppressing allergic symptoms with anti-histamines, steroids and decongestants is not recommended unless symptoms are making life unbearable; the specific homeopathic remedies given under the conditions mentioned above should be tried first.

Broadly speaking, there are two kinds of allergy, fixed allergy and cyclic allergy.

A fixed allergy is one which declares itself before the age of 2. One school of thought attributes this kind of allergy to a 'leaky bowel': the walls of the bowel are such that certain proteins easily pass into the bloodstream, where they are identified as 'foreign' and trigger off antibody production. The bowel may be leaky from birth, or leakiness may develop as a result of inflammation or candida infestation (see THRUSH). The permanent presence in the blood of large numbers of antibodies which would not normally be there seems to encourage allergic reactions. Most fixed allergies involve single substances.

If you suspect a food, a sensible first step would be to restrict consumption and take one of the remedies listed in the Remedy Finder for weight problems and eating disorders (pp. 45–50). If this produces good results, you could then confirm your suspicions by trying the elimination and challenge test (see below). If the results are equivocal and allergic symptoms persist, you should seek constitutional treatment; if appropriate, your homeopath may recommend bowel cleansing and Acidophilus capsules to reduce the permeability of the bowel. If these measures do not work, desensitization may be necessary.

Cyclic allergies tend to occur in older people, and only declare themselves after repeated exposure to certain substances – usually several substances are involved. Exposure may not always cause a reaction because, up to a point, the body develops tolerance; this is known as

'allergy masking'. In the authors' experience, cyclic allergies are often a symptom of much deeper imbalances. In some people, identifying and eliminating one substance or group of substances uncovers a sensitivity to others; it is as if removing one allergy obliges the body to find another way, and sometimes a more unpleasant way, of expressing its imbalances. That is why initial treatment should be constitutional. If this fails, avoidance of specific substances is the logical next step, provided nutrition is not compromised by cutting out too many foods; if this is likely, vitamin and mineral supplements may have to be taken under supervision, and safe foods eaten in strict rotation to prevent new allergies developing. Desensitization, orthodox and homeopathic, is a last resort.

Food allergies may be fixed or cyclic, and can declare themselves in many ways – as rashes, stomach upsets, mood swings, hyperactivity, aggression, general tiredness, apathy, and malaise, and as cravings. If you suspect you have a food allergy the first items to be suspicious of are: foods which upset you; foods which you crave or find difficult to resist; foods you would miss if you were asked to give them up; foods which make you feel better after having eaten them. In this context 'foods' include beverages.

Testing for allergies

Orthodox and complementary medicine offer a number of tests, and there are simple tests which you can do yourself (see Self-help below). Skin tests, also known as patch tests, are a good way of assessing sensitivity to inhaled or contact allergens but not to food substances; a single drop of allergen extract is placed on the skin and the skin is then gently scratched with a needle; if an angry weal develops, there is an allergy. Radio absorption testing (RAST) detects antigen-antibody reactions in a blood sample by means of radioactive isotopes. Cytotoxic testing, which is expensive but accurate in 70–80 per cent of cases, involves taking a small sample of blood and examining the activity of white blood cells when exposed to suspect substances. Sublingual testing involves placing a small amount of the suspected allergen under the tongue to see if it causes a reaction; the allergen is then diluted to see at what dilution the allergic response disappears. Applied Kinesiology and Touch for Health practitioners detect allergies by placing suspect substances on the tongue and then testing the strength of various muscles, sometimes with very clear-cut results, sometimes not; weakness is taken as an indication of allergy. Dowsing with a pendulum can sometimes produce good results, and sometimes yield nothing; much depends on the dowser's ability to keep his or her mind clear.

Self-help
There are a number of simple tests you can do yourself. If you suspect you have a food allergy, test the foods mentioned above, eliminating them one at a time. *Never eliminate more than one food at a time.* This is called 'elimination and challenge' testing. Eliminate each food for at least 4 days, then reintroduce it within 12 days. If you feel better after not eating it and worse when you reintroduce it, you are probably allergic to it. Once you have established which foods are safe, take care to eat them on a rotational basis; if you eat them too frequently, you may develop intolerance to them again.

You might also try the pulse test. This involves taking your pulse before you eat a particular food and again afterwards to see if your pulse rate rises rapidly or not. If it does, you are probably allergic to that food. To take your pulse, place your fingers lightly on the thumb side of the inside of your wrist for 30 seconds, and count the number of beats. This test only works if you are calm and breathing quietly to start with, and if your pulse rate is not too variable. If your pulse rate is more or less the same on five successive occasions when you have been sitting calmly for 15 minutes or so, the test may well work for you.

If you suspect that paints, plastics, or household chemicals may be the culprit, try the 'sniff test'. Go for an hour's walk in the fresh air, and when you get home quickly go round the house sniffing anything which gives out a strong smell. The smell which affects you most may well be the one you are allergic to. Some patients have reported marked benefits from taking selenium, zinc and gamma linolenic acid (as in evening primrose oil).

Amenorrhea
Temporary or permanent absence of periods; may be primary if periods have not started by age of 16 (see DELAYED PUBERTY for specific homeopathic remedies), or secondary if periods have started and then stopped because of ANOREXIA or excessive weight loss (see WEIGHT PROBLEMS), excessive exercise (especially on vegetarian diet), or STRESS; an established menstrual cycle can also be disrupted by HORMONE IMBALANCES (as MENOPAUSE approaches, for example) or by coming off the Pill; after childbirth, periods may be absent or irregular for 6 weeks to several months. In rare cases, amenorrhea may be due to a gross displacement of the uterus (see UTERUS PROBLEMS), although this can be corrected by special exercises. It can also be caused by flying, especially long haul.

If periods have been absent for more than 9 months and woman wishes to get pregnant, GP may prescribe a fertility drug; however, absence of periods cannot be relied on as a method of contraception since ovulation may restart (or start) at any time. Homeopathy offers constitutional treatment in appropriate cases; provided secondary amenorrhea is not due to pregnancy, childbirth, or anatomical problems, remedies below may be of benefit; if periods do not restart within 2 months, see your homeopath.

Specific remedies to be taken every 12 hours for up to 14 days:

- Periods stop suddenly due to great emotional shock or exposure to dry cold *Aconite 30c*
- Periods stop after becoming extremely chilled after strenuous exercise *Dulcamara 30c*
- Feeling tired, giddy, and chilly, with legs as heavy as lead, breasts swollen and painful, nerviness and jumpiness *Calcarea 30c*
- Thinning hair, headaches, constipation, irritability, recent emotional shock *Natrum mur. 30c*
- Periods cease because of grief or loss *Ignatia 30c*
- Dryness of vagina, lower abdominal pain, headache, slightest emotional upset disrupts periods, feeling faint and shivery, weepy and sad *Lycopodium 30c*
- Abnormal vaginal discharge, sallow patches on face, feeling weak, tearful, and irritable *Sepia 30c*
- Weariness, weakness, wanting to sit down all the time, face usually pale, occasional hot flushes *Ferrum 30c*
- Periods stop after exposure to damp cold *Pulsatilla 30c*

Self-help
Take a multivitamin and mineral supplement.

Anaemia
Occurs for various reasons, but essentially means that blood does not carry enough oxygen; classic symptoms are pallor, tiredness, breathlessness, and palpitations.

Iron-deficient anaemia is the most prevalent form, affecting mainly women. Cause is lack of iron, essential for formation of oxygen-carrying pigment haemoglobin. Iron may be lacking in diet or not absorbed properly (as in COELIAC DISEASE) or iron stores may be depleted by pregnancy or blood loss (perhaps because of injury, but also because of periods of internal bleeding from peptic ulcers), damage to stomach (from aspirin, non-steroidal anti-inflammatories and other drugs), PILES or CANCER of gastro-intestinal tract. In conditions such as rheumatoid arthritis or chronic kidney failure the body may not be able to use its iron reserves.

In addition to causing pallor and fatigue, iron deficiency lowers resistance to infection, especially to THRUSH. If you suspect you are anaemic see your GP; it is important that the underlying cause is diagnosed. Iron tablets and injections may solve the problem, but if iron depletion is very severe blood transfusions may be necessary. Provided steps are being taken to remedy iron deficiency, the specific remedies below are recommended.

Specific remedies to be taken every 12 hours for up to 2 weeks:

- Anaemia due to blood loss, oversensitivity, chilliness, exhaustion *China 30c*
- Face pale but flushes easily, generally robust appearance, oversensitivity *Ferrum 30c*
- Constipation, dull or muddy complexion, headache, dry mouth and lips, tendency to cold sores *Natrum mur. 30c*
- Anaemia during growth spurt (during first two years of life or during adolescence), irritability, poor digestion *Calcarea phos. 30c*
- Anaemia coupled with mental overload *Picric ac. 30*

Self-help

Make sure your diet contains plenty of iron-rich foods and vitamin C. This is especially important if you are a vegetarian since wholegrains and pulses bind iron, limiting absorption. Avoid drinking tea at mealtimes – the tannin in it makes iron absorption less efficient. Calc. phos. and Ferrum phos. (see Tissue Salts, p. 24) are also recommended.

Bartholinitis, Bartholin's cysts
see VAGINAL AND VULVAL PROBLEMS

Body odour

Sweat glands in groin and under arms begin to broadcast their special odours around age of 15 or 16 in girls and a year or two later in boys. Most adolescent worries about body odour are related to these unfamiliar smells rather than to excessive sweating; STRESS increases sweating, and many girls find they sweat more during their periods. Fresh sweat does not usually smell unpleasant; odour becomes offensive when bacteria breed in stale sweat; daily washing, and alkalinity of soap, discourage bacteria. If sweating is related to stress, constitutional treatment is recommended; otherwise, one of the remedies below may be helpful.

Specific remedies to be taken hourly for up to 10 doses as required:

- Sour-smelling perspiration, especially during exercise or sleep, woman overweight and feels the cold *Calcarea 6c*
- Cold sweats, worst on feet, woman slim and feels the cold, especially cold draughts around head *Silicea 6c*
- Sweat smells unpleasant, woman tends to sweat in both hot and cold situations, and may produce a lot of saliva *Mercurius 6c*
- Skin looks dirty, odour persists even after washing *Psorinum 6c*

Breast problems
see also CANCER OF THE BREAST

The best insurance against breast cancer and other problems is regular self-examination of breasts; this should be done just after every period or, if periods have ceased, on same date each month; just before a period breasts can be misleadingly lumpy or tender due to activation of milk-producing tissue; it is also quite normal for one breast to be slightly larger than the other. If you detect anything suspicious, see your GP. You are not wasting his or her time.

Undress to waist and stand in front of mirror. Can you see any differences between breasts when you lean forwards, lift breasts upwards, stretch arms above head, press hands on hips? Things to watch for are different 'hang' and 'swing', and areas of dimpling or flattening. This test is based on the fact that between the skin of the breast and underlying muscle are found lots of little elastic fibres, which maintain the shape of the breast in different positions. If a number of these get snagged by a small early cancer they will no longer be capable of expanding, although this may not be visible when the breast is stationary. As you move your arm and the breast moves also, these fibres will *not* move, therefore dragging the skin down, causing characteristic dimpling.

Lie in bath or on bed and feel each breast with flattened fingers. Does one breast feel different from the other? Are there any lumps or areas of thickening or tenderness in breast or armpit? Has one nipple begun to retract or stick out in an odd direction? Is there any discharge from it? Is there any new or persistent pain?

Obviously any lump which you find should be shown to the doctor. Having said that, most lumps and bumps are not cancerous, and will not become so. There are various cyclical changes which occur in the breast which are completely normal, including the following:

1 Breast pain which is usually worse before period in women between 30–50.

2 Nodules which come and go during menstrual cycle in women of all ages.

3 Fluid-filled cysts, which may start as a lump, are very common in women over 35 up to the menopause.

4 Fibroadenomas – small, well-defined, moveable lumps in women aged 15–30.

5 Problems in the ducts which lead to discharge from the nipple, retraction, or abscesses.

6 Breast abscesses; these are usually associated with breastfeeding.

Breast abscess (mastitis) due to milk stasis in the breast glands postnatally. If breastfeeding, continue to do so unless symptoms are very severe; symptoms are red, painful swelling in breast, some tenderness in armpit glands, and possibly mild fever. Homeopathic remedies below are recommended as first resort; if they do not work, see your GP; if antibiotics do not subdue infection, abscess may have to be drained. However, antibiotics are best avoided if you are breastfeeding; tell your GP you are breastfeeding if she proposes antibiotics, for whatever reason.

Specific remedies to be taken every hour for up to 10 doses:

- Abscess brewing, with hardening of breast tissue and pain on slightest movement *Bryonia 6c*
- Symptoms as above, with red streaks on affected breast *Belladonna 6c*
- Pain very localized, area extremely tender, irritability *Hepar sulph. 6c*
- Armpit glands swollen, looking generally pale, feeling shivery *Phytolacca 6c*
- Nipple cracked and discharging pus, general exhaustion *Silicea 6c*

Self-help At first sign of pain bathe breast in hot water or stroke it from the edge towards the nipple with a hot flannel. Use gravity to help drain the affected area of milk by positioning breast and baby so that abscess is uppermost. Apply Calendula ointment to nipple. For other self-help measures see BREASTFEEDING PROBLEMS.

Galactorrhea

Abnormal production of small quantities of breast milk, usually from both breasts, unrelated to childbirth or breastfeeding; discharge is whitish or greenish; causes include excessive production of milk-stimulating hormone prolactin by pituitary, malfunction of hypothalamus, CANCER OF THE BREAST, drugs such as oral contraceptives, tranquillizers, and diuretics, and more rarely injury, burns, or surgery, nervous dis-

orders such as shingles, and problems with cervical part of spine. Problem affects very few women, notably women who suffer from AMENORRHEA, and can occur in men. Milk production ceases once underlying cause is found and treated.

Specific remedies to be taken 4 times daily for up to 7 days:

- Discharge of milk follows injury to breast *Arnica 30c*
- If breast remains swollen after taking Arnica *Bellis 6c*
- Where breast is hard and painful to touch *Conium 6c*

Lumps in breasts

May be due to a cyst (fluid-filled sac of tissue), to fibroadenosis (thickening of milk-producing tissue), to a benign growth, or to cancer (see CANCER OF THE BREAST); pain is rare in such cases, so regular self-examination of breasts is important. Only a breast infection or abscess (see above) can be relied on to cause pain; it is also of sudden onset. If you notice *any* changes in nipple shape, skin colour, skin texture, or 'hang' of breasts, or any hard or tender areas you have not felt before, see your GP as soon as possible. Breasts may feel slightly tender before a period, but this is perfectly normal and due to changing hormone levels.

Cysts are conventionally treated by draining off fluid, provided diagnosis has been determined; otherwise they need surgical removal. Benign tumours are also treated by surgical removal; after such treatments, check-ups are carried out every 2 years. In homeopathic medicine, all of these conditions are treated constitutionally, although the remedies listed below may be used while constitutional treatment is being sought. For conventional and homeopathic treatment of malignant tumours, see CANCER OF THE BREAST.

Specific remedies to be taken 4 times daily for up to 14 days:

- Cyst diagnosed, affected area hard and painful, stitching pains in nipple, and itching inside the breast, discomfort worse just before and during period, wanting to press breast hard with hand *Conium 6c*
- Cysts present, breasts have purplish tinge and feel extra tender before and during period, chill, damp weather and emotional strain make discomfort worse *Phytolacca 6c*
- Pain comes and goes suddenly, reducing you to tears *Pulsatilla 6c*

- Breasts swollen, hard, and thickened, nipples sore, cracked, and blistered *Graphites 6c*
- Breasts painful and engorged with milk at time of period *Mercurius 6c*
- Breasts red, throbbing, and heavy, lying down makes discomfort worse *Belladonna 30c*
- Breast feels hard, slightest movement makes pain worse *Bryonia 30c*

Self-help Reduce intake of animal fats and of tea, coffee, and other beverages containing caffeine. Occasionally substitute oily fish (herring, mackerel, sardines) for meat or dairy products. An 8-week course of vitamin E is also recommended, gradually increasing daily dosage from 100 to 600 units; however, if you have high blood pressure, check with your GP first as extra vitamin E can temporarily raise blood pressure. Extra vitamin B_6, magnesium, and zinc, and also evening primrose oil and kelp, would also be beneficial.

Nipple problems
Dark red discharge from one nipple may indicate a benign tumour called a duct papilloma, which requires surgical removal, or CANCER OF THE BREAST; white or greenish discharge from both breasts, unrelated to childbirth, may be galactorrhea (see above). Brown area around nipple (areola) can be affected by cysts or boils. Eczema only affecting the nipple area may be Bowen's disease, which may lead to cancer. Nipples which do not protrude are said to be retracted or indented; in some women this is quite normal, but may make breastfeeding difficult; recent indentation, however, may be a sign of CANCER and requires prompt investigation by GP. For other nipple problems see POSTNATAL BREAST PROBLEMS.

Specific remedy to be taken every 12 hours for up to 7 days:

- Long-standing indentation of nipples, provided cancer has been ruled out *Silicea 30c*

Painful breasts
General tenderness is quite common before period (see PRE-MENSTRUAL SYNDROME); localized pain may be an abscess (see above) or a lump (see above for possible causes).

Size problems
Except postnatally, when milk glands are working hard, breast tissue is largely fat, laid down and maintained by action of the female sex hormone oestrogen; since fat distribution is determined genetically, losing or putting on weight is not an infallible way of reducing or increasing breast size; however, if you are over-weight and suffer from pain in neck and shoulders because your breasts are too heavy for the muscles which support them, do try to lose weight; if you are underweight, extra calories will enable you to lay down more fat, which will encourage oestrogen production. Breast reduction is occasionally necessary on medical grounds, breast augmentation almost never.

Homeopathy offers a number of remedies for enlarged or shrunken breasts and associated symptoms; if there is no improvement within 1 month, see your homeopath.

Specific remedies to be taken every 12 hours for up to 7 days:

- Breasts large because of fluid retention *Natrum mur. 30c*
- Breasts heavy and pendulous, especially if woman is obese, pale, and prone to sweats and chills *Calcarea 30c*
- Enlargement associated with pain and tenderness *Conium 30c*
- Enlargement associated with darting pains *Carbo an. 30c*
- Small, flaccid breasts which enlarge and harden before period *Conium 30c*
- Gradual loss of fatty tissue, bluish-red lumps in skin of breasts, tendency to feel hot all the time *Iodum 30c*
- Breasts poorly developed or wrinkled and shrunken *Sabal 30c*

Cancer of the breast
see also BREAST PROBLEMS

Most common form of cancer in women, affecting 1 woman in 20, usually between age of 40 and 50; risk is slightly higher if MENOPAUSE is late, if breast cancer runs in family, and in women who have not had children and in smokers. Warning signs are a lump, usually in outer or upper part of breast, which may or may not be painful, dimpling or creasing of skin in region of lump, discharge from nipple, and recent indentation or reorientation of nipple (see self-examination routine, p. 218); usually only one breast is affected. Not all lumps are malignant (see BREAST PROBLEMS) but immediate investigation is essential as even small tumours can quickly spread. Orthodox treatment is to remove the lump ('lumpectomy'), affected breast (simple mastectomy), or affected breast plus adjacent lymph nodes (radical mastectomy), with radiotherapy or chemotherapy as necessary; however, with new radioactive implant techniques, removal of the whole breast is likely to become a less common procedure. In some cases diseased tissue can be replaced by a silicon implant, preserving the shape of the breast. It has recently been reported that women should have breast cancer surgery late in their menstrual cycle.

The psychological effects of losing a breast can be devastating; this is why counselling before and after mastectomy is important; spouses can give enormous reassurance too.

Obviously if your GP is worried she will send you for a mammogram. Routine mammograms are being recommended for women over 50; some authorities think the age should be reduced to 40. A recent survey, however, cast doubt on the wisdom of this. It was found that surgery which follows the discovery of a lump may actually accelerate the cancer instead of eradicating it. This is probably due to a weakening of the immune system from the surgery, anaesthetic and radiotherapy.

Another interesting piece of research in the USSR appears to suggest that sunlight – possibly due to its vitamin D effects – can protect against breast cancer.

See HYSTERECTOMY for post operative remedies and below for general homeopathic approach to cancer.

Cancer

Every day, as part of the continuous growth and repair process which takes place in the human body, some 500 billion new cells are formed. Occasionally defective cells are produced, some of which may escape the policing activities of the immune system and begin to multiply extremely fast. Rapid, uncontrolled growth is a characteristic of cancer cells. A rapidly dividing colony of cancer cells becomes a tumour, invading normal tissue; if cancer cells spread to other parts of the body via the blood or lymph, secondary tumours may develop; this spreading process is known as metastasis.

What causes the formation of defective cells in the first place? Chromosome damage is one possible explanation; inherited or acquired defects in the immune system are another; ageing may also be a factor, because as we age our immune system becomes less efficient and chromosome-copying mistakes occur. Cell function can be altered by: radiation (including strong sunlight), foods, sexual behaviour (the more sexual partners you have the more likely you are to get cancer of the cervix), alcohol, food additives, viruses, tobacco smoke, asbestos fibres and other occupational factors, other airborne irritants, waterlogging by retention of sodium in the cells, toxic wastes which accumulate as result of constipation, etc.

Overall, cancer affects more men than women, and older people rather than youngsters, but there are exceptions; brain tumours and certain forms of leukaemia, for example, are no respecters of youth. Incidence can also be influenced by nutritional habits, climate, and cultural practices.

Although cancer is not a modern disease, its incidence is increasing. This is partly due to external factors such as smoking and pollution, but also to increased life expectancy. We are not dying young from infectious diseases, as we used to, but living to a ripe old age and succumbing to degenerative diseases instead.

The role of the psyche in all this is difficult to assess. For years psychologists have been pointing out that there is a 'cancer personality', rooted in unresolved conflict between mother and child; typically the child deals with his or her frustration by becoming too adult too soon, by repudiating affection and denying his or her own needs. Sooner or later these unsatisfied needs reassert themselves, usually as the result of the loss of a loved object or person. Though cancer is not the only expression of buried needs, diagnoses of cancer in people who have lost a close relative or friend within the previous 18 months are well above chance. It should also be said that the age–cancer link may have something to do with the generally low esteem in which old people are held in our society.

That said, most experts agree that there is no single cause for cancer. At least 2 factors – heredity and diet, for example, or pollution and personality – need to come together in the same individual for cancer to develop.

Early warnings

1 Persistent lump or thickening anywhere on the skin or in the breast.
2 Unexplained swelling in a limb.
3 A mole or wart which starts to bleed, get bigger, itch or changes colour.
4 Sores, scabs, ulcers or bites which do not heal within 3 weeks.
5 Unusual bleeding from mouth, anus, genitals, nipples. Bleeding between periods, altered bleeding during periods, or bleeding more than 6 months after last period of menopause.
6 Persistent indigestion or change in bowel habits unrelated to alterations in diet.
7 Unexplained weight loss of more than 0.5 kg (1 lb) per week.
8 Hoarseness lasting for more than one month.
9 Increasing difficulty in swallowing or in passing urine.
10 Severe or recurrent headaches.
11 Change in size or weight or shape of testicles.

Treatment

No single branch of medicine offers a certain cure for every type of cancer. All forms of therapy should be considered – listen to everyone, take what appeals to you, and avoid fanatics. Depending on the kind of cancer you have and the stage it has reached, you may need several forms of treatment. For example, it might be sensible to buy time with orthodox treatment while you rebuild your immune system with homeopathy.

The homeopathic view of cancer is that it represents a profound breakdown in health at all levels. Home prescribing is not really appropriate in such circumstances. Instead you should seek the help of an *experienced homeopath*, who will probably prescribe specific remedies as well as constitutional treatment. In some cases, injections of potentized mistletoe (iscador) may be given. Some homeopaths also use Bach Flower Remedies as part of cancer treatment. Vitamins and minerals may also have a role to play.

A deficiency of vitamin C has been found in conjunction with certain tumours; high levels of vitamin A have some protective effect against cancer in smokers – high doses of vitamin A are used in therapy but can give rise to toxic side-effects; vitamin E and selenium, both anti-oxidants, are also believed to have protective effects, although in high doses they can weaken the immune system; vitamin B complex, potassium, iron, zinc, magnesium, copper, manganese, and calcium may also be relevant in some cases; digestive enzymes may be given to try to halt the activities of 'trophoblastic' cancer cells.

There are various dietary therapies for cancer, most based on strict vegan or lacto-vegetarian regimes. However, drastic changes in diet are not appropriate except in the early stages of cancer; in the later stages you may be too run down. The Gerson diet – strictly vegan initially, with juices and coffee enemas to detoxify the liver – has shown good results with cancers such as malignant melanoma, which are difficult to treat; it is not suitable if you have already had chemotherapy (see below).

Orthodox medicine offers surgery, radiotherapy, chemotherapy, and hormone treatment as appropriate.

Unfortunately orthodox successes with childhood leukaemia have not been repeated with the more common forms of cancer. Surgery removes malignant tissue and also an area of healthy tissue around it; radiotherapy uses radioactive radium or cobalt to destroy cancer cells *in situ* – cancer cells are more easily destroyed by radiation than normal cells; chemotherapy involves treatment with strong drugs, often called cytotoxic drugs because they interfere with cell reproduction and metabolism – again, normal cells are less interfered with than cancer cells.

Psychological treatment is now regarded as a valuable adjunct to orthodox and alternative treatment. Cancer sufferers are taught to relax and create a vivid mental picture of their cancer being dissolved by the combined energies of their own immune system and whatever treatment they are receiving; this technique is called 'positive visualization'.

To find out more about treatment options, contact Cancer Help Centre, (addresses p. 333).

Cancer of the cervix

see also CERVICAL PROBLEMS

Affects 1 woman in 80, especially after age of 40; usually a late consequence of untreated cervical erosion which has developed into cervical dysplasia (see CERVICAL PROBLEMS); incidence is higher in women who have had many sexual partners or who start having intercourse very young and in smokers; genital warts (see VULVAL WARTS, PENILE WARTS) and a deficiency of vitamin B_6 may also be contributory factors. Symptoms are offensive, watery bleeding between periods, after intercourse, or after MENOPAUSE; cervical polyps (see CERVICAL PROBLEMS) cause similar symptoms. See your GP immediately if you have any suspicions; a cervical smear will indicate if there is likely to be malignancy present. Suspicious smears may be followed up by colposcopy, where the cervix is examined with a telescope-like instrument. Routine treatment, provided cancer has not spread beyond uterus, depends on grading of cancer by cervical smear and biopsy. It may range from laser treatment or local surgery through to HYSTERECTOMY (usually removal of ovaries and Fallopian tubes along with uterus and cervix), backed up by radiotherapy. See CANCER for homeopathic approach.

Cancer of the ovary

Rare and difficult to detect in early stages because ovaries are deep-lying; once symptoms develop – lower ABDOMINAL PAIN and swelling, general malaise, perhaps weight loss (see WEIGHT PROBLEMS) – cancer may be well established and already have spread; occasionally, an untreated OVARIAN CYST becomes cancerous. Routine treatment is to remove ovary, or ovary and uterus (see HYSTERECTOMY); if cancer has spread, its progress can be kept at bay for several years with radiotherapy and chemotherapy. For homeopathic treatment, see CANCER.

Cancer of the uterus

Most common in women aged 50–60 who have not had children; warning signals are period-type pains at abnormal times, spotting of blood between periods, or reappearance of blood after MENOPAUSE, sometimes accompanied by watery pink or brown discharge which smells unpleasant; a cervical smear and a D & C (removal of tissue from inside uterus) are necessary to confirm or rule out presence of cancer; malignant change in lining of uterus is fairly slow, although eventually muscular walls of uterus, Fallopian tubes, ovaries, and other abdominal organs may be affected. If detected early enough, chances of HYSTERECTOMY and radiotherapy effecting a complete cure are very good. For homeopathic treatment, see CANCER.

Cancer of the vulva
see also VAGINAL AND VULVAL PROBLEMS

A very rare, slow-growing form of cancer, most common in women over 60; begins as hard lump on labia or at entrance to vagina, often on site of persistent irritation or infection, and develops into an ulcer with a thick rim and a moist centre; almost always curable, if detected early enough, by surgical removal and radiotherapy; in some cases lymph glands in groin may have to be removed. For homeopathic treatment, see CANCER.

Cervical problems
see also CANCER OF THE CERVIX

Often discovered during a routine check-up rather than as a result of obvious symptoms. Check-up involves manual and visual examination of vagina, and a cervical smear or 'Pap' test, which involves taking a few cells from mouth of cervix for analysis.

Current medical opinion is that all women should have a smear test within 1 year of becoming sexually active, and then at 3–5-year intervals until age of 65–70. More frequent, even yearly, tests are recommended if woman (or her partner) has many sexual partners, has vulval warts (or if partner has penile or anal warts), smokes heavily, or has had a previously abnormal smear.

Cervical dysplasia
Just occasionally, when delicate tissue around tip of eroded cervix (see Cervical erosion, below) reverts to tougher tissue typical of lining of vagina, certain cells become abnormal and may eventually become pre-cancerous; to minimize risk of malignant change, suspect tissue is surgically removed or destroyed by laser or cauterization. Follow-up by cervical smears on a regular basis is recommended. Dysplasia is likely to be symptomless, although its precursor, cervical erosion, may not. Homeopathic treatment is constitutional.

Cervical erosion
Signalled by watery bleeding after intercourse or between periods (see unusual discharge – MENSTRUAL PROBLEMS); cause is extension of delicate, mucus-secreting lining of cervical canal to outer part of cervix during or after pregnancy or as result of taking oral contraceptives; in itself, condition is harmless, although it makes mouth of cervix more vulnerable to infection; if discharge is heavy, cauterization of affected tissue may be recommended. Constitutional homeopathic treatment is advised, but in the meantime the following remedies may lessen discharge and clear up any infection.

Specific remedies to be taken 4 times daily for up to 14 days:

- Burning discharge, worse during day, especially in afternoon *Alumina 6c*
- Profuse, smarting discharge, with bleeding after intercourse *Phosphorus 6c*
- Bloody discharge, lower abdomen feels heavy and sore, intercourse painful *China 6c*
- Copious discharge between periods, feeling drained and weak *Cocculus 6c*
- Brown watery discharge with strands of mucus in it *Nitric ac. 6c*
- Discharge milky and itchy *Calcarea 6c*

Chlamydia infections
These can affect the eye, genitals, lymph nodes or, occasionally, lungs. The offending organism is half-way between a virus and a bacterium. In men it causes NON-SPECIFIC URETHRITIS, with a burning discharge from the penis. Unfortunately for women, however, it appears not to cause any symptoms at all, but is still capable of ascending through the uterus to attack the delicate lining of the Fallopian tubes. There it can then give rise to PELVIC INFLAMMATORY DISEASE (PID), and worse still, INFERTILITY. It is resistant to penicillin and cephalosporin type antibiotics, and needs to be treated with a combination of drugs, especially if PID is present. Along with AIDS, it is another good incentive for using barrier-type contraceptives, and being very choosy about your sexual partners. Whilst homeopathic treatment can be supportive (see VAGINAL AND VULVAL PROBLEMS, unusual discharge), we recommend that you also take antibiotics.

Cholecystitis
see also GALLSTONES

An acute condition in which the gall bladder becomes inflamed and swollen because flow of bile into duodenum is blocked by GALLSTONES; result is biliary colic – intense pain in upper right abdomen or between shoulders, indigestion, especially after fatty food, and nausea with or without vomiting; untreated, condition can lead to jaundice and occasionally, if gall bladder bursts, to peritonitis. If site of pain is as described above, and pain persists for more than 3 hours, ②; painkillers and antibiotics will probably be prescribed, and then surgery recommended to remove the gall bladder; only in exceptional cases are gallstones dissolved *in situ*.

Occasionally, infection elsewhere in the intestines can spread to the gall bladder; treatment is by antibiotics and painkillers.

Specific remedies to be given ½-hourly for up to 6 doses while waiting for medical treatment:

- Obstructed bile duct, radiating, tearing pains made worse by jarring, pale stools, signs of jaundice *Berberis 30c*
- Pains extend from under right ribs to right shoulder blade, especially after eating fatty food *Chelidonium 30c*
- Great flatulence which is not relieved by belching, person feels chilly, especially in draughts, prefers to move around rather than sit still, bending double reduces discomfort *China 30c*
- Cutting pains relieved by bending double, intestines feel as if they are being pinched between two stones, diarrhoea *Colocynth 30c*
- Griping, drawing, bursting, or cutting pains made worse by pressure on abdomen, relieved by bending backwards *Dioscorea 30c*
- Pain markedly better if a hot water bottle is held to abdomen *Magnesia phos. 30c*

Circumcision

In other than developing nations female circumcision appears to be savage butchery. It is estimated that more than 84 million women in 30 countries in the world, particularly in Africa, have had this operation performed. Part or all of the clitoris and labia majora and minora are removed, and sometimes the vaginal entrance itself is narrowed. Complications may include retention of urine, loss of sexual desire and other psychological problems, trauma during sexual intercourse and difficulties in childbearing.

Coeliac disease

Inability of cells lining upper part of small intestine to break down gluten, a protein found in wheat, oats, barley, and rye. At present the disease cannot be positively diagnosed except by biopsy (removing a tiny sample of tissue for analysis); this is not a pleasant procedure, but it is hoped to replace it by blood or urine tests in the future.

Intolerance to gluten seems to run in families, but is less often seen in children who are breast-fed or introduced relatively late to foods containing gluten. In susceptible children, the disease develops by the age of 2, usually 3–6 months after gluten is introduced into the diet. Signs are failure to gain weight (see growth charts p. 156), CONSTIPATION, or on the contrary bulky, offensive-smelling stools passed with great frequency, lack of muscle tone, a blown-out stomach, and general pallor and apathy.

Chronic sufferers, usually adults, may develop a rash called dermatitis herpetiformis – a red itchy rash in symmetrical patterns on parts of the body.

The only effective treatment is to remove gluten from the diet on a temporary or permanent basis. Early constitutional treatment from an *experienced homeopath* may make permanent avoidance of gluten unnecessary.

The above symptoms are not solely those of coeliac disease, however. ALLERGY (especially to cow's milk, soya products, and fish), lactose intolerance in the wake of gastroenteritis, cystic fibrosis, immune deficiencies, and even emotional deprivation can produce similar symptoms. Do not put your child on a gluten-free diet until you are sure of the diagnosis. For further information contact the Coeliac Society of the United Kingdom (address p. 333).

Constipation

Definitions vary, some doctors defining constipation as the failure to pass a stool every day, others regarding a bowel movement every 4 or 5 days as acceptable, provided stools are not too hard or painful to pass. Nevertheless the longer faeces remain in the bowel the more opportunity there is for toxic substances to be reabsorbed into the bloodstream and passed to the liver, causing poor liver function and other problems. Constipation may be caused by anal fissure, hypothyroidism (see THYROID PROBLEMS), or parental over-emphasis on regular bowel habits. Persistent constipation requires constitutional treatment. If the remedies listed below fail to work within 48 hours, 12. Laxatives and suppositories should be used only on your doctor's instructions.

Specific remedies to be taken 4 times daily for up to 14 days:

- Stools difficult to pass even when soft, woman has no desire to pass stool unless rectum is completely full, itchy eyes, dry skin *Alumina 6c*
- Stools large, dry, and hard, mouth and tongue dry, woman very thirsty *Bryonia 6c*
- Woman irritable and chilly, feels urge to pass stool but is unable to, or if able to feels there is more to come *Nux 6c*
- Sudden stomach cramps, urge to pass stool but stool slips back up inside *Silicea 6c*
- Woman feels better when constipated *Calcarea 6c*

- Small, hard stools with ineffectual straining and a lot of wind *Lycopodium 6c*

Diarrhoea

Failure of the large intestine to absorb water from faeces; this can happen with IRRITABLE BOWEL SYNDROME (diarrhoea alternates with constipation), gastroenteritis (diarrhoea and vomiting), ulcerative colitis (blood in faeces), food poisoning (diarrhoea and vomiting), worms and other intestinal parasites, lactose intolerance and other food intolerances, and even anxiety. Certain drugs, especially antibiotics, cause diarrhoea; also antacids because of their magnesium content, and so does a lack of vitamin B_3 or folate; too much vitamin D can cause constipation as well as diarrhoea. Liquid stools can also be the price of eating too many pulses or prunes. Chronic diarrhoea can cause potassium deficiency.

If diarrhoea continues for more than 48 hours, or is accompanied by fever or blood in faeces, ②; regardless of the cause, person may be seriously dehydrated. Orthodox treatment consists of rehydration with electrolyte solutions for 12–24 hours, followed by investigation and, if persistent, antidiarrhoeal agents such as kaolin and morphine or drugs which inhibit peristalsis or cause constipation.

A tendency towards diarrhoea is best treated constitutionally, although in acute attacks the remedies below may be used.

Specific remedies to be taken every ½ hour for up to 10 doses:

- Diarrhoea comes on suddenly after shock or exposure to cold wind, or overheating in summer, abdomen distended, woman feels better after passing stool *Aconite 30c*
- Diarrhoea after a summer chill, after food which disagrees, or after anger outburst, tip of tongue very red, symptoms worse in morning and made worse by eating, painful urination, yellowish-green stools, a lot of wind, difficult to distinguish between wanting to pass stool and wanting to pass wind *Aloe 6c*
- Anxiety and apprehension, belching, craving for salt and sweet things *Argentum nit. 6c*
- Scanty, odourless, brown stools which seem to burn skin around anus, especially after cold drinks, ice creams, ice lollies, or over-ripe fruit, woman finds small sips of hot drinks soothing *Arsenicum 6c*
- Copious and offensive stools the colour of pea soup and the consistency of batter, with a lot of wind and colic, urgency early in morning, empty feeling afterwards *Podophyllum 6c*
- Profuse, watery stools with bits of food in

them, woman feels better after passing them *Phosphoric ac. 6c*
- Need to pass stool propels woman out of bed at 5 am, anus feels hot, piles may be present *Sulphur 6c*
- Profuse stools, vomiting, forehead breaks out in cold sweat, craving for iced water *Veratrum 6c*
- Stools like chopped egg, a lot of wind, made worse by summer chills or fruit, woman very irritable *China 6c*
- Diarrhoea accompanied by spasmodic, griping pains, doubling up or pressing on abdomen lessens pain, stools copious, thin, frothy, and yellowish, attack possibly brought on by anger *Colocynth 6c*
- Diarrhoea comes on in damp weather or as a result of getting chilled after exertion, stools are slimy, green or yellow, and may have blood in them *Dulcamara 6c*
- Diarrhoea worse at night, also made worse by cold drinks, onions, and rich, fatty foods, no two stools alike *Pulsatilla 6c*

Self-help

To combat dehydration, drink plenty of boiled cooled water, with a little honey in it, or rice water, or barley water (water in which rice or barley has been cooked). Once diarrhoea settles down, eat arrowroot, tapioca, semolina, or Slippery Elm Food for a day or two, then gradually revert to your normal diet. If diarrhoea has been caused by antibiotics, take Acidophilus capsules or Acidophilus yoghurt. Take extra folate and vitamin B for 1 month, and cut down intake of vitamin D. Avoid analgesics.

Dizziness in elderly women

Disorders which most often affect balance in old age are Parkinson's disease (degeneration of nerve centres responsible for coordinating movement), arteriosclerosis (hardening and narrowing of arteries, especially those which supply brain), OSTEOARTHRITIS (especially in hips and knees), and cervical spondylosis (bony growths on neck vertebrae which press on spinal cord and blood vessels to head). Treatment of underlying disorder may alleviate balance problem.

Specific remedies to be taken every 8 hours; if no improvement within 2 weeks, see your GP or homeopath:

- Standing up from sitting or lying position causes dizziness, or dizziness which comes on after an injury, dizziness wears off lying down *Arnica 6c*
- Dizziness made worse by movement, with nausea *Theridion 6c*

- Dizziness worse in cold weather, coughing causes seepage of urine *Causticum 6c*
- Poor circulation due to arteriosclerosis, walking out of doors improves circulation, feeling weak and weary and wanting to lie down *Baryta 6c*
- Senile dementia and loss of concentration, dizziness worse between 4 and 8 pm *Lycopodium 6c*
- Poor circulation, dizziness worse in cold weather and when lying on left side *Silicea 6c*
- Dizziness when lying down and turning over in bed *Conium 6c*

Drug addiction

see also ADDICTION

Addictive drugs may be legal and prescribed by a doctor, or illegal and 'recreational' or 'street'. The longer a drug is taken for, the more the body adapts to it; when the drug is stopped, the adaptive mechanisms continue to operate, unopposed by the drug, usually producing unpleasant rebound effects such as restlessness, trembling, nervousness, and anxiety.

Among the prescription drugs the benzodiazepines or Valium-type tranquillizers (especially lorazepam or Ativan) are the most addictive and the most commonly prescribed; they should not be taken for longer than 2–3 weeks; if taken continuously for 3 months or more, the person taking them is likely to have become addicted to them. The main effect of benzodiazepine drugs is abnormal sleepiness or drowsiness. If you suspect an overdose, but the person is still conscious, give first aid and take him or her to your local casualty department; if unconscious, (999), put him or her in the recovery position and take any tablets, powders, or drug-taking equipment along to the hospital for identification.

Illegal drugs include marijuana, LSD, cocaine, crack, ecstasy, opiates such as heroin, and various solvents taken by sniffing. As with alcohol, there is no easy demarcation line between social use and addiction, or casual use and intensive use. Unfortunately in a book of this scope it is not possible to describe each drug and the kind of addiction it causes. But if you are a mother and are worried about your child taking drugs, write to the Department of Health Leaflets Unit (address p. 335) and ask for the leaflet 'Drugs: what you can do as a parent'; it describes the effects of all the commonest substances of abuse, what the symptoms of addiction are, and how to get help.

If you yourself have a problem, seek expert help, initially through your GP or homeopath.

There are many reasons why people turn to drugs, why they 'escape into failure' – they may be insecure and unhappy, bored, fed up with establishment values, or simply copying their peers and unable to resist the urge to experiment.

Whether a drug is regarded as 'soft' or 'hard', 'recreational' or 'social', or taken casually or intensively, it is illegal. Some of the consequences of taking drugs – the hassle, the fines, the imprisonment, the social stigma – may well endorse the user's low opinion of society, but it is the user, and his or her family and friends, who will be damaged, not society. Also, drugs popularly seen as harmless may be more damaging than was once thought; recent reports suggest that frequent marijuana abuse causes irreversible brain damage.

Coming off prescription drugs

If you feel you are becoming addicted to a drug, go and see your doctor and explain your feelings. If he or she advises you not to come off it, ask why (the effects of coming off some prescription drugs, Ativan for example, can be very unpleasant). If you are not satisfied with the explanation, you are entitled to seek a second opinion, but make sure the person you seek it from is medically qualified. There may be a tranquillizer addicts' support group in your area (Citizens' Advice Bureau will give you the address) through which you can find sympathetic help, or perhaps assurance that the symptoms you are experiencing are nothing to worry about. A medically qualified homeopath may or may not recommend constitutional treatment, but will almost certainly prescribe vitamins and mineral supplements (especially vitamins B and C, and calcium and magnesium) to aid recovery from the drug.

To put your system in a fit state to do without the drug, reduce your consumption of tea, coffee, cigarettes, and alcohol before you start to come off; come off the drug gradually rather than suddenly, unless you are on a very small dose; and take more exercise – it will increase the general efficiency of your metabolism.

Coming off illegal drugs

Living without drugs, once the habit has developed, takes a lot of courage, discipline, and perseverance, and the chances of coming off and staying off are better with professional help than without it. This is especially true of opiate drugs such as heroin. However, there is great controversy as to whether the short-term 'cold turkey' (detoxification) approach or the long-term 'maintenance' approach is more effective/ ethical/socially responsible. Maintenance, on synthetic opiates such as methadone, may cut down burglary and theft as a means of financing drug-taking, but it does not 'cure' addiction; in fact many addicts find methadone harder to kick than heroin. Detoxification treatment is given on an in-patient basis, maintenance by a GP or a local drug clinic. Most large towns have a branch of Narcotics Anonymous, which offers support and counselling to anyone who has a drug problem; Families Anonymous is a sister organization which offers support to the relatives and friends of addicts. Addresses for both are on p. 335.

Addiction cannot be treated homeopathically, but constitutional treatment can prevent drug-taking progressing beyond the experimental stage. There are also a number of specific remedies which antidote the effects of first time use. However, if a person becomes violent, suicidal, or appears to be losing consciousness, ⑨⑨⑨; if possible, gently restrain the person, but without putting yourself in danger, or, if appropriate, put him or her in the recovery position.

Specific remedies to be taken every 15 minutes for up to 10 doses or until the effects of first time use wear off:

• Great anxiety, restlessness, fear of being alone *Arsenicum 6c*
• Woman depressed or very talkative, feeling persecuted *Lachesis 6c*
• Sudden panic, fear of dying, feeling chilly *Aconite 30c*
• Woman depressed, dizzy, disorientated, having hallucinations *Absinthium 6c*
• Marked paranoia (woman feels persecuted or controlled by external forces), muttering, obscene talk and behaviour *Hyoscyamus 6c*

Self-help
A course of multivitamins and minerals is recommended.

Fibroids

Non-cancerous growths in or on walls of uterus, sometimes on a stalk and varying in size from a pea to a large plum; tend to occur severally rather than singly and may take a few or many years to develop; small fibroids are often symptomless, but large ones can give rise to heavy, prolonged periods (see MENSTRUAL PROBLEMS), PAINFUL INTERCOURSE, and CYSTITIS (because they press on bladder and prevent it emptying properly); they may also prevent conception, cause MISCARRIAGE or pain during pregnancy, or obstruct delivery; if stalk of fibroid becomes twisted, cutting off blood supply, result is severe PAIN IN LOWER ABDOMEN; appropriate action is ② and Aconite 30c every 15 minutes for up to 10 doses.

Fibroids are especially common in women aged 35–40, but cause is not known, although it has been speculated that oestrogens in oral contraceptives may encourage condition. Small fibroids seldom require treatment and tend to disappear after age of 45; troublesome fibroids can be removed surgically following a D & C (scraping of uterus) to confirm diagnosis; sometimes HYSTERECTOMY is advised. Homeopathic treatment is constitutional, although in the short term the remedies below should be tried.

Specific remedies to be taken 4 times daily for up to 3 doses:

• Small fibroids, profuse yellow discharge from vagina *Calcarea iod. 6c*
• Swollen uterus, urge to bear down, watery brown discharge from vagina, painful cramps during periods *Fraxinus 6c*
• Menstrual flow heavier than usual, body feels icy cold, bleeding between periods *Silicea 6c*
• Continuous bleeding *Thlaspi 6c*
• Short scanty periods as menopause approaches, great pain eased by menstrual flow, abdomen very sensitive to tight clothing *Lachesis 6c*
• Where menstrual blood is bright red *Phosphorus 6c*
• Uterus feels as if it is being squeezed during periods *Kali iod. 6c*
• Uterus feels swollen and painful, spasmodic contractions of vagina *Aurum mur. 6c*

Fright
see also PANIC ATTACKS

An extreme reaction to a threatening event. Breathing rate speeds up, sometimes leading to HYPERVENTILATION; adrenaline pours into the bloodstream, speeding up heartbeat, felt in extreme cases as palpitations; digestion slows down, causing a churning sensation in the stomach; blood vessels in the skin constrict, causing the skin to turn pale.

If any of the above symptoms follows injury, or is accompanied by nausea and vomiting, severe pain, fainting, or clouding of consciousness, the person may be in shock, in which case ⑨⑨⑨ and give first aid.

Specific remedies to be given 4 times daily for up to 14 days, or ½-hourly for up to 10 doses in extreme cases:

• Marked palpitations, fear of dying *Aconite 30c*
• Woman scared stiff, numb and dozy with fright *Opium 6c*
• Woman hysterical, weeping one minute and laughing the next *Ignatia 6c*
• Inability to get to sleep because mind is racing *Coffea 6c*

Galactorrhea

see BREAST PROBLEMS

Gallstones

Solid accretions of various substances present in bile, including calcium and cholesterol; may be few and large, or many and small, and cause few symptoms while they remain in gall bladder; in fact, many gallstones are discovered during routine scans or X-rays. However, if a stone blocks exit from gall bladder or becomes stuck in duct leading to duodenum, gall bladder becomes swollen with trapped bile and fats in duodenum pass into small intestine undigested, causing pain and tenderness under right rib cage, nausea with or without vomiting, and discomfort after eating fatty food – all the symptoms in fact of acute CHOLECYSTITIS.

Women are more at risk than men, especially women who take or have taken oral contraceptives, and risk increases with age and being overweight; gallstones also seem to increase risk of acute pancreatitis. Cause may be underproduction of bile by the liver, excessive elimination of toxins through the liver, food ALLERGY, or abnormally high blood cholesterol levels.

Conventional treatment for gallstones is removal of the gall bladder, even if symptoms are not those of full blown CHOLECYSTITIS on the 'better safe than sorry' principle. This can now sometimes be done through a tiny hole in the abdominal wall by laporoscopy, rather than by a full operation. It may also be possible to shatter the stones with lithotripsy, using shock waves, or to dissolve them chemically *in situ*, or just take the stones out via laparoscopy; in all the latter there is a risk of recurrence. If stones are present but causing no symptoms consult your homeopath.

Specific remedies to be taken 4 times daily for up to 14 days while seeking homeopathic treatment:

• *Berberis 6c*
• If Berberis is not effective, and woman is nervy, chilly, and oversensitive *China 6c*

Self-help
Both as a preventive and after removal of the gall bladder, cut rich fatty foods, fried foods, and refined carbohydrates down to a minimum, and eat plenty of vegetables, fruit, and fibre. The possibility of a food allergy would also be worth investigating.

If gallstones have been diagnosed, and *provided no symptoms of cholecystitis* are present, it is possible to flush out the stones yourself using the following method, called a liver and gall bladder flush. In the five days leading up to the flush, eat a normal diet but drink as much fresh-pressed apple juice as possible; on the day of the flush, eat a normal lunch but for supper have only citrus fruit or juice.

Take a pint of purest olive oil and eight or nine lemons. (If lemons are not available, then use pure lemon juice.) You should begin the treatment at about 7 pm. Take four tablespoonsful of the olive oil immediately followed by one tablespoonful of neat, unsweetened lemon juice. After 15 minutes, repeat this pair of doses in exactly the same way. Continue repeating the pair of doses at intervals of 15 minutes until all of the oil has been taken; finish off the treatment by drinking any remaining lemon juice. Then go to bed and lie on your right side, with your knees pulled up to your chest for the first 30 minutes. When you open your bowels the next day, the gallstones will appear as irregular, gelatinous, green objects in the stools. If you are constipated, take 2 dessertspoons Epsom salts in warm water 4 hours before taking the oil/lemon mixture, and repeat the Epsom salts the next morning.

There is a theoretical risk that flushing may cause stones to lodge in the bile duct rather than pass into the duodenum, but in the authors' experience this has never happened; if the oil/lemon mixture can be kept down, and not vomited up, flushing can be extremely effective.

Glandular fever (infectious mononucleosis)

Viral infection, spread by personal contact, which begins rather like influenza (fever, sore throat, headache, general achiness); within a day or two glands become swollen and painful, tonsils enlarge and become dirty-looking, and jaundice or a rash similar to that of rubella may develop. Though these symptoms wear off in 2–3 weeks, full recovery may take some time (see CHRONIC FATIGUE SYNDROME). Since antibiotics are ineffectual against viruses, only treatment is rest and plenty of fluids. Your GP will do a blood test to confirm diagnosis, but this is not always reliable as glandular fever can involve many viruses, not just one. Constitutional homeopathic treatment is recommended if condition drags on.

Specific remedies to be taken every 4 hours for up to 10 doses during acute phase:

• Sudden onset of high fever, woman excited, incoherent, and red in the face *Belladonna 30c*
• Feeling chilly and shivery, sticking tongue out makes glands in neck feel painful, cold air and mental exertion make symptoms worse *Cistus 6c*
• Headache, weakness, muscular pains, ulcers in throat make swallowing difficult *Ailanthus 6c*
• Dark red tonsils, swallowing causes pains which shoot up towards ears, food and hot

drinks make swallowing more painful *Phytolacca 6c*
- Glands distinctly swollen, especially if sufferer is a child and a late developer *Baryta carb. 6c*
- Chilliness, sweating, sour taste in mouth, feeling mentally and physically worn out *Calcarea 6c*
- Offensive perspiration, glands feel tender *Mercurius 6c*
- Weepy, can't stand stuffy rooms, thirstless even with fever *Pulsatilla 6c*

Prevention

Glandular fever nosode 30c, taken once a day for up to 10 days, would be a sensible precaution if family, friends, or colleagues are affected.

Self-help

Rest is the best medicine – avoid strenuous exercise and do only 75 per cent of what you are actually capable of (see CHRONIC FATIGUE SYNDROME). Take extra vitamin C, B complex, and zinc, and evening primrose oil.

Headache

see also MIGRAINE

Most headaches are due to strain on the muscles in the neck or head, or congestion of the blood vessels which supply them; the brain itself cannot feel pain because it contains no pain receptors.

Headaches can be a symptom of anxiety, STRESS, physical tension (especially in the back and shoulders), lack of sleep, over-consumption of caffeine in tea or coffee or suddenly cutting down caffeine intake, food ALLERGY, eyestrain, fever, HYPOGLYCAEMIA (low blood sugar, especially if you have not eaten for some time), MIGRAINE (recurrent one-sided headaches, with nausea, vomiting, and bivisual disturbances), drug side-effects (especially if you have started a new drug), sinusitis (especially after a cold, if there is dull pain or tenderness in the cheeks or around the eyes which gets worse when you bend forwards), cervical spondylosis (stiff neck, an ache which extends from spine to top of head, headache made worse by lifting, driving, or turning head slowly) and other spinal problems, PRE-MENSTRUAL SYNDROME (headache comes on before a period), post-herpetic neuralgia following shingles, mal-occlusion or sepsis after dental treatment (see your dentist), and high blood pressure. That very common form of headache, the hangover, is caused mainly by dehydration (alcohol is a powerful diuretic). Temporal arteritis (dull, throbbing headache behind one or both temples) is caused by inflammation of the arteries which supply the scalp.

Headaches can also be a symptom of damage to the blood vessels in and around the brain itself, or of infection to the tissues surrounding the brain and spinal cord. In such cases prompt action and close observation are required.

If a headache follows a head injury, and the person is drowsy, nauseous, and vomiting, the cause may be an extradural brain haemorrhage; if there has been no injury, but symptoms are headache, nausea, vomiting, drowsiness, and intolerance of light, cause may be a subarachnoid brain haemorrhage; in either case (999) and give Arnica 30c every 15 minutes until help arrives.

A bad headache, with a temperature of more than 100°F or 38°C and intolerance of light, may be meningitis; pain behind one eye, with blurred vision, may be acute glaucoma or iritis; if any of these conditions is suspected, (2).

Where a headache has lasted for several days, seems worse in the mornings, and is accompanied by nausea or vomiting, 12; high blood pressure, STRESS, or a brain tumour may be the cause.

Constitutional treatment is recommended for recurrent headaches caused by stress, anxiety, or tension. However, if you know or suspect that a headache is a symptom of another condition, one which does not require prompt medical attention, look up the remedies for that condition, then compare the symptoms listed with those given against the remedies below. If you still draw a blank, refer to the General Remedy Finder (pp. 269–96). Remedies for severe, one-sided, sick headaches are given under MIGRAINE.

Specific remedies to be taken every 10–15 minutes for up to 10 doses:

- Headache comes on suddenly, feels worse in cold or draughty surroundings, woman apprehensive, headache feels like a tight band around head or as if brains are being forced out of head *Aconite 30c*
- Head feels bruised and aching, pain occasionally sharp, made worse by stooping *Arnica 30c*
- Stinging, stabbing or burning headache, rest of body feels bruised and tender, symptoms worse in hot, stuffy surroundings *Apis 30c*
- Throbbing, drumming headache, flushed face, dilated pupils, distinctly worse in hot sun *Belladonna 30c*
- Head feels bruised, sharp, stabbing pain made worse by slightest eye movement *Bryonia 30c*
- Head feels full and swollen, face purple and congested-looking, expression dull and heavy, dilated pupils, limbs weak and shaky *Gelsemium 6c*
- Violent headache in which every heartbeat sets up an answering thump and throb in the head, made worse by stooping or shaking head *Glonoinum 30c*

- Bursting, aching headache, hypersensitive scalp, worse in damp, foggy weather *Hypericum 30c*
- Headache described as tight band across forehead or as nail being driven out through side of head *Ignatia 6c*
- Woman often irritable, prone to dull, dizzy, bruising headaches which are rather like being beaten around the head, worse first thing in morning but better when person gets up *Nux 6c*
- Pressing, bruising headache associated with fatigue, made worse by reading, alleviated by rest *Ruta 6c*

Specific remedies for hangovers, to be taken hourly for up to 6 doses, with copious glasses of water between doses (where headache is main feature, see also ALCOHOLISM):

- For the proverbial 'bear with a sore head' who wants to be left alone *Chamomilla 6c*
- Head feels super-sensitive, mind in overdrive, tea and coffee make things worse *Coffea 6c*
- Head aches as if it has been beaten, feeling dull, dizzy, and irritable *Nux 6c*
- Feeling weepy and miserable, hangover due to rich food as well as alcohol *Pulsatilla 6c*

Self-help
If taking supplements of vitamin A, stop them for a while and see if the headaches stop – overdosing with vitamin A does occasionally cause headaches. Take extra vitamin B_3 and potassium for a while. Osteopathy, in particular cranial manipulation, would be well worth trying.

Hormone imbalances
Hypothalamus, pituitary, and ovaries carry out a delicate balancing act in order to maintain fertility, nourish new life, and ensure that body chemistry is biased towards femaleness; if balance is upset, ovulation and periods are the first processes to go awry (see MENSTRUAL PROBLEMS). Function of hypothalamus can be disturbed by severe illness, by drastic weight changes, by STRESS and very strong emotions, and by coming off the Pill; these in turn affect function of pituitary, although most common cause of pituitary malfunction is a tumour; underproduction of FSH (follicle stimulating hormone) or LH (luteinizing hormone) by pituitary can affect oestrogen- and progestogen-producing activities of ovaries, although OVARIAN CYSTS and CANCER OF THE OVARY can have similar effects; low oestrogen levels mean that testosterone (male hormone) produced by adrenal glands exerts greater influence, perhaps resulting in spotty skin, more facial and body hair, a deeper voice, and weight gain (see WEIGHT PROBLEMS). If you have any of these symptoms, and also have period problems or are approaching the MENOPAUSE, see your GP. Homeopathic treatment is constitutional.

Hyperventilation
Caused by rapid and irregular breathing which fails to push air deep into the lungs where gaseous exchange takes place. The stomach muscles as well as the diaphragm should be used. Excessive loss of carbon dioxide causes body fluids to become alkaline, increasing excitability of nerves, causing tingling sensations in arms and legs and sometimes tetany (muscles go into spasm, beginning with those of forearm and face). Some experts believe that this is the mechanism responsible for palpitations, angina-type chest pains, dizziness, ALLERGY, phobic symptoms (see PHOBIA), and anxiety attacks.

Chronic shallow breathing is associated with a combination of fatigue and over-arousal (lack of sleep plus stress, for example); it may also stem from organic problems in the brain (after a stroke, for example), diabetes, kidney failure or in the lungs themselves (see CHRONIC FATIGUE SYNDROME).

Chronic hyperventilation is diagnosed by a 3-minute provocation test. Acute attacks are a reaction to emotional or physical trauma (childbirth, being in an accident, receiving bad news, etc.).

In an acute attack, breathe into a paper bag (this helps to re-establish acid-alkaline balance of blood) and take Aconite 30c every 5 minutes for up to 6 doses.

Chronic hyperventilation requires constitutional homeopathic treatment, attention to sleep patterns, and measures to improve breathing and reduce stress.

Hypoglycaemia
Low level of glucose in blood, causing a variety of symptoms in different people; these include sweating, dizziness, trembling, weakness, hunger, slurred speech, blurred vision, tingling in hands or lips, HEADACHE, irritability, aggressiveness, even unconsciousness. All body cells, especially those in the brain, require energy in the form of glucose to function properly, hence the variety of symptoms. Blood glucose level can be lowered by alcohol, paracetamol, progesterone, and oral contraceptives; Addison's disease, hypopituitarism, THYROID PROBLEMS, and cancer of the pancreas can also lead to low glucose levels; more commonly, low blood sugar is a symptom of taking too much insulin to correct insulin-dependent diabetes or of overdosing with hypoglycaemic drugs to correct insulin non-dependent diabetes. In emergencies, orthodox

treatment is to give an injection of glucagon (a pancreatic hormone which stimulates liver to release stored glucose) or of glucose; a spoonful of honey or a small glass of milk will boost blood sugar level almost as quickly. However, long-term solution is dietary (see Self-help below), plus treatment of the underlying cause.

Naturopaths, most homeopaths, and a few GPs also recognize a phenomenon called *spontaneous, functional,* or *reactive hypoglycaemia* in which none of the causative factors mentioned above is present, blood sugar level appears to be normal, yet the woman suffers from typically hypoglycaemic symptoms. In addition to those mentioned above, the person may suffer from confusion, forgetfulness, lack of concentration, DEPRESSION, purposelessness, anxiety, PHOBIA, or think and behave in a suicidal or anti-social way; on the physical plane, headaches, dizziness, numbness, staggering, fainting or blackout, twitching of muscles, convulsions, fatigue, bloating, abdominal spasm, muscle and joint pain, backache, colitis and cold sweats. These symptoms often manifest themselves before breakfast, 2 hours after exercise or emotional stress. They are always of sudden onset. One possible explanation of this form of hypoglycaemia is that although blood glucose level may be normal, the level of glucose in brain may be low. Symptoms seem to be helped by eating foods which have a relatively low glycaemic index (low rate of conversion into glucose); these are precisely the foods recommended in the BLOOD SUGAR LEVELLING DIET on pp. 265–6. Causes of reactive hypoglycaemia appear to be STRESS, excessive consumption of caffeine or refined carbohydrates, food ALLERGY, and smoking.

Hypoglycaemia is conventionally diagnosed by an extended glucose tolerance test over 5 hours. Fasting blood samples are taken first thing in the morning, followed by a sugar load. Blood samples are then taken at half-hourly intervals for 5 hours. Hypoglycaemia is diagnosed if the blood sugar level falls below a certain level, or if the rate of decline is very sharp. The authors believe that even with this test the results can be normal for 2 reasons. Firstly the dips in blood sugar can occur quite suddenly, and be remedied equally suddenly due to release of stores of sugar from the liver. Unless the blood test is actually taken at the time of the drop in blood sugar therefore, it will not show up. Secondly, many people may become hypoglycaemic under conditions of stress or exercise. The glucose tolerance test, however, is done under laboratory conditions, with the patient usually seated in the waiting room reading magazines, which is stressful neither from a mental nor a physical point of view. The authors therefore consider that the change in diet (see BLOOD SUGAR LEVELLING DIET p. 265), should be used as a diagnosis as well as a treatment, although we recognize that benefit could also be psychological.

See PRE-MENSTRUAL SYNDROME for effects of oestrogen and progesterone on blood sugar.

Homeopathic treatment for both true and functional hypoglycaemia is constitutional.

Self-help

If you are prone to hypoglycaemic attacks, make sure your family and work colleagues know what to do if you pass out. Always carry glucose tablets or barley sugar, but keep these strictly for emergencies. Make sure you eat something every 2 hours or so, especially before strenuous exercise, and stick to those foods permitted under the BLOOD SUGAR LEVELLING DIET. Take extra vitamin C and B complex, and also chromium, magnesium, potassium, zinc and manganese. Get a full 8 hours sleep a night, avoid getting overtired, and exercise regularly, slowly increasing exercise periods.

Hysterectomy

Surgical removal of uterus and cervix, and sometimes Fallopian tubes and ovaries as well, through horizontal incision ('bikini incision') in lower abdomen or through the vagina; convalescence can take up to 2 months, depending on age and general state of health. It is not uncommon after hysterectomy for some women to experience a temporary depression. This is a natural reaction to the feeling of loss of a very important part of you, and the loss of potential for having more children. Don't try to put a brave face on it. Find someone to talk to, and don't be afraid to break down and cry. Once vaginal and lower abdominal scars have healed, intercourse can be resumed and sexual enjoyment and the ability to have orgasm should not be impaired. You will then be able to enjoy intercourse without the hassle of contraception or periods. A word of warning, however. You may still have a cycle, due to fluctuating hormones, and experience the symptoms of PRE-MENSTRUAL SYNDROME, which may be difficult to recognize as there is no period at the end of it. Perversely, your ovaries may start to fail and you may go into an early MENOPAUSE.

Unfortunately, for CANCER OF THE UTERUS or CANCER OF THE OVARY, and for FIBROIDS which occupy space equivalent to that occupied by a 12-week-old foetus, hysterectomy may be the only effective treatment. However, an alternative operation is now being developed, which may lead to reduction in number of hysterectomies performed for HEAVY OR PAINFUL PERIODS. In all other cases, hysterectomy should be a last resort.

Homeopathic remedies below alleviate post-operative pain and promote healing.

Specific remedies to be taken after operation:

- Immediately after operation as soon as anaesthetic wears off *Arnica 30c* hourly for up to 3 doses, then every 12 hours for up to 5 days
- If healing is slow or there are complications *Staphisagria 6c* every 4 hours for up to 5 days

Irritable bladder (urge incontinence)

Sudden contraction of the bladder causing instant urge to pass urine regardless of time or place, often associated with STRESS INCONTINENCE (see CYSTITIS), or PROLAPSE OF THE UTERUS, in which the pelvic floor muscles are weak, or with urinary tract infections such as CYSTITIS (frequency, burning sensation on passing urine). Orthodox treatment depends on cause, but if nervous control is faulty drugs may be prescribed to suppress nervous impulses to bladder or relax bladder muscles.

For homeopathic treatment, look up whichever of the above conditions is most appropriate; if none of the remedies mentioned seems suitable, select one from the list below.

Specific remedies to be taken every 4 hours for up to 7 days:

- Great urge to pass urine but nothing comes, chilliness, irritability *Nux 6c*
- Non-stop urge to pass urine, straining produces only a few drops at a time, burning pain at neck of bladder and in urethra, especially in older women *Copaiva 6c*
- Involuntary passage of urine when coughing or sneezing *Causticum 6c*
- Involuntary passage of urine on sitting down, walking, coughing, or passing wind *Pulsatilla 6c*

Self-help

See STRESS INCONTINENCE or MENOPAUSE for exercises to strengthen pelvic floor muscles; nervous control of bladder muscles may also be improved by not instantly answering the urge to urinate, but holding on for as long as possible.

Irritable bowel syndrome (spastic colon)

Also known as functional or nervous diarrhoea, colon or vegetative neurosis, or mucous colitis; main symptoms are CONSTIPATION and DIARRHOEA, turn and turn about, occasional cramping pains in lower abdomen, and sometimes pain on defecating. Muscular contraction in the colon or ileum is uncoordinated and spasmodic, though not for any reason which can be detected by X-rays or endoscopy; causes are as likely to be psychological – family, marital, or work problems, cancer PHOBIA, in fact STRESS in general – as dietary. However, a low-fibre diet, or intolerance to wheat, corn, dairy products, citrus fruit, tea, coffee, apples, pears, and salads – in that order – is sometimes the culprit (see food ALLERGY). Less often, spasms can be triggered off by a bowel infection, bowel parasites (threadworms, tapeworms, amoebae, etc.), overgrowth of bowel flora, THRUSH (candidiasis), spinal maladjustment, or excessive use of laxatives. Twice as many women are affected as men.

The diagnosis is mainly made by excluding other conditions, but if the symptoms mentioned above are accompanied by persistent weight loss (see WEIGHT PROBLEMS), [48]; if there is also fever or blood in faeces, [12]. Prompt investigation is especially important in people over 50, if only to rule out CANCER. Anti-spasmodic drugs may be prescribed, and also a high-fibre diet (although bran may aggravate problems if there is intolerance to wheat).

The homeopathic approach to irritable bowel syndrome is constitutional, although the remedies given below may be tried first. The remedies listed under ABDOMINAL PAIN and DIARRHOEA would also be appropriate.

Specific remedies to be given 4 times daily for up to 14 days:

- Great flatulence, constipation alternating with diarrhoea, pain in upper left abdomen, mucus in stools, fluttery, tense feeling in stomach *Argentum nit. 6c*
- Burning pains in abdomen, great thirst, nausea and vomiting, woman also has cystitis *Cantharis 6c*
- Watery stools, tearing pains, and nausea made worse by smell of food *Colchicum 6c*
- Griping pains relieved by doubling up or pressing on abdomen, attack associated with or brought on by anger *Colocynth 6c*
- Constipation following acute emotional stress, e.g. death of a loved one *Ignatia 6c*

Self-help

If a particular food is suspect, eliminate it from your diet for 4 days, then reintroduce it and see if problems recur. If the results are inconclusive, consult a dietary therapist. If problem is due to a trapped spinal nerve, consult a physiotherapist, chiropractor, or osteopath.

If no other treatment is working try the LIVER DIET (p. 264) and COLON CLEANSE (p. 267) for 1 month.

Mastitis

see BREAST PROBLEMS

Migraine

Occasional severe headaches usually confined to one side of the head, associated with nausea and vomiting, blurred vision and other visual disturbances, intolerance to light and occasionally numbness and tingling in the arms. In a severe attack the only thing to do is lie in a darkened room until symptoms wear off. In 1 out of 4 cases attacks are heralded by an 'aura' which consists of abnormal tiredness, nausea, and flashing, shimmering or distortion of objects in the visual field; speech disturbance or pins and needles all over the body; once a headache comes on these symptoms seem to disappear.

The major cause of migraine headaches is constriction then swelling of the arteries which supply the brain, but why the arteries behave in this way is not known. It is thought that a chemical substance is released into the bloodstream which may affect them. Trigger factors for this include STRESS, HYPOGLYCAEMIA, VDUs, lack of exercise, FATIGUE, high blood pressure, hot baths, travel, dental, eye, sinus or jaw problems. Migraines are often aggravated by oral contraceptives, but alleviated in pregnancy. This miserable complaint affects 1 person in 12, of which two thirds are women. Most often worse around period time. Frequency of the attacks tends to tail off in middle age, although they may worsen during the menopause.

Taken early enough, vasoconstrictors, antihistamines, and anti-emetics can minimize the symptoms of an attack; alternatively, combinations of anti-hypertensives, tranquillizers and anti-depressants can be taken on a permanent basis to prevent attacks. A few hospitals offer biofeedback treatment, in which sufferers are trained to control their blood pressure and body temperature by relaxation. Osteopathy, in particular cranial manipulation, may also offer relief.

A dental check-up is also worthwhile, as migraines may be due to grinding teeth at night, misplaced, worn or missing teeth, or gum disease leading to non-alignment of the jaw; the latter causes spasm of the neck and face muscles during sleep, especially when patient is tired or stressed, causing her to wake with a severe headache. One hospital has been experimenting with stroboscopic goggles which seem to give relief in an actual attack.

Homeopathic treatment of migraine is constitutional; however, the remedies listed below are recommended for use in emergencies.

Specific remedies to be taken ¼-hourly for up to 10 doses, if possible at the first signs of an attack:

- Blurring of vision before headache comes on, tight feeling in scalp, headache right-sided but less insistent if woman moves around, vomit mostly bile *Iris 6c*
- Headache worse on right side, feels as if temples are being screwed into each other, trying to concentrate makes pain worse, dizziness *Lycopodium 6c*
- Throbbing, blinding headache, warmth and moving around make headache worse, head feels overstuffed and congested, attack preceded by numbness and tingling in lips, nose, and tongue *Natrum mur. 6c*
- Headache worse in evening or during a period, aggravated by rich, fatty food, head feels as if it is about to burst, woman easily bursts into tears *Pulsatilla 6c*
- Headache worse in morning, bursting pain which is right-sided and seems to start at back of head, with pain extending into right shoulder, some improvement later in day *Sanguinaria 6c*
- Pain starts at back of head, then shifts and settles above one eye, aggravated by cold, alleviated by wrapping head up warmly and tightly, woman prone to head sweats *Silicea 6c*
- Sharp, darting, severe pain over left eye, pain seems to pulse with every heartbeat, stooping or moving suddenly makes pain worse *Spigelia 6c*
- Left-sided headache, as if head is being pierced by a nail *Thuja 6c*

Self-help

In addition to avoiding stress, tension, and tiredness, and learning some form of relaxation or meditation, try eliminating certain foods from your diet and then reintroducing them, to see what effect they have. Foods known to trigger off migraines are, in order of their attack-producing potential: chocolate (and other forms of concentrated sugar), cheese and dairy products, citrus fruit, alcohol (especially red wine), greasy fried foods, some vegetables (especially onions, broad beans, and sauerkraut), tea, coffee, cocoa, and cola (all of which contain caffeine), wheat and yeast extracts, meat (especially pork, liver, sausages, and cured meats such as bacon and salami), and shellfish. Stay off these, one at a time, for about 4 weeks, then reintroduce them. Alternatively, consult a dietary therapist; he or she may be able to help you pinpoint the offending food more quickly.

Food additives – notably E101, E210-219, E321, and E621 – can also act as migraine triggers, as can smoking, perfumes, and some oral contraceptives. Excessive TV watching is not a good idea either.

Positive measures include taking extra vitamin B_6, C, and E, and also evening primrose oil, and also adding fresh root ginger to cooking.

Some sufferers swear by the herb feverfew, but in the opinion of the authors it should only be taken on a 5 days out of 7 basis, and then only if constitutional treatment is not working; feverfew can cause griping abdominal pain, heavier than normal periods, mouth ulcers, and swelling of the tongue if taken too enthusiastically.

If you sense an attack coming on, splash your face with cold water for a few minutes, then lie down somewhere quiet for an hour or so; for some sufferers this has the effect of fending off an attack altogether. For more information about research and treatment write to the Migraine Trust (address p. 334).

Nipple problems
see BREAST PROBLEMS

Osteoarthritis (osteoarthrosis)

With age, injury, or overuse, cartilage covering articulating surfaces of bones breaks down; underlying bone becomes thickened and distorted, restricting joint movement and sometimes causing episodes of inflammation, pain, and swelling; joints most commonly affected are the load-bearing ones – hips, knees, and spine; 90 per cent of people over 40 have some degree of osteoarthritis in one or more joints. Condition can be aggravated by being overweight, by an over-acid diet, and by laxative abuse. Conventional treatments include painkillers, anti-inflammatory drugs, steroid injections into joints, physiotherapy to prevent muscles wasting, and replacement of worn joints, especially hips, with artificial ones; hip replacements have a high success rate, but may themselves have to be replaced within about 20–30 years.

Homeopathy offers constitutional treatment if osteoarthritis is chronic, but for isolated flare-ups the remedies below should be tried; if they do not improve matters, consult your GP or homeopath. Many sufferers get great benefit from osteopathy, chiropractic and physiotherapy, naturopathy and acupuncture.

Specific remedies to be taken 4 times daily for up to 2 weeks:

- Pain relieved by heat but aggravated by cold and damp, more insistent when resting but wears off with continued movement, stiffness worse in morning Rhus tox. 6c
- Severe pain, made worse by heat and movement, relieved by cold applications Bryonia 30c
- Heat and warm rooms make joint pains worse, feeling weepy Pulsatilla 6c
- Affected joints feel cold and numb, pain and stiffness increase when weather changes, weakness on climbing stairs Calcarea phos. 6c

- For after-effects of steroid injections, or for small joints, especially toes, which give pain and make cracking noises, joint pains seem to progress up the body, pain relieved by cold applications Ledum 6c
- Joint pains a consequence of, or made worse by, injury Arnica 30c
- Severe flare-up in cold dry weather Aconite 30c

Self-help

Two-thirds of osteoarthritis sufferers find the Alkalinizing Diet (see p. 262) beneficial; stick strictly to the diet for 1 month, and see if it helps you. Take some of the weight off your joints by using a stick or by losing weight. Sleep on a firm bed and take several short rest periods during the day. Don't give up on exercise – your muscles need regular exercise to keep them strong. If you are severely disabled, contact the Disabled Living Foundation (address p. 335) for information on special equipment – long-handled dustpans, retrieving sticks, electrical plugs with handles on them, etc. Some sufferers say that green lipped mussel extract, devil's claw, and extra vitamin B_5 help. Vitamins A, B, C and E, and also iron, zinc, copper, selenium, and manganese would certainly be beneficial.

Ovarian cysts
see also CANCER OF THE OVARY

Fluid-filled outgrowths of tissue which develop on or near ovaries; often symptomless unless large enough to press on bladder or cause visible swelling in lower abdomen or pain on intercourse; if production of ovarian hormones is affected (see HORMONE IMBALANCES), menstrual cycle may become irregular, but this is rare; risk of cancerous change is small, the greater risk being peritonitis (sudden, severe abdominal pain, nausea, fever, abdominal distension) if cyst bursts. Where possible, especially in younger women, cyst is removed without damaging ovary; in other cases removal of ovary and Fallopian tube may be advised. Constitutional homeopathic treatment is usually required, but the remedies given below may be of some benefit.

Specific remedies to be taken 4 times daily for up to 14 days:

- Left ovary affected, local pain which is worse in morning but wears off during period Lachesis 6c
- Lower abdominal pain which feels like a wedge being driven through ovary and womb Iodum 6c
- Right ovary affected, sore, stinging pains locally, painful periods with tenderness in lower abdomen Apis 6c

- Small, round cysts which cause pain which seems to bore through lower abdomen, bending double and pressing fists into abdomen gives some relief *Colocynth 6c*

Ovulation pain

Ovulation occurs, on average, 12–14 days before onset of menstruation, but it is an event of which many women are unaware, unless they practise natural contraception; some women, however, experience what is called 'mittelschmerz', lower ABDOMINAL PAIN which is more localized and qualitatively different from period pain. If the homeopathic remedies below prove ineffective, see your homeopath; if pain is part of a wider picture, constitutional treatment may be recommended.

Specific remedies to be taken every hour for up to 10 doses:

- Nervy pains, relieved by warmth, by bending double, or by pressing fists into lower abdomen, often worse on left side, and often associated with anger *Colocynth 6c*
- Violent, cramping pains, worse on left side, ovary feels as if it is being dragged up towards heart *Naja 6c*
- Right-sided pain, worse between 4 and 8 am, constipation and wind, apprehensiveness *Lycopodium 6c*
- Right-sided pain which shoots up to breast, alleviated by pressure, abdomen feels bloated *Palladium 6c*

Pain in lower abdomen

Menstrual pain occurs just before and during first 2 or 3 days of period, with lower abdominal pain often accompanied by dull, aching pain in small of back (see painful periods – MENSTRUAL PROBLEMS). Pain due to PELVIC INFECTION is sometimes accompanied by heavy, unpleasant discharge from vagina. Burning or scalding pain while urinating suggests CYSTITIS. OVARIAN CYSTS and CANCER OF THE OVARY can also cause lower abdominal pain. If pain occurs during sexual intercourse, possible cause may be FIBROIDS, ENDOMETRIOSIS, or RETROVERSION OF THE UTERUS. Severe pain and abnormal bleeding from vagina suggests ECTOPIC PREGNANCY.

Some women who suffer from unexplained pelvic pains may have abnormally wide and congested veins in the pelvis. This could be a result of ovaries producing too much oestrogen, probably due to emotional stress – caused by problems at home or at work – or due to stressful backgrounds going back to childhood. The stress reflects through the hypothalamus and pituitary gland to stimulate the ovaries. If this is the case try relaxation techniques. For other causes, see ABDOMINAL PAIN, p. 211.

Pelvic infection [also known as salpingitis, pelvic inflammatory disease or PID]

Acute or chronic infection of uterus, Fallopian tubes, ovaries, or surrounding tissue by germs which enter through vagina, especially during intercourse, although sometimes infection follows abortion (see TERMINATION), MISCARRIAGE, or fitting of an IUD. For unknown reasons, the Pill appears to protect against PID. Condition is related to frequency of intercourse, and is most common in younger women. Symptoms include early or heavy periods (see MENSTRUAL PROBLEMS), profuse and smelly vaginal discharge between periods (see VAGINAL AND VULVAL PROBLEMS), PAINFUL INTERCOURSE, and PAIN IN LOWER ABDOMEN; if infection is acute, pain is likely to be severe and persistent, and temperature higher than normal. Early treatment is essential, since infection can lead to abscess formation, peritonitis, and even blood poisoning; INFERTILITY is also a risk if delicate membranes of reproductive tract become scarred. This may occur without other symptoms (see CHLAMYDIA). Routinely treated with antibiotics and, if necessary, painkillers.

Homeopathic treatment is constitutional, designed to boost general resistance to infection; in acute cases, specific remedies given below should relieve pain and inflammation, but if there is no improvement within 24 hours or if temperature suddenly rises, see your GP.

Specific remedies to be taken every 2 hours for up to 10 doses in acute cases:

- Sudden onset, mild fever, anxiety, symptoms aggravated by emotional shock or exposure to cold *Aconite 30c*
- Stinging, burning pains, mainly on right side of abdomen, lack of thirst *Apis 30c*
- Sudden onset, severe abdominal pain made worse by slightest jarring, face bright red and burning hot *Belladonna 30c*
- Cramping pains, relieved by doubling up and pressing fists hard into abdomen *Colocynth 6c*
- Alternate chills and sweats, sweat smells unpleasant, rest makes you feel better *Mercurius corr. 6c*

Self-help

Rest in bed until symptoms wear off, and refrain from intercourse for 4 weeks. Take a multivitamin and mineral and extra zinc (see NUTRITIONAL SUPPLEMENTS).

Polycystic ovary syndrome

also known as Stein-Leventhal Syndrome

(see OVARIAN CYSTS)

Due to a hormone imbalance, resulting in periods becoming very light or absent altogether. Affected women may become abnormally hairy and over-weight, and infertile, because ovulation no longer occurs. There are usually numerous ovarian cysts which can be seen on ultrasound.

Homeopathic treatment is constitutional. In the meantime, if there is a strong craving for sweets and sudden drops in energy, try the BLOOD SUGAR LEVELLING DIET for 1 month.

Prolapse of the uterus or vagina

Occurs when ligaments and muscles which hold uterus and vagina in place become weak or slack with age or as a result of childbirth, allowing the uterus to bulge into vagina and press on bladder or rectum; this causes a heavy, uncomfortable feel-ing in lower abdomen generally, backache, STRESS INCONTINENCE or difficulty emptying bladder, or straining and discomfort when passing stools. If prolapse is complete, a large part of the vagina or uterus may actually protrude through the vaginal opening, causing soreness or ulceration and encouraging infection. Surgery to tighten pelvic floor may be necessary if exercises do not restore muscle tone; a ring pessary, fitted behind pubic bone, may be advised if person is elderly. If symptoms are not too severe, homeopathic remedies below may be of benefit; if there is no improvement within a week or two, see your homeopath.

Specific remedies to be taken 4 times daily for up to 14 days:

- Dragging sensation in lower abdomen, made worse by doing jobs which involve bending or lifting, scanty periods, pain on intercourse, depression *Sepia 6c*
- Vagina very hot and dry, pain in lower back, leaden feeling in abdomen and just below ribs, as if abdominal and pelvic contents are about to drop out *Belladonna 6c*
- Sharp spasms of pain, constant urge to pass urine or stool, irritability *Nux 6c*
- Sensation of downward pressure in lower abdomen, pain in small of back, nausea, weepi-ness, heat and periods make symptoms worse *Pulsatilla 6c*
- Nervousness, irritability, pain and tenderness in lower abdomen, bladder affected, urgent desire to pass stool, itchy vulva which feels as if it needs external support, rest alleviates symptoms *Lilium 6c*

Self-help

To strengthen muscles of pelvic floor, try stopping and starting flow of urine several times each time you urinate; this may be difficult at first, but persevere (see Pelvic Floor Exercises under MENOPAUSE). These exercises are a vital part of orthodox and homeopathic treatment, and particularly important after childbirth. If you are heavier than you should be, try to lose weight.

Pruritis ani

Intractable itching around the opening of the anus. External causes include excessive sweating due to wearing woollen or nylon knickers or tights, lack of cleanliness, irritants in washing powders and possibly in coloured toilet paper, and liquid paraffin used to relieve constipation; discharge from PILES, an anal fissure or anal fistula, or from the vagina can also cause it, and so can diabetes (diabetes mellitus), THRUSH, thread-worms, and DIARRHOEA (particularly in children with alactasia, in which milk sugars cannot be digested). Other causes include citrus fruit and sugar and cigarette smoking, or the itching may have a psychological component.

Specific remedies to be taken 4 times daily for up to 14 days:

- Itchiness of vulva which seems to get worse in company *Ambra 6c*
- Violent itching and a crawling sensation around anus, made worse by warmth *Ignatia 6c*
- Itching worse when walking outdoors or after passing stool *Nitric ac. 6c*
- Itching feels like lots of pin pricks, burning sensation in anus, stools soft but passed with difficulty *Alumina 6c*
- Itching due to threadworms, continuous irrita-tion, especially on going to bed, restlessness, crawling sensation in rectum after passing stool *Teucrium 6c*
- Where sufferer is a girl who takes unreasonable hatreds to people, itching worse at night, grinding of teeth in sleep *Cina 6c*
- Itchiness and smarting worse at night, alter-nate constipation and diarrhoea, especially if woman is elderly, mucous discharge from anus, heat, wine, acid foods, and water make itching worse *Antimonium 6c*
- Anal area red and sore, burning diarrhoea worse in morning *Sulphur 6c*

Self-help

Try not to scratch – this only damages the skin and makes it easier for particles of faeces to cause further irritation – and wear cotton underwear. Do not use toilet paper. First thing in the morning and last thing at night, and after passing stool, wash anal area with warm soapy water, rinse with clean warm water, and pat dry with a towel reserved for the purpose. Then rinse your hands and apply Hamamelis ointment, or Wheatgerm oil.

Pruritis vulvae
see VAGINAL AND VULVAL PROBLEMS

Retroversion of the uterus
In 20 per cent of women the uterus lies close to rectum rather than just behind bladder; this is perfectly natural, and has no effect on conception, carrying a baby, or giving birth, but a few women experience backache because of it, especially during periods, or find that deep penetration during intercourse causes pain because the penis strikes an ovary (see PAINFUL INTERCOURSE). Uterus can be repositioned temporarily by inserting a device called a ring pessary into the vagina, or permanently by an operation called a ventro-suspension. See PAINFUL INTERCOURSE for suitable homeopathic remedies.

Self-help
Try different love-making positions so that penetration is shallower.

Sleep problems
The purpose of sleep is not fully understood; certainly lack of sleep, especially of dreaming sleep, leads to lapses in concentration, irritability, irrationality, hallucinations, and even death. Though sleep seems to be essential to the brain, it seems less so to the body. What sends us to sleep is also a puzzle; it could be a decrease in oxygen supply to the brain, a decrease in sensory input to the brain, fluctuation of certain chemicals in the brain, or simply a conditioned response. Most adults need 7–8 hours sleep, even as we get older. With increasing age we tend to sleep for less time and go into less of a deep pattern, tending to have more disturbed nights.

Insomnia is not a single night or even several nights of disturbed sleep, but a persistent pattern of short-sleeping which leaves the sufferer feeling unrested, worn out, and ragged round the edges. Most people who complain of insomnia do in fact get some sleep, but clearly not enough. Insomnia can be due to physical problems such as breathlessness brought on by heart or lung disease, discomfort during pregnancy, or having to get up during the night to pass urine; or the cause may be too many late meals, too much caffeine, a food ALLERGY, over-indulgence in alcohol or drugs, or something as simple as an airless or overheated bedroom. More often the causes are emotional – anxiety caused by pres-

sure of work or financial problems, DEPRESSION, GRIEF, too much excitement. Coming off sleeping pills or tranquillizers can also cause insomnia. In fact one of the commonest causes of insomnia is fear of not being able to sleep. The drugs most commonly used to treat insomnia today are the benzodiazepines, which have a sedative, anti-anxiety, muscle relaxing action; they also have side-effects, and may interact with alcohol. People tend to develop a tolerance after between 3 and 14 days of continuous use, and they may lead to falls in old people.

Menopausal women tend to have long sleeps. This is restless sleep, however, and is associated with daytime sleepiness and general lack of energy. A small proportion of people have never slept well since childhood (see SLEEP PROBLEMS IN CHILDREN).

Other sleep disorders include nightmares, night terrors, sleepwalking, sleep-talking, rocking, head banging, grinding teeth, paralysed wakefulness, restless legs (a creeping sensation under the skin of the legs, or twitching of the leg muscles, which disturbs sleep but does not necessarily cause the person to wake), and disturbed breathing (breathing may cease for anything from 10 seconds to 3 minutes, occurring perhaps hundreds of times a night, followed by snorts or gasps for breath, during which the person partially wakes).

Nightmares and night terrors are more common in children than adults, possibly because adults have developed other mechanisms for coping with anxiety than insomnia; during a nightmare heart rate climbs from about 64 beats per minute to 80, or during a night terror to 150, often causing the person to wake up; as well as being manifestations of anxiety, bad dreams can be a symptom of mental exhaustion, fever, over-indulgence in food or alcohol, withdrawal from sleeping tablets, or a side-effect of certain prescription drugs.

Sleepwalking, sleep-talking, and making repetitive movements during sleep are also less common in adults than children. The muscles and senses concerned are, as it were, on automatic pilot, the person's conscious mind not being involved; she has no memory of the night's activities. Psychologists believe that dissociation of behaviour from consciousness is an attempt to resolve conflict. Interestingly, this kind of behaviour does not occur during dreaming, when all muscle movements, except those around the eyes, are inhibited. The important thing is to prevent the person concerned from coming to harm.

Paralysed wakefulness is an unpleasant state in which the person is awake but cannot move; it most often occurs, very briefly, on waking, but is not a cause for worry.

Chronic sleep problems require constitutional treatment, but in the short-term the remedies below may help. If no improvement is discernible within 3 weeks, consult your GP or homeopath.

Specific remedies to be taken 1 hour before going to bed for 10 nights running; repeat dose if woken by a nightmare or if you wake and cannot get to sleep again:

- Mind overactive as the result of good or bad news, inability to switch off *Coffea 30c*
- Sleeplessness due to great mental strain, over-indulgence in food or alcohol, or withdrawal from alcohol or sleeping tablets, woman wakes around 3 or 4 am then falls asleep just as it is time to get up, has nightmares, is irritable during day *Nux 30c*
- Woman restless in first sleep, feels too hot and throws covers off, then feels too cold and lies with arms above head, not thirsty, insomnia worse after rich food *Pulsatilla 30c*
- Sleep problems worse after shock or panic, restlessness, nightmares, fear of dying *Aconite 30c*
- Feeling wide awake and irritable during first part of night, especially if person is a child and wants to be carried around *Chamomilla 30c*
- Mind very active at bedtime, going over and over work done during day, woman aware of dreaming a lot, talks and laughs in sleep, wakes around 4 am *Lycopodium 30c*
- Woman used to being up at night, perhaps looking after an invalid, feels too tired to sleep, giddy, irritable *Cocculus 30c*
- Woman yawns a lot but cannot sleep, dreads not being able to sleep, especially after emotional upset; when sleep comes nightmares come too *Ignatia 30c*
- Bed feels too hard, woman over-tired, fidgety, dreams of being chased by animals *Arnica 30c*
- Feeling sleepy but unable to get to sleep, senses feel so sharp a fly can be heard walking on the wall, bed too hot, or else sleep comes but is so heavy that the person snores and cannot be roused *Opium 30c*
- Waking between midnight and 2 am, restless, worried, apprehensive, foreboding dreams of fire or danger *Arsenicum 30c*
- Woman cannot sleep, is irritable, restless and walks about, especially if there is pain or discomfort *Rhus tox. 30c*
- Dreams about dying, hunger, or problems at work, descent into profound depression *Aurum 30c*

Self-help

Insomnia is one ailment that can be very successfully tackled by self-help methods. Try whichever of the following measures seem most appropriate.

1 Stop working an hour before bedtime and read something light.
2 Take more exercise, preferably earlier in the day.
3 Avoid meals late at night and eat at the same times each day to establish body rhythms.
4 As a bedtime drink, try a herbal infusion (chamomile, valerian, passionflower, skullcap) or a hot milky drink which contains tryptophan (thought to help sleep); but avoid cocoa, tea, and coffee, and over-the-counter sleep remedies.
5 Take a warm bath.
6 Sexual release has a tension-reducing effect.
7 Learn some form of relaxation or meditation.
8 Don't lie tossing and turning if you cannot get to sleep; switch the light on and read, or do the ironing, then go back to sleep; resist tea, coffee, and other stimulants.
9 If you are over-tired when you go to bed, take an afternoon nap (no longer than 15 minutes) to try to break the cycle, and go to bed 15 minutes earlier every second or third night until you go into a deeper pattern of sleep and get off to sleep quickly. Use some relaxation or meditation techniques at least twice daily.
10 Get your partner to give you a massage.
11 Wake up at the same time each day.
12 Remove the clock from your bedroom.
13 Make sure the room is not too hot or too cold (15–19°C [59–66°F] is about right) and minimize noise and light.
14 Increase your intake of vitamin C, B$_1$, biotin, folate, and zinc, and if you are taking supplements of vitamin A reduce your intake. Also check for excess lead and copper in your diet or environment.

Stress incontinence

see also IRRITABLE BLADDER

A very common and embarrassing complaint, almost unique to women, in which small quantities of urine are involuntarily passed when coughing, sneezing, laughing, lifting things, etc. Because the muscles of the pelvic floor are weak – often as the result of childbirth, being overweight, or general loss of muscle tone after the menopause – the urethral sphincter does not close properly. If incontinence occurs frequently, ask your GP to refer you to a specialist for assessment; the options, depending on the severity of the problem, are pelvic floor exercises, wearing special briefs, or an operation to tighten the pelvic floor muscles. We have included specific remedies and self-help below; the latter will help if the problem occurs only once in a while.

Specific remedies to be taken 4 times daily for up to 3 weeks while waiting for specialist treatment:

- Problem made worse by coughing, laughing, sneezing, excitement, person unaware that leakage is occurring *Causticum 6c*
- Problem made worse by sitting down, walking, passing wind, desire to pass urine increases when lying down *Pulsatilla 6c*
- Problem worse during day, with tickling sensation in urethra and bladder, especially if sufferer has pale complexion *Ferrum 6c*
- Incontinence associated with 'bearing down' sensation, as if abdominal contents are escaping through vagina, stream of urine slow to start *Sepia 6c*

Self-help
The pelvic floor muscles can be strengthened by alternately tightening and relaxing them as you urinate, so that stream of urine stops and starts, and stops and starts, or by tightening the muscles around the anus, as if controlling the passage of a stool; this last exercise can be done sitting or standing, reading the paper or waiting for a bus! If you are overweight, try to lose weight; this will relieve some of the downward pressure of the abdominal organs on the bladder and pelvic floor. See also exercise in MENOPAUSE.

Tenosynovitis (repetitive strain injury or RSI)

RSI used to be associated with assembly lines, food packaging, sewing and tennis ball production, for instance. It is now affecting computer keyboard users because computers can be used so much faster than the ordinary typewriter keyboard; an additional problem is that the same keying action is constantly repeated, without a break for other movements as with a typewriter. It has become well publicized for the very good reason that journalists are one of the main professions affected. However, the people most typically affected by it are low-paid, easily replaced women involved in companies who provide key-to-disk and key-to-tape services, whereby data is typed in via computer to a storage medium, the faster the better. The risk of getting tenosynovitis is increased by stress. It appears that provided the number of key strokes employed is under 10,000 an hour (or about 1,600 words an hour) the risk of RSI drops off significantly.

Among the dos and don'ts given by the Repetitive Strain Association (see Useful Addresses), are:

1 If you develop RSI, don't rush back to work and resume the activity that caused it to happen in the first place; make sure it is gone completely.
2 Do not aggravate the condition by continuing to perform the tasks that caused it.
3 Do not accept conditions or relate your pay to key stroke work rates or incentive bonuses to maximize output.
4 Do not bend the hands upwards or overstretch your fingers; do not over-practise if you are a musician, or rush back to your instrument before the symptoms have disappeared.
5 Be careful about using drugs, having cortisone injections and strenuous physiotherapy, although hydrotherapy can be helpful.

Remember that the only known cure for RSI is rest; splints may be used as a last resort, but should be custom-made.

Specific remedies to be taken every 2 hours for up to 10 doses in acute cases:

- Affected fingers hot and swollen, with stinging pains *Apis 30c*
- Condition caused by injury *Arnica 30c* followed by *Ruta 6c*
- Slightest movement makes fingers hurt *Bryonia 30c*
- Affected fingers swollen, movement more painful after rest and in cold damp weather, eased by warmth and gentle movement *Rhus tox. 6c*

Specific remedy to be taken 4 times daily for up to 14 days if condition is chronic; if no improvement within 14 days, see your GP or homeopath:

- *Causticum 6c*

Self-help
Pay close attention to the design of any keyboard you are asked to use. Desks and chairs should provide an appropriate comfortable posture. In addition we recommend ensuring that keying is limited to 4 hours a day, and that the lighting for your working environment is correct. These questions should be taken up with your employer. Try learning the Alexander Technique. We also suggest that you get a copy of 'Tackling Teno' from the GMB trade union.

Thyroid problems
Under- or over-production of thyroid hormone (thyroxine) can slow down or speed up all chemical processes in the body.

Thyrotoxicosis
This thyroid problem (also referred to as hyperthyroidism, toxic goitre, or Graves' disease) occurs when the whole thyroid gland is overactive,

usually because the pituitary gland is producing too much thyroid stimulating hormone, or because there is a 'nodule' (a fluid-filled cyst, a small haemorrhage, or a benign or malignant growth) in part of it; a nodule may be visible as a lump at front of neck, general enlargement as a sizeable swelling. Large amounts of thyroxine are continuously produced and released into the bloodstream, causing a wide variety of symptoms: restlessness, a high level of anxiety, inability to relax or sleep properly (see SLEEP PROBLEMS), shakiness and poor control of fine hand movements, sweating, feeling hot even on cold days, rapid heart rate, palpitations, breathlessness, weight loss (see WEIGHT PROBLEMS) despite a ravenous appetite, DIARRHOEA, bulging eyes, etc. Accelerated metabolism places extra strain on heart, especially if person already has high blood pressure or arteriosclerosis, and increases risk of angina and heart failure. Orthodox treatment consists of anti-thyroid drugs, destruction of part of thyroid gland with radioactive iodine, or surgical removal of nodule or large part of gland; blood thyroxine levels must also be checked regularly to ensure that hypothyroidism (see below) does not set in. The homeopathic remedies below may help to bring acute symptoms under control; however, if condition dramatically worsens, 12 .

Specific remedies to be taken every hour for up to 10 doses:

- Woman who is obsessive, feels very hot, can't stop hurrying, especially if she is dark-haired and dark-eyed *Iodum 30c*
- Constipation, palpitations, earthy complexion *Natrum mur. 30c*
- Flushed face and staring eyes *Belladonna 30c*
- Heart pounding and racing, exophthalmos *Lycopus 30c*

Hypothyroidism

This is underactivity of the thyroid gland, due in some cases to lack of iodine in the diet or lack of thyroid stimulating hormone from the pituitary; in other cases thyroid defect may be congenital or gland may be missing altogether; in Hashimoto's disease, an autoimmune response develops which destroys thyroid tissue. In adults, the symptoms of low thyroxine production are tiredness, abnormal sleepiness or drowsiness, aches and pains, slow heart rate, CONSTIPATION, feeling cold most of the time, weight gain (see WEIGHT PROBLEMS) despite poor appetite, myxoedema (thick, dry, swollen skin), lifeless hair, deep or hoarse voice, loss of hearing, numbness and tingling in hands, and LACK OF DESIRE FOR SEX;

women tend to have heavy periods (see MENSTRUAL PROBLEMS). Babies who are hypothyroid are very torpid, uninterested in food, and may develop jaundice shortly after birth; since thyroxine is essential for growth and mental development, lack of it at this young age can cause cretinism and stunted growth.

Both adults and babies are treated with thyroxine tablets; most babies develop normally if treatment is started before age of 3 months. However, if hypothyroidism is mild, thyroid gland extract (which contains all the constituents of thyroid tissue, including thyroxine) may be preferable to thyroxine itself; if thyroid gland recovers, thyroid gland extract is more easily discontinued than thyroxine. Constitutional homeopathic treatment is recommended in addition to orthodox treatment.

Specific remedy to be taken every 12 hours for up to 5 days while constitutional treatment is being sought:

- *Arsenicum 30c*

Self-help Avoid thiourea-containing foods such as broccoli, cabbage, carrots, kale, peaches, peanuts, pears, soya beans, spinach and strawberries. Also general foods such as sugar, salt, red meat, eggs and fat.

Eat plenty of high iodine-containing foods such as kelp, dulse, algae, melons, beets, radishes, parsley, potato, fish and kidney beans. Use hot and cold showers and compresses to the thyroid area in the front of the neck – 90 seconds hot, 30 seconds cold.

Avoid electric blankets. Exercise regularly, and use the 'plough' Yoga technique unless you have a neck or back problem.

Toxic shock syndrome

This is a severe and sometimes fatal illness caused by a toxin in the bacterium staphylococcus aureus. It was first recognized in the late 1970s, and there were many cases in the early 80s. Most of these occurred in women using vaginal tampons of a particular brand, which have now been taken off the market. Other cases have been linked to the use of cap, diaphragm or sponge, but toxic shock can come from infection by the same organism in other places in the body. Symptoms are high fever, vomiting and DIARRHOEA, dizziness, disorientation, HEADACHE, muscular pains and rash resembling sunburn on the palms and soles which peels within 1 or 2 weeks. In more serious cases blood pressure can drop dramatically and shock develop. Other serious problems include kidney and liver failure. Although this condition is rare, women who have had it should never wear tampons, caps, diaphragms or sponges, and should treat wound infections promptly. If you suspect this condition ② and take Aconite 30c, 1 tablet every quarter hour.

Self-help

Avoid high absorbency tampons; change tampons every 4–6 hours; use towels and tampons alternately; use towels at night; remember to remove last tampon at end of period; never use tampons except when menstruating.

Toxoplasmosis

An infection caught from contact with faeces of dogs and cats; microorganism responsible is toxoplasma, which invades digestive and nervous system, and can affect developing foetus; in rare instances, infection can cause meningitis and hydrocephalus; more commonly, it causes vague ABDOMINAL PAIN and slightly swollen glands, or no symptoms at all. Your GP will prescribe a course of drugs to kill toxoplasma, but to boost general immunity constitutional homeopathic treatment is also recommended. It is estimated that 2 in every 2,000 pregnant women will contract a primary infection each year; 480 babies will be born infected.

Prevention Discourage pets from licking you, wash your hands thoroughly after grooming them, wash their eating utensils separately from your own, and always wash your hands before eating or preparing food. Do not allow children to play in parks or gardens fouled with faeces.

Trophoblastic tumours

Benign or malignant growths which develop in placental tissue, causing MISCARRIAGE, or in fragments of placenta remaining in uterus after abortion (see TERMINATION OF PREGNANCY) or CHILDBIRTH; symptoms are irregular bleeding and severe MORNING SICKNESS; diagnosis is by ultrasound scan and by checking urine for excessive levels of HCG (human chorionic gonadotrophic) hormone. Benign tumours, also known as hydatidiform moles, are rare, and malignant tumours extremely rare; the former are removed by D & C (scraping placental tissue out of womb), but the latter may require HYSTERECTOMY and chemotherapy. For homeopathic approach to malignancy, see CANCER. The remedies given below are for tumours diagnosed as benign; they offer symptom relief until a D & C can be arranged.

Specific remedies to be taken every 4 hours for up to 2 weeks:

- Where constitution is strong *Pulsatilla 6c*
- Where constitution is weak *Secale 6c*
- Penetrating pain from base of spine to pubic bone, shooting pains in vagina, bleeding, slightest movement makes symptoms worse *Sabina 6c*
- Where urination is painful *Cantharis 6c*

Vaginal and vulval problems

Best insurance against infection is to wash vulva daily with plain water – no soap or bath salts – and avoid vaginal deodorants and medicated douches. Underwear should be changed daily, and sanitary towels and tampons every 6 hours at least; towels are preferable to tampons if periods are heavy after childbirth or if CYSTITIS is a recurrent problem. Infections occur when acid environment of vagina and its population of healthy bacteria are disturbed – by antibiotics, deodorants, irritants in contraceptive creams, etc.

Bartholinitis

Acute infection of Bartholin's gland, which lies at entrance to vagina and secretes fluid which lubricates vagina during intercourse. Symptoms are extreme tenderness, followed by discharge of pus or formation of abscess; conventionally treated with antibiotics. If homeopathic remedies below do not improve matters, see your GP.

Specific remedies to be taken every 2 hours for up to 10 doses:

- Early stage of infection, entrance to vagina hot, red, and swollen *Belladonna 30c*
- Discharge of pus, extreme tenderness *Hepar sulph. 6c*
- Symptoms accompanied by fever and chill, feeling hot and cold by turns *Mercurius 6c*

Bartholin's cyst

Condition in which exit from Bartholin's gland (see above) becomes blocked, resulting in swelling and tenderness at entrance to vagina. If the homeopathic remedy below produces no improvement, see your GP; if surgical removal of gland is recommended, constitutional homeopathic treatment should be sought after the operation.

Specific remedy to be taken 4 times daily for up to 3 weeks:

- *Baryta carb. 6c*

Dryness of vagina

May be due to lack of foreplay before intercourse, to MENOPAUSE, or to HORMONAL IMBALANCES. See MENOPAUSE for suitable homeopathic remedies.

KY jelly, obtainable from chemist, is a safe lubricant.

Pruritis vulvae

Intense itching or irritation of whole vulval area due to skin problems generally (see ITCHING), HORMONAL IMBALANCES (especially in elderly women), anxiety about intercourse (especially in very young women), use of tampons, irritants in spermicidal creams, vaginal deodorants, talcum powder, traces of detergent in underwear, etc. Other contributory factors may be a lack of B vitamins, especially B_{12}, poor hygiene, excessive exercise or exertion, and spending too much time sitting down. Condition is not uncommon in diabetes, and can be an after-effect of rape. If slightly thickened, whitish patches of skin (leucoplakia) develop in itchy areas, see your GP; there is a very small risk of their becoming malignant (see CANCER OF THE VULVA). Where orthodox treatment relies on steroid creams, homeopathic medicine treats pruritis vulvae constitutionally; however, the specific remedies and self-help measures given below should be tried first.

Specific remedies to be taken 4 times daily for up to 14 days:

- Vulva itches, crotch very sweaty and smelly, matters made worse by heat and washing *Sulphur 6c*
- Increased desire for sex, creeping sensation in vulva which wears off during daytime naps but gets worse at night or when moving around *Caladium 6c*
- Labia visibly swollen, local veins distended *Carbo veg. 6c*
- Localized itching, skin very red, itching relieved by heat *Rhus tox. 6c*
- Itching aggravated by suppressed desire for sex or by frequent sex *Conium 6c*
- Itchiness worse immediately before and after period, general sweatiness and chilliness, especially if woman is overweight *Calcarea 6c*
- Itchiness soothed by hot baths and by moving around out of doors, most uncomfortable first thing in morning *Radium brom. 6c*

Self-help Try not to scratch. Apply Calendula and Urtica ointment to vulva 4 times a day, or bathe vulva with Thuja solution (10 drops of mother tincture to 0.25 litre [½ pint] boiled cooled water). For other local measures, see PRURITIS ANI. To reduce friction during intercourse, lubricate vagina with KY jelly (obtainable from chemist).

Trichomoniasis

Vaginal infection caused by single-celled trichomonas organism; symptoms are similar to those of THRUSH but vaginal discharge smells unpleasant and is usually copious and greenish. Conventionally treated with drugs such as metronidazole. For homeopathic remedies and self-help measures, see Unusual discharge (below).

Unusual discharge

Vagina and cervix are naturally wetter and more slippery around time of ovulation; at other times mucus secreted by walls of cervix is stickier and slightly cloudy. If vaginal discharge is due to THRUSH, it is thick, curdy, causes itching or intense soreness, but does not smell unpleasant; vaginal deodorants, medicated douches, antibiotics, oral contraceptives, and diabetes can produce similar symptoms. Trichomonas infection (see above) causes quite heavy greenish-yellow discharge which is irritant and smells unpleasant; if LOWER ABDOMINAL PAIN is present as well, this type of discharge suggests PELVIC INFECTION. Heavy, greyish discharge with an offensive smell to it suggests a bacterial infection called gardnerella.

Organisms responsible for genital infections flourish in damp, airless conditions, and are often transmitted by sexual intercourse (see SEXUALLY TRANSMITTED DISEASES), but self-infection is also common, especially if hygiene is poor (leaving tampons in too long, allowing caps to get dirty, inserting barrier devices or checking IUD threads with dirty fingers). Conventional medicine treats such infections with antifungal drugs or antibiotics, as appropriate.

If you suspect you have an infection, select a suitable homeopathic remedy from the list which follows, take it for up to 5 days, and at the same time implement the self-help measures described below; if discharge does not return to normal, see your homeopath or GP.

Specific remedies to be taken 6 times daily for up to 5 days:

- Frequent, copious, straw-coloured discharge which causes vulva to itch and smart and stiffens underwear, itchiness relieved by washing in cold water, discharge worse before and after period *Alumina 6c*
- Discharge transparent like egg white and highly irritant, scalded feeling on inside of thighs *Borax 6c*
- Itchy, milky discharge which smells like rye bread, preceded by flushed face and pains in small of back, great weakness *Kreosotum 6c*

- Watery, cloudy discharge which causes smarting and soreness, worse before and after periods and when lying down *Pulsatilla 6c*
- Yellowish, smarting discharge, itchy vulva, sharp stinging sensation in uterus, walking adds to discomfort, abdomen distended, worse during day *Sepia 6c*
- Yellowish, burning discharge *Carbo an. 6c*
- Milky discharge which makes vulva itch, worse after passing urine and before periods *Calcarea 6c*
- Greenish discharge which smarts and stings, suspected trichomonas infection *Bovista 6c*
- Stinging discharge with foul smell, containing some solid matter, feeling chilly and sweaty by turns, trichomonas infection suspected *Mercurius 6c*
- Stringy mucus which is greenish or pinkish and more copious after period, trichomonas infection suspected *Nitric ac. 6c*
- Corrosive, greenish discharge, especially before period, trichomonas infection suspected *Carbo veg. 6c*
- White or yellowish discharge which burns and stings, cramping pains in abdomen or pinching sensation around navel, pain and discharge worse in week before period *Sulphur 6c*

Self-help In general, coffee, alcohol, and sweets are to be avoided; constipation and lack of exercise are not helpful either. Wear cotton underwear and change it every day, and do not use vaginal deodorants, perfumed bath salts, or talcum powder.

If vaginal douching does not put you off, there are several simple ways to soothe vagina and restore its natural acidity (harmful organisms flourish when populations of beneficial acid-producing bacteria are decimated). First, douche vagina with Hypericum and Calendula solution (5 drops of mother tincture of each to 0.25 litre [½ pint] boiled cooled water); do this 3 times a day, and last thing at night apply a cold water compress to lower abdomen. As soon as itchiness and soreness abate, douche vagina 3 times a day with yoghurt solution (1 pot natural live yoghurt to 1.75 litres [3 pints] boiled cooled water) or with a weak solution of fresh lemon juice or vinegar (1 tablespoon to 0.25 litre [½ pint] boiled cooled water); a preparation called Aci-gel is also available from chemists. Obstinate cases of thrush may respond to extra iron, zinc, vitamins C and B, and evening primrose oil, and cutting down on carbohydrates and products containing yeast.

Vaginitis
Irritation of vagina in absence of infection; sometimes part of a general skin condition (see ITCHING), sometimes a reaction to spermicidal creams, medicated douches, or vaginal deodorants; in younger women it may be a reaction to a difficult sexual relationship; vagina feels sore and itchy. See Unusual discharge (above) for self-help measures and homeopathic remedies.

Vulval warts
Localised viral infections on labia or around entrance to vagina, often associated with pregnancy or with vaginal infections such as THRUSH, during which vaginal discharge increases; like penile warts (see PENIS PROBLEMS), vulval warts should not be neglected because they are moderately contagious, easily transmitted to sexual partners, and can become malignant (see CANCER OF THE VULVA), although this is rare; it has also been suggested that they play a part in development of CANCER OF THE CERVIX, so have a yearly smear. GP may prescribe special wart paint or recommend removal of warts by freezing or cauterization. Homeopathic treatment is constitutional; in the meantime select a remedy from the list below, one for yourself and one for your sexual partner.

Specific remedies to be taken 4 times daily for up to 3 weeks:

- Fleshy warts, especially if they develop in weeks following orthodox immunizations *Thuja 6c*
- Warts are itchy, tendency to suffer from catarrh, shakiness or flutteriness *Medorrhinum 6c*
- Warts associated with sores or ulcers *Nitric ac. 6c*
- Intense itchiness and smarting *Sabina 6c*

Self-help Genital warts can easily spread from warts elsewhere on body; so if you have warts, especially on your hands, always wash your hands before touching your own or your partner's genitals.

Varicose veins
A sign that valves in affected veins are weak and unable to prevent backflow of blood; veins become lumpy and distended with blood, and smaller veins and capillaries show as twisted, purplish lines on skin; poorly drained tissues may develop brown staining. Condition mainly affects legs, but also rectum and anus (see PILES); legs tend to ache or swell, and become tender and itchy. Valves may be naturally weak, or become so as result of prolonged sitting or standing, deep vein thrombosis, CONSTIPATION, OBESITY, or pregnancy; complications include varicose ulcers and thrombophlebitis. Orthodox treatment is to 'strip' or remove varicosed sections of veins, or give injections to close them; surrounding

smaller veins rapidly enlarge to compensate. Support stockings are also prescribed.

Homeopathy offers the remedies below; if there is no improvement within 3 weeks, or if condition becomes dramatically worse, see your GP.

Specific remedies to be taken every 12 hours for up to 7 days:

- Varicose veins feel bruised and sore, person may also suffer from piles *Hamamelis 30c*
- Warmth and allowing legs to hang down make varicose veins worse, especially during pregnancy, woman feels chilly *Pulsatilla 30c*
- Legs look very pale but redden easily, walking slowly makes weak, achy feeling wear off *Ferrum 30c*
- Skin mottled and marbled *Carbo veg. 30c*

Self-help
Sit with feet raised above hip level whenever you can, and spend as little time standing as possible. Always wear support stockings. If a vein bursts and bleeds, apply a pad and bandage it on tightly, and keep leg raised until bleeding stops; if it doesn't, see your GP as soon as possible. Guard against constipation by eating more fibre, and increase your intake of vitamins E and C, and bioflavinoids.

PART 4
NUTRITION

General Nutrition

The subject of nutrition is vast, but we will try to answer some basic questions: How has our diet changed in recent times – and for worse or better? What should we eat? How should food be produced, stored and cooked? How is food absorbed by the body – and do we need to take supplements?

Our evolutionary past

Some 40,000 years ago our ancestors were probably mainly vegetarian, eating roots and seeds and fruits, with meat only occasionally. These hunter-gatherers would have been continually on the move; they picked their food fresh, they shared it and did not store it. This situation had its advantages. Modern examples of hunter-gatherers, such as the Bushmen of Botswana, are rarely obese, have few signs of malnutrition or high blood pressure, and have low blood cholesterol levels and no tooth decay.

Gradually, hunting took over from gathering. More meat was included in the diet, and the extra protein, especially, was linked with an increase in stature (as it is today). Remember that the fat content of the meat from wild animals, at about 4 per cent, is much lower than that of today's domestic animals – which can be up to 30 per cent. But the diet at this time was still high in fibre, calcium and vitamin C, and low in fats, sugar and salt.

By about 10,000 years ago, people were beginning to grow and store crops and rear animals in one place. The resulting development of the structured society encouraged increasingly concentrated human populations and a reduced variety of food.

The modern diet

The majority of the world today is still predominantly vegetarian, for economic, ecological, philosophical, religious and even political reasons. The diseases linked with over-consumption of refined carbohydrates and animal fats are mainly confined to the 'developed' societies: obesity, degenerative diseases, dental decay, coronary artery disease, diabetes, gallstones and diverticular diseases. But there is also a high level of malnutrition among the poor of the developed world.

Although there has been a marked change in diet over the last 40,000 years, there has been little change in our bodies to cope with it. Physical and biochemical evolution simply does not work that fast. In order to avoid the diseases of over-nutrition, the World Health Organization has redefined the ideal diet to conform more closely to that of our hunter-gatherer forefathers – indeed, the very diet our bodies are designed for.

Two studies bear this out.

1 Members of a tribe in Kenya who left their villages for Nairobi developed a significant rise in blood pressure within a month, mainly due to a change in diet, particularly higher salt intake. This rise in blood pressure could also be due to an increase in weight, or stress.

2 In a report from Bahrain in the Arabian Gulf it was found that when the diet was changed from traditional foods such as fish, rice, dates and vegetables to more red meat, chicken, eggs, milk, fat, sugar, prepared and packaged foods, there was an increase in heart disease, diabetes, obesity, dental caries and some forms of cancer. The World Health Organization now recommends that people should eat 5 fruits and vegetables a day.

There are 4 main categories of diet. Vegans eat no animal protein of any kind; lacto-vegetarians include milk products and sometimes eggs in their diet; an omnivore wholefood diet includes all types of wholefoods (foods not processed, treated or refined by industry); while a western omnivore diet includes refined and processed foods.

Heart disease and diet

It is important to cut down on salt as much as you can. It has been concluded that using ½ tsp less per day of salt can prevent 1 in 5 people having a stroke, 1 in 6 from heart disease and halve the number of people needing drugs to reduce blood pressure; if food manufacturers reduced the salt content of processed foods, blood pressure could be lowered by twice the number achieved by drugs and prevent 70,000 deaths annually in the UK.

In addition cut down on full-fat milk and cheese, cream, butter, eggs, fatty meat, lard, dripping, and hydrogenated vegetable fats; look for margarines and oils high in polyunsaturates (those based on sunflower, safflower, and corn oil are best), and don't heat them above 120°C (250°F). Eat oily fish (herring, mackerel) twice a week. Add garlic to your food and take brewer's yeast (containing B vitamins and chromium); these will help to reduce cholesterol levels. Add fresh ginger to your cooking; this will help to reduce stickiness of blood platelets and prevent clotting. Cut down on refined carbohydrates, at their most concentrated in sugar, sweets, chocolate, biscuits, cakes, and soft drinks. Other items to be wary of are shellfish and salt; avoid salty foods and don't add salt to your food. If you cannot wean yourself off caffeine and alcohol entirely, make them a twice-a-week treat only. Make sure you eat plenty of unrefined, high-fibre foods – principally that means wholegrain cereals, leafy vegetables, and pulses. Take extra vitamin B_6, C, and E (if you have high blood pressure or are taking anticoagulants, check with your GP before taking extra vitamin E). Take fish oils, e.g. Max EPA, evening primrose oil and recommended daily amounts of manganese, calcium, selenium, magnesium, iodine, lecithin, and rutin.

The 'twice a week' rule This memory aid helps you to simplify diet planning and include in your diet the right proportions of the various types of food. Foods are divided into groups and you should eat foods from each group no more than twice a week.
Group 1 – meat and poultry
Group 2 – fish
Group 3 – eggs
Group 4 – cheese
Group 5 – sugar in concentrated form (sweets, cakes)

In addition, keep milk to an average of less than 250 ml (about ½ pint) per day but be careful to keep up your general level of fluid intake to keep your kidneys well flushed out. Drink semi-skimmed or skimmed milk.

The rest of your diet should be made up of wholemeal bread and flour, cereals, grains, nuts and seeds, vegetables, legumes and fruit, organically grown if possible. You will then be eating a well-balanced diet which your digestive system is designed for and which satisfies your body's nutritional needs.

Organic foods are grown in humus-rich soils without artificial fertilizers and pesticides. Demand for organically grown vegetables is increasing and some supermarkets are now promoting their organic ranges. Vegetables with split stalks, cracked skins or an unnaturally bright green or pasty yellow colour are unlikely to be organically grown.

If you have any bad habits, nutritional or otherwise, indulge them only twice a week – though preferably not at all. Use small amounts of salt, Lo Salt, or Ruthmol for cooking, if at all. Do not add salt to your food at the table. If you have a sweet tooth, eat muesli bars, dried fruit, carob chocolate or cakes and biscuits made with un-refined sugars.

Remember that even if you are eating a pesticide-free, organically grown, additive-free diet, you are still in danger if your diet is very restricted and you eat too much of one particular food. Variety is the spice of life!

Children's food
Old habits die hard, and eating habits are moulded in childhood. Try to educate children in the ways of a good diet. Many of the factors associated with heart disease, such as poor diet, start when we are young. Use the twice-a-week rule (above), but increase the amount of protein from animal and vegetable sources. Avoid salt and too much fat. Read labels on foods and avoid additives if possible. The additives E250, E251, E310, E311, E312, E320, E321 and Ethoxyquin are not allowed in foods meant for children, but they are sometimes found in adult foods that children eat. Some children are especially susceptible to certain foods or to additives, and food allergy may lead to behavioural problems.

Children often go through 'faddy' phases of refusing to eat, or eating only certain things. There appears to be no medical basis for this, unless they are actually ill. The problem usually resolves itself if you pay it as little attention as possible. The child may well be trying to get a reaction, and if an emotional battle develops, it can be very difficult to overcome. Continue to serve food only at normal meal times, even when it is not eaten. Try serving the same food in different guises, puréed or cut into interesting shapes. Give only small amounts. Encourage the child to eat a small piece of everything on the plate, not just one item. Make sure he or she has not eaten sweets or biscuits or had a large drink before a meal. No one can eat when the stomach is already full!

To reassure yourself, try keeping a diary of everything that your child eats over a 2-week period. Food intake over a day may not be adequate, but you will probably find that the diet averages out. Children will not starve themselves to death, and their metabolism is much more efficient than an adult's.

The tongue bears taste buds that are sensitive to salt and sugar. In ancient times these flavours were probably provided by fruits, wild honey and vegetables. Today there is salt or sugar in many processed foods. Children readily develop a taste for them, so try to avoid using junk food as a treat. A recent research project involved removal of sugar, food colourings and preservatives from the meals served in a residential school. Fresh, unrefined foods were substituted. The startling results included higher academic achievements, less fighting and better behaviour.

Healthy alternatives to junk food are not difficult to find. Instead of fizzy drinks and adulterated squash, give mineral water, unsweetened fruit juices or non-additive squash. Ice cream and yogurt can be bought without additives and with a low fat content. Sweets and snacks can be replaced by muesli bars, dried or fresh fruits, and carob can be used instead of chocolate. Make your own cakes, biscuits and puddings using low-sugar recipes, wholemeal flour, fresh and dried fruits and yoghurt. Burgers, sausages and fish-fingers can also be made at home or bought as low-fat, additive-free products. Soya products can replace meat, but beware of colouring chemicals. Choose additive-free crisps or try tortilla chips and corn chips.

Children can be raised on vegetarian diets. But great care must be taken, especially on vegan diets, that the combinations of foods give adequate amounts of nutrients. Expert planning is needed. Contact the Vegan Society (address p. 336).

The elderly and food

Elderly people need less energy, and so they tend to eat less: but their food should still be of a high nutritional quality. Yet because of poverty or an unwillingness to cook when living alone, the reverse is often the case. Older people should avoid too much fat, salt, sugar and red meat, and eat plenty of wholegrain bread, cereals, vegetables, fruit and fish. It is best to eat several small meals and healthy snacks rather than one large daily meal. Elderly people who rarely get out in the fresh air may need to take vitamin D supplements. Go easy on tea and coffee, since they contribute to insomnia. Some drugs interfere with absorption of nutrients, so consult a doctor about your diet if you are taking medication.

Fasting

see also FASTING on p. 262

Eating nothing, on occasions, can be good for you, provided your general health is satisfactory. Complete abstinence from solid food rests the digestive system and allows the body to cleanse itself of toxic residues. Also, any unknown allergens in your diet will cease to bother you. If you are in any doubt about your fitness to fast, consult a homeopath or doctor. When you fast, take plenty of additive-free fruit juices, herb teas or mineral water. Do not fast for longer than 3 days without supervision. After a fast, gradually introduce easily digested foods such as yoghurt, fruit and vegetable stew.

Digestion

Digestion is the process that changes food into a form which the cells of the body can use. The mouth, stomach and intestines, and the organs associated with them, form the digestive system. Digestive capabilities vary from person to person and deteriorate as we get older. The liver is the central organ for the breakdown of digested nutrients (catabolism) and the building, from them, of chemicals required by the cells of the body (anabolism). Collectively the processes of body chemistry are called metabolism.

In order to eat enjoyably and healthily, it is necessary to understand what is in the food we eat, and why the body needs it – or not.

What is food?

Energy

Food contains energy, usually measured in calories. One calorie is the amount of heat required to raise the temperature of 1 g of water by 1°C. The 'calorie' of the nutritionist is in fact equivalent to one kilocalorie (1,000 calories) of the physicist, and is written Calorie (capital C). This is the convention we adopt here. In addition, very up-to-date energy measurements are sometimes given in joules (J). One Calorie equals about 4.2 joules.

The body needs energy for all its processes, physical, mental and chemical. The number of Calories the body requires varies according to age, sex, build, and activity level (which is closely linked to occupation).

Average daily Calorie requirements

Child	varies greatly, 1,000–3,000 at school age
Teenager	varies greatly, 2,000–3,000
Woman	sedentary, 2,000 active, 2,300–4,000
Man	sedentary, 2,500 active, 3,000–5,000
Elderly person	1,000–2,000

If the energy in food is not used by the body, by being converted into growing tissue or movement or warmth, then it is stored, generally as fat. This is what makes people overweight (see OBESITY, p. 35).

Carbohydrates

These are the chief source of energy for bodily functions and muscular exertions. Carbohydrates come in the form of sugar, for example in fruit and vegetables, or starch, for example cereals, potatoes and bread. It is better to take carbohydrates in their unrefined or wholefood form, when the foods rich in them also contain fibre, vitamins and minerals, and the digestive system is better able to cope with them.

Snacks containing high levels of refined carbohydrates (such as chocolate bars) lead to a sudden rise in blood sugar level. When the level begins to drop again there is often a craving for sugar, dizziness, trembling and headaches. Long-term over-indulgence in refined carbohydrates leads to obesity and caries and may be involved in such diseases as diabetes, high blood pressure, atherosclerosis, cancers of the digestive tract, gastric ulcer, anaemia and kidney disorder.

Fats

Fats in food are the most concentrated forms of energy, producing twice the number of Calories per gram as carbohydrates and proteins. The substances that give fats their flavours, textures and melting points are called fatty acids and these may be 'saturated', 'unsaturated' and 'poly-unsaturated'. These names derive from the nature of the chemical bonds within the molecules. Suffice to say that 'saturated' fatty acids come mainly from animal sources (lard, dripping) and are usually solid at room temperature. They are less healthy than 'unsaturated' and 'polyunsaturated' fatty acids, which come from vegetable sources and are usually liquid. They can be solidified by a process called hydrogenation to give the familiar vegetable-oil margarines.

Three fatty acids, linoleic, arachidonic and linolenic, are essential in the diet because the body cannot make them itself. They are necessary for the transport and breakdown of cholesterol and lowering the blood pressure, and they are involved in blood clotting and inflammation.

Fat deficiency is rare in the West today, but it can lead to deficiency of fat-soluble vitamins. Signs include dry skin and eczema, sterility in men, retarded growth and poor vision. Too much fat in the diet is much more likely and so animal fats, processed foods and fried foods should be kept to a minimum. Over-indulgence in fats leads to obesity and atherosclerosis which can in turn be involved in kidney failure, angina, stroke and heart attack.

Proteins

These are the 'building blocks' in food, the construction materials for growth and repair of cells. The body needs proteins throughout life, but the need is greatest during infancy, pregnancy and after illness or injury.

Protein may also be used as an energy source. If carbohydrates or fats are lacking in the diet, protein is converted to fat by the liver and burned to provide energy, or burned directly. It yields the same amounts of energy, weight for weight, as carbohydrate.

During digestion, proteins are broken down into units called amino acids. The body requires 22 different amino acids, but it can make 13 itself from other amino acids. The remaining 9 are called essential amino acids because they must be present in the diet. Meat and dairy products contain all the essential amino acids, but individual vegetable foods may contain only some of them. It is important, therefore, in a vegetarian diet, to eat a variety of fruits, nuts, cereals, legumes and vegetables that provides all the essential amino acids.

While proteins are obviously essential to the healthy body, they are dangerous in excess. Obesity, kidney disorders and gout are linked to a diet too high in certain proteins. A diet rich in animal proteins leads to diseases such as kidney stones, high fat levels in the blood, high blood pressure and the formation of cancer-inducing agents in the bile.

Dietary fibre

The indigestible parts of plants such as cellulose, lignin and pectin are known as 'fibre', 'roughage' or non-starch polysaccharides (NSP). They cannot be broken down by our digestive system and therefore pass through it. On the way, fibre aids digestion, absorbs water and makes the stools larger and softer, so preventing constipation. It takes up wastes such as toxins and bile salts and removes them in the stools.

Bowel problems such as diverticular disease, IRRITABLE BOWEL and some cancers of the bowel may be caused by lack of fibre. However, too much fibre can lead to blockage of the intestine, poor absorption of vitamins and minerals, and grain-sensitive bowel inflammations such as coeliac disease. About 30 g (approximately 1 oz) per day of fibre is suitable for the average person: you should manage this easily if you eat wholefoods.

Vitamins

These are organic substances which the body cannot make, but which it requires in small amounts (the exception to this is vitamin D, which can be made from sunlight). Vitamins are either fat- or water-soluble. The fat-soluble vitamins, A, D, E and K, can be stored in the body, but the water-soluble B group and C are quickly excreted. Vitamins often work together or with minerals, and their absorption in the gut may be aided or prevented by certain minerals. (See NUTRITIONAL SUPPLEMENTS for more details of individual vitamins and minerals.)

In an ideal world you should not need extra vitamins and minerals if you are eating a well balanced diet with plenty of whole grains, raw fresh fruits and vegetables. Unfortunately, nowadays it is virtually impossible to obtain anything which is 100 per cent natural. Even if it is grown under organic conditions there will be some traces of pesticides and herbicides in the rain which waters it. There is therefore some argument for taking an anti-oxidant mixture to combat any free radicals which cause damage to cells produced by these substances (see NUTRITIONAL SUPPLEMENTS). There are also conditions where supplements may be recommended, such as alcohol abuse, smoking, taking the oral contraceptive pill, pregnancy, dieting, illness and exposure to radiation. Supplements may also be required by bottle-fed babies, lactating mothers and elderly people. See ARE SUPPLEMENTS NECESSARY?

Additives
Food has probably always been mixed with other things – herbs, salts, spices, for example – to make it more appealing to eat. In the past 30 years, however, there has been a massive explosion in the chemical adulteration of food. It probably represents the biggest uncontrolled experiment ever performed. However, the results will be hard to analyse. We know some of the short-term effects on the body of individual chemicals added to food, but there is no way of telling what the combined long-term effects will be.

Additives in food are used to colour, flavour, preserve, sweeten, emulsify, stabilize, acidify, thicken, anti-oxidize . . . and of course increase the profits of the growers and processors and sellers. Meat carcasses are sometimes injected with polyphosphates to increase water intake, in order to make them heavier. Antibiotics and even hormones are routinely fed to animals to speed up growth rates. There are 1,200 legal additives for ice cream! Some people – especially children – are extremely allergic to many of them (see Children's food, above, p. 248).

Pesticides
After 2 decades of isolation from mainstream orthodox opinion, the role of pesticides in the causation of disease is now being taken increasingly seriously. A card system has been set up to report acute poisoning episodes, and concern is growing that chronic exposure to pesticides may be linked to cancer, problems in the foetus, allergy and other effects on the immune system, nervous system damage and damage to genetic material. The ideal solution is obviously to eat organically prepared food as much as possible. You can also get rid of 85 per cent of residues by peeling, but that leaves some 15 per cent which is still going into the food. Taking an anti-oxidant formula will help too (see NUTRITIONAL SUPPLEMENTS).

Naturally occurring toxins
As well as the additives we put in food, there may also be natural toxins (poisons). Some plants produce toxins to avoid being eaten by animals. These are often destroyed by cooking, are not dangerous to humans in small amounts, or are chemically neutralized in the whole plant. Examples include bananas, legumes (especially red beans), potatoes, mushrooms, brassicas, rhubarb, cheese, almonds, quail and certain fish. There are also foods which often seem to cause allergies in certain people. For example, wheat causes the digestive disorder known as COELIAC DISEASE. Anaflatoxins are present in some nuts.

Infections and parasites are often present in foods: salmonella in chickens, listeria in certain cheeses, brucellosis in meat, tuberculosis in milk, and worms and flukes in meat and fish. Fresh vegetables may have fluke eggs or moulds on their surfaces. Infections such as dysentery and gastroenteritis may be caught from food because of bad hygiene.

Better livestock health and the introduction of pasteurized milk should have removed these risks, although it is possible they have increased the risks for other usually better adapted parasites. The use of antibiotics and overcrowding of animals for slaughter has increased the risk of salmonella. If, however, you eat untreated products from untested animals, take care to prepare and cook the food properly. Thorough washing of food, cooking to adequate temperatures, correct storage, good hygiene and not reheating food will prevent most infections from being transferred.

Preserving food
From earliest times people have preserved food by heating, drying, pickling and salting, in sugar or vinegar or alcohol. Modern methods include canning, cooling or freezing, chemical preservation, and more recently, irradiation. Food decomposes because of the enzymes in it or because bacteria or fungi contaminate it, and preservation kills or slows the contaminants.

Preservation has become essential for city living. It has also removed seasonal and regional restrictions on availability. In some cases it may not be harmful: research has shown that a diet based on modern canned foods gives no adverse effects.

Irradiation uses gamma-rays to kill bacteria in foods. It is already in use in certain countries such as South Africa, the Netherlands, Japan and the USA. Irradiation gives a longer shelf-life, it leaves no taste, and no chemicals are introduced. It destroys vitamins, however, and the long-term effects are not known. Because the word 'radiation' has negative associations, there are moves to call the process by another name, such as 'picowaving'.

Cooking food

When buying and preparing food, select the best quality food possible and bear in mind its origins, production and processing.

Take care when storing, preparing and cooking food, that the nutrients are not damaged and toxic chemicals are not introduced. For instance, avoid preparing vegetables in advance, since they will lose their vitamins if allowed to soak for long in water.

Microwave cooking causes a loss of nutrients, but whether this is greater than any other form of cooking is not yet known. There is also evidence that microwave cooking causes a breakdown of fats, with release of free radicals which can harm cells. Again it is not yet known if this damage is greater than in any other form of cooking. If you do use a microwave do not stand in front of it when it is on and do not cover food with clingfilm to cook.

Toasting and browning alters the chemical composition of the surface layers and may destroy amino acids and vitamins. Frying is to be avoided if possible; not only does it increase the amount of fat in the diet, but high temperatures can produce carcinogens in fats.

Food, cooked or raw, should always be kept covered in the fridge. Frozen food should be defrosted thoroughly and as quickly as possible before cooking. In a recent survey it was found that some 12 per cent of pre-cooked, ready-to-eat poultry and 18 per cent of cook/chill meals contained listeria. As a result of the danger to pregnant women of LISTERIA the government issued the following recommendations in February 1989:

1 Keep foods for as short a time as possible, following the storage instructions carefully, and observe the 'eat by' and 'best by' dates on the label.
2 Do not eat under-cooked meat or poultry products, and be sure to reheat chilled meals thoroughly according to the instructions on the label. Wash salads, fruit and vegetables that will be eaten raw.
3 Make sure your refrigerator is working properly, and is keeping food stored in it cold.
4 Store cooked foods in the refrigerator away from raw foods and cheeses.
5 When reheating food make sure it is piping hot all the way through, and do not reheat more than once.
6 When using a microwave oven to reheat food, observe the standing time recommended by the oven manufacturer to ensure food obtains an even temperature before it is eaten.
7 Throw away left-over reheated food.
8 Cooked food which is not to be eaten straight away should be cooled as rapidly as possible and then stored in the refrigerator.

Utensils

Even the implements you use when cooking can affect health. Rinse detergents thoroughly from kitchenware, since experiments have linked them with eczema and damage to the intestinal lining. Iron utensils are recommended since they distribute heat evenly for thorough cooking, and they may also be a source of iron in the diet! Earthenware pots are sometimes glazed with lead or cadmium, which can be dangerous; white porcelain or glass containers are more suitable. Copper, brass and aluminium pans should be avoided. Aluminium, especially, may be associated with digestive-system complaints ranging from mouth ulcers to piles. Non-stick teflon coatings may lead to gut trouble when they start to peel off.

Nutritional Supplements and Special Diets

Dosage Doses advised are deliberately on the safe side and may not be high enough to give benefit, but it is recommended that higher dosages should only be taken under the care of a practitioner experienced in nutritional medicine.

Side-effects refer to effects of much larger doses on the whole than those recommended in this book.

Are supplements necessary?

Supplements should not be needed provided that one is eating a good, well-balanced, wholegrain diet with plenty of raw, organically grown vegetables and fruit. There is concern, however, that certain agricultural processes have led to losses of specific nutrients in the food chain. There are also specific times when supplementation may be required, such as when taking certain drugs, oral contraceptive pills, during pregnancy and while lactating, during and after weight loss, and if you are elderly. If you feel that you are generally under par, i.e. physically low in energy or mentally lethargic, there is no harm in taking a multivitamin and mineral supplement for a month. We recommend that you take one that is not time-released, which contains less than 25 mg of each of the major B vitamins (B_1, B_5, B_6) and has a zinc to copper ratio of not less than 14 to 1. Choose one that is free of additives and colourings. Children's chewable vitamins and minerals are available.

The quality of supplements

Nutritional supplements are available from one of four sources: chemists, health food shops, your doctor and specialist mail order companies. Supplements from the chemist are very strictly controlled as to their content but chemist's shops tend not to include such a wide range of vitamins and minerals in their multivitamin preparations as health food shops, and they frequently contain tartrazine and other additives which may upset people who are prone to allergies.

Some companies are introducing a range of vitamins and minerals which are described as being in a food state. These are grown in a yeast culture after which the yeast is killed and spray dried, and the resulting mixture made into tablets. It is said that these food-state vitamins and minerals are absorbed more efficiently in the body as they are bound in a more organic form.

Whilst there are intellectual arguments against this view the figures for magnesium do bear out this contention; it deserves wider exploration, especially in view of possible limiting of dosage by the EC.

Rules for prescribing supplements

Deficiencies When you read through 'Ailments and Conditions', or 'A–Z of Other Conditions', you may find under certain complaints that there may be a need for certain nutrients, such as vitamin C or zinc. This means either that the ailment is thought to be due to a deficiency of these nutrients or that it responds to increasing their intake in the diet, although you are not necessarily deficient in them.

If you have this complaint, turn to the nutrient section which follows. This will tell you which foods contain the recommended nutrient, and you should increase your intake of those foods for one month. If this does not help, then take a supplement, in the amount equal to, or less than, that which is advised as a maximum for another month. If there is still no improvement, see your GP, a nutritionally trained physician or a dietician. If you do feel better then you may continue taking the supplement, but stop for 2 days a week. We have deliberately erred on the cautious side when advising dosages of nutrients. However, except with fat-soluble vitamins and certain minerals like selenium, it is rare to find side-effects occurring even if you are taking up to 100 times more than the RDA. Any supplement not mentioned below may also be taken, but stop for 2 days a week after one month, and watch the health press for possible hazards.

In EC countries there is considerable debate at present about the dosage of vitamins and mineral supplements that should be available over the counter. This will probably result in some of the higher potency vitamins and minerals no longer being available. Common sense would state, because of the difficulties in fixing RDAs or DRVs (see below), that apart from some water-soluble vitamins, such as vitamin C, supplements should not contain more than 10 times the DRV or RDA.

DRVs and food labelling

You may have seen recommended daily allowance (RDA) requirements for various nutrients. These are based on whether a nutrient is essential for the body's health, and the amount required to prevent deficiency and disease. RDAs have varied considerably from country to country, and although not ideal, they seem to work reasonably well to prevent nutritional disease. The Government Committee of Medical Aspects of Food Policy (COMA) has recently published new dietary reference values for foods, and has introduced the following new terminology.

EAR: the Estimated Average Requirement of a group of people for energy, protein, vitamins and minerals. About half of us usually need more EAR, and about half need less than the LRNI (or the Lower Reference Nutrient Intake) for protein, vitamin and minerals; this is an amount of the nutrient that is enough for only the few people in a group who have low needs.

RNI: a Reference Nutrient Intake for protein, vitamins and minerals. It is the amount of the nutrient that is enough, or more than enough, for about 97 per cent of people in a group. If the average intake of a group is at RNI, then the risk of deficiency in the group is very small.

Safe Intake: a term used to indicate intake, or range of intake, of a nutrient for which there is not enough information to estimate the RNI, EAR or LRNI. It is an amount that is enough for almost everyone but not so large as to cause undesirable effects.

DRV (Dietary Reference Value): a term used to cover LRNI, EAR, RNI and Safe Intake.

The report containing this information is complex, and mainly for professional nutritionists. Nevertheless, it may lead to further recommendations, most of which we have tried to incorporate in this book by giving the new DRVs.

Dangerous supplements

Recently 4 nutritional supplements have had health warnings issued against them, or have been banned in the UK.

Tryptophan was banned from sale in September 1990 by the Department of Health because it was found to be causing a condition known as Eosinophilia Myalgia Syndrome (EMS). This consisted of a rise in certain white cells, severe muscle pains and pains in the joints, fever, swelling and rash. It is still not known whether this is due to tryptophan itself or to some contaminant.

Germanium was marketed as a product to boost the immune system, but in October 1989 all doctors were warned that it could cause diseases of the kidney which could lead to renal failure, and it was then banned.

Niacin has been used for some time to lower cholesterol levels, but it was found that moderately high doses may alter liver function tests; high doses can cause actual liver damage, and can also aggravate diabetes and depression.

Vitamin A see below for effects on pregnant women.

EFAs (essential fatty acids – linoleic and linolenic acids)

Required for integrity of cell walls and the production of potent chemicals such as prostaglandins.

Found in: vegetables, grains, wheat, beans, spinach, fish, especially oily fish like mackerel.

Supplements available as: oil-filled capsules. These should be taken orally or broken open and the oil rubbed into unbroken skin, on the inner arms or legs, for example. Trade names are Glanolyn, Efamol, Oil of Evening Primrose (containing gammalinoleic acid).

Max EPA contains docosahexaenoic and eicosapentanoeic acid.

DRV: Not given. Maximum dosage – less than 1 g a day of Efamol. Up to 4 capsules a day of Max EPA.

N.B. Always take supplements of zinc, magnesium, vitamins C, E and B complex and selenium when taking EFAs.

Avoid Oil of Evening Primrose if you are epileptic and Max EPA if you have a bleeding disorder, except under medical supervision.

Vitamin A

Important for the functioning of the eyes and cell membranes. Too little may lead to night blindness, scaly skin and poor growth. Vitamin A may also be involved in resistance to certain diseases.

Found in: offal, cheese, eggs, butter, margarine, fish oils, green, yellow and orange vegetables, e.g. carrots, cabbage and spinach.

Supplements available as: tablets, oil-filled capsules, bottles of oil, e.g. cod liver oil, all of which are taken orally. Maximum dose 15,000 IUs daily unless you are pregnant – see below.

DRV: Children 350–500 mcg
        Women 600 mcg
        Pregnant women 700 mcg
        Lactating mothers 950 mcg
        Men 700 mcg

Side-effects: If you take a supplement of more than 9,000 mcg or 30,000 IU, you may suffer nausea, vomiting, dizziness, dry scaly skin, hair loss, fatigue or headaches, liver or bone damage or double vision.

N.B. Vitamin A can harm the unborn foetus. It has been suggested that there is a relationship between the incidence of birth defects and vitamin A intakes of more than 3,300 mcg per day during pregnancy. For this reason women in the UK who are or might become pregnant are advised not to take supplements containing vitamin A unless directed to do so by a doctor or antenatal clinic. If you are taking a general multivitamin and mineral supplement, check with your doctor first that it does not contain too much vitamin A. It is also wise to avoid eating liver in pregnancy as this can cause damage too.

Beta-carotene supplements are not toxic, although high intakes lead to a yellow appearance.

Vitamin B₁ (thiamine)

Needed for carbohydrate metabolism; deficiency may cause irritability, depression, loss of concentration, fatigue and insomnia. In alcoholics and the elderly, deficiency can cause loss of memory and heart failure.

Found in: whole cereals, nuts, beans, peas, pulses, yeast, pork, beef, liver, wholemeal bread.

Supplements available as: capsules or tablets, usually found in combination with other B vitamins.

DRV: Children 0.2–0.7 mg
 Women 0.7–0.8 mg
 Pregnant women 0.9 mg in last 3 months
 Lactating mothers 1.0 mg
 Maximum dose under 50 mg/day

Side-effects: An excess of 3 g a day may cause headache, irritability, insomnia, rapid pulse, weakness, contact dermatitis, pruritis – and in one case has led to death.

Vitamin B₂ (riboflavin)

Aids in the metabolism of fats, carbohydrates and proteins. Deficiency can lead to soreness of the lips and tongue, and photophobia (intolerance of bright light).

Found in: liver, offal, milk, cheese, eggs, fish, green vegetables, yeast extract.

Supplements available as: pills or tablets, usually with other B vitamins.

DRV: Children 0.4–1 mg
 Women 1.1 mg
 Pregnant women 1.4 mg

 Lactating mothers 1.6 mg
 Men 1.3 mg

Side-effects: Supplements containing B₂ may cause urine to become yellow.

N.B. The level of B₂ in milk decreases on exposure to light.

Vitamin B₃ (niacin, nicotinic acid or nicotanamide)

Involved in general metabolism. Deficiency can lead to irritability, loss of memory and dementia, dermatitis and headache.

Found in: meat, fish, pulses, wholegrains, offal, nuts.

Supplements available: in many forms, usually in combination with other B vitamins.

DRV: Children 3–12 mg
 Women 12–14 mg
 Lactating mothers 14–16 mg
 Men 15–18 mg
 Maximum under 100 mg a day

Side-effects: Moderate to high doses may alter liver function tests and can aggravate diabetes and cause depression. High doses may cause actual liver damage. These effects wear off after stopping the supplements. It can also cause uncomfortable flushing of the skin, but this usually passes off.

N.B. The B₃ in maize corn has to be liberated with alkali or hot ash before it is available to the body.

Vitamin B₅ (pantothenic acid)

Helps with the metabolism of fats, carbohydrates and proteins. Deficiency leads to fatigue, emotional swings and numbness.

Found in: a wide variety of foods. High levels in eggs, wholegrain cereals and meat.

Supplements available in: mainly B complex tablets.

DRV: Infants 1.7 mg
 Adults 3.7 mg

Vitamin B₆ (pyroxidine)

Also involved in the metabolism of all three main types of nutrients, and of minerals and certain body chemicals called neuro-transmitters. Deficiency leads to irritability, insomnia, dermatitis, and reduced resistance to infection.

Found in: liver, wholegrain cereals, nuts, seeds, bananas, most fruits, green leafy vegetables and avocados.

Supplements available in: many forms, usually but not always in combination with other B vitamins.

DRV: Children 0.2–1 mg
          Women 1.2 mg
          Men 1.2–1.5 mg

Side-effects: B_6 can aggravate a B_2 deficiency and very large doses of over 2,000 mg a day have been reported to cause nerve damage. Doses of over 100 mg have been reported to produce an increase in dreaming and wakefulness. Even doses of 50 mg a day have been known to cause peripheral nervopathy (nerve damage) but patients recover after stopping the vitamin.

Vitamin B_{12} (cobalamine)

Necessary for both haemoglobin production and the functioning of the nervous system. Deficiency results in anaemia and lack of co-ordination; it may not always be caused by lack of B_{12} in the diet, but by inadequate absorption of the vitamin from the intestine.

Found in: offal, fish, pork, eggs, cheese, yoghurt, milk and brewer's yeast.

Supplements available in: tablets from health food shops and chemists. Injections from doctor.

DRV: Children 0.3–1 mg
          Women 1.2–1.5 mg
          Lactating mothers 1.7–2.0 mg
          Men 1.2–1.5 mg

Folic acid (folate)

Closely linked to B_{12} and the workings of the nervous system. Anaemia and mental problems may result from its deficiency. Inadequate intake is especially common in pregnancy and may contribute to the risk of spina bifida.

Found in: liver, spinach, broccoli tops, asparagus, beets, kidney, cabbage, lettuce, avocados, nuts and wheatgerm.

Supplements available in: tablets from health food shops or chemists.

DRV: Children 50–150 mcg
          Women 200 mcg
          Pregnant women 300 mcg
          Lactating mothers 60 mcg
          Men 200 mcg

Side-effects: Avoid if on certain drugs used to treat epilepsy, or if you have an oestrogen-dependent breast tumour. It should not be taken on its own for too long without B_{12} in case a B_{12} deficiency is masked and damage results to the central nervous system. Toxicity can result if more than 15 mg per day is taken, causing distension and flatulence, nausea, loss of appetite, sleep disturbances, vivid dreams, malaise and irritability. High intake may reduce zinc absorption.

Choline

Involved in nerve impulse conduction. Part of lecithin.

Dose 5–20 mg daily

PABA (paramino-benzoic acid)

Thought to be involved in melanin production.

Dose 5–10 mg daily.

Biotin

One of the lesser known B vitamins. Helps to prevent mycelial extension of fungi, i.e. candida.

Found in: meats, dairy products and wholegrain cereals.

Possible to become deficient in it when on long-term antibiotics, and by eating large amounts of raw egg; this contains substance which counteracts biotin.

Supplements available in: tablets.

Dose 500 mcg daily.

RDA: not known; *safe intake* set at 180–200 mcg a day.

Vitamin C (ascorbic acid)

Has a central role in cell metabolism and helps to prevent infection and repair injury. It also aids absorption of iron. Deficiency results in the bleeding gums and bruised, dry skin of scurvy. Extra vitamin C may be required by the elderly, heavy smokers and drinkers, women taking the contraceptive pill, and those on other medications such as aspirin, antibiotics or steroids.

Found in: most fruit and vegetables – preferably raw; milk, liver and kidney and new potatoes.

Supplements available in: powder, soluble tablets, pills. It is probably best to give a natural vitamin C which usually comes from Acerola cherries. Synthetic ones are usually described as ascorbic acid. Natural vitamin C preparations usually also contain bioflavonoids, thought to be necessary for its proper functioning. A form of bioflavonoids (oxyrutin) is available on prescription only for varicose veins.

DRV: Children 25–30 mg
          Women 35–40 mg
          Pregnant women 45–55 mg
          Lactating mothers 65–70 mg
          Men 35–40 mg
Maximum dose on or under 500 mg a day.

Side-effects: See your GP if you are taking it as a supplement. It may react with drugs such as PAS, salycilates, amphetamines, anti-depressants and Warfarin. Over 50 g a day there is shown to be an increase in the excretion of calcium, iron and manganese in the urine, with reduced availability of zinc, copper and increased uric acid and oxalic acid excretion. You should avoid vitamin C supplementation if you suffer from glucose-6-dehydrogenase deficiency (an inborn error of metabolism).

Taking vitamin C with the Pill can increase availability of oestrogen, and so convert a low contraceptive pill into a high dose one. Take 500 mg/day or less if on the Pill.

There has been shown to be an increase in excretion of calcium, iron and manganese in the urine, with reduced availability of zinc, copper, and increased uric acid and oxalic acid excretion; this may cause kidney stones in susceptible individuals. Therapeutically, vitamin C is given in increasing doses until onset of diarrhoea, and then cut back.

N.B. If you suddenly stop supplementation of large doses of vitamin C, it may precipitate scurvy, so gradually cut it down over a period of a few weeks. Suddenly stopping supplementation has also been reported to cause sleeplessness, sore tongue, constipation, diarrhoea, canker sores, pain on passing urine, reduced fertility in women, and abortion in large doses (over 6 g).

Vitamin D (calciferol)

Needed for the absorption and metabolism of calcium. Its deficiency may lead to rickets or osteomalacia. It can be synthesized by the body when skin is exposed to sunlight. This is the major source for the body.

Found in: fish liver oils, vegetable and animal oils and dairy products.

Supplements available in: capsules of cod or halibut liver oil, bottled cod liver oil and tablets.

DRV: Children 8.5–7 mcg
   Women over 65 10 mcg
   Pregnant and lactating women 10 mcg
   Men over 65 10 mcg
No DRV for others, providing exposed to sunlight.

N.B. Amounts drop as you get older.

Side-effects: Usually caused by taking more than 100,000 units a day – high blood levels of calcium with stone formation in the kidney, joints, blood vessels, heart and lungs; loss of appetite, nausea and vomiting, thirst, increased production of urine, constipation or diarrhoea, pains in the head and weakness. Avoid supplementation if you have sarcoidosis and high blood calcium and are often exposed to sunlight.

Vitamin E (tocopherol)

Involved in the breakdown of fats. It is especially necessary for women on the contraceptive pill, or those who are pregnant or menopausal.

Found in: vegetable oil, wheatgerm, sunflower seeds, safflower oil, eggs, butter and wholemeal cereals. (Destroyed by rancid oils and deep-freezing.)

Supplements available as: Capsules, pills, tablets, oils. It may be found as naturally derived vitamin E – usually expressed as amounts in IUs, or as synthetic vitamin E, usually expressed in mg. Also available in droplet form for better absorption from specialized manufacturers.

DRV: Calculated as the percentage of polyunsaturated fats (see p. 250) in the diet, and no absolute levels are given. The more polyunsaturated fats you eat the more vitamin E you should take.

Maximum dose for adults 100 mg.

Side-effects: Can interfere with iron absorption so it should be given at different meals. It should not be given to patients on anticoagulants without medical supervision. Dosages of 300 mg interfere with the immune system, 600 mg causes lowering of the triglyceride and thyroid levels, 900 mg depression and fatigue, 3,200 mgs diarrhoea, headache, blurred vision, cramps, dizziness, skin rash, irritability of the gastro-intestinal tract, increase in blood pressure, gynaecomastia (swelling of the breasts), vaginal bleeding, hypoglycaemia, stomatitis, chapped lips and reproductive disturbances. Diabetics should be aware of hypoglycaemia attacks if taking large doses of vitamin E.

Vitamin K

Plays a role in the clotting of blood at the site of a wound. It is especially important in newborn babies.

Found in: spinach, cabbage, lettuce, wheatgerm, tomatoes, oil, eggs, liver.

DRV: None.

Safe intake: Children 10 mcg a day
    Adults 1 mcg per kilogram of weight

Supplements: not recommended because of its toxicity. Injectable, vitamin K is used in hospitals to prevent haemorrhagic disease of the newborn which is particularly common in premature babies, and babies of mothers who are on anti-epileptic drugs. It is now given routinely as the disease can cause permanent brain damage. It also interacts with drugs which stop the blood clotting (anticoagulants).

Calcium

Found in bones, teeth, muscles, nerves and blood; there is more than 1 kg (2¼ lb) in the body. Its absorption in the digestive system is affected by vitamin D, magnesium, bran (which can inhibit absorption), phosphorus, fats, the oestrogen hormones and the parathyroid glands. Deficiency results in osteoporosis (brittle bones). Growing children and older women need a lot of calcium.

Found in: milk (particularly skimmed milk), cheese, wholemeal bread, sesame seeds, soya flour, haricot beans, almonds, parsley, spinach, broccoli, turnip, hard water, herring roe and fish.

Supplements available in: soluble and non-soluble tablets.

DRV: Infants 525 mg
       Children 350–550 mg
       Women 800–700 mg
       Lactating mothers 1,350–1,250 mg
       Men 1,000–700 mg

N.B. Amounts drop as you get older.

Side-effects: It has been suggested by some authorities that milk is not a good source of calcium to rely on, partly because of the commonness of allergic reactions and also because it lacks magnesium, which can lead to a magnesium deficiency, especially in children drinking large quantities. It is usually not toxic in healthy persons. Do not give at the same time of day as magnesium and manganese. Ensure stomach acidity is satisfactory.

Magnesium

Necessary for metabolism of proteins and carbohydrates. There is a long list of deficiency conditions which includes mental problems, heart rhythm disturbances, menstrual problems, high blood pressure and constipation.

Found in: green vegetables, wholegrain cereals and nuts, shrimps, soya beans and hard water.

Supplements available in: powders, tablets or in combination with amino acids or B vitamins.

DRV: Infants 55–80 mg
       Children 82–200 mg
       Women 300–270 mg
       Lactating mothers 350–320 mg
       Men 280–300 mg

N.B. Some requirements decrease with age.

Side-effects: Rare.

N.B. Don't take after meals, can cause diarrhoea. If taking calcium as well take 2 parts of calcium to 1 of magnesium.

Phosphorus

Found in bones and in all cells, especially those of the nervous system. Deficiency may result in muscle weakness and anaemia.

Found in: foods rich in calcium and protein.

Supplements: are rarely necessary as this mineral is widespread in foods.

RDA: Should be equal to calcium intake (measured in mmols).

Side-effects: None known unless large doses lead to increased requirements of calcium and magnesium.

Iron

Necessary for the formation of the haemoglobin which carries oxygen in red blood cells. Deficiency leads to anaemia.

Found in: sausage, liver, fish, eggs, pulses, oatmeal, millet, barley, wheat, cane molasses, wholemeal bread, nuts and seeds and green vegetables.

Supplements available in: tablets, usually bound to another substance to help absorption and sometimes combined with vitamins or folic acid. Take with vitamin C.

DRV: Infants 1.7–7.8 mg
       Children 6.1–8.7 mg
       Women (unless heavy menstrual loss, may need supplement) 14.8–8.7 mg
       Men 11.3–8.7 mg

N.B. Some requirements decrease with age.

Side-effects: Siderosis, which is a condition usually developed as a result of taking supplements or cheap wine, causing iron to be deposited in the liver, pancreas, lungs, spleen or heart causing damage, with symptoms of dizziness, weight loss, headache, shortage of breath and fatigue.

N.B. Tannin, e.g. in tea, inhibits absorption of iron, so limit your tea intake.

Zinc

Involved in the absorption and metabolism of vitamins, carbohydrates and phosphorus. In the short term, 30 mg of zinc daily interferes with the metabolism of both iron and copper. Larger amounts, over 75 mg, lead to features of copper deficiency such as anaemia and low white cell counts. It is found especially in the reproductive organs. Deficiency can slow growth and bring on infertility. It is also associated with skin disorders, impaired hearing, loss of taste or smell, and white spots on nails.

Found in: oysters, meat, ginger, wholegrains, nuts and seeds, green vegetables, yeast, legumes, milk and eggs.

Supplements available in: capsules, soluble tablets, sometimes combined with other substances to aid absorption.

DRV: Infants 4–5 mg
      Children 5–7 mg
      Women 9–7 mg
      Lactating mothers 15–11 mg
      Men 9–9.5 mg

N.B. Some requirements decrease with age.

Side-effects: Over 150 mgs daily for 6 weeks may cause weakening of the immune system and over 200 mg a day may cause collapse. If on more than 15 mg a day, don't take within 1 hour of food.

N.B. Zinc has been found to alleviate acne in some cases.

Iodine

Essential for the production of the hormone thyroxine, which is responsible for regulating the metabolic rate, ensuring normal growth and maintaining skin and hair. A deficiency may lead to goitre, a swelling of the thyroid gland which is located in the neck.

Found in: seafood, seaweed, kelp, lava bread, iodized salt and fish liver oils.

Supplements available in: kelp or iodine tablets or solution, capsules of fish oils from chemists, health food shops or on prescription.

DRV: Infants 50–60 mcg
      Children 70–110 mcg
      Women 130–140 mcg
      Men 130–140 mcg

Sodium

Involved in the body's fluid balance and nerve and muscle function. Deficiency may lead to cramps, exhaustion, nausea and circulatory problems.

Found in: salt, meat, fish, yeast extract, bread, butter, vegetables, margarine, biscuits and cheese.

Supplements available in: salt.

DRV: Infant 210–250 mg
      Children 500–1,200 mg
      Women 1,600 mg
      Men 1,600 mg

Side-effects: May cause high blood pressure or loss of potassium.

Potassium

Plays an important role in water balance and nerve and muscle function. Deficiency symptoms include cramps, fatigue, heart irregularities and headache.

Found in: milk, beef, soya flour, dried fruits, vegetables, cereals. A vegetarian diet has a better sodium and potassium balance than an omnivorous one.

Supplements available in: tablets of potassium chloride and other salts, salt substitutes such as ruthmol, also found combined with diuretic tablets.

DRV: Infants 850–700 mg
      Children 800–2,000 mg
      Women 3100–3,500 mg
      Men 3,100–3,500 mg

Side-effects: Weakness and heart problems. High doses in the elderly can seriously affect kidney function.

N.B. Use salt substitutes containing potassium such as ruthmol, but don't take more than you would if using ordinary salt. Take it with or after food to avoid stomach irritation.

Copper

Found in many enzymes and is essential for healthy blood cells and bones. Anaemia and skeletal defects, raised blood cholesterol and lowered fertility are among the symptoms of deficiency.

Found in: liver, kidney, nuts, shellfish, legumes, stone fruits, yeast, cocoa, wholemeal cereal, water.

Supplements: are rarely needed, as copper is found in many foods.

DRV: Infants 0.2–0.3 mg
      Children 0.4–0.7 mg
      Women 0.8–1.2 mg
      Lactating mothers 1.1–1.5 mg
      Men 0.8–1.2 mg

Manganese

Involved in growth, nervous system function, and hormonal, fat and vitamin metabolism. Symptoms of deficiency include cartilage problems, low fertility and birth defects, growth retardation.

Found in: fresh vegetables, nuts, spices, wholegrains, tea.

Supplements available in: tablets prepared in conjunction with amino acids and other substances to help absorption.

DRV: Infants and children 16 mcg
    Adults 1.4 mg

Side-effects: Irritability, tremor, muscle rigidity.

Fluoride

Contributes to strong bones and teeth and helps to prevent dental decay.

Found in: China tea, sea food, hard water, wheat, carrots, beets, currants, cabbage leaves.

DRV: Infants 0.05 mg per kg of weight a day

Side-effects: Mottling of teeth, hardening of bone.

Chromium

Involved with blood-sugar regulation and the hormone insulin. Clouding of the cornea, athero-sclerosis and low fertility are symptoms of deficiency.

Found in: blackstrap molasses, honey, brewer's yeast, wholewheat bread, nuts, shellfish, kidney, liver, grape juice, black pepper.

Supplements available in: brewer's yeast, solution of chromic chloride.

DRV: Children and adolescents 0.1–1 mcg per kg of weight a day
    Adults 25 mcgs
    Maximum dose 200 mcg

Side-effects: Very large doses may be cancer-forming. Glucose tolerance factor chromium preparations are more active but are yeast derived and people with yeast allergies should avoid them.

Selenium

Necessary for healthy liver, heart and white blood cells. Liver disease, skin problems, cancer and arthritis may indicate deficiency.

Found in: brewer's yeast, sesame seeds, garlic, eggs, fish, shellfish, offal and vegetables.

Supplements available in: tablets or solution.

DRV: Infants 10–13 mcg
    Children 15–30 mcg
    Women 45–60 mcg
    Lactating mothers 60–75 mcg
    Men 45–75 mcg
    Maximum dose 200 mcg

Side-effects: Dental decay in children under 12, hair loss, brittle nails, fatigue, skin rash, loss of appetite, sour taste in mouth, possibly congenital malformations.

Silicon

Important for healthy teeth, arteries and growth generally.

Found in: unrefined grains. Used as an additive to stop foods clogging up or foaming.

Do not supplement.

Nickel

May be involved in regularizing blood sugar levels and fat metabolism. Congenital defects have been linked to its deficiency.

Found in: most nickel enters the system from environment as nickel is widespread in coins, jewellery, kitchen appliances, etc.

RDA: Unknown.

Side-effects: May cause dermatitis and lung cancer.

Formulae for special needs

1 Anti-oxidant formula – recommended for anyone who has been exposed to PESTICIDES and other toxic chemicals, or who lives or works in a very smoky atmosphere. It is also suitable for people who smoke until they give it up. Dose is 1 per day with meals. The formulation is beta-carotene 15 mg (equivalent to 8,333 units vitamin A activity), vitamin C 1,000 mg, vitamin E 100 units, selenium 25 mcg.
2 Women on oral contraceptives – a multi-vitamin and mineral such as Optivite.
3 Women on HRT – a multivitamin and mineral such as Gynovite plus.
4 Women in the menopause – special supplement – a multivitamin and mineral such as Gynovite plus.
5 Women with PMS – special supplement – a multivitamin and mineral such as Optivite.
6 Women wishing to become pregnant (and their partners too) – special supplement – Foresight vitamins and minerals.

Pro-biotics

Pro-biotics is the process of re-populating the bowel with healthy bacteria which are meant to be living there, called *Lactobacillus acidophilus.* It counters yeast growth by preventing mycelial extensions, and is also capable of producing natural antibiotics which are effective against food-borne organisms. The obvious problem is that any tablet, powder or capsule or pill will be attacked by all the digestive enzymes and killed by the time it gets to the bowel. However, it seems that women, who need this most, do not usually produce adequate amounts of acid in the stomach and enzymes from the pancreas in the first place; this may be part of the problem. Some products appear to be more effective than others; in many cases it is worth having one carton a day of a BA yoghurt (containing *Bulgaricus acidophilus*) in addition to the supplement. One or two women have had reactions from taking acidophilus, such as nausea, disturbing flatulence and wind. In these cases the supplement should be stopped. In the USA it has been suggested that taking acidophilus cultures for too long can pre-dispose to cancer of the bowel. Like all other supplements, it should therefore be stopped at weekends after being taken for one month. It should probably not be continued for longer than 3–4 months.

Toxic or excess effects of vitamins and minerals

On reading the ailments section you may have found that your ailment could be due to an excess of certain nutrients or toxic vitamins. If it is a mineral or vitamin, check the mineral supplement that you are taking and if it contains this particular nutrient then stop taking it. If it is a toxic metal, look at the toxic sources and remove them, then get a hair analysis done. If it is positive see your nutritionist or your GP, who may test your blood and advise on which steps to take.

General points about avoiding toxic metals

1 Avoid tobacco smoke at home and at work, exhaust fumes, cooking in unsuitable containers.
2 Eat plenty of fibre and nutrient-rich vegetables and fruit.
3 Don't buy fruit and vegetables from displays on stalls or outside shops where they may have been exposed to leaded exhaust fumes.
4 Correct any nutritional deficiencies you may have by improving your diet.
5 Don't allow young children to suck lead toys.

Lead

There are over 10,000 papers on the toxicity of lead. High levels of lead are known to produce potentially fatal results such as anaemia, and other symptoms may include colicky abdominal pains, damage to the peripheral nerves or brain; however, many authorities are now convinced that lower levels than originally thought can cause sub-acute poisoning, leading to stillbirths and congenital abnormalities, learning and behavioural problems, cancer, heart disease and high blood pressure, kidney and metabolic disease, immune dysfunction, and vague symptoms such as lethargy, depression, muscular aches and pains and frequent infections.

Sources: traffic fumes, unlined copper food pans, dust, polluted water from flaking lead pipes, or lead alloy sealed copper piping, cracked lead-glazed earthenware, lead soldiers, dust and dirt, vegetables grown by the roadside or exposed to traffic fumes, bone meal, dolomite, cigarette ash and tobacco, and occupational exposure.

N.B. Since 1986, no white interior paints have contained lead, nor since 1987 have any coloured interior paints.

Mercury

As with lead, high levels of mercury contamination are known to cause problems, mainly with the nervous system. It is said that hatters suffered from mercury poisoning as a result of the mercury used in the old days in hat production (hence the expression 'mad as a hatter'). However, it is now thought that even quite small quantities of mercury may cause problems. Symptoms may include a muscular sclerosis type of degeneration.

Sources: tuna fish, fish from water polluted by effluent, especially from papermaking factories, drinking water, weed killers, dental amalgam, seed wheat and thermometers.

Cadmium

Cadmium displaces zinc from the enzyme system. The effect on the body is mainly centred around the kidney and it may cause high blood pressure.

Sources: cigarette smoke, plumbing alloys, soil, people living in cadmium hotspots near industrial works; it is also widespread in many foods and in rubber tyres, old plaster and carpet backing. It is particularly dangerous to pregnant women and children.

Aluminium

This mainly affects the central nervous system, bone metabolism, liver and kidneys. It may be involved in child hyperactivity and joint problems, and has been incriminated in Alzheimer's disease.

Sources: aluminium pans – especially when used to cook vegetables or fruit (e.g. rhubarb, apples), pressure cookers, teapots, cake tins, pie tins, roasting pans, baking foil, foil saucers, Coffeemate, water, antacids, domestic water and water boilers, yoghurt pot lids, fruit juice containers, TV dinners in foil, etc. It is released from the soil by acid rain. It is aggravated by a deficiency of magnesium and calcium.

Arsenic

This poison is found in shellfish, insecticides and animal feed additives, wallpaper and ceramics. Very large doses can be fatal. It is also found in the ground near tin mines, e.g., in Cornwall, and a degree of tolerance can be built up by eating vegetables grown there.

Therapeutic diets

One of the criticisms thrown at orthodox doctors is that they treat people like they treat cars. In one sense this is true. Like a car, a body will only run properly if it is given the right fuel at the right time. It is clear, however, that great variations exist and what is a good way of eating for one person may be disastrous for another. We believe that everybody should look at the food they eat and the way they eat it at least once in their lives, preferably when they are in good health. This should be done in the spirit of taking general responsibility for your own health. Part of this is to find out the most efficient fuel supply for your body and should be part of a total programme including exercise, attention to lifestyle and avoidance of stress, etc. If you feel you could do with a cleanout, try a limited fast (see below); this could be followed by a LIVER DIET (p. 264) over one month, but remember to substitute permitted for forbidden foods and eat enough quantity and variety of foods. Chew carefully and try to be in a quiet frame of mind at mealtimes.

Allergies

It is not the intention of any of these diets to unmask allergies but several of them may exclude certain foods or complete food groups altogether. If you find when you start the diet that you get a severe reaction, or that when stopping the diet and going back to your usual eating habits, the symptoms which have disappeared whilst you were on the diet come back suddenly, it is possible that you do have an allergic reaction to something you are eating. This may need to be evaluated further by elimination diets. We suggest you read the section on ALLERGY (p. 215) and, if necessary, consult a book which deals more extensively with exclusion diets such as Stephen Davies and Allan Stewart's *Nutritional Medicine*, or see a nutritionally qualified physician.

Fasting

Sheldon, a respected naturopath, defined the difference between starvation and fasting like this – as long as hunger is lacking it is fasting, but when hunger returns you are starving. Fasting results in the resting of the digestive tract, mobilization of the detoxification mechanism and an increase in the activity of the healing powers. It is an excellent introduction to observing the effects that certain foods have on you, and of course the effects of not eating at all. One of these is the release of toxins, previously stored in deposits of fat, into the system. This can mean that the liver, which is responsible for sifting out toxins, becomes overworked. To avoid this, it is advised that you take fruit juices, not just water, when you're fasting, as these can help to stimulate the body's own detoxification powers, while slowing down the rate of toxin release. You should not go into a fast straight from your usual diet, but have a day or two on raw vegetables and fruit, and similarly when you break the fast, have a couple of days on fruit and vegetables before going on to carbohydrates and then proteins. It is better to start gradually with fasting, so maybe do it for one day the first time, 2 days the next and so on. Fasting on a regular basis of, say one day a week, is probably better than a long fast once a year. Apart from prevention of certain illnesses, fasting can be helpful in cases of acute febrile illnesses, skin rashes, gastroenteritis, rheumatism, asthma, sinusitis, cholecystitis and colitis. When used as a preventive it is not uncommon to go through a healing crisis somewhere between the third and fourth day, where there is a drop in blood sugar, loss of appetite, coating of the tongue and acetone on the breath. After this healing crisis there is a gradual return to appetite. The tongue becomes clean and you feel generally better, almost as if you were walking on air.

There are, however, certain points to remember before starting a fast:

1 Only do so when you can be sure of being relaxed, and not under pressure – physical or mental.
2 Accept that you will not be able to smoke during the fasting period as it would make you very lightheaded (as well as being a pollutant to the body).
3 Obtain your doctor's clearance if you are known to have a severe allergy, or are taking a course of prescribed drugs.
4 If you are seriously ill or very run down you'd do better to wait until you're stronger before fasting.
5 *Do not fast* if you are hypoglycaemic or dependent on alcohol or drugs.

Notes for people undertaking the diets

On reading through the ailments and diseases section you may be referred to one of the diets from the following pages. These diets should not be undertaken as a punishment but as a challenge to you to find new foods to eat and new ways of cooking. If, however, you are suffering from a severe illness or are on orthodox drugs, it is better to ask your physician if it is all right to start the diet. However, it is very unlikely that any of these diets will lead to problems, provided that a wide enough variety of foods is eaten and that you eat them in sensible quantities. Remember that to get sufficient protein you need to mix grains and pulses in a ratio of 2 : 1, and of that mixture you only need ¾ of the weight of meat that you'd normally eat.

Tips for cooking pulses
Never add salt to pulses while they're boiling as this toughens the skins.

Always boil red kidney beans *vigorously* for 10 minutes at the start of cooking to destroy the natural toxins they contain, and remember to throw away the cooking liquids afterwards.

Pulses and legumes will cook more quickly if you first soak them overnight in plenty of cold water.

The arthritis diet
This is an alkaline diet used for the treatment of osteoarthritis and rheumatoid arthritis and other conditions where over-acidity is thought to play a part. Naturopaths believe that arthritis is caused by the accumulation of toxic acids in the joints. These acids are thought to come naturally from the intestine, and from a failure of the body's metabolism to detoxify them when in excess in the diet. Time limit – maximum – of the diet is one month and it should then be relaxed either by introducing forbidden foods one at a time or by having any of the foods previously not permitted on two occasions during the week.

Opinions on the efficacy of this diet in the treatment of arthritis and other 'acid' conditions vary from ridicule from the orthodox medical profession to claims of miraculous cures from naturopaths. The dietary recommendations given here represent a cross section of those opinions. They should be adhered to until the condition has stabilized. Remember to relax the restrictions after one month; then they can be relaxed further – although certain items should be avoided for life, such as white bread, junk food etc., except on very rare occasions. The dietary advice that follows on these pages should be followed strictly unless otherwise directed by your practitioner. These recommendations are an adjunct to individual homeopathic prescriptions and are designed to give your body the best possible chance to heal itself.

Foods to avoid	Foods allowed
A Red meat (beef, lamb, pork).	A White fish. Pulses (peas, beans, lentils, etc). Chicken – two meals a week only. Egg – two meals of two eggs a week only.
B Cow's milk, cheese and yoghurt.	B Goat's milk, cheese and yoghurt. Soya milk.
C Brown and white wheat flour, bran. (Do not use any produce where wheat starch, edible starch, cereal binder, cereal filler or cereal protein are listed as ingredients.)	C Oats, brown rice, corn (maize), buckwheat pasta, millet, 100% rye crispbread e.g. Ryvita, sugar-free oatcakes, sugar-free muesli e.g. Waitrose's.
D Citrus fruit, fruit covered in wax, such as imported apples.	D All other fruit. Dried fruit. Tomatoes twice a week only.
E	E All vegetables.
F Dry roasted nuts.	F All other nuts especially hazel, almond, cashew and walnut.
G Sugar and foods containing sugar. Syrup, treacle and honey.	G Sugar cane molasses, dried fruit, sugar-free jams such as Nature's Store, Robertsons and Whole Earth products.
H Coffee, decaffeinated coffee, cocoa, tea, alcohol.	H Grain coffees (Caro Extra for example), herbal teas, maté and Rooibosch teas, suitable unsweetened fruit juices, unsalted instant soup, vegetable juices.
I Salt, pepper, vinegar.	I Ruthmol salt, Martlett salt-free salad cream, Vecon vegetarian stock cubes.
J Butter and margarine – use as little as possible.	J Vegetable margarine (Vitaseig, Vitaquell, Tomor), vegetable oil.
K Chocolate.	K Carob.

Hay diet
This is a variation of the ARTHRITIS DIET which was developed by Dr Hay, an American physician who cured himself of kidney disease in the early part of the twentieth century. It is a food combination diet based on digestive requirements because different dietary constituents need different conditions to be digested.

Along with dietary changes, Dr Hay also advised fresh air, exercise and general lifestyle changes. The basic rules of his diet are: starches and sugar should not be eaten with proteins and acid fruits at the same meal; vegetables, salads and fruits should play a major part in the diet; proteins, starches and fats should be eaten in small quantities and only wholegrain unprocessed starches should be used; and finally at least 4 to 4½ hours should elapse between meals of different food groups.

It is particularly useful in patients with chronic digestive disorders such as flatulence, constipation, indigestion and obesity, and we would advise you to read *Food Combining for Health* by Doris Grant.

Yeast and mould free diet

This could be called the anti-candida diet; it should be combined with low carbohydrate diet and followed for a month but be careful to substitute permitted for forbidden foods, eat proper quantities of food and do not do the diet if you are on drugs without first consulting your GP or nutritionally trained physician. If after a month the symptoms have disappeared but return when you go on to an ordinary diet, you should seek the help of your homeopath or nutritionally trained physician.

For further information read *Candida Albicans* by Leon Chaitow.

Yeasts and fungi are used in many food preparation processes, and can be introduced into foods inadvertently. Brewer's and baker's yeasts are two strains of the organism: mostly people who react to one will react to the other. Yeast and wheatgerm are the two major sources of B-group vitamins. Persons who react to yeast may also react to mushrooms and truffles. No list can be comprehensive but yeast is certainly found in the following:

Bakery products All bread, buns, cakes, biscuits, rolls containing yeast and any food dressed in breadcrumbs. Also Twiglets, pizzas and bread pudding. Soda or unleavened bread is acceptable unless an allergy to wheat is suspected.

Alcoholic beverages All alcoholic drinks depend on yeasts to produce the alcohol – they are all risky. So is root beer.

Other beverages Citrus fruit drinks and juices – only home-squeezed are yeast-free. Malted milk, malted drinks and tea and coffee.

Cereals Malted cereals, malted dairy foods for babies, cereals enriched with vitamins.

Condiments Pickles and pickled foods, salad dressings, mayonnaise, horseradish sauce, tomato sauce, barbecue sauce, French dressing etc. Mustard, ketchup, sauerkraut, olives, chilli peppers, tamari and soy sauce, vinegar and Worcester sauce.

Dairy products All cheese including cottage cheese and cheese spreads, buttermilk, milk enriched with vitamins.

Fungi Mushrooms, mushroom sauce, truffles, etc. contain organisms closely related to yeast.

Meat products Hamburgers, sausages and cooked meats made with bread or breadcrumbs.

Yeast extracts Bisto, Marmite, Oxo, Bovril, Vegemite, gravy browning and all similar extracts.

Vitamins All B-vitamin preparations are likely to be derived from yeast unless otherwise stated, but most manufacturers do make some B-vitamin preparations free of yeast. Some selenium-rich foods.

Mould foods These foods either belong to the mould family, encourage moulds, or are prepared with them: buttermilk, sour cream, cheese snacks, peanuts, sour milk products, cheese dressings, cream cheese, pistachios, tinned and packet sauces, hydrolysed vegetable proteins and antibiotics. Many dairy products, eggs and meat contain antibiotics in small quantities. Eat sparingly.

Sugar foods Sugar, sucrose, fructose, maltose, lactose, glycogen, glucose milk, sweets, chocolate, sweet biscuits, cakes, candies, cookies, puddings, desserts, canned food, packaged food, hamburgers, honey, mannitol, sorbitol, galactose, monosaccharides, polysaccharides, date sugar, turbinado sugar, molasses, maple syrup, most bottled juices, all soft drinks, tonic water, milkshakes, raisins, dried apricots, dates, prunes, dried figs, other dried fruit.

N.B.:

1 Food labels should be checked carefully for hidden sugar and yeast. Avoid MSG (monosodium glutamate) also.
2 Shop or restaurant beef or hamburgers may contain added sugar.
3 Fruit should be avoided in the first few weeks due to its high content of natural sugars (fructose). Very sweet melons should probably be avoided altogether.
4 Milk is also best avoided initially, although live natural yoghurt is allowed because of its lactobacilli content, which will help to re-balance the gut flora.
5 Fibre content should be as high as possible to increase the absorptive surface of food in the gut and hasten the elimination of toxic waste. This is best achieved by high content of fresh vegetables, raw and cooked, or using cereal and pulse mixtures as a high fibre source to replace some meat meals. Oatbran or linseed may be added to the diet for this purpose as well.
6 Red meat should be avoided unless organically produced, in order to avoid antibody and steroid residues. White meat and fish is preferable.
7 To avoid development of candida-related food allergy it may be wise to try and eat foods in

rotation, so that no one food is eaten every day, but food groups are eaten twice a week (see twice-a-week rule p. 248). Many candida sufferers develop an allergy to grains, especially wheat.
8 Sugar substitutes i.e., saccharin and aspartame, are acceptable in small amounts in the short-term, but their long-term effects are not yet known.

Liver diet

This diet has been used to good effect by a naturopath and by a homeopathic doctor in the treatment of a variety of conditions where malfunction of the liver is suspected. Its purpose is to avoid those foods which the liver finds it difficult to process. Time limit: one month. Then have 'forbidden' foods twice weekly.

Foods to avoid	Foods to be eaten in unlimited quantities
A Meat, fowl.	A Fish (white preferred, limited tinned fish with oil washed off). Pulses – beans, peas and lentils.
B Eggs.	B Tofu – a soya milk product also known as bean curd, available from Chinese food shops.
C Refined bread and cereals.	C Wholemeal bread, unsweetened whole-grain cereals and wholegrains – brown rice, wholewheat pasta.
D Sugar, foods containing sugar, syrup, treacle, honey.	D Molasses, unsweetened jams (refrigerate after opening), Marmite.
E Cow's and goat's milk and products e.g. cheese.	E Soya milks.
F Tomatoes, citrus fruit, bananas, avocados.	F Vegetables, pineapples, grapes, melons. Suitable fruits tinned in natural juice.
G Nuts (except almonds).	G Almonds, sunflower and sesame seeds.
H Coffee, cocoa, alcohol, 2 cups of tea only a day.	H Grain coffees, herb teas, suitable unsweetened fruit juice, Rooibosch and maté teas.
I Chocolate.	I Carob powder.
J Fried food.	J Food can be sautéed using cold-pressed margarine or oil or vegetable butter.

Restricted foods: Berries (strawberries, raspberries, gooseberries, etc.) and apricots, peaches, sultanas, raisins and dates can be eaten twice a week in unlimited quantities. Less than ⅛ teaspoon salt can be taken daily.

Suggested menu plan

Uncooked breakfast – muesli or breakfast cereal and soya milk or some suitable fruit juice. Wholemeal toast and suitable margarine or spread.
Cooked breakfast – Mushrooms on toast or white fish. Porridge and soya milk.
Main meal – white fish/pulse dish/textured vegetable protein. TVP is available from health food shops – two meals weekly only. Wholemeal pasta/brown rice/potatoes. Fresh vegetables, some uncooked if possible i.e. as a side salad with the meal.
Desserts – suitable fruits, with or without wholemeal pastry or crumble. Desserts based on soya milk. Brown rice puddings with soya milk.
Smaller meals – wholemeal sandwiches with a suitable filling i.e. Marmite, pear/apple spread, tahini spread, lentil or bean spread. Salad. Suitable fresh or stewed fruit. Home-made soup and wholemeal bread.

Blood sugar levelling diet

This is used in the treatment of diabetes and HYPOGLYCAEMIA (p. 230), with a time limit of one month. After this if the diet has been successful in helping the symptoms you should keep off tea, coffee, sugar and alcohol except for the odd occasion and be careful to keep up your 2-hourly snacks. You can now have bread and potatoes as often as you like but not as snacks. In other words only have sandwiches or crisps as part of a light meal; and always have them with slow burning foods e.g., lentil soup.

On this diet you may feel slightly worse before you feel better, but that should not last for more than a few days. You may have a headache caused by caffeine withdrawal. If you are concerned or on drugs or insulin see your own doctor or a nutritionally qualified physician. Make sure that you substitute permitted for forbidden foods and that you have a wide variety of food and eat the proper amount, chew well and eat in a quiet frame of mind. You should also rest and get plenty of sleep.

Recent research regarding the glycaemic index of food, which gives an indication of the rate at which food is converted into glucose, suggests that the higher the index, the greater the rate of conversion and the less desirable these foods may be for those with a blood sugar problem. These are the foods which are avoided in this diet. There appear to be many differences between very similar foods and their ability to affect the index, and all the previous rules about simple and complex carbohydrates have now been proven to be unreliable. One point, however, which is probably valid is that like anthracite coal, small packages seem to burn slowly whilst large ones seem to burn quickly. When food is in its natural state, wheat for example, it will have a low glycaemic index, but as soon as the package is broken i.e. by grinding it into flour, the glycaemic index rises. For this reason, legumes such as lentils, kidney and soya beans are extremely good for patients who have blood sugar problems.

It is important on this diet to eat little and often. You should eat 3 meals a day but these should not be large meals. Between each meal you should take a snack – *so that you are eating something every 2 hours* or before you get a drop in energy or a gnawing hunger. Snacks should consist of raw nuts or seeds (such as pumpkin or sunflower), a glass of milk, yoghurt, Bombay mix or unsweetened oatcakes, e.g. Patersons. If you are getting very bored with these after a few weeks you can add more animal proteins as snacks, e.g., cold chicken, sardines, tuna etc. It is probably easiest to work out a menu for 2 weeks in advance to ensure that the restrictions on certain foods (see below) are adhered to. If weight is a problem, you may include protein powder or capsules once or twice daily instead of a snack.

Foods to avoid completely	*Substitutes which can be eaten in unlimited quantities*
A All refined and processed food.	A Unsweetened oatcakes, 100% rye crispbread, wholemeal pasta, pulses – all types of beans, peas, lentils etc., brown rice.
B All forms of sugar, honey, all sweets and confectionery, all products containing sugar, glucose, glucose syrup, honey, dextrose, fructose, etc.	B Sugar-cane molasses may be used for sweetening in cooking. As a honey substitute, use unsweetened jams such as those made by Robertsons, Nature's Store and Whole Earth.
C Cereals containing sugar.	C Unsweetened muesli, porridge, nut butters, e.g. cashew nut butter.
D Cakes and biscuits, pies, puddings, bananas, custard.	D Fruit including citrus fruit, fresh or stewed without sugar, yoghurt, cottage cheese, raw nuts, seeds, pancakes.
E Tea, coffee, alcohol, soft drinks, hot chocolate, Ovaltine.	E Cow's milk, grain coffee, e.g. Caro Extra, herb teas, maté and Rooibosch teas, unsweetened fruit juice, vegetable juice.
F Potatoes.	F All other vegetables, wholemeal pasta, pulses, etc.
G Cough syrups, laxatives, medications with caffeine or sugar, relish, ketchup, mustard, sauces.	G Olive oil, sunflower oil.

And no smoking!

Foods which may be eaten in limited quantities Each week you may eat 2 meals using white fish, 2 meals using meat, and 2 meals using eggs (2 eggs to each meal), while pasta may be eaten twice a week. 1–2 slices of rye bread may be eaten every day or 1 slice of wholemeal bread. Wholemeal flour may be used for cooking pastry and flans which may be eaten twice a week. Only ⅛ teaspoon salt is allowed daily. Butter or margarine in small amounts is permitted on bread, etc. Cook with oil. Raisins and other dried fruits are allowed in small quantities twice a week only. Full fat cheese may be eaten twice a week.

Suggested meal pattern
Uncooked breakfast: Grapefruit segments fresh or canned in natural juice. Muesli, rye crispbread, fresh fruit.
Cooked breakfast: Poached or boiled eggs, pancakes, porridge, unsweetened baked beans, mushrooms or tomatoes on toast.
Lunch or supper: Meat, white fish, cheese or eggs. Vegetable purées can be used to replace gravy or other sauces. Wholemeal pasta, pulse dishes. Vegetables, salads.
Uncooked lunch or evening meal: Salads, bread or toast, rye crispbread, with suitable spread – lentil paste, cottage cheese, unsweetened jam, vegetable pâté, etc.
Desserts: Fresh or stewed fruit, baked apples, nuts, yoghurt, fruit fools made with stewed fruit and yoghurt. Pancakes made with wholemeal flour.

Colon diet
There are basically two circumstances under which dietary regimes which act specifically on the colon may be employed. The first, and most common, is having a disease actually affecting the colon, such as irritable bowel syndrome or a form of colitis. If you are suffering from a severe form of colitis, such as Crohn's disease, or if you

are on any drugs, then you should not use any of the following diets without asking your GP or nutritionally qualified physician. The most common diet for the colon is a high fibre diet which aims to give more than 30 g of fibre a day. This is done by a) eating less refined carbohydrate, b) eating plenty of fresh fruit and vegetables, c) eating wholegrain cereals and d) eating larger than usual quantities of pulses and legumes such as peas, lentils, beans, etc. Once again, the twice-a-week rule, page 248, applies.

Then there is the food exclusion diet for the colon. Researchers in Cambridge have found that the five most common food groups to cause irritable bowel syndrome, as measured by levels of prostaglandins in the rectum, are reflected in the colon diet which avoids wheat, corn, dairy products, tea, coffee, citrus fruits. These can either be stopped all at once, or one at a time, then reintroduced to see whether previous symptoms disappear when these foods are excluded, and return when they are included again. If you find that any one food seems to make the irritable bowel worse, then you can cut it down, say to twice a week, but remember to find a substitute. If you find that it is causing problems even when you are having it only twice a week, then you should consult your homeopath or nutritionally qualified physician about it.

Natural laxatives
Linseed tea: dissolve 1 dessertspoon of linseeds in 0.5 litre (1 pint) water. Simmer for 10 minutes, strain and drink 1 cup 10 minutes before food.
Linseed meal: dissolve 1 dessertspoon of linseeds in water and take up to 3 times a day. For best results, allow to soak overnight.
Blackstrap molasses: take 1 dessertspoon 3 times a day.

Colon cleansing
The other way in which nutrition can be used to help the colon is if it is felt that toxins are being absorbed from the colon and going up in the portal system to the liver where they are causing sluggishness of the liver, leading to such symptoms as headaches, irritability, hang-over feelings, general lack of energy and mild depression. There may also be other specific symptoms such as joint pains. The colon plan is best carried out along with the liver diet, which should not be attempted by anyone with bowel trouble or who is on drugs, without the consent of their GP or nutritionally qualified physician. The ingredients of the colon cleanse are:

1 *Alfalfa tablets:* start with one tablet 3 times a day after meals, followed by water, and build up to 4 tablets 3 times a day.
2 *Acidophilus capsules:* which are a concentrate of a healthy bacteria normally found in the colon: take one capsule a day, building up to one capsule 3 times a day 10 minutes before food. These capsules should be kept in the refrigerator once the package is opened. Each capsule should be around 500 mg, and if you cannot obtain acidophilus capsules, have one carton of live plain yoghurt daily.
3 *Psyllium husks:* start with half a teaspoon a day building up to 3 teaspoonfuls a day taken in a small amount of water. Drink 2 cups of water immediately afterwards. The husks do not dissolve well and you may find it easier to take them in soda water or other aerated drinks as the bubbles appear to help them stay dispersed, thus making them easier to swallow. Psyllium husks are also available in capsules; dose is 3–9/day. If you cannot obtain psyllium husks, use linseeds in the same manner, but starting with half a dessertspoon and building up to 3 dessertspoons.

All these products are natural and should not cause problems such as pain, constipation or diarrhoea. Should you feel, however, that they are upsetting you, stop everything and then reintroduce them one by one to find out what is causing the trouble. Discuss the problem with your homeopath or nutritionally qualified physician. The bowel programme can be continued for up to 3 months providing it is not causing any problems. If you experience a lot of flatulence it may be that the alfalfa is clearing out the toxins faster than the psyllium husks or linseeds can remove them; stop the alfalfa for a few days to see if this helps.

Appendix A
General Remedy Finder

Note: see How to Use This Book, PART 1, for help on how to use the General Remedy Finder.

Body

Appetite
see WEIGHT PROBLEMS,
pp. 35–50

Breathing

Difficulty in breathing
Apis
Arsenicum
Bryonia
Cactus
Carbo veg.
Causticum
Chelidonium
China
Cina
Croton tig.
Cuprum
Ferrum
Hepar sulph.
Ipecac.
Kali ars.
Kali carb.
Kali iod.
Lachesis
Lycopodium
Mercurius corr.
Naja
Natrum sulph.
Nux mosch.
Opium
Phosphorus
Pulsatilla
Selenium
Silicea
Spongia
Squilla
Stannum
Sulphur
Tarentula
Veratrum

Gasping for breath
Apis
Lycopodium

Irregular breathing
Ailanthus
Angustura
Belladonna
Cuprum
Digitalis
Opium

Rapid breathing
Aconite
Antimonium
Arsenicum
Belladonna
Bryonia
Carbo veg.
Chelidonium
Cuprum
Gelsemium
Ipecac.
Lycopodium
Phosphorus
Sepia
Sulphur

Sighing frequently
Bryonia
Caladium
Calcarea phos.
Carbo veg.
Digitalis
Ignatia
Ipecac.
Opium
Secale
Selenium
Stramonium

Wheezy breathing
Arsenicum
Carbo veg.
Ipecac.
Kali carb.

Clothing

Intolerance of clothing
Argentum nit.
Calcarea

Lachesis
Lycopodium
Nux
Onosmodium
Spongia

Wanting to loosen clothing
Calcarea
Lachesis
Lycopodium
Nitric ac.
Nux

Uncovering makes symptoms worse
Arsenicum
Hepar sulph.
Kali ars.
Kali carb.
Lycopodium
Magnesia phos.
Nux
Nux mosch.
Rhododendron
Rhus tox.
Sambucus
Silicea
Squilla
Zinc

Complexion
see Remedy Finder for Face
under Beauty Care Problems

Drinking
see THIRST, WEIGHT PROBLEMS

Eating
see WEIGHT PROBLEMS

Symptoms get worse while eating
Ammon. carb.
Carbo an.
Carbo veg.

Conium
Kali carb.
Nitric ac.
Sulphur

**Eating to satiety alleviates
symptoms**
Arsenicum
Iodum
Medorrhinum
Phosphorus

**Eating to satiety makes
symptoms worse**
Calcarea
Lycopodium
Pulsatilla
Sulphur

Facial expression

Anxious
Aconite
Aethusa
Ailanthus
Arsenicum
Borax
Camphora
China sulph.
Lac can.
Veratrum

Confused
Aesculus
Arsenicum
Bufo
Lycopodium

Distressed
Ailanthus
Arsenicum
Cactus
Croton
Iodum
Nux mosch.
Stramonium

Frightened
Aconite
Baptisia
Cantharis
Stramonium

Haggard
Arsenicum
Camphora
Capsicum
Carbo veg.

Hydrastis
Hyoscyamus
Kali carb.
Lachesis
Natrum mur.
Phosphorus
Silicea
Veratrum vir.

Old-looking
Argentum nit.
Calcarea
Conium
Guaiacum
Natrum mur.
Opium

Sickly
Arsenicum
Cina
Lachesis
Lycopodium

Stupid, stupefied
Argentum nit.
Arnica
Arsenicum
Cannabis ind.
Ferrum
Gelsemium
Helleborus
Hyoscyamus
Nux mosch.
Stramonium

Sleepy
Cannabis ind.
Nux mosch.
Opium

Suffering
Arsenicum
Cactus
Kali carb.
Lyssin
Manganum
Silicea
Sulphur

Faeces

**Symptoms worse before
bowel movements**
Aloes
Argentum nit.
Dioscorea
Kali carb.
Magnesia carb.
Mercurius

Rheum
Veratrum

**Symptoms worse during
bowel movements**
Arsenicum
Chamomilla
Iris
Kali bichrom.
Mercurius
Pulsatilla
Sulphur

**Symptoms better after bowel
movements**
Bryonia
Colchicum
Nux
Spigelia

**Symptoms worse after bowel
movements**
Alumina
Causticum
Ignatia
Iris
Mercurius corr.
Nux
Phosphorus
Selenium

Frequent bowel movements
Arsenicum
Capsicum
Chamomilla
Mercurius
Mercurius corr.
Nux
Phosphorus
Podophyllum
Veratrum

Dry faeces
Bryonia
Lac deflor.
Lycopodium
Natrum mur.
Nitric ac.
Nux
Opium
Phosphorus
Silicea
Zinc

Foul-smelling faeces
Argentum nit.
Arsenicum
Asafoetida

Baptisia
Benzoic ac.
Bryonia
Carbo veg.
Carbon sulph.
Crotalus
Graphites
Kali ars.
Kali phos.
Lachesis
Mercurius corr.
Natrum sulph.
Nux mosch.
Opium
Podophyllum
Psorinum
Silicea
Squilla
Sulphur
Tuberculinum

Greenish faeces
Argentum nit.
Calcarea phos.
Chamomilla
Colocynth
Croton
Gratiola
Ipecac.
Magnesia carb.
Mercurius
Mercurius corr.
Natrum mur.
Natrum sulph.
Phosphorus
Plumbum
Podophyllum
Pulsatilla
Secale
Sulphur
Veratrum

Hard faeces
Alum
Alumina
Ammon carb.
Ammon mur.
Antimonium
Bryonia
Calcarea
Carbon sulph.
Carduus
Collinsonia
Graphites
Kali brom.
Lac deflor.
Lachesis
Lycopodium

Magnesia mur.
Mezereum
Natrum mur.
Nitric ac.
Nux
Opium
Phosphorus
Plumbum
Selenium
Sepia
Silicea
Sulphur
Veratrum
Verbascum
Zinc

Pale-coloured faeces
Arsenicum
Borax
Calcarea
Carduus
Chelidonium
China
Digitalis
Lycopodium
Mercurius
Phosphoric ac.
Sanicula
Silicea
Tabacum

Pasty-looking faeces
Bryonia
Chelidonium
Colocynth
Croton
Mercurius
Mercurius corr.
Podophyllum
Rheum
Sulphur

Faeces like sheep's droppings
Alum
Alumina
Chelidonium
Magnesia mur.
Mercurius
Natrum mur.
Nitric ac.
Opium
Plumbum
Sulphur

**Faeces containing
   undigested food**
Arsenicum
Bryonia

Calcarea
China
China ars.
Ferrum
Graphites
Magnesia mur.
Phosphoric ac.
Phosphorus
Podophyllum

Watery faeces
Agaricus
Antimonium
Apis
Apocynum
Argentum nit.
Asafoetida
Benzoic ac.
Calcarea
Carbon sulph.
Chamomilla
Colchicum
Conium
Dulcamara
Iris
Kali bichrom.
Magnesia carb.
Mercurius
Natrum mur.
Natrum sulph.
Nux
Opium
Phosphorus
Picric ac.
Podophyllum
Psorinum
Pulsatilla
Secale
Sulphur
Thuja
Veratrum
Veratrum vir.

Hearing
   see NOISE

Left side/right side
   see also MOVEMENT AND
   POSTURE p. 275

Symptoms worse on left side
Argentum nit.
Asarum
Capsicum
Cina
Clematis
Crocus
Euphrasia

Graphites
Kreosotum
Lachesis
Mezereum
Oleander
Phosphorus
Selenium
Sepia
Squilla
Stannum
Sulphur

Worse on left then right
Lachesis

Symptoms worse on the right
Apis
Argentum
Arsenicum
Aurum
Baptisia
Belladonna
Borax
Colocynth
Conium
Crotalus
Lycopodium
Lyssin
Nux
Pulsatilla
Ratanhia
Sarsaparilla
Secale
Sulphuric ac.

Mouth

Bad breath
Arnica
Arsenicum
Arsenicum iod.
Carbo veg.
Chamomilla
Chelidonium
Kali phos.
Kreosotum
Lachesis
Mercurius corr.
Natrum mur.
Nitric ac.
Nux
Plumbum
Psorinum
Sulphur
Tuberculinum

Dry lips
Antimonium
Bryonia

Hyoscyamus
Nux mosch.
Pulsatilla
Rhus tox.
Sulphur
Veratrum vir.

Pale lips
Arsenicum
Ferrum
Kali ars.
Medorrhinum

Red lips
Sulphur

Cracked lips
Arsenicum
Alum tri.
Bryonia
Calcarea
Carbo veg.
Carbon sulph.
China
Graphites
Lachesis
Natrum mur.
Sulphur

Mouth feels dry
Aconite
Arsenicum
Baryta
Baryta mur.
Belladonna
Borax
Bryonia
Cannabis ind.
Capsicum
Carbo veg.
Chamomilla
China
Hyoscyamus
Ignatia
Kali bichrom.
Lachesis
Laurocerasus
Lycopodium
Mercurius
Muriatic ac.
Naja
Natrum ars.
Natrum mur.
Natrum sulph.
Nux
Nux mosch.
Phosphoric ac.
Phosphorus

Rhus tox.
Sepia
Silicea
Sulphur
Veratrum
Veratrum vir.

More saliva produced than usual
Ammonium carb.
Arum
Baryta
Borax
Fluoric ac.
Iodum
Ipecac.
Kali carb.
Lyssin
Mercurius
Mercurius corr.
Natrum mur.
Nitric ac.
Nux
Veratrum

Increased saliva production at night
Argentum nit.
Mercurius
Natrum mur.
Rhus tox.

Tongue looks black
Carbo veg.
China
Mercurius
Phosphorus

Tongue feels dry
Aconite
Agaricus
Ailanthus
Apis
Arsenicum
Belladonna
Bryonia
Calcarea
Camphor
Causticum
Chamomilla
China
Cocculus
Cuprum
Helleborus
Hyoscyamus
Lachesis
Mercurius
Muriatic ac.

Nux mosch.
Psorinum
Pulsatilla
Rhus tox.
Sulphur
Terebinth
Veratrum vir.

Tongue red all over
Apis
Arsenicum
Belladonna
Mercurius
Nitric ac.
Phosphorus
Rhus tox.

Tongue red on tip only
Argentum nit.
Arsenicum
Phytolacca
Rhus tox.
Rhus ven.
Sulphur

Tongue red around edges
Arsenicum
Chelidonium
Mercurius
Sulphur

Tongue looks swollen
Aconite
Apis
Belladonna
Crotalus
Mercurius

Tongue white and coated
Antimonium
Arsenicum
Belladonna
Bryonia
Calcarea
Hyoscyamus
Kali bichrom.
Mercurius
Nitric ac.
Pulsatilla
Spigelia
Sulphur
Taraxacum

Tongue looks yellow
Antimonium
Chelidonium
Mercurius
Nux mosch.

Rhus tox.
Spigelia

Teething problems
Aconite
Arsenicum
Borax
Calcarea
Calcarea phos.
Chamomilla
Mercurius
Silicea
Staphisagria
Sulphur

Movement and posture

Moving around alleviates symptoms
Aurum
Aurum mur.
Capsicum
Cyclamen
Euphrasia
Ferrum
Kali sulph.
Pyrogenium
Pulsatilla
Sabadilla
Sambucus
Sulphur
Taraxacum
Tarentula
Valerian

Moving around makes symptoms worse
Belladonna
Bismuth
Bryonia
Chelidonium
China
Cocculus
Colchicum
Colocynth
Guaiacum
Ledum
Mercurius
Nux
Ranunculus
Sabina
Silicea

Constant movement alleviates symptoms
Capsicum
Conium
Euphrasia
Ferrum

Fluoric ac.
Pulsatilla
Rhododendron
Rhus tox.
Sambucus
Syphilinum

Starting to move makes symptoms worse
Capsicum
Conium
Euphrasia
Ferrum
Lycopodium
Pulsatilla
Rhus tox.

Rapid or vigorous movement alleviates symptoms
Arsenicum
Bryonia
Ferrum
Sepia

Rapid or vigorous movement makes symptoms worse
Arsenicum
Bryonia

Sudden movement makes symptoms worse
Cocculus
Ferrum
Kali carb.

Bending backwards alleviates symptoms
Antimonium
Drosera

Bending backwards makes symptoms worse
Chamomilla
Colchicum
Platina
Pulsatilla
Rheum
Rhus tox.
Sepia
Staphisagria

Bending forward alleviates symptoms
Manganum

Bending forward makes symptoms worse
Belladonna
Coffea

Bending double alleviates symptoms
Calcarea
Colocynth
Kali carb.
Magnesia phos.
Rheum
Rhus tox.
Sulphur

Changing position alleviates symptoms
Ignatia
Natrum sulph.
Phosphoric ac.
Rhus tox.
Sepia
Valerian

Changing position makes symptoms worse
Capsicum
Euphrasia
Ferrum
Ignatia
Lycopodium
Pulsatilla
Rhus tox.
Syphilinum

Downward motion makes symptoms worse
Borax
Gelsemium

Physical exercise makes symptoms worse
Alumina
Arnica
Arsenicum
Arsenicum iod.
Bryonia
Calcarea
Calcarea sulph.
Cocculus
Conium
Digitalis
Ferrum iod.
Gelsemium
Iodum
Laurocerasus
Lilium tig.
Natrum ars.
Natrum carb.
Natrum mur.
Picric ac.
Rhus tox.

Selenium
Sepia
Spigelia
Spongia
Stannum
Staphisagria
Sulphur
Teucrium
Tuberculinum

Jarring or vibration makes symptoms worse
Arnica
Belladonna
Bryonia
Cicuta
Conium
Lachesis
Nitric ac.
Rhus tox.
Silicea
Theridion

Kneeling makes symptoms worse
Cocculus

Lifting things makes symptoms worse
Arnica
Bryonia
Calcarea
Carbo an.
Conium
Graphites
Rhus tox.
Ruta
Silicea

Drawing up limbs makes symptoms worse
Rhus tox.
Sabina

Drawing up limbs makes symptoms better
Calcarea
Sepia
Sulphur
Thuja

Limbs hanging down alleviates symptoms
Conium

Limbs hanging down makes symptoms worse
Belladonna
Calcarea

Lying down makes symptoms worse
Apis
Arsenicum
Aurum
Capsicum
Chamomilla
Conium
Drosera
Euphrasia
Ferrum
Hyoscyamus
Kali carb.
Lycopodium
Menyanthes
Natrum sulph.
Phosphorus
Platina
Pulsatilla
Rhus tox.
Rumex
Sambucus
Sanguinaria
Taraxacum

Lying down makes symptoms better
Ammonium mur.
Asarum
Belladonna
Bryonia
Calcarea
Ferrum
Manganum
Natrum mur.
Nux
Picric ac.
Squilla

Lying on back alleviates symptoms
Ammonium mur.
Bryonia
Calcarea
Mercurius corr.
Pulsatilla
Rhus tox.

Lying on back makes symptoms worse
Ignatia
Nux
Phosphorus

Lying on left side makes symptoms worse
Phosphorus
Pulsatilla

**Lying on right side makes
symptoms worse**
Mercurius

**Lying on right side makes
symptoms better**
Phosphorus
Pulsatilla

**Lying on painful side makes
symptoms better**
Bryonia

**Lying on painful side makes
symptoms worse**
Baryta carb.
Caladium
Cyclamen
Hepar sulph.
Iodum
Lachesis
Magnesia mur.
Nux mosch.
Ruta
Silicea

**Lying on unaffected side
makes symptoms worse**
Bryonia
Colocynth
Fluoric ac.
Pulsatilla
Secale

**Lying with head high
alleviates symptoms**
Arsenicum
Kali nit.

**Lying doubled up alleviates
symptoms**
Colocynth

**Lying on abdomen alleviates
symptoms**
Belladonna

**Rising up from sitting or lying
position makes symptoms
worse**
Aconite
Belladonna
Bryonia
Carbo veg.
Cocculus
Digitalis
Lycopodium
Nux

Opium
Rhus tox.
Silicea
Spigelia
Sulphur

**Rising up makes symptoms
better**
Ammonium carb.
Arsenicum
Calcarea
Capsicum
Cyclamen
Dulcamara
Platina
Sambucus
Sepia
Verbena
Viola

**Rising up from bed alleviates
symptoms**
Phosphoric ac.
Pulsatilla

**Sitting makes symptoms
worse**
Agaricus
Ammonium mur.
Arsenicum
Capsicum
Conium
Cyclamen
Dulcamara
Euphrasia
Lycopodium
Phosphorus
Platina
Pulsatilla
Rhus tox.
Sepia
Sulphur
Valerian
Verbena
Viola
Zinc
Zinc phos.

Sitting alleviates symptoms
Bryonia
Colchicum
Digitalis
Nux

Urgent need to sit down
China
Conium
Graphites

Nux
Phosphorus
Squilla

**Standing makes symptoms
worse**
Cocculus
Conium
Cyclamen
Lilium
Pulsatilla
Sepia
Sulphur
Valerian

**Standing up makes symptoms
better**
Arsenicum
Belladonna

**Stooping makes symptoms
worse**
Bryonia

**Stretching makes symptoms
worse**
Arsenicum
Causticum
Chamomilla
Nux
Pulsatilla
Rhus tox.

**Travelling makes symptoms
worse**
Cocculus
Helonius
Petroleum
Sepia
Tabacum

**Travelling makes symptoms
better**
Nitric ac.

Walking aggravates symptoms
Aesculus
Belladonna
Bryonia
Calcarea
Calcarea sulph.
Causticum
China
Cocculus
Colchicum
Conium
Fluoric ac.
Ledum

Magnesia phos.
Nitric ac.
Nux
Phosphorus
Rhus tox.
Sepia
Spigelia
Stannum
Sulphur

Walking makes symptoms better
Aurum
Conium
Cyclamen
Dulcamara
Euphrasia
Ferrum
Kali iod.
Pulsatilla
Rhus tox.
Sabadilla
Sambucus
Sulphur
Taraxacum
Valerian

Muscles

Tired or aching
Aconite
Antimonium
Arnica
Causticum
Cimicifuga
Colchicum
Dulcamara
Gelsemium
Ranunculus
Rhus tox.
Ruta
Veratrum
Veratrum vir.

Pain

Pain appears gradually and disappears gradually
Platina
Sanguinaria
Stannum
Syphilinum

Pain appears suddenly
Belladonna
Nitric ac.

Pains appear suddenly and disappear suddenly
Belladonna
Kali bichrom.
Nitric ac.

Pain in bones
Asafoetida
Eupatorium
Ipecac.
Mercurius
Nitric ac.
Phosphoric ac.
Pulsatilla
Ruta

Pain in ligaments
Fluoric ac.
Guaiacum
Rhus tox.
Ruta

Pain in glands
Arnica
Belladonna
Lycopodium
Mercurius
Phosphorus
Thuja

Pain in joints
Argentum
Arnica
Bryonia
Calcarea phos.
Ledum
Nux
Plumbum
Pulsatilla
Rhus tox.

Painful lining of the bones (periostium)
Ammonium carb.
Arnica
Asafoetida
Aurum mur.
Kali iod.
Phosphoric ac.
Ruta

Pain which appears in small spots
Arnica
Ignatia
Kali bichrom.
Lachesis
Sabadilla
Sulphur

Pain in tendons
Rhus tox.

Pain before thunderstorms
Rhododendron

Pain which disappears as suddenly as it comes on
Belladonna
Kali bichrom.
Nitric ac.

Pain which comes on and wears off gradually
Platina
Stannum

Biting pain
Carbo veg.
Nux
Petroselinum
Sulphur
Zinc

Boring, penetrating pain
Argentum nit.
Aurum
Belladonna
Bismuth
Pulsatilla
Spigelia

Burning pain – external
Apis
Arsenicum
Arum
Bryonia
Carbo veg.
Carbon sulph.
Causticum
Euphrasia
Iris
Mercurius
Natrum mur.
Nux
Phosphoric ac.
Phosphorus
Ratanhia
Secale
Sepia
Silicea
Stannum
Sulphur

Burning pain – internal
Aconite
Arsenicum
Arum

Belladonna
Berberis
Bryonia
Cannabis
Cantharis
Carbon sulph.
Graphites
Kali bichrom.
Mercurius
Mercurius corr.
Mezereum
Nitric ac.
Nux
Phosphorus
Prunus
Pulsatilla
Rhus tox.
Sabadilla
Sanguinaria
Secale
Sepia
Spigelia
Spongia
Sulphur
Zinc

Constricting pain – external
Platina
Pulsatilla

Constricting pain – internal
Ambra
Ignatia
Phosphoric ac.
Platina

Cutting pain – external
Belladonna
Calcarea
Conium
Drosera
Natrum carb.
Petroleum

Cutting pain – internal
Belladonna
Calcarea
Cantharis
Colocynth
Conium
Dioscorea
Hyoscyamus
Kali carb.
Lycopodium
Mercurius
Natrum mur.
Nux
Pulsatilla

Silicea
Sulphur
Veratrum
Zinc

Digging or gouging pain
Dulcamara
Rhododendron
Spigelia

Dragging or pulling pain
Carbo veg.
Chelidonium
Graphites
Nitric ac.
Valerian

Flitting, shifting pain
Kali bichrom.
Kali sulph.
Lac can.
Ledum
Pulsatilla

Gnawing pain
Arsenicum
Causticum
Mercurius
Silicea
Staphisagria
Sulphur

Sudden cramping pain – external
Asafoetida
Calcarea
Causticum
Menyanthes
Natrum mur.
Nux
Pulsatilla
Rhus tox.
Taraxacum
Valerian

Sudden cramping pain – internal
Belladonna
China
Ignatia
Kali carb.
Nitric ac.
Pulsatilla
Silicea
Sulphur
Thuja

Numbing pain
Chamomilla
Oleander
Platina
Sabadilla
Verbascum

Paralysing pain
Belladonna
Cina
Cocculus
Colchicum
Cyclamen
Nux
Sabina

Pinching pain
Arnica
Belladonna
Nux

Pressing, persistent pain – external
Agaricus
Apocynum
Cannabis ind.
Causticum
China sulph.
Drosera
Eupatorium
Ferrum
Kali bichrom.
Moschus
Nitric ac.
Nux
Phosphorus
Podophyllum
Pulsatilla
Rhododendron
Rhus tox.
Ruta
Sepia
Silicea
Spigelia
Stannum
Staphisagria
Sulphur

Pressing, persistent pain – internal
Argentum nit.
Arnica
Arsenicum
Asafoetida
Belladonna
Bromium
Calcarea
Cantharis

Carbo veg.
China
Cimicifuga
Colocynth
Cuprum
Hamamelis
Lachesis
Lilium
Lycopodium
Menyanthes
Natrum mur.
Nux
Opium
Petroleum
Phosphorus
Pulsatilla
Ranunculus
Rhus tox.
Ruta
Sanguinaria
Secale
Senega
Sepia
Silicea
Spigelia
Spongia
Stannum
Sulphur
Valerian
Veratrum
Zinc

Heavy, pressing pain
Aconite
Belladonna
Bromium
Bryonia
Ipecac.
Lilium
Menyanthes
Nux
Pareira
Phosphorus
Ranunculus
Rhus tox.
Sepia
Sticta
Sulphur

Inward-pressing pain
Anacardium
Platina
Stannum

Outward-pressing pain
Asafoetida
Bryonia
Cimicifuga

Pulsatilla
Sulphur
Valerian

Scraping pain
Bryonia
Drosera
Nux
Pulsatilla
Sulphur
Veratrum

Sore, bruised feeling
Argentum
Arnica
China
Cicuta
Cimicifuga
Drosera
Hamamelis
Platina
Pyrogenium
Rhus tox.
Ruta
Silicea

Splinter-like pain
Agaricus
Argentum nit.
Hepar sulph.
Nitric ac.

Squeezing pain
Alumina
Asarum
Cocculus
Nux
Platina
Sulphur

Stitch-like pain – external
Asafoetida
Belladonna
Bryonia
Calcarea
Carbon sulph.
Cicuta
Conium
Kali carb.
Kali sulph.
Ledum
Mercurius
Nitric ac.
Pulsatilla
Ranunculus
Rhus tox.
Spigelia
Staphisagria

Sulphur
Taraxacum
Thuja
Zinc

Stitch-like pain – internal
Asafoetida
Berberis
Borax
Bryonia
Cannabis ind.
Cantharis
Carbon sulph.
Chelidonium
China
Ignatia
Kali carb.
Kali sulph.
Lachesis
Ledum
Mercurius
Mercurius corr.
Nitric ac.
Phosphorus
Plumbum
Pulsatilla
Ranunculus
Sepia
Silicea
Spigelia
Squilla

Tearing pain – external
Aconite
Arnica
Belladonna
Berberis
Bryonia
Carbon sulph.
China
Colchicum
Hypericum
Kali carb.
Kali phos.
Kali sulph.
Ledum
Lycopodium
Natrum mur.
Natrum sulph.
Nitric ac.
Pulsatilla
Sepia
Silicea
Sulphur
Zinc

Tearing pain – internal
Belladonna
Berberis

Bryonia
Carbo veg.
Conium
Kali sulph.
Ledum
Lycopodium
Mercurius
Nux
Pulsatilla
Sepia
Silicea
Spigelia
Sulphur

Absence of pain in conditions which are usually painful
Helleborus
Opium
Stramonium

Perspiration

Sweat smells offensive
Arnica
Baryta mur.
Carbo an.
Carbon sulph.
Graphites
Hepar sulph.
Lycopodium
Mercurius
Nitric ac.
Nux
Petroleum
Pulsatilla
Sepia
Silicea
Sulphur
Thuja

Sour
Arsenicum
Bryonia
Colchicum
Hepar sulph.
Iodum
Lycopodium
Mercurius
Nitric ac.
Psorinum
Sepia
Silicea
Sulphur
Veratrum

Sweet
Arsenicum
Caladium

Sepia
Uranium nit.

Rest

Rest makes symptoms worse
Aurum
Capsicum
Conium
Cyclamen
Dulcamara
Euphrasia
Ferrum
Lycopodium
Magnesia mur.
Pulsatilla
Rhus tox.
Sabadilla
Sambucus
Sepia
Taraxacum
Valerian

Rest makes symptoms better
Belladonna
Bryonia
Colchicum
Gelsemium
Ledum
Nux
Sepia

Sex
see also LIBIDO p. 296

Aversion to
Asarum
Causticum
Natrum mur.
Sepia

Lack of enjoyment during intercourse
Causticum
Sepia

Ailments from coitus interruptus
Bellis

Pain on intercourse
Argentum nit.
Lyssin
Natrum mur.
Platina
Sepia

Tingling voluptuous sensation in vagina as if having intercourse
Platina

Sight
see Specific Remedy Finder under Eyes in BEAUTY CARE PROBLEMS

Skin
see Specific Remedy Finder under Skin in BEAUTY CARE PROBLEMS

Sleep

Sleep makes symptoms worse
Lachesis
Selenium
Spongia
Stramonium
Sulphur

Sleep makes symptoms better
Phosphoric ac.
Phosphorus

Symptoms worse before sleeping
Arsenicum
Bryonia
Calcarea
Carbo veg.
Mercurius
Phosphorus
Pulsatilla
Rhus tox.
Sepia
Sulphur

Symptoms get worse in first stages of sleep
Arsenicum
Belladonna
Bryonia
Crotalus
Kali carb.
Lachesis
Pulsatilla
Sepia

Symptoms get worse during sleep
Arnica
Arsenicum
Belladonna
Borax
Bryonia
Chamomilla
Hepar sulph.
Hyoscyamus
Lachesis

Mercurius
Opium
Pulsatilla
Silicea
Stramonium
Sulphur
Zinc

Loss of sleep makes symptoms worse
Cocculus
Nux
Phosphorus

Symptoms worse on waking
Ambra
Ammonium mur.
Arsenicum
Calcarea
Causticum
Hepar sulph.
Lachesis
Nux
Phosphorus
Pulsatilla
Rhus tox.
Sepia
Sulphur

Overpowering need for sleep
Antimonium
Nux mosch.
Opium

Overpowering need for sleep, especially in afternoon
Pulsatilla

Sleeplessness before midnight
Ambra
Arsenicum
Calcarea
Calcarea phos.
Carbo veg.
Coffea
Conium
Kali carb.
Lycopodium
Magnesia mur.
Mercurius
Natrum ars.
Natrum carb.
Phosphorus
Picric ac.
Pulsatilla
Rhus tox.
Sepia
Silicea
Sulphur

Sleeplessness after midnight
Arsenicum
Capsicum
Coffea
Hepar sulph.
Kali ars.
Kali carb.
Nux
Phosphoric ac.
Silicea

Sleeplessness after 1 or 2 am
Kali carb.

Sleeplessness from anxiety
Arsenicum
Cocculus

Difficulty in falling asleep in a dark room
Pulsatilla
Stramonium

Sleeplessness during diarrhoea
Bufo
Phosphorus

Sleeplessness after eating supper
China

Sleeplessness due to over-excitement
Coffea
Hyoscyamus
Nux

Sleeplessness after mental study and mental work
Arsenicum
Hyoscyamus

Sleeplessness from fear
Aconite

Sleeplessness after fright
Aconite

Sleepy before you go to bed, sleepless in bed
Ambra

Sleeplessness from grief
Natrum mur.

Sleeplessness with headache
Aurum

China
Sulphur

Sleeplessness from homesickness
Capsicum

Sleeplessness from irritability
Hyoscyamus

Sleeplessness from itchiness
Psorinum

Sleeplessness from jerking
Belladonna

Sleeplessness because of excessive joy
Coffea

Sleeplessness from pain
Chamomilla

Sleeplessness with sweating
Conium

Sleeplessness due to racing thoughts
Arsenicum
Calcarea
Coffea
Hepar sulph.
Nux
Opium
Pulsatilla

Sleeplessness with twitching of the limbs
Arsenicum
Pulsatilla

Over-tiredness preventing sleep
Arsenicum

Sleeplessness after drinking alcohol
Nux

Inability to get back to sleep after waking up
Arsenicum
Lachesis
Magnesia carb.
Natrum mur.
Silicea

Talking during sleep
Belladonna
Kali carb.
Lachesis

Unusual sleepiness in the morning (unrefreshing sleep)
Calcarea
Calcarea phos.
Carbon sulph.
Graphites
Nux
Sepia
Sulphur
Tuberculinum

Sleepiness in the afternoon
China
Nux
Rhus tox.
Sulphur

Sleepiness after eating
Agaricus
Calcarea
Nux

Sleepiness after dinner
Agaricus
Lycopodium
Nux
Tuberculinum

Abnormal sleepiness while eating
Kali carb.

Abnormal sleepiness in hot weather
Antimonium

Abnormal sleepiness during periods
Nux mosch.

Sleepiness after mental exertion
Arsenicum

Swellings

Swellings generally
Apis
Arsenicum
Belladonna
Bryonia
Kali bichrom.
Mercurius
Nux
Pulsatilla
Rhus tox.

Swelling of affected part only
Aconite
Actaea spic.
Belladonna
Bryonia
Crotalus
Euphrasia
Gelsemium
Kali carb.
Mercurius
Mercurius corr.
Pulsatilla
Rhododendron
Rhus tox.
Sepia
Silicea
Spongia
Sulphur

Tobacco

Aversion to tobacco
Calcarea
Ignatia
Nux
Pulsatilla

Desire for tobacco
Tabacum

Tobacco makes symptoms worse
Arsenicum
Ignatia
Nux
Pulsatilla
Spigelia
Spongia
Staphisagria

Touch and Pressure

Touch makes symptoms worse
Agaricus
Apis
Argentum
Asafoetida
Belladonna
Bryonia
Chamomilla
China
China sulph.
Cocculus
Coffea
Colchicum
Cuprum
Guaiacum
Hamamelis
Hepar sulph.
Hyoscyamus
Kali ars.
Kali carb.
Lachesis
Lycopodium
Magnesia phos.
Manganum
Nitric ac.
Nux
Ranunculus
Rhododendron
Rhus tox.
Sabina
Sepia
Silicea
Spigelia
Staphisagria
Sulphur

Touch makes symptoms better
Asafoetida
Calcarea
Cyclamen
Thuja

Firm pressure makes symptoms worse
Agaricus
Apis
Baryta
Cina
Hepar sulph.
Iodum
Lachesis
Lilium
Lycopodium
Mercurius corr.
Silicea

Firm pressure makes symptoms better
Bryonia
China
Colocynth
Conium
Drosera
Ignatia
Lilium

Magnesia mur.
Magnesia phos.
Menyanthes
Natrum carb.
Plumbum
Pulsatilla
Silicea
Stannum

Rubbing makes symptoms worse
Anacardium
Conium
Pulsatilla
Sepia
Sulphur

Rubbing makes symptoms better
Calcarea
Cantharis
Carbolic ac.
Natrum carb.
Phosphorus
Plumbum
Sepia
Terebinth
Veratrum

Urethral discharges

Burning and scalding
Argentum nit.
Mercurius
Mercurius corr.

Jelly-like
Kali bichrom.

White or milky-looking
Natrum mur.
Sepia

Yellowish
Mercurius
Natrum sulph.
Nitric ac.
Pulsatilla
Selenium
Sepia
Thuja

Urine
see also CYSTITIS

Urine cloudy
Apis
Berberis
Bryonia

Cantharis
Carbo veg.
Carbon sulph.
Chamomilla
Chelidonium
China
Cina
Conium
Graphites
Mercurius
Myristica
Phosphoric ac.
Phosphorus
Sabadilla
Sepia
Sulphur

Colourless urine
Cannabis ind.
Gelsemium
Natrum mur.
Sepia

Offensive-smelling urine
Apis
Arnica
Baptisia
Benzoic ac.
Calcarea
Carbo veg.
Dulcamara
Nitric ac.
Sepia
Sulphur
Viola

Dark-coloured urine
Aconite
Antimonium tart.
Apis
Belladonna
Benzoic ac.
Bryonia
Calcarea
Chelidonium
Colchicum
Crotalus
Equisetum
Helleborus
Lachesis
Lactic ac.
Mercurius
Mercurius corr.
Plumbum
Selenium
Sepia
Terebinth
Veratrum

Vaginal discharge

Burning
Borax
Calcarea
Calcarea sulph.
Kreosotum
Pulsatilla
Sepia
Sulphur

Creamy
Pulsatilla

Excoriating, causing skin to blister
Alumina
Arsenicum
Borax
Carbon sulph.
Caulophyllum
Chamomilla
Ferrum
Ferrum ars.
Fluoric ac.
Graphites
Kreosotum
Lycopodium
Mercurius
Nitric ac.
Phosphorus
Pulsatilla
Sepia
Silicea

Greenish
Carbo veg.
Mercurius
Natrum mur.
Natrum sulph.
Nitric ac.
Sepia

Gushing
Calcarea
Kreosotum
Sepia

Worse in the menopause
Graphites
Sepia

Offensive
Carbolic ac.
Kali ars.
Kali phos.
Nitric ac.
Nux
Psorinum
Sepia

Worse during pregnancy
Alumina
Kreosotum
Sepia

Worse at puberty
Sepia

Stringy or ropey
Hydrastis
Kali bichrom.
Kali mur.
Nitric ac.
Sabina

Thick
Arsenicum
Calcarea
Hydrastis
Kali bichrom.

Like egg white
Borax
Hydrastis
Natrum mur.
Sepia

Watery
Graphites
Nitric ac.
Pulsatilla

Yellowish
Arsenicum
Calcarea
Chamomilla
Hydrastis
Kreosotum
Sepia
Sulphur

Worse before periods
Bovista
Calcarea
Graphites
Kreosotum
Sepia

Washing, getting wet
see also COLD, WARMTH AND
HEAT p. 290

**Symptoms made worse by
washing**
Ammonium carb.
Calcarea
Calcarea sulph.
Clematis

Rhus tox.
Sepia
Sulphur

**Symptoms made better by
washing**
Asarum
Ledum
Pulsatilla

**Cold baths make symptoms
worse**
Ammonium carb.
Antimonium tart.
Calcarea
Clematis
Ignatia

**Hot baths make symptoms
worse**
Apis
Gelsemium
Iodum
Kali iod.
Lachesis
Natrum mur.

**Hot baths make symptoms
better**
Arsenicum

**Wet applications make
symptoms worse**
Ammonium carb.
Antimonium
Calcarea
Chamomilla
Clematis
Rhus tox.
Sulphur

**Wet applications make
symptoms better**
Asarum
Pulsatilla

**Getting wet makes symptoms
worse**
Alumina
Calcarea
Causticum
Natrum sulph.
Pulsatilla
Rhus tox.
Sepia

**Wet feet make symptoms
worse**
Nux
Pulsatilla
Silicea

Yawning

**Yawning makes symptoms
worse**
Cina
Ignatia
Kreosotum
Nux
Rhus tox.

**Yawning makes symptoms
better**
Staphisagria

Environment

Cold

**Cold in general makes
symptoms worse**
Arsenicum
Baryta
Calcarea ars.
Calcarea fluor.
Calcarea phos.
Calcarea sil.
Capsicum
Causticum
China
Dulcamara
Graphites
Hepar sulph.
Hypericum
Kali ars.
Kali carb.
Kali phos.
Lycopodium
Magnesia phos.
Moschus
Natrum ars.
Nitric ac.
Nux
Phosphorus
Psorinum
Pyrogenium
Ranunculus
Rhus tox.
Rumex
Sabadilla
Sepia

Silicea
Spigelia
Strontium

Cold air improves symptoms
Aloe
Ambra
Amyl nit.
Bryonia
Fluoric ac.
Gelsemium
Glonoinum
Iodum
Natrum sulph.
Picric ac.
Pulsatilla
Sanguinaria
Secale

Cold air makes symptoms worse
Agaricus
Allium
Arsenicum
Aurum
Badiaga
Baryta
Calcarea
Calcarea phos.
Camphora
Causticum
Cimicifuga
Cistus
Dulcamara
Helleborus
Hepar sulph.
Hypericum
Kali ars.
Kali carb.
Lycopodium
Magnesia phos.
Moschus
Nux
Nux mosch.
Psorinum
Ranunculus
Rhododendron
Rhus tox.
Rumex
Sabadilla
Sepia
Silicea
Strontium

Tendency to catch cold
Aconite
Alumina
Baryta

Bryonia
Calcarea
Chamomilla
Dulcamara
Hepar sulph.
Kali carb.
Kali iod.
Lycopodium
Mercurius
Natrum ars.
Natrum mur.
Nitric ac.
Nux
Psorinum
Rumex
Sepia
Silicea
Tuberculinum

Becoming cold improves symptoms
Iodum
Lycopodium
Pulsatilla

Becoming cold makes symptoms worse
Arsenicum
Aurum
Baryta
Hepar sulph.
Kali ars.
Kali bichrom.
Kali carb.
Lycopodium
Moschus
Nux
Phosphoric ac.
Pyrogenium
Ranunculus
Rhus tox.
Sabadilla
Sepia
Silicea
Sulphuric ac.

Symptoms come on after catching cold
Arsenicum
Baryta
Belladonna
Bryonia
Calcarea
Calcarea phos.
Chamomilla
China
Dulcamara
Hepar sulph.

Hyoscyamus
Mercurius
Nux
Phosphorus
Pulsatilla
Pyrogenium
Ranunculus
Rhus tox.
Sepia
Silicea
Spigelia
Sulphuric ac.

Cold bathing and cold applications improve symptoms
Aloe
Amyl nit.
Apis
Argentum nit.
Arnica
Aurum
Bryonia
Fluoric ac.
Glonoinum
Iodum
Ledum
Natrum mur.
Picric ac.
Pulsatilla
Secale

Cold bathing and cold applications make symptoms worse
Actaea
Antimonium
Antimonium tart.
Apocynum
Baryta
Belladonna
Capsicum
Causticum
Chimaphila
Kreosotum
Lachesis
Magnesia phos.
Muriatic ac.
Nitric ac.
Phosphorus
Rhus tox.
Ruta
Sepia
Spigelia

Change from cold to warm air makes symptoms worse
Bryonia

Kali sulph.
Psorinum
Sulphur
Tuberculinum

Entering a cold place makes symptoms worse
Arsenicum
Kali ars.
Ranunculus
Sepia

Draughts

Draughts make symptoms worse
Belladonna
Calcarea
Calcarea phos.
Kali carb.
Pulsatilla
Rhus tox.
Selenium
Silicea
Sulphur

Being fanned alleviates symptoms
Apis
Carbo veg.
Sulphur

Heat and cold
see also COLD p. 285,
WARMTH AND HEAT p. 290

Extreme heat and cold make symptoms worse
Antimonium
Causticum
Fluoric ac.
Graphites
Ipecac.
Lachesis
Lycopodium
Mercurius
Natrum carb.
Natrum mur.
Nitric ac.
Phosphoric ac.
Psorinum
Sepia
Silicea
Sulphur

Humidity

Damp air alleviates symptoms
Aconite

Belladonna
Bryonia
Causticum
Hepar sulph.
Ipecac.
Nitric ac.
Nux
Platina
Spigelia
Spongia
Zinc

Damp air makes symptoms worse
Actaea
Bryonia
Dulcamara
Gelsemium
Hypericum
Sanguinaria
Thuja
Urtica

Damp house or cellar makes symptoms worse
Arsenicum
Dulcamara
Natrum sulph.
Nux mosch.
Rhus tox.
Terebinthum
Thuja
Veratrum

Dry air alleviates symptoms
Ammonium carb.
Calcarea
Dulcamara
Lycopodium
Manganum
Mercurius
Natrum sulph.
Nux mosch.
Rhododendron
Rhus tox.
Ruta

Dry air makes symptoms worse
Aconite
Belladonna
Bryonia
Causticum
Hepar sulph.
Nux

Light and dark
see also TIME OF DAY p. 289

Light makes symptoms worse
Calcarea
Colchicum
Glonoinum
Natrum carb.

Symptoms better in dark
Calcarea
Cicuta
Hepar sulph.
Natrum carb.
Nux
Sepia

Symptoms worse in dark
Cannabis ind.
Causticum
Phosphorus
Pulsatilla
Rhus tox.
Stramonium

Moon

Full moon makes symptoms worse
Calcarea
Crocus
Graphites
Natrum carb.
Natrum mur.
Silicea
Spongia

New moon makes symptoms worse
Ammonium carb.
Calcarea
Causticum
Crocus
Cuprum
Sepia
Silicea
Staphisagria

Waxing moon alleviates symptoms
Clematis

Waxing moon makes symptoms worse
Alumina
Arnica
Calcarea
China
Clematis

Noise

Sensitivity to noise
Aconite
Asarum
Belladonna
Borax
China
Coffea
Conium
Kali carb.
Nitric ac.
Nux
Opium
Sepia
Silicea
Theridion
Zinc

Sensitivity to music
Aconite
Ambra
Chamomilla
Graphites
Kreosotum
Lycopodium
Natrum carb.
Natrum mur.
Natrum sulph.
Nux
Phosphoric ac.
Sabina
Sepia
Tarentula

Noise makes symptoms worse
Aconite
Arnica
Belladonna
Cannabis ind.
China
Cicuta
Coffea
Conium
Ipecac.
Ignatia
Kali carb.
Natrum carb.
Natrum mur.
Nux
Phosphoric ac.
Phosphorus
Picric ac.
Silicea
Spigelia
Stramonium
Zinc

Open air

Being out of doors improves symptoms
Alumina
Argentum nit.
Arsenicum
Cannabis ind.
Crocus
Kali iod.
Magnesia carb.
Magnesia mur.
Natrum sulph.
Pulsatilla
Rhus tox.
Sabadilla
Sabina

Being out of doors makes symptoms worse
China
Cocculus
Guaiacum
Hepar sulph.
Kali carb.
Mercurius
Nitric ac.
Nux
Nux mosch.
Rumex
Silicea
Sulphur

Desire to be in open air
Aurum
Aurum mur.
Calcarea iod.
Carbo veg.
Crocus
Iodum
Kali iod.
Kali sulph.
Lycopodium
Pulsatilla
Sulphur

Dislike of open air
Ammonium carb.
Baptisia
Calcarea
Calcarea phos.
Chamomilla
Cocculus
Coffea
Ignatia
Kali carb.
Natrum carb.
Nux

Petroleum
Rumex
Silicea
Sulphur

Becoming warm in open air makes symptoms worse
Bryonia
Iodum
Lycopodium
Pulsatilla

Sea

Seaside air makes symptoms worse
Arsenicum
Kali iod.
Magnesia mur.
Natrum mur.
Natrum sulph.
Sepia

Air at sea improves symptoms
Bromium
Medorrhinum
Natrum mur.

Swimming in sea makes symptoms worse
Arsenicum
Magnesia mur.
Rhus tox.
Sepia
Zinc

Seasons

Symptoms worse in spring
Ambra
Bromium
Crotalus
Iris
Kali bichrom.
Lachesis
Lycopodium
Pulsatilla

Symptoms better in summer
Aesculus
Causticum
Silicea

Symptoms worse in summer
Antimonium
Argentum nit.
Bromium
Gelsemium
Glonoinum

Kali brom.
Lachesis
Natrum carb.
Natrum mur.
Nux
Podophyllum

Symptoms worse in autumn
Baptisia
Dulcamara
Iris
Kali bichrom.
Mercurius
Rhus tox.

Symptoms worse in winter
Aesculus
Causticum
Ipecac.
Mezereum
Nux mosch.
Rhus tox.
Silicea

Time of day

Symptoms worse during day
Sepia
Stannum
Sulphur

Symptoms worse in morning
Agaricus
Ammonium mur.
Argentum
Arsenicum iod.
Aurum
Bryonia
Calcarea
Calcarea phos.
Carbo an.
Carbo veg.
Carbon sulph.
Chamomilla
Chelidonium
Cina
Crocus
Kali bichrom.
Kali nit.
Lachesis
Natrum ars.
Natrum mur.
Natrum sulph.
Nitric ac.
Nux
Onosmodium
Petroleum
Phosphoric ac.
Phosphorus

Podophyllum
Pulsatilla
Rhododendron
Rhus tox.
Rumex
Sepia
Spigelia
Squilla
Sulphur
Sulphuric ac.
Valerian

Symptoms worse just before noon
Natrum carb.
Natrum mur.
Podophyllum
Sabadilla
Sepia
Stannum
Sulphur
Sulphuric ac.

Symptoms better in late morning
Lycopodium

Symptoms worse around 10 am
Natrum mur.

Symptoms worse around 11 am
Sulphur

Symptoms worse at noon
Argentum

Symptoms worse in afternoon
Belladonna
Kali nit.
Lycopodium
Pulsatilla
Rhus tox.
Sepia
Silicea
Thuja
Zinc

Symptoms worse around 3 pm
Belladonna

Symptoms worse around 4 pm
Lycopodium

Symptoms worse between 4 and 8 pm
Lycopodium

Symptoms better in evening
Alumina
Aurum
Medorrhinum
Sepia

Symptoms worse in evening
Alumina
Ambra
Ammonium carb.
Antimonium
Antimonium tart.
Arnica
Belladonna
Bryonia
Calcarea
Capsicum
Carbo an.
Carbo veg.
Carbon sulph.
Causticum
Chamomilla
Colchicum
Cyclamen
Euphrasia
Helleborus
Hyoscyamus
Kali nit.
Lachesis
Lycopodium
Magnesia carb.
Menyanthes
Mercurius
Mezereum
Natrum phos.
Nitric ac.
Phosphoric ac.
Phosphorus
Platina
Plumbum
Pulsatilla
Rumex
Ruta
Sepia
Silicea
Stannum
Strontium
Sulphur
Sulphuric ac.
Valerian
Zinc

Symptoms worse at twilight
Pulsatilla

Symptoms worse around 9 pm
Bryonia

Symptoms worse at night
Aconite
Argentum nit.
Arnica
Arsenicum
Arsenicum iod.
Calcarea
Calcarea iod.
Calcarea phos.
Calcarea sulph.
Carbo an.
Carbon sulph.
Chamomilla
China
Cinnabar
Coffea
Colchicum
Conium
Cyclamen
Dulcamara
Ferrum
Graphites
Hepar sulph.
Hyoscyamus
Iodum
Ipecac.
Kali ars.
Kali bichrom.
Kali carb.
Kali iod.
Lachesis
Lilium
Magnesia carb.
Magnesia mur.
Manganum
Mercurius
Nitric ac.
Phosphorus
Plumbum
Psorinum
Pulsatilla
Rhus tox.
Rumex
Sepia
Silicea
Strontium
Sulphur
Zinc

Symptoms worse before midnight
Argentum nit.
Arsenicum
Carbo veg.
Chamomilla
Coffea
Kali ars.
Ledum

Lycopodium
Phosphorus
Pulsatilla
Rumex
Sabadilla
Stannum

Symptoms better after midnight
Lycopodium

Symptoms worse after midnight
Arsenicum
Drosera
Kali carb.
Kali nit.
Natrum ars.
Nux
Phosphorus
Podophyllum
Rhus tox.
Silicea
Thuja

Symptoms worse around 1 am
Arsenicum

Symptoms worse between 2 and 4 am
Kali carb.

Warmth and heat

Warmth makes symptoms worse
Alumina
Apis
Arsenicum iod.
Glonoinum
Iodum
Kali sulph.
Lachesis
Ledum
Mercurius
Pulsatilla
Secale

Warm rooms make symptoms worse
Apis
Calcarea sulph.
Carbon sulph.
Crocus
Graphites
Iodum
Kali iod.
Kali sulph.
Lycopodium

Pulsatilla
Sabina
Secale
Senega
Sulphur

Warmth of bed improves symptoms
Arsenicum
Bryonia
Hepar sulph.
Kali carb.
Lycopodium
Nux
Nux mosch.
Rhus tox.
Silicea
Tuberculinum

Warmth of bed makes symptoms worse
Apis
Chamomilla
Drosera
Ledum
Mercurius
Opium
Pulsatilla
Sabina
Secale
Sulphur

Warm applications make symptoms worse
Apis
Iodum
Kali sulph.
Ledum
Lycopodium
Pulsatilla
Secale
Sulphur

Radiant heat improves symptoms
Arsenicum
Hepar sulph.
Ignatia
Kali carb.
Magnesia phos.
Nux
Rhododendron
Rhus tox.
Silicea

Radiant heat makes symptoms worse
Antimonium

Apis
Argentum nit.
Bryonia
Cocculus
Glonoinum
Iodum
Kali iod.
Ledum
Natrum mur.
Pulsatilla
Secale

Becoming overheated improves symptoms
Aurum
Phosphoric ac.
Sepia

Becoming overheated makes symptoms worse
Antimonium
Bromium
Bryonia
Colchicum
Graphites
Kali sulph.
Lycopodium
Pulsatilla
Thuja

Stuffy rooms make symptoms worse
Apis
Argentum nit.
Bromium
Bryonia
Lachesis
Lilium
Lycopodium
Magnesia carb.
Natrum mur.
Pulsatilla
Sepia
Sulphur

Weather

Changes in weather make symptoms worse
Dulcamara
Nux mosch.
Phosphorus
Psorinum
Ranunculus
Rhododendron
Rhus tox.
Silicea
Tuberculinum

Cold, dry weather makes symptoms worse
Aconite
Asarum
Causticum
Hepar sulph.
Kali carb.
Nux

Cold, wet weather makes symptoms worse
Ammonium carb.
Arsenicum
Badiaga
Calcarea
Calcarea phos.
Colchicum
Dulcamara
Medorrhinum
Natrum sulph.
Nux mosch.
Pyrogenium
Rhododendron
Rhus tox.
Silicea
Tuberculinum

Both cold and hot weather make symptoms worse
Fluoric ac.

Warm, wet weather makes symptoms worse
Carbo veg.
Gelsemium
Iodum
Kali bichrom.
Lachesis
Natrum sulph.
Silicea

Wet weather makes symptoms worse
Ammonium carb.
Arsenicum
Badiaga
Calcarea
Dulcamara
Natrum sulph.
Nux mosch.
Pulsatilla
Rhododendron
Rhus tox.

Cloudy weather makes symptoms worse
Rhus tox.

Foggy weather makes symptoms worse
Bryonia
Gelsemium
Hypericum
Manganum
Nux mosch.
Plumbum
Rhododendron
Rhus tox.
Sabina
Silicea

Snow makes symptoms worse
Calcarea
Conium
Lycopodium
Phosphorus
Phosphoric ac.
Pulsatilla
Rhus tox.
Sepia
Silicea
Sulphur

Sun makes symptoms worse
Antimonium
Glonoinum
Natrum carb.
Natrum mur.
Pulsatilla

Symptoms worse before thunderstorm
Agaricus
Calcarea
Gelsemium
Manganum
Medorrhinum
Natrum carb.
Natrum mur.
Petroleum
Phosphorus
Pulsatilla
Rhododendron
Rhus tox.
Sepia
Sulphur
Syphilinum

Symptoms worse during thunderstorm
Gelsemium
Natrum carb.

Petroleum
Phosphorus
Psorinum
Rhododendron
Silicea
Syphilinum

Wind makes symptoms worse
Chamomilla
Lycopodium
Nux
Pulsatilla
Rhododendron
Phosphorus

Cold wind makes symptoms worse
Belladonna
Hepar sulph.
Nux
Spongia

Windy and stormy weather makes symptoms worse
Aconite
Badiaga
Chamomilla
China
Hepar sulph.
Lachesis
Magnesia phos.
Muriatic ac.
Nux
Nux mosch.
Phosphorus
Psorinum
Pulsatilla
Rhododendron
Sepia

Mind and Emotions

see also BREATHING p. 271,
FACIAL EXPRESSION p. 272

Anger
Aconite
Anacardium
Arsenicum
Aurum
Bryonia
Chamomilla
Hepar sulph.
Ignatia

Kali carb.
Kali sulph.
Lycopodium
Natrum mur.
Nitric ac.
Nux
Petroleum
Sepia
Staphisagria
Sulphur

Anxiety
Aconite
Argentum nit.
Arsenicum
Arsenicum iod.
Aurum
Belladonna
Bismuth
Bryonia
Cactus
Calcarea
Calcarea phos.
Calcarea sulph.
Camphora
Cannabis ind.
Carbo veg.
Carbon sulph.
Causticum
China
Conium
Digitalis
Iodum
Kali carb.
Kali iod.
Kali phos.
Kali sulph.
Lycopodium
Mezereum
Natrum ars.
Natrum carb.
Nitric ac.
Phosphorus
Psorinum
Pulsatilla
Rhus tox.
Secale
Sulphur
Veratrum

Apprehension
Bryonia
Calcarea
China sulph.
Cicuta
Phosphorus

Brooding, tendency to dwell on things
Ambra
Benzoic ac.
Chamomilla
China
Cocculus
Conium
Natrum mur.
Platina
Sepia
Sulphur

Desire for company
Argentum nit.
Arsenicum
Bismuth
Hyoscyamus
Kali carb.
Lac can.
Lycopodium
Phosphorus
Pulsatilla

Not in mood for company
Anacardium
Baryta
Carbo an.
Chamomilla
Cicuta
Gelsemium
Ignatia
Natrum mur.
Nux

Criticism makes symptoms worse
Staphisagria

Delusions, hallucinations, overactive imagination
Argentum nit.
Belladonna
Cannabis ind.
Cocculus
Hyoscyamus
Ignatia
Lachesis
Petroleum
Phosphoric ac.
Sabadilla
Stramonium
Sulphur

Depression
Aconite
Arsenicum
Arsenicum iod.

Aurum
Aurum mur.
Calcarea
Calcarea ars.
Calcarea sulph.
Carbo an.
Carbon sulph.
Causticum
Chamomilla
China
Cimicifuga
Ferrum
Ferrum iod.
Gelsemium
Graphites
Helleborus
Ignatia
Iodum
Kali brom.
Kali phos.
Lac can.
Lachesis
Lilium
Lycopodium
Mercurius
Mezereum
Murex
Natrum ars.
Natrum mur.
Natrum sulph.
Nitric ac.
Platina
Psorinum
Pulsatilla
Rhus tox.
Sepia
Stannum
Sulphur
Thuja
Veratrum
Zinc

Despair
Arsenicum
Aurum
Calcarea
Coffea
Helleborus
Ignatia
Psorinum

Discontent, dissatisfaction
Anacardium
Calcarea phos.
Mercurius
Natrum mur.
Sulphur

Disappointment which makes symptoms worse
Ignatia

Dullness, sluggishness, difficulty understanding what is going on
Argentum nit.
Baptisia
Baryta
Baryta mur.
Belladonna
Bryonia
Calcarea
Calcarea phos.
Calcarea sulph.
Carbo veg.
Gelsemium
Graphites
Guaiacum
Helleborus
Hyoscyamus
Kali brom.
Kali carb.
Lachesis
Laurocerasus
Lycopodium
Natrum ars.
Natrum carb.
Natrum mur.
Nux mosch.
Opium
Phosphoric ac.
Phosphorus
Picric ac.
Plumbum
Pulsatilla
Senega
Silicea
Staphisagria
Sulphur
Tuberculinum
Zinc

Embarrassment or shame makes symptoms worse
Colocynth
Ignatia
Lycopodium
Natrum mur.
Palladium
Phosphoric ac.
Staphisagria

Emotional exhaustion, apathy, and indifference due to grief
Phosphoric ac.

Enthusiasm makes symptoms worse
Phosphorus

Excitement, excitability
Aconite
Argentum nit.
Aurum
Belladonna
Chamomilla
Coffea
Graphites
Hyoscyamus
Kali brom.
Kali iod.
Lac can.
Lachesis
Moschus
Natrum mur.
Nitric ac.
Nux
Opium
Phosphoric ac.
Phosphorus
Pulsatilla

Ailments brought on by too much excitement or joy
Aconite
Coffea
Opium
Pulsatilla

Fear
Aconite
Aurum
Belladonna
Borax
Calcarea
Calcarea phos.
Carbon sulph.
Cicuta
Digitalis
Graphites
Ignatia
Kali ars.
Lycopodium
Natrum carb.
Phosphorus
Platina
Psorinum
Sepia
Stramonium

Ailments brought on by fright
Aconite
Ignatia
Lycopodium

Natrum mur.
Opium
Phosphoric ac.
Phosphorus
Silicea

Easily frightened
Argentum nit.
Arsenicum
Baryta
Borax
Graphites
Lycopodium
Natrum ars.
Natrum carb.
Sepia
Stramonium

Grief
Aurum
Causticum
Ignatia
Natrum mur.
Pulsatilla

Ailments brought on by grief
Aurum
Causticum
Cocculus
Ignatia
Lachesis
Natrum mur.
Phosphoric ac.
Staphisagria

Guilt
Alumina
Ammonium carb.
Anacardium
Arsenicum
Aurum
Carbo veg.
Causticum
Chelidonium
Cocculus
Conium
Digitalis
Ferrum
Graphites
Hyoscyamus
Ignatia
Medorrhinum
Mercurius
Natrum mur.
Nux
Psorinum
Rhus tox.
Silicea
Sulphur

Thuja
Veratrum
Zinc

Feeling harassed makes symptoms worse
Anacardium
Cina
Colocynth
Ignatia
Ipecac.
Phosphorus
Staphisagria

Hallucinations
    see DELUSIONS

Haste and hurry
Lilium
Medorrhinum
Mercurius
Natrum mur.
Sulphur
Sulphuric ac.
Tarentula

Homesickness
Aurum
Capsicum
Carbo an.
Ignatia
Phosphoric ac.
Pulsatilla

Impatience
Chamomilla
Ignatia
Nux
Sepia
Sulphur

Indifference, lack of interest in people or things
Apis
Carbo veg.
China
Helleborus
Lilium
Mezereum
Natrum carb.
Natrum mur.
Natrum phos.
Onosmodium
Opium
Phosphoric ac.
Phosphorus
Platina
Pulsatilla
Sepia
Staphisagria

Indignation
Arsenicum
Calcarea phos.
Colocynth
Ignatia
Nux
Staphisagria

Irritability
Aconite
Alumina
Antimonium
Apis
Aurum
Belladonna
Bovista
Bryonia
Calcarea
Calcarea sulph.
Carbo veg.
Carbon sulph.
Causticum
Chamomilla
Graphites
Hepar sulph.
Kali carb.
Kali iod.
Kali sulph.
Lilium
Lycopodium
Magnesia carb.
Natrum carb.
Natrum mur.
Nitric ac.
Nux
Petroleum
Phosphoric ac.
Phosphorus
Platina
Pulsatilla
Ranunculus
Rhus tox.
Sepia
Silicea
Staphisagria
Sulphur
Sulphuric ac.
Thuja
Veratrum vir.
Zinc

Jealousy
Apis
Calcarea sulph.
Hyoscyamus
Lachesis
Lycopodium

Medorrhinum
Pulsatilla
Stramonium

Can't bear to be looked at
Antimonium
Antimonium tart.
Arsenicum
Chamomilla
China
Cina
Iodum
Natrum mur.

Mental exhaustion, perhaps from studying too hard
Picric ac.

Mental exhaustion and memory problems while studying for exams
Anacardium

Can't bear to be opposed or contradicted
Aurum
Bryonia
Cocculus
Ferrum
Ignatia
Lycopodium
Nux
Sepia
Silicea

Oversensitiveness, crying when others are hurt or in trouble
Causticum
Ignatia
Natrum carb.
Natrum mur.
Nitric ac.
Nux
Phosphorus

Excessive pride
Calcarea
Lachesis
Palladium
Platina
Silicea
Sulphur

Punishment makes symptoms worse
Argentum nit.
Capsicum

Chamomilla
China
Ignatia

Restlessness, nervousness
Aconite
Anacardium
Argentum nit.
Arsenicum
Arsenicum iod.
Baptisia
Belladonna
Calcarea
Calcarea phos.
Camphora
Cimicifuga
Colocynth
Cuprum
Ferrum
Helleborus
Hyoscyamus
Lycopodium
Mercurius
Plumbum
Pulsatilla
Rhus tox.
Sepia
Silicea
Staphisagria
Stramonium
Sulphur
Tarentula
Zinc

Rudeness
Hyoscyamus
Lac can.
Lycopodium
Nux
Stramonium
Veratrum

Rudeness makes symptoms worse
Staphisagria

Sympathy relieves symptoms
Pulsatilla

Sympathy makes symptoms worse
Ignatia
Natrum mur.
Sepia
Silicea

Can't bear being spoken to
Arsenicum

Arsenicum iod.
Carbon sulph.
Chamomilla
Gelsemium
Graphites
Hyoscyamus
Iodum
Natrum sulph.
Sulphur
Tarentula

Symptoms worse in presence of strangers
Ambra
Baryta
Bryonia
Sepia
Stramonium
Thuja

Suppressed, bottled up emotions
Aconite
Bryonia
Conium
Cuprum
Graphites
Lachesis
Natrum carb.
Natrum mur.
Opium
Secale
Sepia
Staphisagria
Sulphur
Zinc

Tearfulness
Apis
Calcarea
Calcarea sulph.
Carbon sulph.
Causticum
Cicuta
Graphites
Ignatia
Kali brom.
Lac can.
Lycopodium
Natrum mur.
Palladium
Platina
Pulsatilla
Rhus tox.
Sepia
Sulphur
Veratrum

Aversion to thinking
Baptisia
Carbo veg.
China
Gelsemium
Lycopodium
Phosphoric ac.
Phosphorus

**Thinking about ailments
   tends to make them better**
Camphora
Helleborus

**Thinking about ailments
   tends to make them worse**
Alumina
Baptisia
Baryta
Calcarea phos.
Causticum
Gelsemium
Helleborus
Lachesis
Medorrhinum
Nitric ac.
Nux
Oxalic ac.
Ranunculus
Sabadilla
Spongia

Timidity
Baryta
Calcarea
Calcarea sulph.
Gelsemium
Kali carb.
Lycopodium
Natrum carb.
Petroleum
Phosphorus
Plumbum
Pulsatilla
Sepia
Sulphur

**Ailments brought on by
   unhappy love affair**
Aurum
Hyoscyamus
Ignatia
Natrum mur.
Phosphoric ac.

Upset by bad news
Apis
Calcarea
Gelsemium

Ignatia
Medorrhinum
Natrum mur.
Palladium
Sulphur

Libido

Diminished libido
Agnus
Baryta
Graphites
Lycopodium
Silicea
Staphisagria

Excessive libido
Phosphorus
Stramonium
Zinc

Increased libido
Baryta mur.
Calcarea
Calcarea phos.
Cannabis
Cantharis
Conium
Lycopodium
Lyssin
Nux
Picric ac.
Platina
Pulsatilla
Silicea
Staphisagria
Tuberculinum
Zinc

Desire for sex unsatisfied
Apis
Camphora
Conium
Lyssin
Pulsatilla

Talking

Talking very fast
Hepar sulph.
Hyoscyamus
Lachesis
Mercurius

Talking incoherently
Bryonia
Cannabis ind.
Hyoscyamus
Lachesis
Phosphorus

Rhus tox.
Stramonium

Talking obscenely
Belladonna
Hyoscyamus
Lilium
Nux
Stramonium

Extreme talkativeness
Anacardium
Bryonia
Hyoscyamus
Lachesis
Stramonium

Talking very slowly
Argentum nit.
Helleborus
Kali brom.
Lachesis
Opium
Phosphoric ac.
Phosphorus
Plumbum
Secale
Sepia
Thuja

Talking unintelligibly
Belladonna
Hyoscyamus
Mercurius
Phosphoric ac.
Stramonium

**Straying from the point,
   losing the thread**
Belladonna
Hyoscyamus
Lachesis
Lycopodium
Nux
Stramonium

No desire to talk
Aurum
Carbo an.
Cocculus
Glonoinum
Natrum sulph.
Phosphoric ac.
Phosphorus
Platina
Pulsatilla
Sulphur
Veratrum
Zinc

APPENDIX B
HOMEOPATHIC REMEDIES AND THEIR SOURCES

Listed below are all the remedies mentioned in this book, with their Latin and common names. The majority are derived from living organisms, sometimes from specific parts of them. Note that only very small numbers of animals and plants need to be culled to satisfy homeopathic requirements.

Abies can. **Abies canadensis** hemlock spruce, Canada pitch (fresh bark and young buds)

Abies nig. **Abies nigra** black or double spruce (gum)

Abrotanum **Artemisia abrotanum** southernwood, lad's love, old man (fresh leaves and stem)

Absinthium **Artemisia absinthium** absinth, common wormwood (fresh young leaves and flowers)

Acetic ac. **Aceticum acidum** acetic acid

Aconite **Aconitum napellus** wolfsbane, blue aconite, blue monkshood (whole plant, including root, as it comes into flower)

Actaea **Actaea spicata** baneberry, herb Christopher (root in autumn)

Aesculus **Aesculus hippocastanum** horse chestnut (ripe conkers)

Aethusa **Aethusa cynapium** fool's parsley (whole plant when in flower)

Agaricus **Agaricus muscarius** fly agaric (fresh fungus, or dried cap)

Agnus **Agnus castus** chaste tree (ripe berries)

Agraphis **Agraphis nutans** bluebell, wild hyacinth (fresh plant and growing shoots)

Ailanthus **Ailanthus glandulosa** Chinese sumach, tree of heaven (flowers as they begin to open)

Aletris **Aletris farinosa** stargrass, unicorn root, blazing grass, colic root (root)

Allium **Allium cepa** red onion (whole fresh plant in July/August)

Allium sat. **Allium sativa** garlic (fresh bulb)

Aloe **Aloe socotrina** common aloe (gum)

Alum **Alumen** double sulphate of aluminium and potassium

Alumina **Alumina** aluminium oxide

Ambra **Ambra grisea** ambergris, yellow-grey fatty substance from whale's intestine

Ambrosia **Ambrosia artemisiaefolia** ragweed, Roman wormwood, hogweed (fresh flower heads and young shoots)

Ammonium brom. **Ammonium bromatum** ammonium bromide

Ammonium carb. **Ammonium carbonicum** ammonium carbonate

Ammonium mur. **Ammonium muriaticum** sal ammoniac, ammonium chloride

Amyl nit. amyl nitrite

Anacardium **Anacardium occidentale** cashew nut (black juice between outer and inner shell of nut)

Anacardium or. **Anacardium orientale** marking nut (layer between shell and kernel)

Angostura **Angostura vera** bark of *Galipea cusparia*

Anthemis **Anthemis nobilis** Roman chamomile (flowers)

Anthrax **Anthracinum anthrax** poison from spleen of affected sheep

Antimonium **Antimonium crudum** black sulphide of antimony

Antimonium tart. **Antimonium tartaricum** tartar emetic, potassium antimony tartrate

Apis **Apis mellifica** honey bee (whole bee, or venom from sting)

Apocynum **Apocynum cannabinum** Indian or American hemp (whole fresh plant, including root)

Argentum **Argentum metallicum** silver

Argentum nit. **Argentum nitricum** silver nitrate

Arnica **Arnica montana** leopard's bane, fallkraut (whole fresh plant, dried flowers or root)

Arsenicum **Arsenicum album** arsenic trioxide

Arsenicum iod. **Arsenicum iodatum** arsenic iodide

Artemisia **Artemisia vulgaris** mugwort (fresh root)

Arum **Arum triphyllum** Indian turnip (fresh tuber)

Arundo **Arundo mauritanica** an Italian grass (root sprouts)

Asafoetida **Narthex asafoetida** stinkasand (gum)

Asarum **Asarum europaeum** European snakeroot, hazelwort, wild nard (whole fresh plant, including root)

Asclepias   Asclepias cornuti or *A. syriaca* silkweed, milkweed (root)

Astacus   Astacus fluviatilis freshwater crayfish (whole animal)

Asterias   Asterias rubens red starfish (whole animal)

Atropine   Atropinum atropine, poisonous alkaloid found in deadly nightshade, see **Belladonna**

Aurum   Aurum metallicum gold

Aurum mur.   Aurum muriaticum gold chloride

Avena   Avena sativa oat (fresh plant when in flower)

Bacillinum nosode prepared from sputum of patient with tuberculosis

Badiaga   Badiaga Spongia palustris freshwater sponge (dried sponge collected in autumn)

Baptisia   Baptisia tinctoria wild indigo (fresh root and bark)

Baryta   Baryta carbonica barium carbonate

Baryta mur.   Baryta muriatica barium chloride

Belladonna   Atropa belladonna deadly nightshade (whole fresh plant as it comes into flower)

Bellis   Bellis perennis common daisy (whole fresh plant)

Benzoic ac.   Benzoicum acidum benzoic acid

Berberis   Berberis vulgaris common barberry (bark or root)

Bismuth   Bismuthum precipitated sub-nitrate of bismuth

Blatta   Blatta orientalis Indian cockroach (whole live insect)

Boracic ac.   Boracicum acidum boracic acid

Borax   Borax veneta sodium borate

Bothrops   Bothrops lanceolatus yellow viper, fer-de-lance from Martinique (venom)

Bovista   Lycoperdon bovista warted puffball (whole fungus)

Bromium   Bromium bromine

Bryonia   Bryonia alba or *B. dioica* white or common bryony (root before flowering)

Bufo   Bufo rana common toad, Brazilian toad (venom from skin glands)

Cactus   Cactus grandiflorus night-blooming cereus (youngest, tenderest shoots and flowers in summer)

Cadmium   Cadmium sulphuratum cadmium sulphate

Cadmium met.   Cadmium metallicum cadmium

Caladium   Caladium sequinum American arum, dumb cane (whole fresh plant)

Calcarea   Calcarea carbonica calcium carbonate from middle layer of oyster shells

Calcarea ars.   Calcarea arsenicosa calcium arsenite

Calcarea fluor.   Calcarea fluorata fluorspar, calcium fluoride

Calcarea hypophos.   Calcarea hypophosphorica calcium hypophosphite

Calcarea iod.   Calcarea iodata calcium iodide

Calcarea phos.   Calcarea phosphorica calcium phosphate

Calcarea sil.   Calcarea silicata calcium silicate

Calcarea sulph.   Calcarea sulphurica gypsum, plaster of Paris, calcium sulphate

Calendula   Calendula officinalis pot marigold (leaves and flowers)

Camphora   Laurus camphora camphor (gum)

Cannabis ind.   Cannabis indica Indian hemp, hashish, bhang bhanga (young leaves and twigs)

Cannabis sat.   Cannabis sativa European or American hemp (tops of male and female flowers)

Cantharis   Cantharis (Lytta) vesicatoria Spanish fly (whole live beetle)

Capsicum   Capsicum annuum cayenne pepper (dried pods)

Carbo an.   Carbo animalis animal charcoal, made from charred oxhide

Carbo veg.   Carbo vegetabilis vegetable charcoal made from beech, birch or poplar wood

Carbolic ac.   Carbolicum acidum phenol, carbolic acid

Carbon sulph.   Carbonum sulphuratum carbon bisulphide

Carduus   Carduus mariana St Mary's thistle, silybum (seeds)

Caulophyllum   Caulophyllum thalictroides blue cohosh, squaw root (root)

Causticum   Causticum hahnemanni calcium oxide and potassium bisulphate

Ceanothus   Ceanothus americanus New Jersey tea, red root (fresh leaves)

Chamomilla   Chamomilla vulgaris German chamomile (whole fresh plant)

Chelidonium   Chelidonium majus greater celandine (whole fresh plant when in flower, or root)

Chenopodium   Chenopodium anthelminticum Jerusalem oat, wormseed (whole fresh plant, or extracted oil)

Chimaphila   Chimaphila umbellata umbellate wintergreen, ground holly, pipsissewa, prince's pine (root and leaves, or whole fresh plant when in flower)

China   China officinalis Peruvian bark, quinine (dried bark of *Cinchona calisaya*)

China ars.   China arsenica quinine arsenate

Chininum sulph.   Chininum sulphuricum quinine sulphate

Chionanthus   Chionanthus virginica fringe tree (bark)

Cicuta   Cicuta virosa   water hemlock, cowbane (fresh root when plant is in flower)

Cimicifuga   Cimicifuga racemosa   black snakeroot, black cohosh (root or resinoid)

Cina   Cina artemisia maritima   sea southernwood, wormseed (unopened flower heads)

Cinnabar   Cinnabaris   mercuric sulphide

Cistus   Cistus canadensis   frostweed, Canadian rock rose (whole plant)

Clematis   Clematis erecta   virgin's bower (leaves and stems)

Cocculus   Cocculus indicus   Indian cockle (seeds, which contain picrotoxine, a powerful poison)

Coccus   Coccus cacti   cochineal beetle (dried bodies of females)

Codeinum   prepared from codeine, an alkaloid of opium

Coffea   Coffea cruda   unroasted coffee (raw berries)

Colchicum   Colchicum autumnale   meadow saffron, autumn crocus (bulbs in spring)

Collinsonia   Collinsonia canadensis   stoneroot, horsebalm, richweed (fresh root)

Colocynth   Citrullus colocynthis   bitter apple, bitter cucumber (pulp of fruit)

Conchiolinum   mother of pearl from oyster shells

Conium   Conium maculatum   hemlock (fresh plant when in flower)

Convallaria   Convallaria majalis   lily of the valley (whole plant)

Copaiva   Copaifera officinalis   balsam of copaiva (seed pods)

Corallium   Corallium rubrum   red coral from *Gorgonia nobilis* (whole coral)

Crataegus   Crataegus oxycantha   hawthorn (ripe berries)

Crocus   Crocus sativa   saffron crocus (dried stigmas)

Crotalus   Crotalus horridus   N. American rattlesnake (venom)

Croton   Croton tiglium   (oil from seeds)

Cuprum   Cuprum metallicum   copper

Cuprum ars.   Cuprum arsenicosum   Scheele's green, copper arsenate

Cyclamen   Cyclamen europaeum   sowbread (root in spring)

Digitalis   Digitalis purpurea   red foxglove (second year's leaves)

Dioscorea   Dioscorea villosa   wild yam (fresh root or resinoid)

Drosera   Drosera rotundifolia   common or round-leaved sundew (active fresh plant)

Dulcamara   Solanum dulcamara   bittersweet, woody nightshade (fresh green stems and leaves just before plant comes into flower)

Echinacea   Echinacea angustifolia   purple coneflower (whole fresh plant)

Elaps   Elaps corallinus   Brazilian coral snake (venom)

Equisetum   Equisetum hyemale   scouring rush, horsetail (fresh plant, chopped and pulped)

Eupatorium   Eupatorium perfoliatum   boneset, thoroughwort (whole plant)

Euphorbium   Euphorbium officinarum   gum euphorbium (resinous juice)

Euphrasia   Euphrasia officinalis or E. sticta   common eyebright (whole plant)

Ferrum   Ferrum metallicum   iron

Ferrum ars.   Ferrum arsenicum   iron arsenate

Ferrum iod.   Ferrum iodatum   iodide of iron

Ferrum phos.   Ferrum phosphoricum   iron phosphate

Ferrum pic.   Ferrum picricum   iron picrate

Ferrum sulph.   Ferrum sulphuricum   ferrous sulphate

Fluoric ac.   Fluoricum acidum   hydrofluoric acid

Fraxinus   Fraxinus americanus   white ash (bark)

Fucus vesic.   Fucus vesiculosus   bladder wrack

Gelsemium   Gelsemium sempervirens   yellow jasmine (bark or root)

Gentiana   Gentiana lutea   yellow gentian (root)

Glonoinum   Glonoinum   nitroglycerine

Gnaphalium   Gnaphalium polycephalum   sweet-scented everlasting flower (whole fresh plant)

Graphites   Graphites   black lead from finest English drawing pencils

Gratiola   Gratiola officinalis   hedge hyssop (fresh bulb before plant flowers)

Guaiacum   Guaiacum officinale   resin from lignum vitae tree

Gunpowder   a mixture of saltpetre, sulphur, and charcoal

Hamamelis   Hamamelis virginica   common witch hazel (fresh bark of twigs and roots)

Hecla   Hecla lava   volcanic ash from Mt Hecla in Iceland

Helleborus   Helleborus niger   black hellebore, snow rose, Christmas rose (juice of fresh root)

Hepar sulph.   Hepar sulphuris calcareum   calcium sulphide

Hydrastis   Hydrastis canadensis   golden seal (fresh root)

Hyoscyamus   Hyoscyamus niger   henbane (whole fresh plant)

Hypericum   Hypericum perforatum   St John's wort (whole fresh plant)

Iberis *Iberis amara* bitter candytuft (seeds)

Ignatia *Ignatia amara or Strychnos ignatia* St Ignatius' bean (seed pods)

Iodum *Iodum* iodine

Ipecac. *Cephaelis ipecacuanha* ipecacuanha (dried root)

Iris *Iris versicolor* blue flag (fresh root in early spring or autumn)

Iris ten. *Iris tenax or I. minor* beardless iris (whole plant)

Jaborandi *Pilocarpus pinnatifolius* a S. American tree (fresh or dried leaves and stems)

Jacaranda *Jacaranda caroba* Brazilian caroba tree (fresh flowers)

Juglans *Juglans cinerea* butternut (bark or root)

Kali ars. *Kali arsenicosum* potassium arsenite ('Fowler's solution')

Kali bichrom. *Kali bichromicum* potassium bichromate

Kali brom. *Kali bromatum* potassium bromide

Kali carb. *Kali carbonicum* potassium carbonate

Kali iod. *Kali iodatum* potassium iodide

Kali mur. *Kali muriaticum* potassium chloride

Kali nit. *Kali nitricum* potassium nitrite

Kali phos. *Kali phosphoricum* potassium phosphate

Kali sulph. *Kali sulphuricum* potassium sulphate

Kalmia *Kalmia latifolia or Ledum floribus bullatis* mountain laurel or calico bush (fresh leaves when plant is in flower)

Kreosotum *Kreosotum* creosote, oil distilled from beechwood tar

Lac can. *Lac caninum* dog's milk

Lac defl. *Lac vaccinum defloratum* skimmed cow's milk

Lachesis *Trigonocephalus lachesis* bushmaster, surucucu snake (venom)

Lacnanthes *Lacnanthes tinctoria* red root (whole plant)

Lactic ac. *Lacticum acidum* lactic acid

Lathyrus *Lathyrus sativa* chick pea (flowers or green seed pods)

Latrodectus *Latrodectus mactans* American spider (live spider)

Laurocerasus *Prunus laurocerasus* cherry laurel (young leaves)

Ledum *Ledum palustre* marsh tea, wild rosemary (leaves and small twigs dried and collected as plant comes into flower)

Lilium *Lilium tigrinum* tiger lily (fresh stalks, leaves and flower, or pollen)

Lobelia *Lobelia inflata* Indian tobacco (fresh plant when in flower, also seeds)

Lycopodium *Lycopodium clavatum* wolfs claw club moss (spores)

Lycopus *Lycopus virginicus* bugleweed (fresh plant in flower)

Lyssin *Lyssin hydrophobinum* saliva of dog with rabies

Magnesia carb. *Magnesia carbonica* magnesium carbonate

Magnesia mur. *Magnesia muriatica* magnesium chloride

Magnesia phos. *Magnesia phosphorica* magnesium phosphate

Magnesia sulph. *Magnesia sulphurica* magnesium sulphate

Magnetis arct. *Magnetis polus arcticus* north pole of magnet

Magnetis austr. *Magnetis polus australis* south pole of magnet

Mancinella *Hippomane mancinella* manchineel, manzanilla (fruit, leaves and bark)

Manganum *Manganum metallicum* manganese

Medorrhinum *Medorrhinum* urethral discharge from patient with gonorrhea

Melilotus *Melilotus officinalis or M. alba* sweet clover, yellow and white varieties (fresh plant when in flower)

Menyanthes *Menyanthes trifoliata* buckbean (whole plant)

Mercurius *Mercurius solubilis hahnemanni* mercury, quicksilver

Mercurius corr. *Mercurius corrosivus* corrosive sublimate of mercury

Mercurius cyan. *Mercurius cyanatus* mercurous cyanide

Mercurius dulc. *Mercurius dulcis* calomel, mercurous chloride

Mezereum *Daphne mezereum* spurge olive, mezereon (fresh bark before plant flowers)

Millefolium *Achillea millefolium* yarrow, milfoil (whole fresh plant)

Morbillinum *Morbillinum* nasal discharge from measles patient

Moschus *Moschus moschiferus* musk deer (musky secretion of foreskin)

Murex *Murex purpurea* purple fish, a mollusc (dye)

Muriatic ac. *Muriaticum acidum* hydrochloric acid

Myristica *Myristica sebifera* ucuuba tree (red, acrid, poisonous gum from bark)

Naja   Naja tripudians   hooded snake of Hindustan (venom)

Natrum ars.   Natrum arsenicum   sodium arsenate

Natrum carb.   Natrum carbonicum   sodium carbonate

Natrum mur.   Natrum muriaticum   salt, sodium chloride

Natrum phos.   Natrum phosphoricum   sodium phosphate

Natrum sulph.   Natrum sulphuricum   Glauber's salts, sodium sulphate

Nitric ac.   Nitricum acidum   nitric acid

Nux   Strychnos nux vomica   poison nut tree (seeds)

Nux mosch.   Nux moschata   nutmeg, seed of *Myristica fragrans* (whole nutmeg)

Ocimum   Ocimum canum   Brazilian alfavaca (fresh leaves)

Oenanthe   Oenanthe crocata   hemlock dropwort (fresh root when plant is in flower)

Oleander   Nerium oleander   oleander, rose laurel (leaves)

Onosmodium   Onosmodium virginianum   false bromwell (whole fresh plant)

Opium   Opium   milky juice from unripe seed capsule of opium poppy, *Papaver somniferum*

Oxalic ac.   Oxalicum acidum   oxalic acid

Paeonia   Paeonia officinalis   paeony (fresh root in spring)

Palladium   Palladium   palladium, a rare metallic element

Pareira   Pareira brava   virgin vine (fresh root)

Paris   Paris quadrifolia   herb Paris, true love (whole plant when fruit is ripe)

Parotidinum   Parotidinum   sputum from mumps patient

Petroleum   Oleum petrae   rock oil, coal oil (purified oil)

Petroselinum   Petroselinum sativum   common parsley (whole fresh plant as it comes into flower)

Phellandrium   Phellandrium aquaticum   water dropwort, horsebane (fresh ripe fruit)

Phosphoric ac.   Phosphoricum acidum   phosphoric acid

Phosphorus   Phosphorus   phosphorus

Physostigma   Physostigma venenosum   Calabar bean (whole bean)

Phytolacca   Phytolacca decandra   poke root (fresh leaves or ripe berries, or root in winter)

Picric ac.   Picricum acidum   picric acid, trinitrophenol

Pilocarpin mur.   Pilocarpin muriaticum   hydrochlorate of pilocarpine (an anti-glaucoma drug)

Plantago   Plantago major   greater plantain, ribwort (root)

Platina   Platina metallica   platinum

Plumbum   Plumbum metallicum   lead

Podophyllum   Podophyllum peltatum   May apple (ripe fruit, root after fruit has ripened, or whole fresh plant)

Psorinum   Psorinum   discharge from scabies blister

Pulsatilla   Pulsatilla nigricans   wind flower, pasque flower (whole fresh plant when in flower)

Pyrogenium   Pyrogenium   substance extracted from rotting meat

Quercus   Quercus robur   English oak (acorns)

Radium   Radium   radium, a radioactive metallic element

Radium brom.   Radium bromatum   radium bromide

Ranunculus   Ranunculus bulbosus   bulbous buttercup, bulbous crowfoot (whole plant)

Raphanus   Raphanus sativus   black radish (fresh roots before plant flowers in spring)

Ratanhia   Ratanhia krameria triandra   mapato, a legume (root)

Rheum   Rheum officinale or R. palmatum   rhubarb (dried root)

Rhododendron   Rhododendron chrysanthum   Siberian rhododendron, yellow snow rose (fresh leaves)

Rhus tox.   Rhus toxicodendron   poison ivy (fresh leaves gathered at sunset just before plant comes into flower)

Rhus ven.   Rhus venenata   poison sumach (fresh leaves and stem)

Robinia   Robinia pseudoacacia   black locust acacia, North American locust tree (beans)

Rumex   Rumex crispus   yellow or curled dock (fresh root)

Ruta   Ruta graveolens   rue (whole fresh plant)

Sabadilla   Sabadilla officinarum   seed of *Asagraea officinalis*

Sabal   Sabal serrulata   saw palmetto (juice of fresh green berries)

Sabina   Juniperus sabina   savin juniper (new leaves at tips of branches)

Salicylic ac.   Salicylicum acidum   salicylic acid, main ingredient of aspirin

Sambucus   Sambucus niger   common or black elder (fresh leaves and flowers)

Sanguinaria   Sanguinaria canadensis   bloodroot (fresh root)

Sanicula   Sanicula aqua   mineral spring water of Ottawa, Illinois, USA

Santoninum Santoninum santonin, substance extracted from wormseed, see **Cina**

Sarsaparilla Sarsaparilla smilax officinalis wild liquorice (dried root)

Scutellaria Scutellaria laterifolia skullcap (whole fresh plant)

Secale Secale cornutum ergot, disease caused by fungus *Claviceps purpurea* (affected ears of rye before harvesting)

Selenium Selenium selenium, a non-metallic element

Sempervivum Sempervivum tectorium house leek (fresh leaves)

Senecio Senecio aureus (variety Gracilis) golden ragwort, squaw-weed (fresh plant in flower)

Senega Senega polygala seneca, snake root (dried, powdered root)

Sepia Sepia officinalis cuttlefish ink

Silicea Silicea terra flint

Sol Sol lactose sugar solution exposed to concentrated sunlight

Solidago Solidago virgaurea common golden rod (whole fresh plant)

Spigelia Spigelia anthelmia pinkroot (dried plant)

Spongia Spongia tosta toasted common sponge

Squilla Squilla maritima sea onion (fresh bulb)

Stannum Stannum metallicum tin

Staphisagria Delphinium staphisagria stavesacre (seeds)

Sticta Sticta pulmonaria or Pulmonaria officinalis lungwort (whole plant)

Stramonium Datura stramonium thorn apple (fresh plant in flower, also seeds)

Strontium Strontium metallicum strontium

Sulphur Sulphur sublimated sulphur

Sulphur iod. Sulphur iodatum sulphur iodide

Sulphuric ac. Sulphuricum acidum sulphuric acid

Symphytum Symphytum officinale common comfrey, knitbone (whole fresh plant)

Syphilinum Syphilinum secretion from chancre of person with syphilis

Tabacum Nicotiana tabacum tobacco (fresh leaves before plant comes into flower)

Tamus Tamus communis black bryony, ladies' seal (fresh root or berries)

Taraxacum Taraxacum officinale dandelion (whole plant as flowers open)

Tarentula Lycosa tarentula Spanish spider (live spider)

Tarentula cub. Tarentula cubensis, also Mygale cubensis Cuban tarantula (live spider)

Tellurium Tellurium the element tellurium

Terebinth Terebinthinae oleum turpentine, oleo-resin from various species of pine

Teucrium Teucrium marum verum cat thyme (whole fresh plant)

Theridion Theridion curassavicum orange spider from Curacao and W. Indies

Thiosinaminum alkyl sulphocarbamide, derived from mustard seed oil

Thlaspi Capsella bursa-pastoris shepherd's purse (fresh plant when in flower)

Thuja Thuja occidentalis tree of life, *arbor vitae*, white cedar (fresh green twigs)

Tuberculinum Tuberculinum of Koch culture of tuberculosis bacilli

Tuberculinum bov. Tuberculinum bovum cultivation of cow's tubercular baccilli

Uranium nit. Uranium nitricum uranium nitrate

Urtica Urtica urens small nettle (fresh plant when in flower)

Ustilago Ustilago maidis corn smut (whole fungus)

Uva ursi Arctostaphylos uva-ursi bearberry (fresh leaves in autumn)

Vaccinninum Vaccinninum smallpox vaccine

Valeriana Valeriana officinalis common valerian, all-heal (fresh root)

Variolinum Variolinum discharge from smallpox lesion

Veratrum Veratrum album white or false hellebore (roots before plant comes into flower)

Veratrum vir. Veratrum viride American white hellebore (fresh root in autumn)

Verbascum Verbascum thapsus great mullein, Aaron's rod (whole plant as it comes into flower)

Verbena Verbena hastata iron weed (fresh plant)

Viburnum Viburnum opulus bark elder, water elder, cramp, high cranberry (fresh bark)

Vinca Vinca minor lesser periwinkle (whole fresh plant)

Viola Viola tricolor pansy, heartsease (fresh plant when in flower)

Vipera Vipera communis common viper (venom)

Viscum Viscum album mistletoe (ripe berries, bruised leaves, or whole plant)

Wyethia Alarconia helenoides or Melarhiza inuloides poison weed (tincture of root)

Zinc Zincum metallicum zinc

Zinc sulph. Zincum sulphuricum zinc sulphate

APPENDIX C
60 REMEDY PICTURES

All homeopathic remedies have a double personality. On the one hand they are known to *cause* a range of symptoms in perfectly healthy people. On the other hand, by the law of similars, they are known to *alleviate* the same symptoms in people who are unwell. However, remedies which match physical symptoms only may not be enough to provoke a return to health. Ideally, to provoke the greatest healing, a remedy should match the physical symptoms, the mental symptoms, and the constitution of the person concerned.

So if you have selected, from the lists of remedies in PART 2: 'Ailments and Conditions' or in the General Remedy Finder, a remedy which seems to fit the physical symptoms of the person you wish to treat, look it up in this section of the book and see if it also fits the mental symptoms and general constitution of that person. If it does, it is likely to be very effective. If 2 or more remedies appear suitable on physical or mental grounds, check which is most suitable on constitutional grounds; again, the remedy which most closely matches the constitutional picture will be the most effective. This is why none of the remedies mentioned in this book is, of itself, homeopathic. For example, Antimonium tart. 6c is a homeopathic remedy, homeopathically prepared by successive dilution and succussion, but it will have little effect unless the person it is prescribed for is young, elderly, or very weak.

The following pages describe 60 of the most commonly used homeopathic remedies. Each has a distinct personality, as you will see. Many of them have 'complementary' remedies, remedies whose actions are similar or compatible, and likely to complete a cure once the primary remedy has done its work. Others have 'antidoting' remedies or substances which effectively cancel out their effects. If you need to antidote the effects of a remedy, choose the antidote which best matches your unwelcome symptoms. Still others have 'incompatible' or 'inimical' remedies which, when taken in conjunction with them or in close succession, have the effect of thoroughly confusing the Vital Force. Obviously, antidoting and incompatible remedy combinations should be avoided. One or 2 of the remedies described are also 'specifics', routinely prescribed for certain ailments whatever the constitution of the patient.

The remedy pictures in this book have been compiled from the writings of Hahnemann himself, and from those of James Tyler Kent, Margaret Tyler, and J. H. Clark. Also woven into them are the author's own observations and notes made during absorbing lectures by Margery Blackie, George Vithoulkas, and Francisco Eizyaga.

Aconite

From *Aconitum napellus*, blue monkshood, blue aconite, wolfsbane. The homeopathic remedy is prepared from the whole fresh plant as it comes into flower and is traditionally used to relieve states of acute or chronic tension just before they manifest as inflammation before they result in unusual discharge.

Constitutional indications Adults who respond well to Aconite are usually full-blooded, strong and healthy-looking. Aconite babies tend to be rosy and chubby.

Mental symptoms alleviated Many aspects of behaviour dictated by fear; fear of dying, even predicting hour of own death; agoraphobia; feeling of haste and hurry; specific or free-floating anxiety, which shows itself in the face; restlessness, tossing and turning in sleep.

Physical symptoms alleviated Eye pain or inflammation caused by injury; congested blood vessels in eye; fever which comes on suddenly, with skin hot, dry and angry-looking; tingling sensation in hands and feet; hollow-sounding, crowing cough; great thirst.

The above symptoms are often brought on by shock, fright, exposure to dry, cold winds, and occasionally by intensely hot weather. They are generally made worse by warm rooms, cigarette smoke, music and lying on the affected side; they also tend to be worse in the evening and at night. Fresh air is usually beneficial.

Remedies which follow well Arnica, Belladonna, Ipecac., Bryonia, Silicea, Sulphur.

Complementary remedy Sulphur.

Antidoting remedies/substances Nux, Coffea; acid fruits, wine, coffee, lemonade.

Allium

From *Allium cepa*, the red onion. The homeopathic remedy is made from the whole fresh plant in July/August. Onion contains an acrid, volatile principle which stimulates the tear glands and the mucous membranes of the upper respiratory tract. At one time it was used to cure worms, earache, and bites from mad dogs.

Constitutional indications None in particular.

Mental symptoms alleviated Fear of pain.

Physical symptoms alleviated Headache centred behind forehead; earache in children; streaming eyes, with bland discharge; streaming nose, with discharge which makes nostrils and upper lip sore; stuffed up nose, with discharge from alternate nostrils; toothache in molar area, shifting from left side to right or from one tooth to another; hoarseness, early stages of laryngitis; coughing which causes splitting, tearing sensation in throat – person clutches throat in alarm; coughing brought on by cold air; neuralgic pains; in babies, abdominal colic.

The above symptoms are aggravated by warm rooms, cold or damp, and the smell of flowers; they also tend to start on the left side and move to the right. Cool rooms and fresh air usually improve things.

Complementary remedies Phosphorus, Thuja, Pulsatilla.

Antidoting remedies Arnica, Chamomilla, Veratrum.

Alumina

The homeopathic remedy is prepared from aluminium oxide. Aluminium, absorbed in significant amounts from cooking utensils, causes mental processes to slow down. Its homeopathic derivative is used to treat sluggishness generally.

Constitutional indications Alumina is most effective with people who are confused or senile; those who respond best are usually thin, with dried-up, greyish skin and dry, sore mucous membranes.

Mental symptoms alleviated Confusion, sense of unreality, of time slowing down; feeling pressured and hurried inside despite outward slowness; apprehension, feeling that something awful is about to happen; feeling as if one is talking, hearing, smelling, and seeing through someone else's mouth, ears, nose, and eyes; deep despair, feeling that everything is dark; suicidal or homicidal thoughts at sight of knives or blood.

Physical symptoms alleviated Dizziness on closing eyes; sensation of cobwebs over face; dry skin which feels as if ants are crawling beneath it; sluggish reactions to nervous stimuli; numbness in legs; feeling of heaviness, possibly followed by paralysis; difficulty swallowing solids, with constricted feeling in throat; craving for fruit and vegetables, and for indigestible items such as pencils, chalk, tea leaves, coffee grounds; aversion to meat and beer; difficulty passing urine – stomach muscles have to work hard to empty bladder; in women, profuse, irritant vaginal discharge; lazy bowels – great straining to pass stools, even when stools are soft and rectum is full, with stomach muscles rather than rectal muscles doing the straining; feeling that there is still something to come even when bowels have been opened.

The above symptoms are not improved by cold air, or by items such as wine, vinegar, pepper, salt or potatoes and other starchy foods; discomfort is usually worst in the morning.

Complementary remedy Bryonia.

Antidoting remedies Ipecac., Chamomilla.

Anacardium

From *Anacardium orientale*, the marking nut tree. The homeopathic remedy is made from cardol, a blackish juice extracted from the pith between the shell and the kernel of the nuts. The juice is used, in India and elsewhere, to mark linen and to etch away moles on the skin.

Constitutional indications Anacardium is highly beneficial to people who have an inferiority complex and are trying hard to prove themselves; they suffer from extreme inner conflict and have, as the saying goes, 'a devil on one shoulder and an angel on the other'. Children who suddenly give up studying for exams, saying they can't remember what they are reading, are candidates for Anacardium. Anacardium is also the homeopathic remedy which most closely corresponds to the Chinese concept of possession. This can be simply a feeling that you are not quite yourself – you are observing yourself doing things, or writing the book of your life as you go along. In extreme cases it can feel like possession by another being.

Mental symptoms alleviated Lack of self-confidence, perhaps masked by callous, cruel or sadistic behaviour; confusion between reality and fantasy; extreme suspicion and mistrust of others; a persecution complex; tendency to swear a lot.

Physical symptoms alleviated Tight 'bandaged' feeling around leg or arm; duodenal ulcers which cause intense discomfort two hours after eating but improve immediately after eating.

The above symptoms are made worse by hot baths, showers, or compresses.

Remedy which follows well Platina.

Antidoting remedies Coffea, Rhus tox.

Antimonium

The source of this remedy is antimony sulphide. Antimony poisoning causes headaches, coughing and wheezing, loss of libido, painful urination, abdominal pain, skin eruptions and general debility.

Constitutional indications Antimony is most useful in children and in elderly people. Greediness, sentimentality, a great susceptibility to the charms of moonlight, and a propensity for falling madly in love are often encountered among Antimony types. Physically, such people are often fat, despite a chronic loss of appetite, and may suffer from deformed feet or sores around the mouth.

Mental symptoms alleviated In children, an aversion to being looked at or touched; in adults, bursts of lunatic behaviour, wanting to shoot oneself, finding life unbearable.

Physical symptoms alleviated Itchy scalp, falling hair; red, inflamed eyelids; sore nostrils; coughing, made worse by staring into fire; painful corns or calluses on feet; chronic loss of appetite; belching which smells of food just eaten; in old people, alternate bouts of constipation and diarrhoea.

The above symptoms are exacerbated by heat (from the sun or from the fire) and by eating, and specifically by wine, acid beverages, bread, pastry and pork; they also tend to get worse in the evening, at night and in moonlight. Rest is usually beneficial.

Complementary remedy Sulphur.

Antidoting remedy Hepar sulph.

Antimonium tart.

This remedy is made from potassium tartrate of antimony, also known as tartar emetic, which is both an irritant, causing excessive production of phlegm, and a depressant.

Constitutional indications Antimonium tart. is most beneficial to the very old and very young, and to people who are too weak to cough up phlegm.

Mental symptoms alleviated Drowsiness; irritability, especially when disturbed.

Physical symptoms alleviated Headache which feels like a tight band around the head (made worse by coughing); face pale or cyanosed (bluish), and cold to the touch; tongue thickly coated, but red in centre and around edges; wheezing, with a rattling sound in the chest; inability to cough up phlegm; nausea, relieved by vomiting; lack of thirst, or if thirsty a craving for things which are sour or acidic; legs puffy with retained fluid.

All of these symptoms are aggravated by warm rooms, damp cold, movement or lying down, and tend to become worse between 3 and 4 am. Milk and sour foods are also aggravating. Cold air and sitting up usually offer relief.

Antidoting remedies Pulsatilla, Sepia.

Apis

From *Apis mellifica*, the honey bee. The remedy is prepared from whole bees dissolved in alcohol. Bee stings, as many people know to their cost, cause rapid, watery swellings which smart and burn; anaphylactic reactions can involve the heart and brain.

Constitutional indications None in particular.

Mental symptoms alleviated Depression; irritability; sudden jealousy, suspicion, over-sensitivity.

Physical symptoms alleviated Watery swellings on mouth or eyelids; swelling which spreads to throat and hinders breathing; oedema; fever accompanied by dry skin and a violent headache, with shivering in late afternoon; fever with lack of thirst; any head pain which causes sudden, piercing screams; scanty urination (increased urination indicates that Apis is working well).

The above symptoms tend to start on the right side, then shift to the left; they are aggravated by sleep, touch, pressure, heat and stuffy rooms, and generally get worse in the late afternoon. Fresh air, cold bathing and undressing bring relief.

Complementary remedies Natrum mur. and, if lymph system is involved and glands are swollen, Baryta carb.

Warning: Because of its action on the kidneys, Apis is not recommended in a lower potency than 30c during pregnancy.

Argentum nit.

The source of this remedy is silver nitrate, once known as Hell Stone or Devil's Stone because of its corrosive and sometimes lethal effect. Chronic silver nitrate poisoning causes the skin to turn permanently blue and damages the kidneys, liver, spleen and aorta. Acute poisoning – not uncommon in the days when silver nitrate was used to cauterize wounds after surgery – causes severe respiratory difficulties.

Constitutional indications Argentum nit. is especially good for people who do jobs which call for quick thinking and a good memory, where the emphasis is on performance. Into this category come actors, singers, business executives, lecturers, students, etc. Most Argentum nit. types are extroverts, but much of their behaviour is motivated by a fear of failure.

Mental symptoms Confusion and loss of mental control under stress, head full of irrational thoughts; feeling that one is only just able to resist dangerous impulses, such as throwing onself in front of a train or leaping from a high window; mental exhaustion; sense of hurry and pressure, of going faster and faster; insecurity, forcing oneself to do things because one is afraid of failing; forming irrational notions about things; fear of crowds, fear of heights, fear of being late for trains, appointments, etc., fear of being crushed by tall buildings; always expecting something unpleasant to happen around the next corner; anxiety when faced with the unusual or unexpected, sometimes accompanied by diarrhoea.

Physical symptoms alleviated Headaches which come on gradually but disappear suddenly, brought on by excitement, overwork, travel, sugary foods, etc., and associated with sore, tense neck muscles – pain, usually centred in left temple, wears off in fresh air or if pressure is applied, but becomes more intense if one talks, stoops or moves about; dizziness when looking up at or down from tall buildings; epilepsy; conjunctivitis; stringy mucus in mouth; asthma, relieved by moist air and warmth; warts; sweating brought on by anxiety; palpitations brought on by anxiety, and made worse by lying on left side; craving for salt, sugar and cold food; flatulence, not relieved by belching; vomiting and diarrhoea (greenish stools) brought on by anxiety, worse in hot weather; in babies, diarrhoea during weaning; in women, bearing down sensation in womb, or prolapse of womb.

The above symptoms are not helped by warmth, sugary foods, eating, or emotional problems; they also tend to be worse at night, when there is a moon, and during menstruation. Fresh air and cold usually bring relief.

Antidoting remedy Natrum mur.

Arnica

From *Arnica montana*, leopard's bane or fallkraut. The homeopathic remedy is made from the whole fresh plant or just the root, or from the dried flowers, and is traditionally used to minimize the immediate effects of shock, falls, bruising, bleeding, and injuries caused by blunt objects. It also helps traumatized tissues to heal.

Constitutional indications Those who derive most benefit from Arnica tend to be rather morose and morbidly imaginative. No matter how ill they feel, they are likely to deny that anything is wrong with them and refuse to see a doctor.

Mental symptoms alleviated Wanting to be left alone; hypochondriac tendencies; hopelessness; indifference; restlessness; tossing and turning in bed at night and blaming it on hardness of bed; nightmares about robbers, muddy waters, horrible incidents in the past, etc., from which one wakes mortally afraid and clutching heart; impatience; absentmindedness; inability to concentrate, because one is easily distracted and startled; fear of sudden death.

Physical symptoms alleviated Head feels hot, body cold; concussion; black eyes; eyestrain; cold nose; bad breath; sore gums after dentistry; fever which causes stupor, prostration, even unconsciousness; eczema; boils; broken capillaries internally and on surface of skin, especially after childbirth or injury; sore muscles due to unaccustomed exercise; sprained joints; tennis elbow; in children, whooping cough in which coughing is preceded by crying; aversion to milk and meat; craving for pickles and vinegary foods; foul-smelling stools; faecal incontinence during nightmares.

The above symptoms improve as one starts to move around, then get worse as movement continues. Lying down, with the head lower than the feet, can bring relief. Heat, rest and light pressure generally aggravate matters.

Complementary remedies Aconite, Ipecac.

Antidoting remedy Camphora.

Arsenicum

The source of this remedy is arsenic trioxide, also known as *Arsenicum album*. At one time arsenic was used to treat syphilis, anthrax, yaws and other diseases, and was also widely used in manufacturing processes. It causes weakness, loss of appetite, vomiting, heaviness and discomfort in the stomach, diarrhoea, neuritis, a runny nose, skin eruptions, pigmentation of the skin, and eczema.

Constitutional indications Those who benefit most from Arsenicum are deeply insecure and have an almost insatiable need for comfort and consolation. Arsenicum children are highly strung and delicate, with fine skin and hair; although mentally and physically agile, and often precocious, they get pushed around at school. Arsenicum adults have an anxious, frightened appearance and look as if they are wasting away. Because of their fundamental insecurity, any complaints they have tend to recur.

Mental symptoms alleviated Fear of being alone or going out alone, fear of being burgled, fear of the dark, fear of failure, fear of having an incurable illness – all of which sap the intellect and will; feeling that one is about to die unless the doctor is called; restlessness due to anxiety; thoughts of suicide; great fastidiousness and orderliness in one's dress and habits; irritability; seeing evil omens everywhere and refusing to be reassured; religious mania; possessiveness; hoarding and miserliness; not wanting to meet friends and acquaintances for fear of having offended them; great sensitivity to touch, smell and cold; night terrors; waking at the slightest noise, especially between midnight and 2 am, and getting up and walking about; feeling sleepy but unable to get to sleep.

Physical symptoms alleviated Headaches at 3-weekly intervals, accompanied by dizziness and vomiting, aggravated by pressure and the smell of food or cigarette smoke, but relieved by movement and by cold applications if applied early enough – pain burns and throbs, starting at bridge of nose and extending over entire head, which feels extremely tender; stinging, watering eyes; sneezing, with catarrh which stings and burns, soothed by sniffing warm water up nose; red, swollen lower lip, soothed by hot applications; dry, cracked lips, or pale, bleeding lips; intensely sore mouth ulcers, with a red, glazed-looking tongue; asthma brought on by anxiety, with severe breathlessness between midnight and 2 am which obliges one to sit up to breathe, often improved by warmth and sniffing warm water up nose; early stages of heart failure, with fluid retention, especially around ankles; tendency to bleed easily; veins which feel as if ice-cold or boiling water were flowing through them; rough, scaly, cracked skin; lack of perspiration, or profuse perspiration; vomiting, with vomit which stings; wanting frequent sips of water; wanting to eat only fatty or sour foods; diarrhoea, often accompanied by vomiting, brought on by cold winds or overindulgence in ripe fruit, vegetables, iced foods or alcohol – stools are watery, scant, frequent and foul-smelling, and cause soreness around the anus and burning pains in rectum; dehydration and collapse due to diarrhoea, especially in children.

The above symptoms are often helped by warmth, hot drinks, and an extra pillow when lying down. The sight or smell of food, cold food or cold drinks, and cold dry winds tend to exacerbate them; discomfort is usually worst on the right side and between midnight and 2 am.

Complementary remedies Rhus tox., Carbo veg., Phosphorus, Thuja, Secale.

Antidoting remedies Opium, Camphor, China, Hepar sulph., Nux.

Baryta

The source of this remedy is barium carbonate which, in large amounts, causes nausea, vomiting, convulsions, and diarrhoea.

Constitutional indications Baryta carb. is most effective in the very young and the very old. Children who benefit from it are mentally and physically slow, very skinny for their age, and pot-bellied; they also tend to have wrinkled skin and a vacant expression on their face. Elderly people who respond well tend to be obese. Both groups may also suffer from hormone problems.

Mental symptoms alleviated Extreme shyness; fear of people and situations; lack of concentration; forgetfulness; immature behaviour.

Physical problems alleviated Headaches which improve in open air but get worse in hot sun or in front of fire; swollen tonsils, with swollen lymph glands in neck and abdomen; cough which gets worse in evening but wears off after midnight, relieved by lying on stomach; muscle aches after eating or sleeping; sebaceous cysts; fatty tumours or warts; sore feet due to excessive perspiration and use of foot antiperspirants/deodorants; atherosclerosis, with degeneration of walls of arteries; high blood pressure; aneurysms; palpitations, made worse by exertion; griping pains in stomach, relieved by lying on stomach.

The above symptoms are intensified by cold, damp, rinsing in cold water, hot meals, excitement, raising the arms, dwelling on aches and pains, and by the presence of strangers; they also tend to get worse when lying on the left side. Cold food and being left alone generally improve matters.

Complementary remedies Dulcamara, Psorinum, Silicea.

Incompatible/inimical remedy Calcarea carb.

Belladonna

From *Atropa belladonna*, deadly nightshade. The homeopathic remedy is made from the whole fresh plant, which is highly poisonous, containing the alkaloids atropine, hyoscamine, and scopolamine. The symptoms of deadly nightshade poisoning are giddiness, confusion, increasingly excited, incoherent or violent behaviour, a dry mouth and throat, flushed face, wide staring pupils, and difficulty speaking and swallowing. A high fever develops, sometimes accompanied by convulsions. Drowsiness and coma ensue, and eventually death.

Constitutional indications The kind of person who responds most markedly to Belladonna is sturdily built, apparently in rude health, and vigorous in mind and body.

Mental symptoms alleviated Restlessness; wild, incoherent, excited behaviour; maniacal laughter; racing imagination; hallucinations; jumpiness and fear when approached; feeling dazed and stupid; horrible dreams; feeling sleepy but not able to sleep.

Physical symptoms alleviated Unusual sensitivity to light, noise, touch, pressure, motion, jarring, pain; fits; throbbing headaches which feel as if all the blood in the body has gone to the head (made worse by sun, cold, shock, menstruation, movement, stooping, eye movements); hot, flushed face, with pale mouth and lips; earache, especially on right side (made worse by getting head wet or cold); dilated, staring pupils, and intolerance of light; bright red tongue, sometimes raw around edges but coated in middle; in infants, teething pains; spasms of dry, tickly coughing made worse by talking; sore throat, tender to the touch, and throat pains which cause head and neck to jerk; sudden contraction of throat on swallowing; thirst for lemon juice, not alleviated by drinking it; inflammation of the kidneys; jerking and twitching in sleep; burning, dry, flushed and throbbing skin, with cold hands and feet.

Many of the symptoms above are made worse by jarring, motion, light, noise, pressure, sun, having the hair cut and lying down. They also tend to be worse on the right side and at night from 11 pm onwards. They are often relieved by standing, sitting upright, staying in the warm and applying warmth to the affected parts.

Specific use Scarlet fever.

Complementary remedy Calcarea carb.

Antidoting remedies/substances Camphora, Coffea, Opium, Aconite; acetic acid (in fruit, lemon juice, vinegar), tea, coffee.

Bryonia

From *Bryonia alba* (also known as *B. dioica*), white, red or common bryony. The homeopathic remedy is made from the whole fresh plant. Because it affects fibrous tissues, serous membranes (membranes which secrete fluids), ligaments around joints, the broad part of tendons, and the coating of nerves, all of which can become inflamed and painful with rheumatism, Bryonia is frequently prescribed for rheumatism sufferers, especially if fever is present as well.

Constitutional indications The kind of person who responds to Bryonia is often of rather plodding intelligence, rubicund and well-fleshed, with a dark complexion and dark hair; he or she often gets stitching pains, and is easily angered or irritated.

Mental symptoms alleviated Feeling tired, languid, reluctant to move or speak when spoken to; feeling dull and stupid in the head, as if the head is about to fly to bits, but irritable with it; delusions about being away from home, or wanting to go home, when already at home; wanting something but not knowing what, wanting things impossible to get, or refusing things once they are offered; fear of death, of not regaining health; hopelessness; job or financial worries, especially after a dispute with someone in authority; worry dreams, often about money or job.

Physical symptoms alleviated Bursting headaches, made worse by slightest movement, also by too much food or alcohol, hot drinks, colds and coughing, but relieved by firm pressure and cold; heavy eyelids and stabbing pains in the eyes; dry, sore, itchy lips; foul, coated tongue; dry, constricted throat; extreme thirst at long intervals; vomiting after rich fatty foods and hot drinks; craving for meat and unusual foods; stomach feels as if there is a stone in it – the sensation is made worse by pressure; stools which are large, hard, crumbly, black or burnt-looking; in women, breasts which are hard and inflamed, as if there is an abscess brewing, made worse by slightest movement; chest pains severe enough to make one clutch chest and head when coughing; pains around rib cage, made worse by coughing, drinking and warm rooms, and worse at night; cold hands and feet; in rheumatism sufferers, joints which are hot, swollen and painful, and made worse by cold draughts and slightest movement; profuse, sour-smelling sweat.

Many of the symptoms above are made worse by excitement, bright light, noise, touch, movement, and eating. They are also worse in the mornings, around 9 pm (when delirium and fever tend to reach a peak), and around 3 am. Cold, dry winds and draughts should be avoided. Cool air and firm, cool pressure on affected parts generally bring relief.

Complementary remedies Natrum mur., Natrum sulph. and, to a lesser extent, Alumina.

Antidoting remedies Aconite, Chamomilla, Nux.

Calcarea

The source of this remedy is calcium carbonate derived from oyster shells. Calcium is essential for healthy bones and for the proper functioning of nerves and muscles.

Constitutional indications Adults who respond well to Calcarea are usually fair, flabby and overweight, and have a cold, clammy handshake. Children who respond well tend to be tubby and clumsy, with a chalky pale complexion, coarse skin and coarse, curly hair; they are also prone to head sweats at night. Calcarea types are among the few mortals who actually feel better when they are constipated.

Mental symptoms alleviated Depression; emotional fragility; fear of making a fool of oneself, fear of the dark, fear of losing one's mind; inability to apply oneself after emotional upsets; mania for work, followed by sudden laziness and pre-occupation with oneself and one's ailments; passivity, reluctance to answer questions; resentment; preoccupation with trivia, fiddling with small objects, doodling; feeling sorry for oneself and weeping from self-pity; going over and over details of illness/ailments until others feel like hitting one on the head; poor memory, forgetting what one has just been reading; tendency towards intense religiosity – reading Bible all day, for example; cruelty to people and animals, but shedding tears when relating incidents of cruelty; difficulty getting to sleep, then waking and worrying about what might go wrong; night terrors.

Physical symptoms alleviated Head sweats at night; head which feels cold and damp; in babies, a large head and fontanelles which are slow to close; headaches centred on right temple, brought on by extreme heat or cold, or by becoming overheated; headaches caused by missing breakfast; dizziness; acute eye infections, with redness of white of eyes, especially in right eye; cataract; persistent, unpleasant-smelling discharge from ears; nasal polyps; swollen tonsils and adenoids; late or complicated teething; swollen neck glands; perspiration on chest; coarse skin with large pores; sweaty eczema; chilblains; copious perspiration, with bland or offensive odour; scoliosis or crookedness of the spine; in infants, late walking and unsteadiness on legs due to overweight; hanging feet out of bed at night because soles are burning hot; poor co-ordination, clumsiness; hearty appetite, with craving for eggs, pickles and acid foods, sweet things, and raw potatoes; in children, wanting to eat soap and other indigestible items such as soil and chalk; aversion to coffee, meat and milk (milk tends to aggravate other symptoms); strong-smelling urine; gallstones; piles; feeling better when constipated, worse when bowel movements are soft or loose; in women, early or abnormally heavy periods.

The above symptoms are exacerbated by draughts, cold, cold damp winds, and exertion, and are felt most intensely between 2 and 3 am. They wear off in the morning, improve with constipation, and are generally relieved by lying on the affected side.

Complementary remedies Rhus tox., Belladonna, Lycopodium, Phosphorus, Silicea, Platina.

Antidoting remedies Camphora, Ipecac., Nitric ac., Nux.

Incompatible/inimical remedies Bryonia, Sulphur.

Calcarea phos.

The homeopathic remedy is prepared from calcium phosphate, also used as a Tissue Salt (see p. 24).

Constitutional indications Calcarea phos. suits people who are discontented, uncertain what they want; such people are usually thin (thinner than Calcarea types) and have dark hair, long legs, and a sagging abdomen; as babies they may have been late in walking. Late-developing adolescents with muddy skin also respond well to Calcarea phos.

Mental symptoms alleviated Nervousness, restlessness, fidgeting; dislike of routine; need for stimulation; difficulty getting up in the morning.

Physical symptoms alleviated In babies, delayed closure of fontanelles; headaches in children of school age; numbness or crawling sensations in hands and feet; sweaty scalp; delayed or complicated teething, with rapid tooth decay; painful bones and joints; growing pains; fractures which are slow to heal; craving for bacon rinds and strong-tasting foods; poor digestion, with stomach ache after meals, proneness to vomiting, and upsets after eating ice cream; splattery, greenish stools.

The above symptoms are usually aggravated by damp, cold, changeable weather, melting snow, exertion, lifting things and worrying; grief, bad news, sexual excesses and disappointments in love also have a negative effect. Summer and warm dry weather often produce dramatic improvement.

Complementary remedies Ruta, Hepar sulph.

Cantharis

The source of this remedy is *Cantharis* (or *Lytta*) *vesicatoria*, a species of beetle misleadingly called Spanish fly, which contains a rapid-acting irritant called cantharidin. In traditional medicine Spanish fly was used to cause blistering, increase fluid loss, treat baldness, procure abortion and provoke sexual desire. Patients who took it experienced burning pains in the throat and stomach, difficulty swallowing, nausea, vomiting, diarrhoea and a frantic urge to pass water; the unlucky ones went into convulsions, even into a coma.

Constitutional indications Cantharis should be the remedy of first resort for individuals who look as if they are suffering intensely.

Mental symptoms Paroxysms of rage, made worse by looking at shiny objects or touching throat while drinking; excessive desire for sex, amounting to a frantic itch for intercourse; extreme anxiety; screaming; being insolent, querulous, irritable, even violent; losing consciousness.

Physical symptoms alleviated Seeing things in shades of yellow; burning sensation in throat; urgent thirst, with reluctance to drink because drinking causes spasms of breathlessness; no appetite for food; burning sensation in stomach; loathing for tobacco; pleurisy, accompanied by sweating and palpitations; erysipelas; burns and scalds relieved by cold applications; insect bites with a blackish centre; redness and infection which spreads within 4 hours; swelling and suppurating rashes on hands; ice-cold hands with fingernails which feel red hot; burning sensation on soles of feet at night; severe cystitis, with scalding inflammation which worsens rapidly and cannot be ignored; burning pains in abdomen which feel as if intestinal lining has been stripped raw; severe distension of abdomen; diarrhoea which burns and scalds.

The above symptoms are exacerbated by touch, movement, coffee and cold water, and tend to get worse in the afternoon. However, they respond to warmth and gentle massage, and can be soothed by belching and passing wind; they are least troublesome at night and in the morning.

Complementary remedies Belladonna, Mercurius, Phosphorus, Sepia, Sulphur.

Antidoting remedies Aconite, Pulsatilla, Camphora.

Carbo veg.

The source of this homeopathic remedy is vegetable charcoal, made from beech, birch or poplar wood. Its main action is the removal of excess mucus from the digestive system. In the pre-pharmaceutical era, vegetable charcoal was used to absorb gases and check fermentation.

Constitutional indications Carbo veg. is most beneficial to people who complain of not having felt really well since a particular illness or accident. Mental sluggishness is one of the first symptoms they mention.

Mental symptoms alleviated Slow thought processes and lack of mental energy; patchy, unreliable memory; preferring daylight to darkness; fear of the supernatural; lack of interest in news and current affairs; fixed ideas.

Physical symptoms alleviated Headaches in the morning, especially after overeating – head feels hot and heavy; fainting easily; dizziness and nausea; face which is purplish or has a greenish pallor; red-tipped nose; bitter, salty taste in mouth; cold breath and tongue; hoarseness; spasmodic cough, with gagging, choking and vomiting of mucus; bronchitis, especially in elderly people who smoke; clumsiness, poor coordination; cold, bluish hands and feet; cold, clammy skin; wanting to be fanned because body feels burning hot inside although skin is cold; internal or external bleeding; poor venous circulation, or varicose veins which bleed; gangrene; cold, puffy legs; aversion to meat and milk; craving for salty or acid foods, sweet things and coffee; digestive problems, no matter what kinds of food are eaten; most foods, but particularly fats, cause wind; burning sensation in stomach, heartburn, sour belching and regurgitation of food; indigestion made worse by overeating, eating rich foods, or eating too late in evening.

The above symptoms are generally relieved by cold, fresh air and belching. Fatty foods, milk, coffee and wine only exacerbate discomfort, which is most marked in warm, wet weather, in the evening and when lying down.

Complementary remedies Kali carb., Phosphorus, Pulsatilla.

Antidoting remedies Nux, Camphora, Arsenicum, Ambra.

Causticum

This remedy, made from quicklime (calcium oxide) and potassium bisulphate, was invented by Samuel Hahnemann himself. It is especially good for conditions which involve local paralysis, burning sensations, rawness, soreness or skin eruptions which have been suppressed by steroids, etc.

Constitutional indications Those who derive most benefit from Causticum tend to be dark-haired, dark-eyed, sallow-skinned, weak and rather rigid in their thinking. Children who respond well to Causticum are often very excitable and outgoing, thoroughly involved in everything going on around them and deeply concerned about injustice.

Mental symptoms alleviated Pessimism, depression, anxiety; intellectual laziness; sudden tears and floods of emotion; intense sympathy with people or animals in pain or trouble; lack of self-reliance; irritability; wanting to criticize everything; suspicion and distrust which mask timidity and nervousness; in children, not wanting to go to bed at night.

Physical symptoms alleviated Dizziness when bending forwards or sideways, as if there were an empty space between brain and skull; Bell's palsy; rushing and roaring in ears; hearing echo of own voice; colds which go to the ears; drooping eyelids, dimmed vision, momentary sight loss; soreness inside nose and thick yellow catarrh; post-nasal drip, relieved by cold drinks; dry, tickly cough; hoarseness, especially in morning; scraped feeling in throat, with painless loss of voice; paralysis of vocal cords; rheumatism, with muscular stiffness due to contracted tendons; stiff neck after sitting in a draught; deformed joints, with sharp, tearing pains in them; warts on face or fingers; scars or healed injury sites which become sore again; in women, early periods with scanty flow which stops at night or when lying down; stress incontinence; cystitis, with delayed urination despite intense urging.

The above symptoms are often worse on the right side, but respond to damp and warmth. Cold dry winds, sweet foods, coffee, grief and fright have a deleterious effect.

Complementary remedies Carbo veg., Petroselinum.

Incompatible/inimical remedies Phosphorus, Coffea.

Chamomilla

From *Matricaria chamomilla*, German chamomile. The homeopathic remedy is made from the whole fresh plant. In herbal form, chamomile is used to treat nervous complaints and womb problems.

Constitutional indications Individuals who respond best to Chamomilla have a very low pain threshold and are often bad-tempered and complaining. Complaints often begin with the words 'I can't bear. . .'

Mental symptoms alleviated Inner turmoil; rudeness; spitefulness; being bad-tempered with everyone and everything, including oneself; being impossible to please, rather like a child who is quiet when carried but screams when put down; slightest pain or discomfort at night makes one jump out of bed and walk about.

Physical symptoms alleviated Slightest pain causes sweating and fainting; numb feeling in head; convulsions brought on by anger; throbbing sensation in one half of head, relieved by bending head back; one cheek red, the other pale; severe earache, with congested, blocked feeling in affected ear; tinnitus; teething, especially if accompanied by fever and greenish diarrhoea; toothache which responds to cold rinsing but flares up with hot drinks and also at night; yellow, coated tongue; heartburn; dry, hacking cough; coughing in sleep, and also when angry; feeling sleepy but unable to get to sleep; drowsiness in morning; anxiety dreams which cause one to start out of sleep and get angry; moaning and crying in sleep; skin which feels very hot; sticking feet out of bed at night to cool them; in women, heavy periods accompanied by severe labour-like pains; abdominal pain which causes legs to be drawn up; tearing pains in general; diarrhoea, with thin, slimy, pale green stools; stools which are hot and smell of rotten eggs.

The above symptoms are almost always made worse by bad temper, and also by heat, cold winds, fresh air and belching; they also tend to be worse at night, from 9 pm onwards. Warm wet weather and fasting often improve matters; children feel better if they are carried.

Complementary remedies Belladonna, Magnesia phos.

Antidoting remedies Camphora, Nux, Pulsatilla.

Chelidonium

From *Chelidonium majus*, the greater celandine. The homeopathic remedy is prepared from the whole plant when it is in flower, or from the root only. Its main action is on the liver.

Constitutional indications Chelidonium has an affinity with thin, fair, lethargic people.

Mental symptoms alleviated Depression; anxiety; pessimism and despondency; mental sluggishness, unwillingness to make any effort; tendency to brood; weepiness.

Physical symptoms alleviated Headaches accompanied by great heaviness, lethargy and drowsiness; lead-in-the-head feeling; hangovers which prevent one sitting up or standing up; cataracts; drowsiness during the day; coated tongue, with teeth marks on it; asthma which comes on at night; pain around lower angle of right shoulder blade; upset stomach, with nausea and vomiting; craving for cheese and hot drinks (sometimes aversion to cheese); liverishness, with dizziness and vomiting; distension of upper abdomen.

The above symptoms are generally made worse by movement, heat, touch and changes in the weather; they also tend to affect the right side, and are especially marked early in the morning and around 4 am and 4 pm. Milk, hot drinks, eating and firm pressure usually bring relief.

Complementary remedies Lycopodium, Bryonia.

Antidoting remedy Chamomilla.

China
From *Cinchona calisaya*, an evergreen shrub from South America. The homeopathic remedy is made from the dried bark, also known as Peruvian bark, which yields quinine, used to treat malaria and also to cause abortion. Quinine causes contractions of the bronchi, spleen and uterus, irritation of the stomach, cochlea, and retina, loss of protein in the urine, and heat, fever and sweating. Its homeopathic derivative is very beneficial after debilitating illness or excessive loss of body fluids.

Constitutional indications Individuals of an artistic or poetic nature usually respond well to China.

Mental symptoms alleviated Apathy, indifference; inability to concentrate; emotional fragility, jumpiness, edginess; nervous exhaustion; outbursts of anger despite mild nature; inability to express feelings face to face; building castles in the air, playing the hero in dreams; reliving day's events in dreams.

Physical symptoms alleviated Headaches which wear off by pressing painful area but intensify if hair is combed; neuralgia; dizziness; convulsions; haemorrhages and nosebleeds; tinnitus; weak, jumpy muscles; fever, with alternate bouts of sweating and shivering, refusing to drink during sweats but wanting to drink during chills; profuse sweating; flushing and shivering generally, in absence of fever; sallow, yellowish complexion; skin which is very sensitive to touch; swollen ankles; belching which does not relieve indigestion; sensation of food being stuck behind breastbone; aversion to butter and fatty foods; craving for alcohol; gastroenteritis; gall bladder problems; uncomfortable flatulence, made worse by movement; blood in urine; swollen liver and spleen; frothy, yellow, chopped-egg stools.

The above symptoms are not improved by food, cold, draughts, movement or touching affected areas; they also tend to be worse at night and in the autumn. Sleep, warmth and firm pressure are usually helpful.

Complementary remedies Ferrum, Calcarea phos.

Antidoting remedies Arnica, Arsenicum, Ipecac.

Colocynth
From *Citrullus colocynthis*, the bitter apple or bitter cucumber. The homeopathic derivative is most commonly used to relieve anger and destructive effects of anger, and severe abdominal pain. It is made from the pulp of the fruit, which contains colocynthin, a substance which acts on the bowels, causing great pain and painful straining when stools are passed; the stools themselves become very watery.

Constitutional indications Colocynth is best suited to people who are fair-haired and fair-skinned.

Mental symptoms alleviated Anger and indignation; extreme irritability, made worse by questioning; embarrassment caused by offensive remarks.

Physical symptoms alleviated Dizziness when standing with head to left; headaches which improve by applying warmth or pressure; trigeminal neuralgia; stomach pain, with nausea and vomiting; shooting, nervy pains in kidney area or around ovaries; sciatica; gout; rheumatism; agonizing abdominal pain, alleviated by lying on side with knees drawn up to chin; spasmodic abdominal pain with diarrhoea, relieved by passing wind.

All of the symptoms above are aggravated by anger and indignation, and also by eating, drinking and damp cold; they also tend to be worst around 4 pm. Firm pressure, warmth, sleep, coffee and passing wind usually produce improvement.

Antidoting remedies Coffea, Staphisagria, Chamomilla.

Dioscorea

From *Dioscorea villosa*, the wild yam. The homeopathic remedy is made from the fresh root, which contains a substance called dioscorene, highly irritant to the nerves supplying the bowels.

Constitutional indications None in particular.

Mental symptoms alleviated Calling things by the wrong name.

Physical symptoms alleviated Pain in centre of chest and down both arms, accompanied by breathlessness; sinking feeling in stomach; general discomfort in upper abdomen; belching, especially after drinking tea; pain in liver area (right upper abdomen), radiating to right nipple; constant abdominal pain, punctuated by spasms of acute pain which radiate to other parts of the body, even to fingers and toes.

All the symptoms above tend to get worse in the evening and at night, and are not helped by doubling up or lying down. Standing up, stretching, walking about out of doors and applying pressure usually improve matters.

Antidoting remedies Chamomilla, Camphora.

Dulcamara

From *Solanum dulcamara*, woody nightshade or bittersweet. This plant contains an alkaloid called solanin, which paralyses the vagus nerve and causes the heart to pump faster. The homeopathic remedy is prepared from the stems and leaves of the plant just before it comes into flower, and is traditionally used to treat conditions brought on by changes from warm to cold, or from warm to damp and cold.

Constitutional indications None in particular.

Mental symptoms alleviated None in particular.

Physical symptoms alleviated Paralysis or weakness made worse by cold and damp; sore, itchy, bleeding or encrusted eruptions on face or scalp; ringworm; large, smooth, fleshy or flat warts; urticaria; catarrh which gets worse in warm rooms; hoarseness; coughing up large amounts of phlegm; coughing made worse by lying down; pain around navel; yellow or greenish diarrhoea; difficulty opening bowels or urinating after catching a chill.

Most of the symptoms above improve with warmth and movement. Immobility, damp cold, getting wet and cooling down rapidly after sweating profusely tend to make them worse.

Complementary remedy Baryta carb.

Antidoting remedies Camphora, Cuprum.

Incompatible/inimical remedies Belladonna, Lachesis.

Euphrasia

From *Euphrasia officinalis* (also known as *E. sticta*), common eyebright. The homeopathic remedy is made from the whole fresh plant, traditionally used as a cure for eye ailments. The poet Milton wrote that the Archangel 'Purged with Euphrasy and Rue the visual nerve, for he had much to see'.

Constitutional indications None in particular.

Mental symptoms alleviated None in particular.

Physical symptoms alleviated Bursting headaches; profuse, stinging discharge from eyes; watering eyes; conjunctivitis; intolerance of bright light; dimmed vision; sticky mucus or little blisters on cornea; hot, red cheeks; bland, watery catarrh; early stages of measles; in women, short, painful periods in which flow lasts for only an hour a day, or cessation of periods accompanied by eye problems; in men, prostatitis; constipation.

The above symptoms are generally aggravated by warmth, south winds, bright light and being indoors; they also tend to be worse in the evening. Coffee and darkened rooms often bring relief.

Antidoting remedies Camphora, Pulsatilla.

Ferrum phos.

The homeopathic remedy is prepared from iron phosphate, one of the Tissue Salts (see p. 24). It is most beneficial in the first stages of inflammation, when extra blood flows to affected areas.

Constitutional indications People who respond best to Ferrum phos. are often rather pale, anaemic and complaining, and prone to sudden, fiery congestion of the face.

Mental symptoms alleviated None in particular.

Physical symptoms alleviated Headaches which improve by bathing forehead in cold water; pale face which flushes easily; head colds which begin with nosebleeds; earache; hoarseness; laryngitis; dry, hacking cough with pain in chest; rheumatic joints, with raised temperature and shooting pains which intensify on starting to move but wear off with gentle exercise; fevers which onset slowly, especially if face is pale with red spots on cheeks, if pulse is weak and rapid, and if chill comes on around 1 pm; haemorrhages, especially if blood is bright red; aversion to meat and milk; craving for stimulants; sour belching, and vomiting of undigested food; in women, periods at 3-weekly intervals, with heavy, dragging pain in uterus and pain around apex of head, or dryness of vagina; stress incontinence, with wetting at night; early stages of dysentery, with blood in stools.

The above symptoms are generally made worse by jarring, touching, moving, lying on right side, being too hot, being exposed to the sun, and by not perspiring as one should or suppressing perspiration with antiperspirants; they also tend to be more marked between 4 and 6 am. Cold applications and gentle exercise usually bring relief.

Complementary remedies Kali mur., Kali phos., Calcarea phos.

Gelsemium

From *Gelsemium sempervirens*, yellow jasmine. The homeopathic remedy is prepared from the root of the fresh plant which contains an alkaloid which interferes with nervous control of breathing and movement, causing paralysis, trembling and inflammation.

Constitutional indications Individuals of limited intelligence, who are dull and heavy-looking and have a bluish tinge to their skin, often respond well to Gelsemium. The remedy is also beneficial for heavy smokers.

Mental symptoms alleviated Fears and phobias accompanied by trembling and the need to pass urine; fears often centred around falling, throwing oneself from a great height, going to the dentist, having surgery, heart suddenly stopping if one does not move; dullness and drowsiness; inability to sleep because of excitement; nervousness and a sense of inadequacy.

Physical symptoms alleviated Heavy head which feels as if there is a tight band around it; headaches which wear off after urinating, vomiting or sleeping but which intensify with bright light and movement; dizziness, faintness; scalp which feels sore; face which looks flushed, heavy, hot and sweaty; earache; heavy, drooping eyelids; visual disturbances or double vision; burning pain in right eye; summer colds with mild fever, sneezing and watery catarrh; nasty taste in mouth; numb, trembling tongue with a thick yellow coating; sore throat with red tonsils, with earache and difficulty swallowing, often associated with anxiety and made worse by hot drinks; dry cough; heavy, tired, aching,

trembling limbs, accompanied by pain in neck; twitch or tremor of single muscles, which feel cold and tingly; flu-like chills up and down back, with intermittent waves of heat; lack of thirst; in women, painful periods or pain in uterus unconnected with periods.

The above symptoms are generally worse early in the day and at bedtime; sun, heat, damp, fog, tobacco, impending thunder, excitement, emotional stress, apprehension, worrying about symptoms, and worrying about performing in public tend to make them worse. Open air, exercise, passing urine, taking stimulants or alcohol, applying local heat and bending forward all produce improvement.

Antidoting remedies Coffea, China, Digitalis.

Glonoinum

The source of this remedy is the explosive liquid nitroglycerine. The active principle in nitroglycerine is nitrous oxide or 'laughing gas' which causes blood vessels to dilate, lowering blood pressure.

Constitutional indications Glonoinum is most effective in women who have high blood pressure, especially if they are flushed and overweight.

Mental symptoms alleviated Confusion; loss of sense of place or direction.

Physical symptoms alleviated Bursting sensation in head and neck; dizziness; headaches, especially if caused by extremes of heat or cold, jolting or jarring, strong emotions, or cessation of periods; in women, hot flushes during menopause.

The above symptoms tend to be made worse by heat, exertion, noise, sunlight and bright lights, wine, stimulants, tight or heavy clothing and lying too close to the floor. Cold air and cold applications, firm pressure, bending the head back, and lying with head higher than hips all seem to relieve symptoms.

Antidoting remedy Aconite.

Graphites

The homeopathic remedy is made from plumbago or black lead, a mixture of carbon, iron and silica. At one time black lead was used to treat cold sores.

Constitutional indications Elderly women who are overweight, constipated, chilly and rather melancholy respond well to Graphites. So do coarse-featured, dark-haired individuals with earthy complexions. The Graphites type often does hard manual work in the open air or drives heavy goods vehicles.

Mental symptoms alleviated Indecisiveness, timidity, unresponsiveness to external events; poor short-term memory; awareness that mind is not fully alert and in control causes anxiety; occasional depression; easily startled; tendency to become maudlin and weepy when listening to music.

Physical symptoms alleviated Hair loss; numbness and cramps in hands and feet; intolerance of bright light; deafness which improves with background noise; weepy eczema behind ears; face which feels as if there is a cobweb over it; periodically feeling very hot and sweaty, usually followed by a nosebleed; swollen glands; rough, dry, cracked skin; keloids; cold sores; tendency for slightest cut or abrasion to turn septic; skin lesions which exude thick honey-coloured pus; hardening of old scars; duodenal ulcers, soothed by hot food and by lying down, or duodenal ulcers which alternate with skin complaints; aversion to sweets, fish and salty foods; in women, late periods accompanied by constipation, infrequent or scanty periods, enlarged ovaries or hardening of the breasts; constipation, with large, knotty stools passed with a lot of straining.

The above symptoms tend to wear off in the dark or after sleep, but are aggravated by cold, sweet foods, seafood and suppression of skin eruptions with steroids, etc. Discomfort is often worse during periods and usually located on the left side.

Complementary remedies Hepar sulph, Lycopodium.

Antidoting remedies Nux, Aconite, Arsenicum, China.

Hamamelis
From *Macrophylla dioica* (also known as *M. virginica*), witch hazel. The homeopathic remedy, made from the bark of the twigs and roots which contain a substance which causes veins to haemorrhage, is traditionally used to improve venous circulation and alleviate bruising and soreness.

Constitutional indications None in particular.

Mental symptoms alleviated Depression and withdrawal – wanting to be left alone and not talked to; wanting others to show due respect; restlessness; irritability; grandiose ideas.

Physical symptoms alleviated Headaches, often relieved by nosebleeds, open air, reading, thinking or talking; eyes which are painful and bloodshot; injuries which cause soreness and bruising; tender, rheumatic joints; tickly cough, with blood-flecked phlegm; varicose veins; phlebitis; venous bleeding which is slow to stop; epididymitis; urethritis; in women, inflammation of uterus or ovaries, ovulation pain or heavy menstrual bleeding, with very sore abdomen.

The symptoms above are often made worse by warm damp air, pressure and movement.

Complementary remedy Ferrum.

Antidoting remedy Arnica.

Hepar sulph.
The source of this remedy is calcium sulphide, obtained by heating together the calcareous inner layer of oyster shells with flowers of sulphur. At one time this preparation was used to antidote the effects of the many forms of physic containing mercury.

Constitutional indications Hepar sulph. is best suited to individuals who are overweight, flabby, pale, sluggish and rather depressed; such people tend to look as if they have been through a lot, and gratefully sink into the nearest chair.

Mental symptoms alleviated Irritability with self and others which hides anxiety; great sensitivity to touch, pain, cold dry air, noise, disturbance of any kind; tendency to be hasty, impulsive and to want change for change's sake; taking unreasonable likes and dislikes to people; taking offence easily; outward calm conceals restlessness; feeling hard done by and telling others how everything in the past has gone wrong.

Physical symptoms alleviated Slightest pain causes fainting; sinusitis, with sinus areas very tender, made worse by bending forward but relieved by warmth; corneal ulcers; conjunctivitis; cold sores or ulcers at corner of lips; colds which start with an itchy throat; fish-bone-in-throat sensation; sore throat which causes ear pain when swallowing; hoarseness or loss of voice; choking or intense pain on swallowing, relieved by wrapping something warm around neck; tonsillitis, with swollen glands in neck; dry, hoarse cough brought on by exposure to cold; hollow, crowing cough with loose, rattling phlegm in chest, with retching and vomiting, worse at night; exhausting cough worse between 6 pm and midnight; influenza, with sneezing, fever, sweating and craving for warmth despite high temperature; abscesses or boils, with sour-smelling sweat; constant thirst for sips of fluid (children may not be thirsty at all); craving for fats, condiments and sour, vinegary foods; aversion to alcohol; diarrhoea, made worse by eating ripe, juicy fruit, vegetables, and iced foods.

The above symptoms are generally aggravated by cold air and draughts, undressing and touching affected parts, and are generally most intense in the morning and when lying on the affected side. Eating a meal, staying in the warm, applying compresses and wrapping the head up all improve matters.

Remedies which follow well Calcarea, Calcarea sulph.

Complementary remedy Calendula.

Antidoting remedies Belladonna, Chamomilla, Silicea, Kali iod.

Hyoscyamus

From *Hyoscyamus niger*, henbane. The homeopathic remedy is made from the whole fresh plant and mainly affects the nervous system.

Constitutional indications Hyoscyamus is most effective in the senile and elderly, and in individuals who mutter to themselves or hold conversations with people who are absent or dead. The Hyoscyamus type tends to live in a world of his or her own.

Mental symptoms alleviated Incoherent, excited behaviour not due to infection or fever; obsessional behaviour; fearfulness, jealousy, suspicion; tendency to talk and act obscenely.

Physical symptoms alleviated Involuntary jerking of head, arms and hands; cough relieved by sitting up but worse lying down; twitching in every muscle, with awkward, angular movements; extremely sensitive skin; desire to undress and throw bedclothes off; frequent urge to pass water, though flow is infrequent and scanty; frequent urge to open bowels, with small, infrequent stools.

The above symptoms are generally improved by stooping, but are more troublesome at night, and not improved by eating or lying down.

Antidoting remedies Belladonna, Camphora.

Hypericum

From *Hypericum perforatum*, St John's wort. The homeopathic remedy is made from the whole fresh plant and is mainly used to treat nerve injuries, its principal action being on the central nervous system.

Constitutional indications None in particular.

Mental symptoms alleviated Drowsiness; depression.

Physical symptoms alleviated Concussion; neuralgia; heavy, icy cold sensation in head; head which feels elongated, as if lifted up high into the air; eye injuries; discomfort after going to dentist; toothache, with pulling or tearing pains; coated tongue with a clean tip; severe shooting pains which travel in an upward direction; back pain which travels up or down spine; puncture wounds caused by nails, splinters or bites; crushed fingers or toes; thirst; a craving for wine or hot drinks; nausea; in women, late periods, accompanied by headaches; diarrhoea, with loose yellowish stools; painful, bleeding piles; nervy pains in rectum.

The above symptoms are often relieved by tilting the head back, but tend to get worse in cold, damp or foggy conditions and in warm stuffy rooms; being touched or exposing any part of the body is usually detrimental.

Antidoting remedies Arsenicum, Chamomilla.

Ignatia

From *Ignatia amara*, also known as *Strychnos ignatia*, St Ignatius' bean. The homeopathic remedy is made from the seed pods, which contain the powerful poison strychnine. Strychnine acts on the central nervous system.

Constitutional indications Ignatia is most effective in children who are bright, precocious and highly strung, and in adults who are alert, nervous, rather pale, given to sighing and yawning, and wear a rather strained expression on their face, often with frequent blinking or a facial tic. Ignatia types are very fragile emotionally, inclined to be perverse and unpredictable. Women who respond well to Ignatia are often artistic.

Mental symptoms alleviated Rapid changes of mood; apprehension, fear of going out alone, fear of being seen to take initiative; suddenly bursting into tears; tendency to be self-pitying, self-blaming and hysterical; easily shocked, easily knocked off emotional perch by grief, love, worry; mild depression; little capacity for anger or violence; sensitivity to noise, especially when studying; inability to work; wanting to be socially responsible and well thought of.

Physical symptoms alleviated Headaches which feel as if a nail is being driven into side of head, made more intense by lying on painful side;

nervous headaches in children, relieved by heat but made worse by coffee; fainting in confined spaces; beads of sweat on forehead and upper lip which disappear when eating; sour taste in mouth; hiccups, or spasmodic, irritating cough; febrile convulsions; feeling very thirsty with a chill; red face which is chilly to the touch; inflammation, relieved by firm pressure; extreme sensitivity to pain; pain concentrated in small areas; choking; tickly cough; sore throat which improves on eating solids; feeling as if there is a hard lump in the throat; craving for unusual foods when ill; craving for sour or acidic foods; upper abdominal pain, nausea and vomiting, alleviated by eating; in women, painful spasms of uterus during periods; constipation due to emotional factors; piles; rectal spasms, or prolapse of rectum which causes sharp upward-shooting pains.

The above symptoms are often relieved by eating, urinating, firm pressure, walking as well as resting, lying on the painful side and by external heat. Fear, anxiety, fresh air, cold, being over-dressed, coffee, brandy, tobacco and strong odours are generally irritants; symptoms also tend to be worse in the morning and after meals.

Complementary remedy Natrum mur.

Antidoting remedies Pulsatilla, Cocculus, Chamomilla.

Incompatible/inimical remedies Coffea, Tabacum, Nux.

Ipecac.

From *Cephaelis* (or *Psychotria*) *ipecacuanha,* ipecacuanha. The homeopathic remedy is made from the dried root, whose active principle, emetine, is used in orthodox medicine as an emetic and expectorant. In herbal medicine, ipecacuanha is used to treat dermatitis.

Constitutional indications None in particular.

Mental symptoms alleviated Anxiety; fear of death; contempt for everything around one; moroseness.

Physical symptoms alleviated Fainting; nosebleeds; feeling chilly most of the time; suffocation or difficulty breathing; desire to cough and vomit simultaneously; constant nausea, not relieved by vomiting; asthma, gasping for air; pale, cold, sweaty skin; back pain; profuse bleeding or haemorrhaging, with loss of bright red blood; blood slow to clot; weak pulse; lack of thirst.

The above symptoms tend to come and go, but are usually worse in winter, aggravated by moving about as well as lying down, and can be brought on by embarrassment or stress.

Complementary remedies Cuprum, Arnica.

Antidoting remedies Arsenicum, China, Tabacum.

Kali carb.

The source of this remedy is potassium carbonate.

Constitutional indications Those who benefit most from Kali carb. tend to be sallow-skinned, physically weak, flabby and flat-footed; they are often depressed, dogmatic, inclined to see issues as black or white and have a strong sense of duty; bookkeeping, translating, the law and police work tend to attract the Kali carb. type.

Mental symptoms alleviated Feeling scared stiff, unhappy, irritable, worried about one's future; sense of failure; forgetfulness; nervousness; feeling overwhelmed when alone; sensation of bed sinking into floor as one falls asleep.

Physical symptoms alleviated Headaches behind temples; dizziness brought on by yawning or cold wind; excessive puffiness between eyebrows and upper eyelids; eyes stuck together in morning; stuffed-up nose, worse in warm rooms; watery, yellowish catarrh which causes choking or vomiting; cheesy taste in mouth; throat feels as if there is a lump in it, with a stinging pain on swallowing; backache, especially before periods; stitch-like pains, cutting pains, burning pains, with painful areas clammy or sweaty; asthma which worsens around 3 am, obliging one to sit up; chest pain unrelated to inhaling or exhaling, aggravated by pressure and lying on right side but relieved by leaning forwards; dry, hoarse cough and loss of voice; stomach often affected by shocks and emotional upsets; craving for sweet, starchy, or acid foods, and sour drinks; heavy weight in pit of stomach; nausea followed by sour, watery vomiting; choking on food; bloated abdomen, with griping pains; abdomen distended and full of wind, discomfort relieved by bending over or leaning back but increased by drinking ice cold water; in women, premenstrual weakness and depression, or period pains which feel like labour pains.

The above symptoms are often helped by warmth, moisture and movement, and tend to wear off during the day; they are aggravated by hot drinks, coffee, cold surroundings, changes in the weather, pressure, touch, rest and lying on the affected side, and come on most strongly after sexual intercourse and between 2 and 4 am.

Complementary remedy Carbo veg.

Antidoting remedy Coffea.

Lachesis

From *Lachesis trigonocephalus*, the bushmaster or surucucu snake of South America. The homeopathic remedy is made from the venom which, depending on the size of the victim, inhibits nerve impulses within the heart and causes death very swiftly, or interferes with blood clotting and speeds up the rate at which red blood cells are destroyed, which causes slow death from jaundice, infection or blood loss.

Constitutional indications Lachesis is especially effective in people who are tremulous, rather bloated in appearance and in need of relief from nervous over-stimulation; many such people also have red hair and freckles.

Mental symptoms alleviated Talkativeness, nervousness, restlessness, irritability; tendency to be suspicious and distrustful, sometimes obsessively so; occasional depression; jealousy over petty things; unsociability, especially first thing in morning.

Physical symptoms alleviated Headaches, often made worse by periods, bright light, hot sun; throbbing or bursting headaches aggravated by stooping and by movement generally; *petit mal* epilepsy; fainting; horror of putting things in ears; puffy, purplish face; habit of putting tongue out and flicking it over lips; ropy, foul-tasting saliva; trembling tongue which is dry, red, brown or black and fissured; left-sided sore throat, with pain in left ear when swallowing; throat which feels swollen and constricted, worse for hot drinks, hot applications and tight things around neck, but better for eating hot food; back of throat looks dark purple and inflamed; waking up choking, with swollen neck glands; pneumonia, accompanied by general weakness, a weak heart and fever; hot sweats and shivering, relieved by eating but aggravated by sleep; skin ulcers and wounds which have a bluish margin to them; boils which are red and angry-looking but painless; swollen, engorged veins which make skin look bluish; rapid, weak, irregular pulse; throbbing sensations in various parts of the body, often accompanied by headache; palpitations and fainting; angina and difficulty breathing; swollen glands generally; great thirst; increased appetite; stomach pains with vomiting, made worse by tight clothing; craving for oysters, coffee, and alcohol; appendicitis; anal spasm and bleeding piles; in women, spasmodic, congestive period pains, relieved by flow of blood, pre-menstrual syndrome, or menopausal hot flushes.

The above symptoms are not improved by touch, hot or warm baths, hot drinks, closing eyes, or going to sleep; they also tend to be worse in the spring and more noticeable on the left side. They do improve, however, when there is some sort of discharge.

Complementary remedies Crotalus, Lycopodium, Hepar sulph.

Antidoting remedies/substances Arsenicum, Mercurius; alcohol, salt.

Ledum

From *Ledum palustre*, marsh tea or wild rosemary. The homeopathic remedy is made from the whole fresh or dried plant and is traditionally used to heal puncture wounds and soothe pains which ascend from the lower part of the body.

Constitutional indications None in particular.

Mental symptoms alleviated Anxiety; timidity; moroseness, wanting to be left alone; hatred for fellow human beings; impatience, working oneself into a state of extreme anger.

Physical symptoms alleviated Black eyes; stiff joints which loosen up when bathed in cold water; cold, puffy, purplish skin, especially in cold weather.

The above symptoms are not helped by touch or warmth, and tend to get worse at night. Cold applications are usually beneficial.

Lycopodium

From *Lycopodium clavatum*, wolf's claw club moss. The homeopathic remedy is made from the powdery spores, which have the property of floating on water and flaring up when sprinkled on a naked flame.

Constitutional indications The Lycopodium type usually has a handshake which is so firm that it hurts, and a haughty, unfriendly air; other characteristics are leanness, a stooping posture and an unhealthily sallow skin, often with many lines and wrinkles. Such people tend to gravitate towards politics, teaching, the law and the priesthood.

Mental symptoms alleviated Anxiety, nervousness, insecurity, impatience; cowardice – physical, moral or social; dread of being left on one's own; tendency to be secretive; inability to sleep at night because brain goes over and over day's events; mental fatigue, despite braininess; slow to get into gear in mornings; tightness with money; great sensitivity to noise or smells; hypochondria; memory difficulties; aversion to new challenges; ambition; in children, preferring to bury nose in a book rather than play with other children; talking and laughing in sleep, night terrors, tendency to wake around 4 am, sense of apprehension on waking in morning.

Physical symptoms alleviated Neuralgia-type headaches, alleviated by open air but aggravated by pressure or indigestion; haemorrhaging of blood vessels in eye; early degeneration of retina; chronic catarrh; nostrils which flare on inhaling; mouth which feels dry and swollen; right-sided sore throat, made worse by cold drinks; tracheitis; right-sided pneumonia; obstinate, dry, tickly cough; scalding pain between shoulder blades; slow recovery after flu, or post-viral syndrome; hands and feet hot and dry, or right foot much hotter than left; psoriasis on palms of hands; aneurysms; throbbing sensation in arteries; thyrotoxicosis; craving for sweet foods; aversion to onions; in children, aversion to breakfast due to hatred of school; ravenous hunger, followed by discomfort after a few mouthfuls; getting indigestion if one has to wait for food; often feeling and being sick; in men, increased libido accompanied by inability to achieve or sustain erection, or enlarged prostate; reddish urine with sandy sediment in it; distended abdomen, full of wind; lazy bowels, constipation or spasm of anal sphincter making it impossible to pass stools despite straining; constipation in infants; bleeding piles.

The above symptoms are often relieved by sympathy, movement, undressing, cold surroundings, or a hot meal or a hot drink in the evening; symptoms also tend to wear off after midnight. Stuffy rooms, tight clothing and overeating usually aggravate matters; symptoms are often worse on the right side and cause most discomfort between 4 and 8 pm.

Complementary remedies Calcarea, Sulphur.

Antidoting remedies Camphora, Pulsatilla, Causticum.

Magnesia phos.
The homeopathic remedy is made from magnesium phosphate, one of the Tissue Salts (see p. 24). It has an anti-spasmodic effect.

Constitutional indications Magnesia phos. is most beneficial to people who are thin, dark, nervous, tired, and exhausted.

Mental symptoms alleviated Inability to think clearly; moaning and complaining.

Physical symptoms alleviated Headaches made worse by mental exertion; dizziness brought on by movement; tendency to fall forward when eyes are closed; involuntary, jerky movements of face, hands and arms; in teenage girls, a red, flushed face; neuralgia in right eye or right ear, made worse by washing in cold water; toothache which improves with heat; ulcers on gums, accompanied by swollen neck glands; teething trouble; hiccups; retching; weak or twitching muscles; cramping, nervy pains which improve with warmth and pressure but worsen with cold and strenuous exercise; writer's cramp; belching which does not relieve stomach discomfort; craving for cold drinks; abdominal pain and wind, relieved by warmth and pressure; bloated, distended abdomen, relieved by loosening clothing, walking about or passing wind; period pains, relieved by heat, or early periods, with dark, stringy discharge; constipation.

The above symptoms are almost always relieved by warmth, pressure and bending double; they tend to be worse on the right side and at night, and can be exacerbated by touch, undressing and cold.

Antidoting remedies Belladonna, Gelsemium, Lachesis.

Mercurius
The source of this remedy is black oxide of mercury. Mercury, liberally used in many medicinal preparations at one time, cannot be efficiently eliminated by the body and results in chronic or acute poisoning.

Constitutional indications The Mercurius type is usually light-haired, with slow speech and slow, rather drugged reactions.

Mental symptoms alleviated Feeling dull, slow, muddle-headed; not knowing what to say; nervousness, timidity, suspicion, mistrust, anxiety, restlessness, irritability; sense of haste and hurry; talking very rapidly; poor comprehension and poor memory; lack of willpower; finding that time passes very slowly; weariness and disenchantment with life.

Physical symptoms alleviated Neuralgia; loss of sensation in any part of body; congestive, vice-like headaches; burning pain over left temple; tight band of pain over nose and above eyes; encrusted lesions on scalp, with smelly discharge; profuse discharge of pus from ears, with earache which is made worse by warmth of bed; chronic conjunctivitis, with margins of eyelids red, swollen and stuck together; eyes which sting and water profusely, with a severe ache behind eyeballs, made worse by glare of fire; acrid, watery catarrh; sneezing which makes nose feel raw and scalded, especially in sunshine; open sores on nostrils, aggravated by damp; slimy saliva which stains pillow during sleep; swollen gums; numb or sore gums; trembling tongue, or swollen tongue with teeth marks on it; foul breath; metallic taste in mouth; loose teeth in infected, reddened gums; swollen, raw, dark red throat, or ulcers which constrict throat and make swallowing painful; throat pain accompanied by hot sweats; smarting jaw, worse on right side; cough which produces yellow phlegm, often worse at night and in warm rooms; paroxysms of coughing made worse by warm or damp conditions, smoking and lying on right side; weak, trembling muscles; aching joints; breaking out in hot, drenching sweats, which chill skin as they evaporate; profuse, oily sweats which seem to make other symptoms worse, especially at night; blisters or pus-filled eruptions on skin; open sores; ulcers which itch and sting, especially in bed; low blood pressure; swollen glands; craving for cold drinks or stimulants; stomach upsets, especially after eating sweets and solids; in men, increased production of smegma, with head of penis sensitive and sore; in women, profuse vaginal discharge; alternate bouts of constipation and diarrhoea; chronic dysentery, with raw, sore anus; greenish stools with blood in them; painful urging to pass stools; cutting pains in abdomen; excessive production of urine with protein in it.

The above symptoms tend to improve with rest and wrapping up well. Changes in temperature, heat and cold, being warm in bed, dampness and perspiration are generally aggravating; symptoms also tend to be right-sided and worse at night.

Complementary remedies Badiaga, Sulphur.

Antidoting remedies Hepar sulph., Aurum, Mezereum.

Incompatible/inimical remedy Silicea.

Natrum mur.

The source of this remedy is common salt, sodium chloride.

Constitutional indications Natrum mur. is of most benefit to people of squarish build who tend to walk on their heels; they may be sandy- or dark-haired, but often have greasy skin and a cracked lower lip; although they appear deliberate and self-assured, they can be inward-looking and vulnerable. Skinny children with hard, nodular lymph glands also respond well to Natrum mur.

Mental symptoms alleviated Impatience, clumsiness, touchiness; getting worked up over trivial things; screaming with rage; crying with laughter; often feeling depressed or down in the dumps, especially in morning; anxiety; difficulty expressing true feelings; feeling wounded or humiliated; relieving feelings by locking oneself away and crying; fear of the dark and of thunder; remaining dry-eyed when bereaved; poor sense of humour; sentimentality; brooding over injustice; politeness which hides hardness and ruthlessness; being easy to get on with socially but very difficult to live with – pretending not to want attention, then resentful at not getting it or nasty if one does; expecting others to take an interest in one's problems, and being resentful if they don't.

Physical symptoms alleviated Blinding migraines with zig-zag lines in front of eyes, often brought on by eyestrain, sunlight, travel, crowded public places, emotional trauma, or exercise; migraine headaches which cause sweating; headaches in teenage girls; bursting headaches, or headaches which feel as if inside of head is being attacked by a battery of hammers, often worse between 10 and 11 am; headaches which start at back of head, then radiate all over; left-sided headaches, especially when head is down, alleviated by fresh air; waking up feeling more dead than alive; sensitive scalp; protruding eyes; hot sweaty hands; numb hands; warts on palms of hands; greasy skin; goitre; palpitations and faintness, made worse by lying down; raised blood pressure; anaemia; disorders of the spleen; backache which improves with firm pressure; transparent catarrh; boils in nose; painful spots under nose; nose swollen on one side; cold sores and a higher than normal temperature; cracked lower lip; lips and tongue which feel numb; geographical tongue; hairy tongue; mouth ulcers; increased appetite, or very small appetite; craving for salty foods, fresh milk and beer; aversion to fat, meat, coffee and sour wine; aversion to salt; indigestion, made worse by tobacco; indigestion which is cured by fasting or eating very little; duodenal ulcers which suddenly start to bleed; in women, dry or sore vagina, vaginismus, watery vaginal discharge, amenorrhea caused by stress, shock or grief, irregular periods, feeling unwell just before and just after periods, swollen ankles before periods; bedwetting; constipation, with dry hard stools; an anal fissure which bleeds.

The above symptoms are generally relieved by fresh air, fasting, cold baths, and a firm bed; they tend to worsen around 10 am and in extremely cold or thundery weather, and are not improved by mental or physical exertion, talking, writing, jarring, noise, music, warmth, bright light, hot sun, draughts, seaside air or sympathy.

Complementary remedies Apis, Sepia, Thuja.

Antidoting remedies Arsenicum, Phosphorus.

Natrum sulph.

The source of this remedy is Glauber's salts or sodium sulphate, a constituent of many spa waters and also used as a Tissue Salt (see p. 24).

Constitutional indications Natrum sulph. is especially indicated for people who are pale, tired, ill-looking, and who are sensitive and have been hurt many times.

Mental symptoms alleviated Gloominess and taciturnity; bad temper; emotional turmoil and confusion, often made worse by talking or being spoken to; feeling torn between desire to live and desire to die; suicidal feelings; timidity; anxiety; dreams of running water.

Physical symptoms alleviated Bursting, vice-like headaches at back of head and behind forehead; headaches centred on crown of head; headaches brought on by head injuries; dry mouth, with cracked and blistered lips, ulcers on tongue and palate as if from eating strong spices; copious thin saliva; reluctance to eat; asthma made worse by cold and damp; greenish phlegm; difficulty breathing, especially between 4 and 5 am or on fourth or fifth day of a cold – breathing is not eased by pressure on chest or by warm or wet applications; cough which produces loose phlegm and disturbs sleep, relieved by lying on left side but aggravated by pressure; suddenly sitting up in bed in order to cough up phlegm; pain in left side of chest; empty feeling in chest, with loose phlegm; rheumatic aches and pains on left side; compressed feeling in elbows, especially in damp or stormy weather; tenderness or sharp, stitch-like pains in liver area, aggravated by tight clothing and hot sun; abdomen which rumbles with painful wind, and inability to pass wind; abdominal cramps; bowel movements which oblige one to get out of bed around 5 am; urine scanty and stinging.

The above symptoms are generally relieved by keeping dry and changing position frequently. Damp, cold or wet conditions, sea air, listening to music and lying on left side usually exacerbate symptoms, which tend to be worse in the morning.

Complementary remedies Arsenicum, Thuja.

Nux

From *Nux vomica*, the poison nut tree. The homeopathic remedy is made from the dried, ripe seeds, which contain strychnine, a powerful poison which acts on the central nervous system; in small doses strychnine makes perceptions more vivid and increases production of saliva; in larger doses it causes tetany or muscular spasm, and death from respiratory failure.

Constitutional indications Several physical types respond well to Nux, although self-reliance, efficiency and a liking for hard work tend to be common characteristics, which explains why many Nux types are managers, supervisors, or entrepreneurs. Some Nux types are well-groomed, hearty, and full of life, others slouch as if they have been up all night; many are thin, prematurely bald, suffer from indigestion and irascibility, and aspire to the finer things of life; complexion may be dry, lined and sallow, with rings under the eyes.

Mental symptoms alleviated Fanatical precision and tidiness; irritability; using anger and violence to dominate others; setting high standards which drive others to distraction; craving respect and admiration; pompous, extravagant talk, never expressing worries or doubts; anxiety, hopelessness, weariness; anger and frustration when things go badly; concern for health of others, but not for own; impulsiveness.

Physical symptoms alleviated Hangovers from too much alcohol; waking up with a thick head, or a head which feels very fragile, or a headache which feels like a nail being driven in above the eyes; 24-hour flu, with shivering and stiff, aching muscles; insomnia, made worse by overwork or abuse of alcohol or narcotics; tickly nose which causes sneezing; sneezing which stops out of doors; blocked nose at night, runny nose during the day; nose which feels hot and sore; uncomfortably dry mouth and thickly coated tongue; difficulty swallowing (food goes down then gets stuck); racking cough, with retching; tickly cough, with pain in larynx; backache relieved by sitting up or turning over in bed; when ill, craving fatty foods and finding bread, meat, coffee and tobacco repugnant; occasional cravings for sour foods; a liking for spirits; being very fussy about freshness of food; liking pungent, spicy foods; indigestion and vomiting; in women, early periods which are prolonged and heavy, irregular periods, tendency to faint just before periods, or periods accompanied by urge to pass water and stools; constipation; diarrhoea after eating juicy fruit, vegetables or rice; abdominal cramps, soothed by heat but aggravated by pressure; colicky pains which cause nausea but wear off when bowels are opened; piles which make rectal contractions painful and ineffectual.

The above symptoms are generally relieved by warmth, sleep, firm pressure and washing or wet applications; they also tend to abate in the evening and when the person is left alone. Cold, wind, dryness, noise, spices, stimulants, narcotics, eating, getting angry and being touched tend to make symptoms worse; symptoms are also worse in winter and between 3 and 4 am.

Antidoting remedies Coffea, Ignatia, Cocculus.

Incompatible/inimical remedy Zinc.

Opium

From *Papaver somniferum*, the opium poppy. The homeopathic remedy is made from the dried milky juice which exudes from the green seed capsules. Heroin, morphine and many other drugs are derivatives of opium, which has a vitality-lowering effect.

Constitutional indications None in particular.

Mental symptoms alleviated Apathy, lack of enthusiasm; not complaining when complaint is justified; over-excitement; fright and after-effects of fright.

Physical symptoms alleviated Strokes; delirium tremens; sneezing; irregular breathing; sweaty or clammy skin.

The above symptoms tend to be aggravated by warmth and get markedly worse during and after sleep; they improve in cold surroundings, especially if one keeps moving.

Antidoting remedies/substances Ipecac., Nux, Passiflora; black coffee.

Phosphoric ac.

This remedy is made from phosphoric acid, whose chief action is on the nervous system. Too much phosphoric acid can cause gastroenteritis.

Constitutional indications Phosphoric ac. has most affinity with children or young people who are growing fast and becoming thin and gangly. It is also indicated in people whose constitution, originally strong, has been undermined by a particularly virulent illness, by excessive loss of body fluids, or by grief or depression. Most Phosphoric ac. types have a mild, yielding temperament.

Mental symptoms alleviated Apathy; indifference to people and surroundings; difficulty understanding what is going on.

Physical symptoms alleviated Headaches which are made worse by noise, especially music; during acute illnesss, drowsiness or semi-consciousness; weak chest; coughing; profuse, painless diarrhoea which makes one feel better rather than worse.

The above symptoms are not improved by noise, music, strong odours, bad news, cold draughts, wind, snowy air, or by sitting, standing or being touched. They do respond, however, to walking, fresh air, and sleep, even a short nap.

Antidoting remedy Coffea.

Phosphorus

This remedy is made from amorphous phosphorus.

Constitutional indications Phosphorus is most appropriate in thin children who are tall for their age, delicate and desperate for reassurance; if they appear to stare, it is often because they are scared. Adults who respond best to Phosphorus are usually well-proportioned and have a fine skin which blushes easily, but may be dark or fair, with a coppery tinge to the hair; they are intelligent, gregarious and sometimes artistic, but their passions tend to be shortlived and regretted afterwards; they are drawn towards selling, politics and humanitarian endeavours.

Mental symptoms alleviated Nervous tension, especially from overwork; loathing exams and homework; bottling things up, reluctance to talk about problems; indifference to family and friends when ill; wanting to be in the limelight; fear of dark, thunder, being alone, dying; tendency to see catastrophe around every corner; great sensitivity to atmosphere.

Physical symptoms alleviated Headaches which are made worse by heat but wear off after eating or bathing forehead in cold water; dry skin; extremities often feel very hot; poor circulation in fingers, although plunging hands into hot water causes nausea; red, smarting eyes, made worse by bright light and cold air; print appears red and lights have green haloes around them; hearing echoes of own voice; difficulty picking out human voice from other sounds; beads of perspiration on forehead or upper lip, especially in moments of mental or physical stress; heart noticeably affected by emotion, causing palpitations, faintness or a feeling of suffocation; small, weak pulse; profound anaemia; fever, with alternate bouts of sweating and shivering; nosebleeds, brought on by blowing nose; chronic catarrh; dry mouth and stiff tongue with brownish centre; bleeding gums; sensitive larynx, hoarseness, losing voice; dry, tickly cough made worse by talking, laughing and cold air, possibly causing retching and vomiting; rust-coloured phlegm; pneumonia, made worse by lying on bad side or on back; tight feeling in chest or under breastbone, especially after a chill; acute asthma or bronchitis; laboured breathing; respiratory symptoms which improve in a warm atmosphere but worsen lying down or after eating; hiccups; burning pains in region of spine; numbness or loss of co-ordination; cramps; cold knees, especially at night; craving for salty food, meat, ice cream and cold drinks; aversion to sweet things; heartburn, soothed by eating; sensation of pressure in stomach; nausea; peptic ulcer, signalled by mouth filling with saliva; bleeding from lining of stomach, especially in pregnancy; sexual problems which are vividly felt but not resolved; in women, excessive desire for sex.

The above symptoms are generally improved by sleep, friction, fresh air, lying on right side, drinking and being touched. Physical or mental exertion, hot meals and hot drinks, and lying on painful side make matters worse; symptoms are also more marked between sunset and midnight, and in thundery or changeable weather.

Complementary remedies Arsenicum, Allium, Lycopodium, Silicea.

Antidoting remedies Nux.

Incompatible/inimical remedy Causticum.

Phytolacca

From *Phytolacca decandra*, poke root. The homeopathic remedy is made from the fresh leaves or the ripe berries, or in winter from the fresh root. The active principle on which the remedy depends affects the nervous system, the throat, the digestive system and fibrous tissues throughout the body, including the tissue which sheaths bones.

Constitutional indications None in particular.

Mental symptoms alleviated Indifference to people and things; expecting to die.

Physical symptoms alleviated Shooting pains which feel like electric shocks; dizziness on standing up from sitting position; pain in eyeballs which seems to improve in open air; desire to clench teeth and gums together; swollen, painful throat which makes swallowing difficult, aggravated by hot drinks, with pain in root of tongue and up eustachian tube into ear – on inspection back of throat looks dry, dark red and congested; stiff neck which hurts if moved and gets worse at night (if Bryonia or Rhus tox. fail); hip pain, relieved by rubbing; nausea relieved by vomiting; in women, breasts which feel stony-

hard and painful, but less painful with pressure, or lumpy breasts with discharge from nipples and pain extending backwards from nipple.

The above symptoms tend to be exacerbated by cold, cold damp rooms, bed warmth, movement and menstruation; they are often worse at night and on the right side of the body.

Antidoting remedies Belladonna, Mezereum.

Incompatible/inimical remedy Mercurius.

Pulsatilla

From *Pulsatilla nigricans*, the pasque flower. The homeopathic remedy is made from the whole plant when it is in flower.

Constitutional indications Children who are small, fair, fine-boned, bright and cheerful, but also shy and sensitive and blush easily respond well to Pulsatilla. So do slightly plumper, darker, more languid children who crave affection but find it difficult to give. Adults who are shy, gentle, fair-skinned or fair-haired, and rather plump also benefit from Pulsatilla. The Pulsatilla type is easily led, easily moulded and rather changeable.

Mental symptoms alleviated Depression; tendency to yield and give way to others; preference for a sheltered life; sympathy with people or animals in distress, sometimes to the point of tears; self-consciousness; longing for attention and affection; obliging others by laughing at their jokes and antics; always wanting someone else in room; fear of death and insanity; little obstinacy or determination; rare anger.

Physical symptoms alleviated Headaches centred above eyes, alleviated by firm pressure, aggravated by indigestion, and worse in evening; fainting, especially in hot stuffy rooms; corneal ulcers, styes or conjunctivitis; fever, with lack of thirst; blocked up nose at night, runny nose during day; yellowish, bland catarrh, better in open air and worse in warm; loss of smell; acute sinusitis; nosebleeds; white, coated tongue and bad taste in mouth; dry mouth and lack of thirst; toothache; pricking sensation in gums, relieved by cold air but aggravated by warmth; dry throat; a loose cough, with greenish phlegm in morning; low backache, not improved by movement; flitting joint pains which wear off with exercise and cold applications but get worse with heat; sleeping with hands above head; disturbed sleep due to rich food or overheated bedroom (moderate exercise before bed gives a sound night's sleep); mild anaemia; palpitations; varicose veins; stomach which is tight and tense in morning, and easily upset by rich or fatty food, especially pork; sensation of pressure under breastbone after meals; craving for sweet things; rumbling, gurgling stomach; in women, thick, creamy, smarting discharge from vagina, late periods, or cessation of periods, especially after shock, acute infection or illness; in both sexes, increased desire for sex; bedwetting; bowels loose, with no two stools alike.

The above symptoms are often relieved by crying, raising the hands above the head, gentle exercise, fresh air and cold drinks or cold applications; sympathy also has a positive effect. Sun, heat, changes in temperature, rich or fatty foods and lying on painful side usually intensify symptoms, which are worse in the evening and at night.

Complementary remedies Coffea, Nux, Chamomilla.

Rhus tox.
From *Rhus toxicodendron*, poison ivy, a North American species. The homeopathic remedy is made from the fresh leaves, which are very poisonous if touched, although some people are immune to them. Traditionally Rhus tox. is used to relieve stiffness, whether physical, mental or emotional.

Constitutional indications None in particular, beyond a lack of flexibility in mind and body.

Mental symptoms alleviated Bursting into tears for no particular reason; restlessness, nervousness and irritability; depression or thoughts of suicide; deriving little enjoyment from senses; great mistrust of, and fear of being poisoned by, drugs and other remedies; dreaming of strenuous physical exercise.

Physical symptoms alleviated Dizzy feeling, as if brain were loose inside head, made worse by walking or standing up; head feels heavy, as if hung over; high temperature, accompanied by delirium and confusion, brought down by sweating; fever brought on by a chill; eczema, in which skin is red, swollen and blistered, and burns and itches; patches of red skin, with clear demarcation line between red areas and unaffected areas; eyes swollen, brimming with painful tears; eyelids stuck together; sensitive scalp; violent throbbing sensation in nose, which is blocked in evening; dry, fissured tongue, brownish with red tip; jaws which make a cracking sound when chewing; teeth which feel loose or too long; bitter taste in mouth; swollen throat; irritating cough, which wears off when talking or singing; stiff, painful muscles which seize up with rest but loosen up with exercise and heat; stiffness in lower back; numbness in arms and legs; stitching

pains made worse by cold and damp; craving for cold drinks; nausea and vomiting; drowsiness after eating; in women, early periods, which are heavy and prolonged, or burning pains in vagina, made worse by heat; bedwetting; passing large quantities of urine; frothy, smelly diarrhoea, without abdominal pain; abdominal pain relieved by lying prone.

The above symptoms are generally improved by keeping on the move or changing position frequently, and staying warm and dry. They tend to be aggravated by rest, starting to move after rest, taking clothes off, cold winds and thundery weather; they also intensify at night.

Complementary remedies Bryonia, Calcarea carb., Phytolacca.

Antidoting remedies Anacardium, Croton.

Incompatible/inimical remedies Mezereum, Graphites, Apis.

Ruta
From *Ruta graveolens*, rue, also known as herb-of-grace and herb-of-repentance. The homeopathic remedy is made from the whole fresh plant before it comes into flower. Herbals refer to rue as 'an antidote to all dangerous poisons' and as a defence against witches! In homeopathy Ruta has virtue against restlessness and bruising.

Constitutional indications None in particular.

Mental symptoms alleviated Anxiety; quarrelsomeness, always contradicting people; depression, dissatisfaction with self and others.

Physical symptoms alleviated Headaches due to eyestrain, often brought on by reading fine print and made worse by alcohol; eyes which look red and feel hot; infection of tooth sockets after extraction; weak chest and difficulty breathing, with localized pain over breastbone; tendon injuries and bruised bones; sciatica, often worse at night when lying down; deep aching in the bones; painful bruises; prolapse of rectum, made worse by stooping and crouching; constipation, with large stools which are difficult to pass, alternating with loose stools full of blood and frothy mucus; tearing or stitching pains in rectum.

The symptoms above are generally improved by movement but made worse by cold, damp, rest, and lying down.

Complementary remedy Calcarea phos.

Antidoting remedy Camphora.

Sepia

The source of this remedy is cuttlefish ink. Sepia is used in conditions characterized by stasis, a state of stoppage in which nervous and hormonal impulses seem to be cancelling each other out.

Constitutional indications Those who respond best to Sepia tend to be tall, lean and narrow-hipped, with soft facial features, dark hair, brown eyes, shadows under the eyes, and a sallow complexion (sometimes with a yellow-brown saddle across the nose and cheeks). Although they look tired and low-spirited, they perk up with exercise. Women going through the menopause also respond well to Sepia.

Mental symptoms alleviated Indifference, even to loved ones; irritability and snappiness with family and friends, making one difficult to live with, but cordiality with strangers; inability to conceal thoughts, coupled with wish to hide away physically; selfishness, bottled up anger, despair, fear that something dreadful is about to happen; crying when talking about symptoms or illness; physical and mental torpor, despite ability to be the life and soul of the party; being overwhelmed by life and resentful of one's lot; tendency to be greedy and opinionated; tendency to play the martyr.

Physical symptoms alleviated Headaches accompanied by nausea, especially in evening (often relieved by vomiting or wrapping head, but made worse by stuffy rooms, jarring, noise, tobacco, crowded places and menstruation); dizziness which feels like a ball rolling around in the head; baldness; extreme sensitivity to odours; constant catarrh, which tastes salty; throat which is sensitive to the slightest pressure; pale lips, coated tongue and sour taste in mouth; milk and fatty foods cause indigestion, especially in evening; smell of cooking causes nausea; craving for spicy, pungent foods and for wine and vinegar; aching back and sides, relieved by exercise and pressure but made worse by standing; unbearably itchy skin, with patches of brown-yellow discoloration; vitiligo; smelly foot sweats; low blood pressure; palpitations; flushing hot and cold by turns; congested veins; bedwetting in first stage of sleep; in men, sexual problems or exhaustion after sex; flatulence and tenderness in abdomen, relieved by lying on right side; in women, upsets in menstrual cycle, hot flushes during menopause, sagging or prolapsed womb, pain during intercourse, aversion to sex and to being touched.

The above symptoms tend to wear off after food, sleep, exercise or hot applications, and in thundery weather. They are generally made worse by cold, tobacco, mental fatigue and exertion in hot, damp conditions, and are most marked in the early morning, in the evening, in the build-up to a storm and on the left side.

Remedy which follows well Guaiacum.

Complementary remedies Natrum mur., Phosphorus, Nux.

Inimical remedies Lachesis, Pulsatilla.

Silicea

The source of this remedy is flint, which is primarily silica or silicon dioxide, one of the Tissue Salts (see p. 24). Silica is essential for growth and bone development, is present in connective tissue, and helps to keep cartilage flexible and skin permeable.

Constitutional indications Silicea is of most benefit to children who are puny and lacking in stamina, especially if they have a rather large, sweaty head, delicate skin, sandy hair, blue eyes and small hands and feet. Such children tend to be very lively and friendly, angels if managed properly but devils if they are not. Intellectual adults also benefit from it.

Mental symptoms alleviated Feeling pushed around and taking frustration out on subordinates; self doubts, lack of confidence and assertiveness, fear of failure; overworking or being over-conscientious to point of exhaustion; obstinacy and tenacity balanced by sense of fun, ready wit, gentleness and flashes of courage; occasional spitefulness, especially over small things; disturbed sleep when under stress.

Physical symptoms alleviated Right-sided migraines, worse around midday but relieved by pressure; headaches which are relieved by urination but made worse by mental or physical exertion (pain starts at back of head and extends over one eye); tinnitus; glue ear; sore lower eyelids; chronic catarrh, with cracked skin at side of nose; stuttering; aversion to meat, and to hot foods because they cause sweating; thirst; profuse perspiration, with very smelly feet; unhealthy-looking skin, with spots or pimples; fingers which go dead and icy cold in winter; poor nails with hard skin around them, which tends to split; lack of push when passing stools, so stools slip back inside rectum.

The symptoms above are generally aggravated by lying on the left side, getting pins and needles, undressing, washing and bathing and sudden cessation or suppression of sweat. They also tend to be worse in the morning, in damp or draughty conditions, in cold windy weather, and when the moon is new. Matters often improve in the summer, and in wet or damp conditions; the head needs to be wrapped up well.

Complementary remedies Thuja, Sanicula, Pulsatilla, Fluoric ac.

Incompatible/inimical remedy Mercurius.

Spongia

This remedy is prepared from the common sponge, toasted. The active constituents of sponge are iodine and bromine, which in excessive amounts irritate and inflame the larynx, trachea, thyroid gland, heart and testicles.

Constitutional indications Spongia is most effective in people who are light-haired, blue-eyed, lean and rather dried-up looking. It is especially good if tuberculosis or chest complaints run in the family.

Mental symptoms alleviated Anxiety, apprehension, fear of dying.

Physical symptoms alleviated General feeling of heaviness and exhaustion, with rushes of blood to chest, neck and face; colds which begin with a tickly throat, which is very sensitive to touch; congested feeling in larynx; hoarseness, with sore, burning sensation in larynx; enlarged thyroid gland; dry mucous membranes; dry, sibilant cough which sounds like a saw grating through a plank of wood, made worse by sweating and cold drinks; croup, with marked wheezing during intakes of breath, although chest is clear on examination; waking from sleep feeling as if one is suffocating; palpitations, especially around midnight and during menstruation.

The above symptoms cause most discomfort when talking, swallowing, moving about, lying with the head lower than the feet and touching affected areas; they also tend to be worst around midnight. Warm food, warm drinks and sitting up usually produce some improvement.

Complementary remedies Aconite, Hepar sulph.

Antidoting remedy Camphora.

Staphisagria

From *Delphinium staphisagria*, stavesacre or palmated larkspur. The homeopathic remedy is made from the seeds, which contain a substance used to kill head lice.

Constitutional indications Those who benefit most from Staphisagria tend to suppress their emotions, especially when they are in love.

Though mild and gentle on the surface, there is often great emotional turmoil underneath.

Mental symptoms alleviated Bottled up anger, which tends to make other symptoms worse; impatience, spitefulness; a tendency to dwell on old insults; easily wounded by words; melancholy.

Physical symptoms alleviated Stupefying headache (the 'head-full-of-lead' feeling), made worse by yawning or by excessive sexual activity; styes or lumps on eyelids; bursting pain in eyeballs; itching above and behind ears; toothaches which are aggravated by biting, chewing or touching affected tooth, especially during menstruation; cuts and surgical incisions; eczema; ravenous appetite, even when stomach is full; nausea after abdominal operations; craving for tobacco; urogenital problems, especially after first intercourse – cystitis, painful stretching of vagina.

The symptoms above generally improve with warmth, or after breakfast or a good night's sleep. Anger, indignation, self-denial, grief, sexual excess and being touched, especially on affected parts, tend to make symptoms worse; smoking and dehydration are also aggravating.

Complementary remedies Causticum, Colocynth.

Antidoting remedies Camphora.

Incompatible/inimical remedy Ranunculus.

Sulphur

This remedy is made from flowers of sulphur. Medicinally, sulphur is a purgative and increases the production of urea (from the breakdown of protein) in the liver. It is also a constituent of albumin and epithelial tissue. At one time sulphur was extensively used to treat rheumatism.

Constitutional indications Sulphur is most beneficial to people who have small, red-rimmed eyes and long lashes, a rather dirty-looking complexion, a lean body and stooping shoulders. It may also be appropriate for small, scrawny individuals, or for those who are ruddy-faced and full-bodied. The Sulphur type also tends to be egotistical, a would-be intellectual, a dabbler in philosophy.

Mental symptoms alleviated Shiftless, lazy, couldn't-care-less attitude; lack of energy and willpower; tendency to live by wits rather than hard work; liking to get one's own way; tendency towards melancholy, self-pity, hypochondria; finding crude talk or behaviour distasteful; always professing readiness to help others; daydreaming; dabbling in too many projects at a time and tending to lose heart; suddenly becoming awkward, indecisive and having difficulty understanding what is going on; tendency to wake around 3 am.

Physical symptoms alleviated Headaches which are made worse by fresh air but wear off in warm rooms; hair which is glossy but falls out; dry, scaly skin and scalp; skin which looks dirty even though clean; occasional sweating; palms of hands and soles of feet burning hot (bedclothes may be thrown off at night to cool feet); patches of itchy red skin made worse by warmth, washing or scratching; conjunctivitis or red eyes; chronic greenish catarrh; sensitivity to bad smells; coughing which often ends with sneezing; sore, burning lips; suddenly becoming hot and flushed in the face; giddiness and flushing, especially on getting out of bed in morning; suffocating feeling, especially at night; oppressive, burning sensation in chest, with shooting pains in back, made worse by deep breathing or lying on back; tendency to regurgitate food; irregular meals and ravenous appetite for all the wrong things (fat, salt, sugar, spicy foods, spirits), especially around 11 am and 11 pm; acid stomach and vomiting; sinking feeling in stomach, worse around 11 am; frequent thirst; hypoglycaemia; low back pain, spreading to groin; stiff joints which make a cracking noise; muscle cramps, made worse by bathing; chronic diarrhoea, worse around 5 am, and inflammation around anus; anal fissures.

The above symptoms are generally improved by fresh air, staying warm and dry, or lying on the right side. Immobility, prolonged standing, too many clothes, damp cold, washing, being too warm in bed and drinking alcohol often aggravate matters; symptoms also tend to be worse in the morning and at night, exhibiting a 12-hour cycle.

Complementary remedies Aconite, Aloe, Nux, Psorinum.

Antidoting remedies Camphora, Chamomilla, China, Mercurius, Rhus tox., Sepia, Thuja.

Tarentula

The source of this remedy is *Lycosa tarentula*, a large black spider found in Southern Europe. Its bite was reputed to cause tarantism or dancing mania. The homeopathic remedy is made from the whole live spider and is traditionally used to relieve conditions in which frantic, tormented behaviour is the chief characteristic.

Constitutional indications None in particular.

Mental symptoms alleviated Sudden mood changes; laughter and gaiety which suddenly turn to spitefulness and destructiveness; incredibly quick, foxy reactions; extreme restlessness, wanting everything immediately, never waiting in queues; constant need to busy oneself.

Physical symptoms alleviated Inability to keep still; restless legs, made worse by walking; dizziness; numbness; in women, pruritis vulvae.

The above symptoms are made worse by noise, walking, being touched and seeing other people in trouble. Bright colours, music and open air usually make things better.

Antidoting remedy Lachesis.

Thuja

From *Thuja occidentalis, arbor vitae* or tree of life. The homeopathic remedy is made from the fresh green twigs, which contain a substance which affects the concentration of salt, water and electrolytes in the body. Thuja is most appropriate where areas of pain are small and localized.

Constitutional indications Thuja is most beneficial in people who have a greasy skin and take little interest in their appearance, especially if they are also unattractive, deceitful and manipulative. Small, fine-boned children who are slightly backward or have difficulty expressing themselves also respond well to Thuja.

Mental symptoms alleviated Paranoia (feeling that one is under someone else's influence or always in their presence); reluctance to talk; being very sensitive, easily wounded, often moved to tears by music; conscientiousness; physical activity makes thoughts and emotions less intense; restless sleep, especially on moonlit nights, talking in sleep, dreaming of dead people or of falling.

Physical symptoms alleviated Headaches brought on by overtiredness, over-excitement or stress; chronic greenish-yellow catarrh; clean red tongue; tooth decay; inflamed and swollen gums; asthma; inflamed and swollen joints; brittle bones; warts which weep or bleed; greasy or pale, waxy skin, with exposed areas inclined to sweat; perspiration which smells offensive and stains clothes yellow; left side of body feels cold; fair hair which extends down spine; lack of appetite early in the day; indigestion caused by drinking tea; urinary infections; in women, vaginal and uterine infections, scanty or early periods, severe period pains centred over left ovary, or miscarriages; soft, pale, greasy stools, and grumbling, gurgling bowels.

The symptoms above are generally aggravated by damp cold, vaccination, sunlight and bright lights, bed warmth, fatty foods and coffee; they also tend to be worse on the left side, at night and at the beginning of the day or just after breakfast, and when the moon is waxing. Drawing up the limbs or lying on the affected side often improves matters.

Complementary remedies Sabina, Arsenicum, Natrum sulph., Silicea.

Antidoting remedies Mercurius, Camphora.

Urtica

From *Urtica urens*, the small stinging nettle. The homeopathic remedy is made from the fresh plant when it is in flower. As the old rhyme says, apropos of nettles: 'Cut them in June, come back again soon. Cut them in July and you cut them down truly.' Urtica is traditionally used to alleviate conditions accompanied by burning or scalding sensations.

Constitutional indications Urtica is especially helpful to people who suffer from gout or high uric acid levels.

Mental symptoms alleviated None in particular.

Physical symptoms alleviated Rheumatic pain; neuritis and neuralgia; itchy or blotchy skin, or skin which is hot and blistered; in women, lack of breast milk, or pruritis vulvae.

The symptoms above are generally made worse by touch, cold damp air, water, and snow.

Antidoting substance Dock leaves.

Veratrum

From *Veratrum album*, white hellebore. The homeopathic remedy is made from the roots just before the plant comes into flower, and is traditionally used in cases of collapse, where there is profuse cold sweating.

Constitutional indications None in particular.

Mental symptoms alleviated Excitement, excessive enthusiasm; being overcritical; tendency to brood in silence, but hating to be left alone; melancholy, fear of dying.

Physical symptoms alleviated Extremely cold, sweaty skin, perhaps with a bluish tinge; weak, rapid pulse; violent reactions to pain; muscles which feel weak or paralysed; cramps in calves; extreme thirst; heavy vomiting; cramping pains in abdomen, accompanied by violent diarrhoea.

The above symptoms are often relieved by warmth and by walking, but aggravated by damp cold, drinking, opening bowels, or becoming frightened; they are often worse at night.

Antidoting remedies Camphora, Aconite, China, Staphisagria.

Useful Addresses

Many of the organizations listed below have regional or local branches whose addresses and telephone numbers can be obtained from your local library or Citizens' Advice Bureau. They will also be listed in your local Yellow Pages telephone directory, usually under 'Charitable and benevolent organizations', 'Disabled – amenities and information', or 'Social service and welfare organizations'. The Samaritans and Alcoholics Anonymous are always listed in the local information section at the front of residential and business telephone directories.

Where no telephone number is given, please write. If you are requesting leaflets or printed information, do send a stamped, addressed envelope.

Specific disorders
For more information about national organizations concerned with various diseases and handicaps contact:

AAA (Action Against Allergy), 24–26 High Street, Hampton Hill, Middx TW12 1PD (send s.a.e. for information)

National Ankylosing Spondylitis Society, 5 Grosvenor Crescent, London SW1X 7ER, tel 071 235 9585

Arthritic Association, 1 Little New Street, London EC4A 3TR, tel 071 491 0233

Arthritis Care, 4 Grosvenor Crescent, London SW1X 7ER, tel 071 235 0902

National Asthma Campaign, 300 Upper Street, London N1 2XX, tel 071 226 2660 (Asthma Helpline 0345 010203 1pm–9pm, Monday–Friday)

National Back Pain Association, 31–33 Park Road, Teddington, Middx TW11 0AB, tel 081 977 5474/5

Royal National Institute for the Blind (RNIB), 224 Great Portland Street, London W1N 6AA, tel 071 388 1266

Cancer Help Centre, Grove House, Cornwallis Grove, Clifton, Bristol BS8 4PG, tel 0272 743216

International Cerebral Palsy Society, 5a Netherhall Gardens, London NW3 5RN, tel 071 794 9761

Chest, Heart and Stroke Association, CHSA House, Whitecross Street, London EC1Y 8JJ, tel 071 490 7999

Coeliac Society of the UK, P.O. Box 220, High Wycombe, Bucks, HP11 2HY, tel 0494 437278

National Association for Colitis and Crohn's Disease (NACC), 98a London Road, St Albans, Herts AL1 1NX, Ansaphone 0727 44296

Coronary Prevention Group, 102 Gloucester Place, London W1H 3DA, tel 071 935 2889

Royal National Institute for the Deaf (RNID), 105 Gower Street, London WC1E 6AH, tel 071 387 8033

Depressives Associated, P.O. Box 5, Castletown, Portland, Dorset DT5 1BQ, tel 081 760 0544

British Diabetic Association, 10 Queen Anne Street, London W1M 0BD, tel 071 323 1531

British Dyslexia Association, 98 London Road, Reading, Berks RG1 5AU, tel 0734 668271

Eating Disorders Association (*for help and understanding around anorexia and bulimia*), Sackville Place, 44 Magdalen Street, Norwich, Norfolk NR3 1JE, tel 0603 621414

National Eczema Society, Tavistock House East, Tavistock Square, London WC1H 9SR, tel 071 388 4097

Endometriosis Society, Unit F8A, Shakespeare Business Centre, 245a Coldharbour Lane, London SW9 8RR, tel 071 737 0380

British Epilepsy Association, 40 Hanover Square, Leeds LS3 1BE, tel 0532 439393

Guillain Barre Syndrome Support Group, Foxley, Holdingham, Sleaford, Lincs NG34 8NR, tel 0529 304615

Headway – National Head Injuries Association Ltd, 7 King Edward Court, King Edward Street, Nottingham NG1 1EW, tel 0602 240800

Herpes Association, 41 North Road, London N7 9DP, tel 071 609 9061

British Kidney Patient Association (BKPA), Bordon, Hants GU35 9JZ, tel 0420 472021/2

Lupus UK (*support for sufferers from systemic lupus erythematosus*) Queens Court, 9–17 Eastern Rd, Romford, Essex RM1 3NG, tel 0708 731251

MENCAP (Royal Society for Mentally Handicapped Children and Adults), MENCAP National Centre, 123 Golden Lane, London EC1Y 0RT, tel 071 454 0454

British Migraine Association, 178a High Road, Byfleet, Surrey KT14 7ED, tel 0932 352468

Migraine Trust, 45 Great Ormond Street, London WC1N 3HZ, tel 071 278 2676

Motor Neurone Disease Association, P.O. Box 246, Northampton NN1 2PR, tel 0604 250505/22269

Action for Research into Multiple Sclerosis (ARMS), 4a Chapel Hill, Stansted, Essex CM24 8AG, tel 0279 815553 (Counselling tel nos: London 071 222 3123 Scotland 041 945 3939 Midlands 021 476 4229)

Multiple Sclerosis Society of Great Britain and Northern Ireland, 25 Effie Road, London SW6 1EE, tel 071 736 6267

Muscular Dystrophy Group of Great Britain and Northern Ireland, Nattrass House, 35 Macaulay Road, Clapham, London SW4 0QP, tel 071 720 8055

Myalgic Encephalomyelitis Association, P.O. Box 8, Stanford-le-Hope, Essex SS17 8EX, tel 0375 642466

National Association for the Relief of Paget's Disease, Manchester University Medical Dept., Hope Hospital, Salford M6 8HD

The Pain Society (The British & Irish Chapter of the International Association for the Study of Pain), 9 Bedford Square, London WC1B 3RA, tel 071 631 1650

Parkinson's Disease Society, 22 Upper Woburn Place, London WC1H 0RA, tel 071 383 3513

Phobics Society, 4 Cheltenham Road, Chorlton-cum-Hardy, Manchester M21 1QN, tel 061 881 1937

Positively Women (*for information on women and AIDS*), 5 Sebastian Street, London EC1V 0HE, tel 071 490 5515

Psoriasis Association, 7 Milton Street, Northampton NN2 7JG, tel 0604 711129

The Raynaud's and Scleroderma Association, 112 Crewe Road, Alsager, Cheshire ST7 2JA, tel 0270 872776

Repetitive Strain Association, Communicare, Christchurch, Redford Way, Uxbridge, Middx UB8 1SZ, tel 0895 38663

Schizophrenia Association of Great Britain, International Schizophrenia Centre, Bryn Hyfryd, The Crescent, Bangor, Gwynedd LL57 2AG, tel 0248 354048

Sir Michael Sobell House (Study Centre Coordinator), Churchill Hospital, Headington, Oxford OX3 7LJ

Spastics Society, 12 Park Crescent, London W1N 4EQ, tel 071 636 5020

Spinal Injuries Association, Newpoint House, 76 James's Lane, London N10 3DF, tel 081 444 2121

UK Thalassaemia Society, 107 Nightingale Lane, London N8 7QY, tel 081 348 0437

Tinnitus Support Services, c/o Royal National Institute for the Deaf, 105 Gower Street, London WC1E 6AH, tel 071 387 8033

Women's Nutritional Advisory Service (*for pre-menstrual syndrome and menopausal problems*), P.O. Box 268, Hove, East Sussex BN3 1RW, tel 0273 771366

Children and Parents

National Autistic Society, 276 Willesden Lane, London NW2 5RB, tel 081 451 1114

The International Autistic Research Organisation, 49 Orchard Avenue, Shirley, Croydon, Surrey CR0 7NE, tel 081 777 0095

Children's Hearing Assessment Centre, General Hospital, Nottingham NG1 6HA, tel 0602 412944

Foundation for the Study of Infant Deaths (Cot Death Research and Support), 15 Belgrave Square, London SW1X 8QB, tel 071 235 0965, Helpline 071 235 1721

CRY-SIS HELPLINE (*support group for parents of babies who cry excessively*), BM-CRY-SIS, London WC1N 3XX, tel 071 404 0501

Cystic Fibrosis Research Trust, Alexandra House, 5 Blyth Road, Bromley, Kent BR1 3RS, tel 081 464 7211

National Deaf Children's Society, 45 Hereford Road, London W2 5AH, tel 071 229 9272

Down's Syndrome Association, 155 Mitcham Road, London SW17 9PG, tel 081 682 4001

Foresight (Association for the Promotion of Preconceptual Care), 28 The Paddock, Godalming, Surrey GU7 1XD, tel 0483 427839

Hyperactive Children's Support Group, 71 Whyke Lane, Chichester, Sussex PO19 2LD, tel 0903 725182

La Leche League of Britain (*breastfeeding advice and information*), BM 3424, London WC1N 3XX, tel 071 242 1278

National Childbirth Trust, Alexandra House, Oldham Terrace, Acton, London W3 6NH, tel 081 992 8637

National Council for One-Parent Families, 255 Kentish Town Road, London NW5 2LX, tel 071 267 1361

Association for Improvements in the Maternity Services (AIMS), 40 Kingswood Avenue, London NW6 6LS, tel 081 960 5585

National Society for the Prevention of Cruelty to Children (NSPCC), 67 Saffron Hill, London EC1N 8RS, tel 071 242 1626, Child Protection Helpline 0800 800500 (freephone 24 hrs)

Association for Spina Bifida and Hydrocephalus, ASBAH House, 42 Park Rd, Peterborough PE1 2UQ, tel 0733 555988

Association of Parents of Vaccine Damaged Children, 2 Church Street, Shipston-on-Stour, Warwickshire CV36 4AP, tel 0608 61595

Association of Child Psychotherapists, Burg House, New End Square, London NW3 1LT, tel 071 794 8881

Addiction

Action on Smoking and Health (ASH), 109 Gloucester Place, London W1P 3PH, tel 071 935 3519

Al-Anon Family Groups (also Alateen for teenagers), 61 Great Dover Street, London SE1 4YF, tel 071 403 0888 (*24-hour confidential helpline*)

Alcohol Concern, 275 Gray's Inn Road, London WC1X 8QF, tel 071 833 3471

Alcoholics Anonymous, P.O. Box 1, Stonebow House, Stonebow, York YO1 2NJ, tel 0904 644026

Families Anonymous, Room 8, 650 Holloway Road, London N19 3NU, tel 071 281 8889

Gamblers Anonymous, P.O. Box 88, London SW10 0EL, tel 081 741 4181

Narcotics Anonymous (*support for those wishing to come off drugs*), P.O. Box 417, London SW10 0RS, tel 071 351 6794

SCODA (Standing Committee on Drug Abuse), 1–4 Hatton Place, Hatton Garden, London EC1N 8ND, tel 071 430 2341

The Department of Health publishes various leaflets designed to help drug abusers and their families. These should be available from your local Health Authority (see local Yellow Pages telephone directory under 'Health authorities & services') or you can obtain them direct by writing to:

Department of Health Leaflets Unit, Dept DM P.O. Box 21, Stanmore, Middx HA7 1AY, tel 071 972 2000

The Health Stores (*drug misuse*), No. 2 Site, Manchester Rd, Heywood, Lancs OL10 1PZ

Other Problems

Albany Trust Counselling (*counselling for sexual and relationship problems*), St Paul's Centre, Rossmore Rd, London NW1 6NJ, tel 071 224 9977

Brook Advisory Centres (*national network for young people, offering birth control advice, confidential pregnancy testing, and abortion counselling*), 153a East Street, London SE17 2SD, tel 071 708 1234

National Association of Citizens' Advice Bureaux, Myddelton House, 115–123 Pentonville Road, London N1 9LZ, tel 071 833 2181

Counsel and Care (*advice and help for older people*), Twyman House, 16 Bonny St, London NW1 9PG, tel 071 485 1566

Cruse, Bereavement Care (*support for the bereaved*), Cruse House, 126 Sheen Road, Richmond, Surrey TW9 1UR, tel 081 940 4818

Disabled Living Foundation, 380–384 Harrow Road, London W9 2HU, tel 081 289 6111

Family Planning Association (*advice and information on all aspects of sexuality, birth control and reproductive health*), 27–35 Mortimer Street, London W1N 7RJ, tel 071 636 7866

National Health and Safety Officer, GMB 22–24 Worple Road, London SW19 4DD, tel 081 947 3131

Terrence Higgins Trust (*help and support for people with AIDS and for those who are HIV positive*), 52–54 Grays Inn Road, London WC1X 8JU, tel Admin. 071 831 0330, Helpline 071 242 1010

Medic-Alert Foundation (*Medic-Alert emblem warns police, ambulance and medical services that wearer has a hidden medical condition that may affect emergency care*), 17 Bridge Wharf, 156 Caledonian Road, London N1 9UU, tel 071 833 3034

British Pregnancy Advisory Service (*advice on birth control and pregnancy, pregnancy testing, abortion counselling*), 7 Belgrave Road, London SW1V 1QB, tel 071 222 0985

Rape Crisis Centre (*counselling, medical and legal help, for victims of rape or sexual assault – women only*), P.O. Box 69, London WC1X 9NJ, tel 071 278 3956, 071 837 1600 (24-hr emergency service)

Relate (*marriage guidance*), Herbert Gray College, Little Church Street, Rugby CV21 3AP, tel 0788 573241

Health and Safety Executive (*advice and information on safety in the workplace*), Baynard's House, 1–13 Chepstow Place, London W2 4TF, tel 071 221 0870

Institute for Building Biology, 16 Church St, Saffron Walden, Essex, tel 0799 26575

Samaritans (*help for the suicidal or despairing – telephones at local branches are staffed 24 hours a day, 7 days a week; see local information section at front of local residential or business telephone directory for telephone number*), 10 The Grove, Slough SL1 1QP, tel 0753 532713 (administrative inquiries only)

Sanity (*research into nutritional and biochemical factors in mental illness*), 63 Cole Park Road, Twickenham, Middx TW1 1HT (s.a.e. appreciated), tel 081 892 3924

SPOD (*association to aid the sexual and personal relationships of people with a disability*), 286 Camden Road, London N7 0BJ, tel 071 607 8851

Vegan Society, 7 Battle Road, St Leonards-on-Sea, East Sussex TN37 7AA, tel 0424 427393

Vegetarian Society, Parkdale, Dunham Road, Altrincham, Cheshire WA14 4QG, tel 061 928 0793

Weight Watchers (UK) Ltd, Kidwell's Park House, Kidwell's Park Drive, Maidenhead, Berks SL6 8YT, tel 0628 777077

Women's Health Concern, 83 Earls Court Road, London W8 6EF, tel 071 938 3932 or 071 376 0879

Clinics

BioLab, The Stonehouse, 9 Weymouth Street, London W1N 3FF, tel 071 636 5959/5905

Marigold Treatment Centre (*homeopathic chiropody clinic*), 134 Montrose Avenue, Edgware, Middx HA8 0DR, tel 081 959 5421

Midlands Asthma and Allergy Research Association, 12 Vernon Street, Derby DE1 1ST, tel 0332 362461

Musicians and Keyboard Clinic, 7 Park Crescent, London W1N 3HE, tel 071 436 5961

Park Attwood Clinic (*anthroposophical medical treatment centre*), Trimpley, Bewdley, Worcestershire DY12 1RE, tel 02997 444

Wholistic Research Company (*evaluates and markets equipment designed to make home environment healthier*), Bright Haven, Robins Lane, Lolworth, Cambridge CB3 8HH, tel 0954 781074

Complementary Medicine

Information about acupuncture, chiropractic, homoeopathy, medical herbalism, naturopathy and osteopathy can be obtained from:

Council for Complementary and Alternative Medicine (CCAM), 179 Gloucester Place, London NW1 6DX, tel 071 724 9103

Information about other complementary and alternative therapies, in addition to those mentioned above, can be obtained from:

Institute of Complementary Medicine (ICM), 21 Portland Place, London W1N 3AF, tel 071 636 9543

Postal inquiries, enclosing a large, stamped, self-addressed envelope, would be appreciated. Both CCAM and ICM keep lists of skilled practitioners and also monitor training standards and qualifications.

Information can also be obtained from the organizations listed below, although it should be emphasized that for reasons of space this list is not comprehensive. By including some organizations and not others no recommendation or criticism is intended. Where no telephone number is given, postal contact is preferred.

The Bates Association of Great Britain, 11 Tarmount Lane, Shoreham, West Sussex BN43 6RQ, tel 0273 452623

British Acupuncture Association and Register, 34 Alderney Street, London SW1V 4EV, tel 071 834 1012

College of Traditional Chinese Acupuncture, Tao House, Queensway, Leamington Spa, Warwickshire CV32 5EZ, tel 0926 39347

Council for Acupuncture, 179 Gloucester Place, London NW1 6DX, tel 071 724 5756

British Medical Acupuncture Society,
The Administrator, Newton House,
Newton Lane, Whitley, Warrington, Cheshire
WA4 4JA, tel 0925 730727

Traditional Acupuncture Society,
1 The Ridgeway, Stratford-on-Avon,
Warwickshire CV37 9JL, tel 0789 298798

International Register of Oriental Medicine
(UK), Green Hedges House, Green Hedges
Avenue, East Grinstead, East Sussex
RH19 1DZ, tel 0342 313106/7

Society of Teachers of the Alexander Technique,
Suite 20, 10 London House, 266 Fulham Road,
London SW10 9EL, tel 071 351 0828

Alternate Sitting, P.O. Box 19, Chipping Norton,
Oxfordshire OX7 6NY, tel 0608 658875

British Association for Autogenic Training and
Therapy, 101 Harley Street, London W1N 1DF,
tel 071 935 1811

British Chiropractic Association, Premier
House, 10 Greycoat Place, London SW1P 1SB,
tel 071 222 8866

National Federation of Spiritual Healers,
Old Manor Farm Studio, Church Street,
Sunbury-on-Thames, Middx TW16 6RG,
tel 0932 783164/5

National Institute of Medical Herbalists, 9 Palace
Gate, Exeter, Devon EX1 1JA, tel 0392 426022

British Society of Medical and Dental Hypnosis,
151 Otley Old Road, Leeds LS16 6HN,
tel 0532 613077

European Society of Medical Hypnosis, 3 Troy
Road, Morley, Leeds LS27 8JJ, tel 0532 533494

UK College of Hypnotherapy and Counselling,
10 Alexander Street, London W2 5NT,
tel 071 727 2006 or 071 221 1796

National Register of Hypnotherapists and
Psychotherapists, 12 Cross Street, Nelson,
Lancs, tel 0282 699378

Society of Iridologists, 40 Stokewood Road,
Bournemouth, Dorset BH3 7NE,
tel 0202 529793

Northern Institute of Massage, 100 Waterloo
Road, Blackpool, Lancs FY4 1AW,
tel 0253 403548

West London School of Therapeutic Massage,
41 St Luke's Road, London W11 1DD,
tel 071 229 4672

General Council and Register of Naturopaths,
6 Netherhall Gardens, London NW3 5RR,
tel 071 435 6464

British Society for Nutritional Medicine, P.O.
Box 3AP, London W1A 3AP, tel 071 436 8532

Institute for Optimum Nutrition, 5 Jerdan Place,
London SW6 1BE, tel 071 385 7984

Nutritional Eye Health Centre, Sanctuary House,
Oulton Road, Oulton, Norfolk NR32 4QZ,
tel 0502 583294

The General Council and Register of Osteopaths,
56 London Street, Reading, Berkshire
RG1 4SQ, tel 0734 576585

British Osteopathic Association, 8–10 Boston
Place, London NW1 6QH, tel 071 262 5250

College of Osteopaths, 1 Furzehill Road,
Borehamwood, Herts WD6 2DG,
tel 081 905 1937

Chartered Society of Physiotherapy, 14 Bedford
Row, London WC1R 4ED, tel 071 242 1941

London and Counties Society of Physiologists,
100 Waterloo Road, Blackpool, Lancs
FY4 1AW, tel 0253 403548

British Association for Counselling (*information
about counselling services for personal relationship and psychosexual problems*), 1 Regent
Place, Rugby CV21 2PJ, tel 0788 578328

British Association of Psychotherapists,
37 Mapesbury Road, London NW2 4HJ

Institute of Group Analysis, 1 Daleham Gardens,
London NW3 5BY, tel 071 431 2693

Institute of Psychoanalysis, 63 New Cavendish
Street, London W1M 7RD, tel 071 580 4952

Society of Analytical Psychology, 1 Daleham
Gardens, London NW3 5BY, tel 071 435 7696

London Centre for Psychotherapy (*counselling
and individual or group psychotherapy at
moderate fees*), 19 Fitzjohns Avenue, London
NW3 5JY, tel 071 435 0873

British Reflexology Association, Monks Orchard,
Whitbourne, Worcs WR6 5RB, tel 0826 21207

International Institute of Reflexology,
28 Hollyfield Avenue, Friern Barnet, London
N11 3BY, tel 081 368 0865

Shiatsu Society, 14 Oakdene Road, Redhill,
Surrey RH1 6BT, tel 0737 767896

Yoga for Health Foundation, Ickwell Bury,
Biggleswade, Beds SG18 9EF, tel 0767 27271

British Wheel of Yoga, 1 Hamilton Place, Boston
Road, Sleaford, Lincs NG34 7ES,
tel 0529 306851

Homeopathy

If you are looking for a homeopathic practitioner in your area, or want to know where the nearest homeopathic pharmacy is, the following organizations will be pleased to help you:

Homoeopathic Development Foundation, 19a Cavendish Square, London W1M 9AD, tel 071 629 3205

The Faculty of Homoeopathy, The Royal London Homoeopathic Hospital, Great Ormond Street, London WC1N 3HR, tel 071 837 3091, ext. 72/85

The British Homoeopathic Association, 27a Devonshire Street, London WC1N 1RJ, tel 071 935 2163

The Hahnemann Society, 2 Powis Place, Great Ormond Street, London WC1N 3HZ, tel 071 837 3297

Society of Homeopaths (*has register of non-medically qualified homeopaths*), 2 Artizan Road, Northampton NN1 4HU, tel 0604 21400

Homeopaths who are GPs and working as family doctors within the National Health Service can refer patients to consultants in the following NHS Homeopathic Hospitals:

Bristol Homoeopathic Hospital, Cotham Hill, Cotham, Bristol BS6 6JU, tel 0272 731231

East End Clinic, Buchanan Street, Baillieston, Glasgow, tel 041 771 7396

Glasgow Homoeopathic Hospital, 100 Great Western Road, Glasgow G12 0RN, tel 041 339 0382

Department of Homeopathic Medicine, Mossley Hill Hospital, Park Avenue, Liverpool L18 8BU, tel 051 724 2335

Royal London Homoeopathic Hospital, Great Ormond Street, London WC1N 3HR, tel 071 837 8833 (071 837 7821 for appointments)

Tunbridge Wells Homoeopathic Hospital, Church Road, Tunbridge Wells, Kent TN1 1JU, tel 0892 542977

Most chemists and healthfood shops stock a limited range of homeopathic remedies. For the full range of remedies, however, one has to go to a specialized pharmacy or direct to the manufacturer. All products can be supplied by post.

Ainsworths, 38 New Cavendish Street, London W1M 7LH, tel 071 935 5330

Buxton and Grant, 176 Whiteladies Road, Bristol BS8 2XU, tel 0272 735025

Freeman's Pharmacy, 7 Eaglesham Road, Clarkston, Glasgow G76 7BU, tel 041 644 1165

Galen Homoeopathics, Lewell Mill, W. Stafford, Dorchester, Dorset DT2 8AN, tel 0305 263996

Goulds, 14 Crowndale Road, London NW1 1TT, tel 071 388 4752 or 071 387 1888

Helios, 97 Camden Road, Tunbridge Wells, Kent TN1 2QR, tel 0892 36393

Nelson's Pharmacies Ltd, 73 Duke Street, London W1M 6BY, tel 071 629 3118

A. Nelson and Co Ltd (licensed manufacturer), 5 Endeavour Way, London SW19 9UH, tel 081 946 8527

Weleda (UK) Ltd (licensed manufacturer), Heanor Road, Ilkeston, Derbyshire DE7 8DR, tel 0602 303151

Phials, storage boxes, unmedicated tablets and other homeopathic supplies (but no remedies) can be obtained by post from:

Trevor Cook (Homeopathy) Ltd, 427 Great West Road, Hounslow, Middlesex TW5 0BY, tel 081 577 7781

The Homoeopathic Supply Co, 4 Nelson Road, Sheringham, Norfolk NR26 8BU, tel 0263 824683

Biochemic Tissue Salts and Combination Remedies can generally be obtained from homeopathic pharmacies, healthfood shops, and from some chemists or direct from:

New Era Laboratories Ltd, Marfleet, Kingston upon Hull HU9 5NJ, tel 0482 75234

Bach Flower Remedies are stocked by homeopathic pharmacies and some healthfood shops, or can be bought from:

Dr Edward Bach Centre, Mount Vernon, Sotwell, Wallingford, Oxon OX10 0PZ, tel 0491 34678

Bibliography

Homeopathy

Bannerjee, P. N. *Chronic Diseases: Cause and Cure* Homoeopathy Prachar Karjalaya, Calcutta, 1931

Boericke, W. *Materia Medica with Repertory* Boericke and Tafel, Philadelphia, 1927

Borland, D. M. *Children's Types* British Homoeopathic Association, 1940

Borland, D. M. *Digestive Drugs* British Homoeopathic Association, 1940

Borland, D. M. *Pneumonias* British Homoeopathic Association

Bradford, T. L. *The Life and Letters of Samuel Hahnemann* Royal Publishing House, Calcutta, 1970

Campbell, A. *The Two Faces of Homoeopathy* Robert Hale, 1984

Clark, J. H. *Dictionary of Materia Medica* 3 vols., Homoeopathic Publishing Company, London, 1925

Clark, J. H. *Clinical Repertory* Homoeopathic Publishing Company, London, 1904

Clark, J. H. *The Prescriber* Homoeopathic Publishing Company, London, 8th edition, 1952

Clark, J. H. *Indigestion* James Epps, 7th edition, 1912

Gibson, D. H. *First Aid Homoeopathy in Accidents and Ailments* British Homoeopathic Association, 9th edition, 1982

Haehl, R. *Samuel Hahnemann: His Life and Work* 2 vols., Homoeopathic Publishing Company, London, 1922

Hahnemann, Samuel *The Chronic Diseases* 2 vols., translated by L. H. Tafel from 2nd enlarged German edition of 1835, Winger and Company, Calcutta

Hobhouse, R. W. *The Life of Samuel Hahnemann* World Homoeopathic Links, New Delhi, 1984

Hughes, R. *The Manual of Pharmaco-Dynamics* Leith and Ross, 1899

Jahr, G. H. G. *Diseases of Females* Bhatta-Charrya and Company, Calcutta, 1939

Jouanny, J. *Essentials of Homoeopathic Therapeutics* Laboratoire Boiron, Lyon, 1985

Kent, J. T. *Materia Medica* Sinha Roy, Calcutta, 2nd edition, 1970

Kent, J. T. *Lectures on Homoeopathic Philosophy* Erhart and Carl, Chicago, 4th edition, 1937

Kent, J. T. *Final General Repertory* eds. Chand, D. H. and Schmidt, P. Natural Homoeopathic Pharmacy, New Delhi, 2nd edition, 1982

Lessell, C. B. *Homoeopathy for Physicians* Thorsons, 1983

Nash, E. D. *Leaders in Homoeopathic Therapeutics* Boericke and Tafel, Philadelphia, 1946

Neatby, E. A. and Stoneham, T. G. *A Manual of Homoeopathic Therapeutics* Staple Press, 1948

Ostrum, H. I. *Leucorrhea* Set, Dey and Company, Calcutta, 1937

Panos, Maesimund B. and Heimlich, Jane *Homeopathic Medicine at Home* Corgi, 1980

Pratt, N. *Homoeopathic Prescribing* Beaconsfield Publishers, 1980

Roberts, A. H. *The Principles and Art of Cure by Homoeopathy* Homoeopathic Publishing Company, London, 1936

Royal, G. *Diseases of the Brain and Nerves* Boericke and Tafel, Philadelphia, 1928

Sharma, C. *A Manual of Homoeopathy and Natural Medicine* Turnstone Press, 1975

Smith, Trevor *Homoeopathic Medicine* Thorsons, 1982

Smith, Trevor *Homoeopathic Treatment of Emotional Illness* Thorsons, 1983

Smith, Trevor *A Woman's Guide to Homoeopathic Medicine* Thorsons, 1984

Stevenson, J. H. *Helping Yourself with Homoeopathic Remedies* Thorsons, 1976

Tyler, Margaret L. *Homoeopathic Drug Pictures* Health Science Press, 1952

Tyler, Margaret L. and Weir, Sir John *Acute Conditions, Injuries, etc.* British Homoeopathic Association

Wheeler, C. E. *The Principles and Practice of Homoeopathy* Heinemann, 1940

Yingling, W. A. *The Accoucheur's Emergency Manual* Set, Dey and Company, Calcutta, 1936

General Medicine

Baily and Love's: A Short Practice of Surgery revised by Rains, A. J. and Capper, W. M., H. K. Lewis, 14th edition, 1968

Barker, J. E. *Chronic Constipation* John Murray, 1927

Barnes, B. O. and Galton, L. *Hypothyroidism* Thomas Crowell Company, New York, 1976

Benenson, A. S. *The Control of Communicable Diseases in Man* American Public Health Association, Washington, 1975

Bradford, R. W. and Culbert, M. L. *The Metabolic Management of Cancer* Robert Bradford Foundation, California, 1979

Bradford, R. W. and Culbert, M. L. *International Protocols for Individualized Integrated Metabolic Programs and Cancer Management* Robert Bradford Foundation, California, 1981

Cheraskin, E., Ringsdorf, W. M. and Clark, J. W. *Diet and Disease* Keats Health Science, Connecticut, 1977

Crouch, J. E. and McClintick, J. R. *Human Anatomy and Physiology* John Wiley and Sons, New York, 1976

Davidson's Principles of Medicine ed. McLeod, John, Churchill Livingstone, 12th edition, 1977

Davidson, Sir S., Passmore, R., Brock, J. E. and Trusswell, A. S. *Human Nutrition and Dietetics* Churchill Livingstone, 7th edition, 1979

Dorland's Illustrated Medical Dictionary W. R. Saunders, Philadelphia, 26th edition, 1981

Draper, I. T. *Lecture Notes on Neurology* Blackwell, 2nd edition, 1968

Ellison, W. B. and Mitchell, R.G. *Diseases in Infancy and Childhood* E. and S. Churchill, Edinburgh, 1968

Foxen, E. H. M. *Lecture Notes on Diseases of the Ear, Nose and Throat* Blackwell, 2nd edition, 1968

Fredericks, C. *Psycho-Nutrition* Grosset & Dunlap, New York, 1976

Freed, D. L. J. *The Health Hazards of Milk* Bailliere Tindall, 1984

Fry, L. *Dermatology: An Illustrated Guide* Update Publications, 1973

Gerson, M. *Cancer Therapy* Totality Books, California, 3rd edition, 1977

Glaister, J. *Medical Jurisprudence and Toxicology* Churchill Livingstone, 6th edition, 1930

Herxheimer, A. *Side Effects of Drugs* vol. 7, Excerpta Medica, Amsterdam, 1972

Hutchison, J. H. *Practical Paediatric Problems* 4th edition, Lloyd-Luke, 1975

Jensen, B. *Nature Has the Remedy* Unity Press, California, 1978

Lawrence, D. R. and Bennett, P. N. *Clinical Pharmacology* Churchill Livingstone, 5th edition, 1980

Ledermann, E. K. *Natural Therapy* Watson & Co., 1953

Lindlahr, H. *Practice of Natural Therapeutics* vol. 2, ed. Proby, J. C. P., C. W. Daniel Company, 1981

McLeod, J. *Clinical Examination* Churchill Livingstone, 1967

Paul, A. A. and Southgate, D. A. T. *The Composition of Foods* McCance and Widdowson, HMSO, London, 1978

Pfeiffer, C. *Mental and Elemental Nutrients* Keats Publishing Company, Connecticut, 1975

Roe, D. A. *Drug-Induced Nutritional Deficiencies* AVI Publishing Company, Connecticut, 1976

Schauss, A. *Diet, Crime and Delinquency* Parker House, California, 1981

Schroeder, H. *The Poisons Around Us* Keats Publishing Company, Connecticut, 1974

Tomlinson, H. *Aluminium Utensils* L. N. Fowler & Co., 1967

Tredgold, R. F. and Wolff, B. K. *UCH Notes of Psychiatry* Gerald Duckworth, 1970

Walter, J. W. and Israel, M. S. *General Pathology* Churchill Livingstone, 2nd edition, 1965

Warin, J. F., Ironside, A. G. and Mandal, B. K. *Lecture Notes on Infectious Diseases* Blackwell, 3rd edition, 1980

Williams, P. L. and Warwick, R., eds. *Gray's Anatomy* Churchill Livingstone, 1980

Williams, R. J. and Kalita, D. W., eds. *The Physician's Handbook on Orthomolecular Medicine* Keats Publishing Company, Connecticut, 1977

Journals and Periodicals

Doctor
British Journal of Holistic Medicine
British Homoeopathic Journal
Homoeopathy
Homoeopathy Today
Journal of Alternative and Complementary Medicine
Medicine International
Mimm's Magazine
The Practitioner
Pulse
Update
Communications from the British Homoeopathy Research Group

Books for further reading

Nutrition

Ash, Janet and Robert, Dulcie *Happiness is Junk-free Food* Thorsons, 1986

Ballantine, R. *Diet and Nutrition* Himalayan National Institute, Pennsylvania, 1978

Budd, M. L. *Low Blood Sugar* Thorsons, 1984

Chaitow, L. *Your Own Slimming and Health Programme* Thorsons, 1985

Colgan, M. *Your Personal Vitamin Profile* Blond & Briggs, 1983

Committee on Medical Aspects of Food Policy (COMA) *Dietary Reference Values for Food Energy and Nutrients for the United Kingdom, 1991*

Davies, S. and Stewart, A. *Nutritional Medicine* Pan Books, 1987

Elliot, Rose *Vegetarian Mother and Baby Book* Fontana, 1984

French, Barbara *Coping with Bulimia* Thorsons, 1987

Grant, Doris *Food Combining for Health* Thorsons, 1984

Hall, R. H. *Food for Nought* Vintage Books, New York, 1976

Hanssen, M. *E for Additives* Thorsons, 1984

Hasslam, David *Eat It Up: A Parent's Guide to Problems* Macdonald, 1986

Hirschmann, J. and Munter, C. *Overcoming Overeating* Mandarin, 1989

Lynch, Barry *The BBC Diet* BBC Books, 1988

Marks, J. *A Guide to the Vitamins* Medical and Technical Publishing, 1975

Marshall, Janette *Shopping for Health* Penguin, 1987

Null, G. *The New Vegetarian* William Morrow & Co., New York, 1978

Orbach, Susie *Hunger Strikes* Faber and Faber, 1986

Pleshette, J. *Health on Your Plate* Hamlyn, 1983

Reuben, D. *The Save Your Life Diet* Ballantine, New York, 1981

Shute, Wilfrid *The Vitamin E Book* Keats Publishing Company, Connecticut, 1975

Stanway, A. *Trace Elements* Vandyke Books, 1983

Tatchell, J. *You and Your Food* Usborne, 1985

Templeton, Louise *The Right Food for Your Kids* Century, 1984

Weaver, Gillian *Feeding Time: How to Cope with Your Child's Eating Problems* Columbus, 1985

Wright, Celia *The Wright Diet* Green Library, 1986

General Health

BMA Family Doctor Home Adviser ed. Smith, T., Dorling Kindersley, 1986

Davidson, J. *Subtle Energy* C. W. Daniel Company, 1986

Davis, Adele *Let's Get Well* Unwin, 1966

Dawood, R. *Traveller's Health* Oxford University Press, 1986

Gardner, A. W. and Roylance, P. J. *New Essential First Aid* Pan Books, 1980

Jensen, B. *Tissue Cleansing through Bowel Management* Bernard Jensen, California, 1980

Leach, P. *Baby and Child* revised edition, Penguin, 1989

The Macmillan Guide to Family Health ed. Smith, T., Macmillan, 1982

Physical Fitness: The 11-minute Plan for Men Penguin 1987

Physical Fitness: The 12-minute Plan for Women Penguin 1987

West, R. *The Family Guide to Children's Ailments* Hamlyn, 1983

Ziff, S. *The Toxic Time Bomb* Thorsons, 1984

Zilbergeld, Bernard *Men and Sex* Fontana, 1984

Women's Medicine

Achterberg, Jean *Woman as Healer* Rider Books, 1991

Dickson, Anne and Henriques, Nikki *Menopause: The Women's View* Thorsons, 1987

Evans, Barbara *Life Change* Pan Books, 1979

Greer, Germaine *The Change* Hamish Hamilton, 1991

Heiman, Julia R. and Loppicolo, Joseph *Becoming Orgasmic* Piatkus Books, 1988

Kamen, B. *Startling New Facts About Osteoporosis*

Kilmartin, Angela *Life Change* Pan Books, 1979

Kilmartin, Angela *Victims of Thrush and Cystitis* Arrow, 1986

Melville, Arabella *Natural Hormone Health* Thorsons, 1990

Ojeda, Linda *Menopause Without Medicine* Thorsons, 1989

Schrieve, Caroline *The Pre-menstrual Syndrome* Thorsons, 1983

Schrotenboer, Kathryn *Cystitis* MacDonald Optima, 1987

Specific Problems

Barnes, B. and Gail Bradley, S. *Planning for a Healthy Baby* Ebury Press, 1990

Chaitow, L. *Candida Albicans* Thorsons, 1985

Chaitow, L. *Vaccination and Immunization* C. W. Daniel Company, 1987

Chaitow, L. and Martin, S. *A World Without AIDS* Thorsons, 1988

Cutland, L. *Kick Heroin* Sky Books, 1985

Davidson, J. *Subtle Energy* C. W. Daniel Company, 1986

Davidson, J. *Radiation: what it is, what it does to you, and what we can do about it* C. W. Daniel Company, 1986

Dawes, B. and Downing, D. *Why ME?* Grafton, 1989

Ditzler, James and Ditzler, Joyce *Coming Off Drugs* Papermac, 1986

Franklin, Mike and Sullivan, Jane *Me* Sanctuary, 1989

Grant, E. *The Bitter Pill* Elm Tree Books, 1985

Molton Brown *A Way of Looking* (ed. Lucinda Pearce). Ward Locke, 1987

Randolph, T. G. and Moss, R. W. *Allergies* Turnstone Press, 1981

Stoff, Jesse and Pelegrino, Charles, *Chronic Fatigue Syndrome* Harper and Row, 1989

Trowbridge, John Parker and Walker, Morton *The Yeast Syndrome* Bantam Books, 1989

Woodward, B. *Wired* Faber and Faber, 1984

Homeopathy and Other Therapies

Bach, Edward *Heal Thyself* C. W. Daniel Company, 1931, reprinted 1978

Bach, Edward *The Twelve Healers and Other Remedies* C. W. Daniel Company, 1933, reprinted 1973

Blackie, Margery G. *The Patient Not the Cure: The Challenge of Homeopathy* Macdonald & Jane's, 1976

Blackie, Margery G. *Classical Homoeopathy* Beaconsfield Publishers, 1986

Chancellor, P. M. *Handbook of the Bach Flower Remedies* C. W. Daniel Company, 1971, reprinted 1977

Coulter, C. *Portraits of Homeopathic Medicines* (2 vols.) North Atlantic Books, Berkeley, 1986

Coulter, H. *Divided Legacy* (3 vols.) North Atlantic Books, Berkeley, 1986

Gilbert, P. *A Doctor's Guide to Helping Yourself with Biochemic Tissue Salts* Thorsons, 1984

Hahnemann, Samuel *The Organon of Medicine* tr. Kunli, J., Naude, A., and Pendleton, P., Gollancz, 1986

Inglis, B. and West, R. *Alternative Health Guide* Michael Joseph, 1983

Murray, Michael and Pizzorno, Joseph *Encyclopaedia of Natural Medicine* Macdonald Optima, 1990

Newman-Turner, R. *Naturopathic Medicine* Thorsons, 1984

Tisserand, R. *The Art of Aromatherapy* C. W. Daniel Company, 1977

Ullman, D. *Homeopathy: Medicine for the 21st Century* Thorsons, 1989

Vithoulkas, George *The Science of Homoeopathy* Grove Press, New York, 1980

Vlamis, G. *Flowers to the Rescue* Thorsons, 1986

Index